The Requisites Series

Pediatric Radiology

THE REQUISITES

Pediatric Radiology

FOURTH EDITION

Michele M. Walters, MD
Staff Pediatric Radiologist
Physician Director of Satellite Imaging
Boston Children's Hospital
Instructor in Radiology
Harvard Medical School
Boston, Massachusetts

Richard L. Robertson, MD
Chair, Department of Radiology
Staff Neuroradiologist
Boston Children's Hospital
Associate Professor of Radiology
Harvard Medical School
Boston, Massachusetts

ELSEVIER

ELSEVIER

1600 John F. Kennedy Blvd.
Ste 1800
Philadelphia, PA 19103-2899

PEDIATRIC RADIOLOGY: THE REQUISITES, FOURTH EDITION   ISBN: 978-0-323-32307-9

Notices

Knowledge and best practice in this field are constantly changing. As new research and experience
broaden our understanding, changes in research methods, professional practices, or medical
treatment may become necessary.

Practitioners and researchers must always rely on their own experience and knowledge in
evaluating and using any information, methods, compounds, or experiments described herein. In
using such information or methods they should be mindful of their own safety and the safety of
others, including parties for whom they have a professional responsibility.

With respect to any drug or pharmaceutical products identified, readers are advised to check
the most current information provided (i) on procedures featured or (ii) by the manufacturer of
each product to be administered, to verify the recommended dose or formula, the method and
duration of administration, and contraindications. It is the responsibility of practitioners, relying on
their own experience and knowledge of their patients, to make diagnoses, to determine dosages
and the best treatment for each individual patient, and to take all appropriate safety precautions.

To the fullest extent of the law, neither the Publisher nor the authors, contributors, or editors,
assume any liability for any injury and/or damage to persons or property as a matter of products
liability, negligence or otherwise, or from any use or operation of any methods, products,
instructions, or ideas contained in the material herein.

Previous editions copyrighted 2009 and 1998.

Library of Congress Cataloging-in-Publication Data

Names: Walters, Michele, editor. | Robertson, Richard L., Jr., editor. | Preceded by (work): Blickman,
Johan G. Pediatric radiology.
Title: Pediatric radiology : the requisites / [edited by] Michele Walters, Richard L. Robertson Jr.
Other titles: Pediatric radiology (Walters) | Requisites series.
Description: Fourth edition. | Philadelphia, PA : Elsevier, [2017] | Series: Requisites series | Preceded
by: Pediatric radiology / Johan G. Blickman, Bruce R. Parker, Patrick D. Barnes. 3rd ed. c2009. |
Includes bibliographical references and index.
Identifiers: LCCN 2016030796 | ISBN 9780323323079 (hardcover : alk. paper)
Subjects: | MESH: Diagnostic Imaging | Child | Infant
Classification: LCC RJ51.R3 | NLM WN 240 | DDC 618.92/00757—dc23 LC record available at
https://lccn.loc.gov/2016030796

Executive Content Strategist: Robin Carter
Senior Content Development Manager: Katie DeFrancesco
Publishing Services Manager: Patricia Tannian
Senior Project Manager: Amanda Mincher
Design Direction: Amy Buxton

Printed in the United States of America

Last digit is the print number: 9 8 7 6 5 4

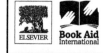 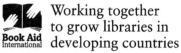

Working together
to grow libraries in
developing countries

www.elsevier.com • www.bookaid.org

For Travis, Jack, and Henry, with love.
Michele M. Walters

Contributors

Rama S. Ayyala, MD
Assistant Professor of Radiology
Department of Pediatric Radiology
Morgan Stanley Children's Hospital
Columbia University Medical Center
New York, New York

Thangamadhan Bosemani, MD
Assistant Professor of Radiology and Radiological Science
Russell H. Morgan Department of Radiology and Radiological
  Science
Johns Hopkins Hospital
Baltimore, Maryland

Micheál Anthony Breen, MB BCh BAO (Hons), BMedSc,
  MRCPI, FFRRCSI
Staff Radiologist
Co-director, Pediatric Radiology Fellowship
Boston Children's Hospital
Instructor in Radiology
Harvard Medical School
Boston, Massachusetts

Stephen D. Brown, MD
Associate Professor of Radiology
Boston Children's Hospital
Harvard Medical School
Boston, Massachusetts

Carlo Buonomo, MD
Radiologist
Boston Children's Hospital
Associate Professor of Radiology
Harvard Medical School
Boston, Massachusetts

Michael J. Callahan, MD
Director, Computed Tomography
Director, Ultrasound
Division Chief, Abdominal Imaging
Department of Radiology
Boston Children's Hospital
Associate Professor of Radiology
Harvard Medical School
Boston, Massachusetts

Sabeena Chacko, MD
Associate in Perioperative Anesthesia
Boston Children's Hospital
Assistant Professor of Anesthesia
Harvard Medical School
Boston, Massachusetts

Patricia Trinidad Chang, MD
Instructor in Radiology
Boston Children's Hospital
Harvard Medical School
Boston, Massachusetts

Jeanne S. "Mei-Mei" Chow, MD
Assistant Professor
Harvard Medical School
Departments of Radiology and Urology
Boston Children's Hospital
Boston, Massachusetts

Stephanie DiPerna, MD
Physician Director of Satellites for Radiology
Boston Children's Hospital
Instructor in Radiology
Harvard Medical School
Boston, Massachusetts

Angela Franceschi, MEd, CCLS
Child Life Specialist
Department of Radiology
Boston Children's Hospital
Boston, Massachusetts

Jamie L. Frost, DO
Staff Radiologist
Advanced Radiology Services
Grand Rapids, Michigan

Thierry A.G.M. Huisman, MD, EQNR, EDiPNR, FICIS
Professor of Radiology, Pediatrics, Neurosurgery, and
  Neurology
Chairman, Department of Imaging and Imaging Science
Johns Hopkins Bayview Medical Center
Director of Pediatric Radiology and Pediatric Neuroradiology
Johns Hopkins Hospital
Russell H. Morgan Department of Radiology and Radiological
  Science
Johns Hopkins Medicine
Baltimore, Maryland

Amy Juliano, MD
Staff Radiologist
Massachusetts Eye and Ear Infirmary
Instructor in Radiology
Harvard Medical School
Boston, Massachusetts

Rajesh Krishnamurthy, MD
Radiologist-in-Chief
Department of Diagnostic Radiology
Nationwide Children's Hospital
Columbus, Ohio

Erica L. Riedesel, MD
Assistant Professor
Pediatric Radiology
University of Wisconsin School of Medicine and Public
  Health
Madison, Wisconsin

Richard L. Robertson, MD
Chair, Department of Radiology
Staff Neuroradiologist
Boston Children's Hospital
Associate Professor of Radiology
Harvard Medical School
Boston, Massachusetts

Caroline D. Robson, MBChB
Operations Vice Chair, Radiology
Division Chief, Neuroradiology
Director, Head and Neck Imaging
Boston Children's Hospital
Associate Professor of Radiology
Harvard Medical School
Boston, Massachusetts

Cassandra Sams, MD
Clinical Assistant Professor of Radiology
University of North Carolina at Chapel Hill
Chapel Hill, North Carolina

Laureen Sena, MD
Staff Radiologist
Boston Children's Hospital
Assistant Professor of Radiology
Harvard Medical School
Boston, Massachusetts

David W. Swenson, MD
Assistant Professor (Clinical)
Department of Diagnostic Imaging
Alpert Medical School of Brown University
Providence, Rhode Island

George A. Taylor, MD
Radiologist-in-Chief Emeritus
Department of Radiology
Boston Children's Hospital
John A. Kirkpatrick Professor of Radiology (Pediatrics)
Department of Radiology
Harvard Medical School
Boston, Massachusetts

Michele M. Walters, MD
Staff Pediatric Radiologist
Physician Director of Satellite Imaging
Boston Children's Hospital
Instructor in Radiology
Harvard Medical School
Boston, Massachusetts

Foreword

The fourth edition of *Pediatric Radiology: The Requisites* brings a new author and editor team to *The Requisites* series. Drs. Walters and Robertson have taken the lead for the fourth edition and have assembled an outstanding group of contributors. Their new volume promises to maintain the philosophy of the series of presenting the core information required for the clinical practice of pediatric radiology without burdening the reader with unnecessary detail or discussion of speculative or unproven concepts. Once again, advancements in radiology have created the daunting challenge of sorting through the new and old to find the right balance to achieve this goal, a challenge ably met by Walters and Robertson and their colleagues. Congratulations to them for adding another outstanding contribution to *The Requisites* series.

There are many special considerations that apply to pediatric radiology with respect to radiation exposure, the need for sedation and/or anesthesia, the need to prepare children to undergo procedures, and the need to communicate with children and their parents, among other issues. An excellent new introductory chapter in the fourth edition of *Pediatric Radiology: The Requisites* addresses these and helps establish context for the rest of the book, including a discussion of the pivotal role of child life specialists who have become integral parts of the pediatric radiology team over the past decade.

Pediatric radiology shares the benefits of major ongoing technical advances in the imaging sciences and the continued increasing importance of high value cross sectional imaging. A critical issue is selecting the best method, which typically requires a balance between information that may be obtained and the costs and risks of respective methods, including relative radiation risks. Drs. Walters and Robertson and coauthors address this head on with a discussion of the Image Gently program. They appropriately point out that when a CT scan is requested, consideration should be given to whether a procedure such as ultrasound or MRI that does not involve ionizing radiation would provide the necessary clinical information.

The basic chapter outline in the fourth edition of *Pediatric Radiology: The Requisites* continues to reflect a logical division of material by organ system with the addition of two new chapters on the spine and on head and neck imaging. These chapters speak to the ongoing need for more subspecialty knowledge in the respective areas. Each chapter has been completely refreshed with a rich mix of contemporary illustrations and updated to reflect current best practices. The liberal use of tables and boxes is a feature of *The Requisites* series that facilitates quick access and review of key material.

The first edition of *Pediatric Radiology: The Requisites* was the very first volume in *The Requisites* to be published. It appeared 25 years ago through the able authorship of Hans Blickman. Since then, 35 books or so have appeared in 11 topical areas. These books have become trusted and valued friends to radiology residents, fellows, and practitioners alike for their efficiency in presenting material and for their authenticity. The books in *The Requisites* series are not intended to be encyclopedic but are intended to be used every day for learning and for practical reference to common topics that arise in clinical practice.

Feedback over the years has been excellent, and the lineup of future new editions is exciting. The fact that every book among the original 10 has undergone revision and republication, with a number of the books in their fourth editions, is a reflection of their wide acceptance and perceived value.

It is my hope that readers of the fourth edition of *Pediatric Radiology: The Requisites* will find that this new volume remains true to the philosophy of the series and meets the high standards for style and substance embodied in the first three editions. I again congratulate Drs. Walters and Robertson in taking the lead in producing this outstanding work.

James H. Thrall, MD

Preface

We are pleased to present the fourth edition of *Pediatric Radiology: The Requisites*. For this edition, we have expanded the content included for all organ systems, revised the text significantly to reflect current knowledge and clinical practice, and included hundreds of new images. Our target audience is the radiology resident, though we feel this book will also serve as a useful resource for pediatric radiology fellows and attending radiologists who practice in a variety of academic and private practice settings. All core areas of general diagnostic body imaging and neuroimaging are covered using an organ systems approach. The content of each chapter is intended to be relevant and manageable, but not exhaustive. We hope that this revision is a welcome addition to *The Requisites* series.

Michele M. Walters and Richard L. Robertson

Acknowledgments

We would like to express our sincere gratitude to Jane Choura for her dedicated, meticulous work in chapter editing. We also extend a heartfelt thank you to Rhonda Johnson and Ethan Bremner for their assistance with manuscript and image preparation. Additional artwork for this edition has been provided by radiologist Dr. Andrew Phelps. We thank Robin Carter and Kathryn DeFrancesco at Elsevier for skillfully guiding us through the editing and layout process.

Contents

Chapter 1

Introduction

Michael J. Callahan, Angela Franceschi, Sabeena Chacko, Stephen D. Brown, and Michele M. Walters

As with other books in *The Requisites* series, this installment is primarily geared toward the radiology resident. It is not intended to provide an exhaustive review of pediatric imaging; rather, the hope is that it will serve as a useful and manageable resource for the topics most commonly encountered in pediatric radiology as a resident completes his or her 3-month rotation covering both the tertiary care and the community settings.

The chapters are organized by organ systems, with six devoted to body imaging and three focusing on neuroimaging. Discussions around imaging modalities and techniques are embedded in the respective chapters. In this first introductory chapter, we have chosen to present a few topics that are particularly important in pediatric imaging and may be somewhat unfamiliar to radiology residents as they begin their first experience in pediatrics. These include radiation dose optimization, the roles of child life and anesthesia/sedation in pediatric imaging, and the unique challenges of communicating effectively with patients and parents in pediatric radiology.

RADIATION DOSE OPTIMIZATION IN PEDIATRIC IMAGING

Medical imaging has a profound impact on the treatment of children and has become an integral part of pediatric patient care in both the inpatient and the outpatient settings. With the exception of magnetic resonance imaging (MRI) and ultrasound, ionizing radiation is an essential element for most common forms of diagnostic medical imaging. Although digital and computed radiographic studies represent a majority of radiologic procedures, they represent a relative minority of the collective effective dose to the pediatric patient population. A large percentage of ionizing radiation in medical imaging is related to the generalized increased use of computed tomography (CT). Despite the fact that CT generates a disproportionately higher dose than radiography and certain fluoroscopic procedures, the clinical value of CT is unquestioned, and this modality is largely regarded as a safe procedure for children provided the study is clinically justified. In general, the amount of ionizing radiation from a single pediatric CT examination is relatively small, particularly if the study is performed properly. The benefits of a clinically indicated diagnostic CT scan are well recognized and documented, and these benefits generally far outweigh the small potential risks for cancer. Even though it is the radiologist's responsibility to perform pediatric imaging studies using the least amount of radiation necessary for a particular clinical question, it is also the responsibility of the pediatric health care professional to ensure that each CT study is indicated and have a general understanding of the relative doses and relative risks of common pediatric imaging studies.

Despite the known virtues of pediatric diagnostic imaging, public perception is often closely linked to the perceived risks of exposure to ionizing radiation. The potential hazards and perceived risks of ionizing radiation in children have been intensely studied and debated for years, and much of the fear associated with the use of ionizing radiation is unjustifiably rooted in the destructive power of nuclear weapons. Although there is no consensus on the true risks of exposure to low-level ionizing radiation, there is a general agreement that exposure to ionizing radiation at doses above a certain threshold can result in a small risk for cancer later in life. More than a decade ago, several articles were published in the February 2001 issue of the *American Journal of Roentgenology* describing the potential risks of ionizing radiation. This raised awareness that many children were receiving a higher dose of ionizing radiation than necessary for CT studies. Although it is challenging to directly demonstrate the potential risks for a single CT examination in an individual patient, some researchers estimate a small number of all cancers in the United States may be attributable to the radiation from CT studies. Until recently, this hypothesis was based largely on data from atomic bomb survivors. Although there is some disagreement within the medical community about the most accurate depiction of risks from ionizing radiation related to CT imaging, it is widely believed in the pediatric radiology literature that dose reduction in children and adherence to the ALARA (as low as reasonably achievable) principle are of paramount importance.

In 2008, the Image Gently campaign (http://www.imagegently .org) was founded and championed by the Society for Pediatric Radiology, the American Society of Radiologic Technologists, the American College of Radiology, and the American Association of Physicists in Medicine. The collaborative campaign is a dynamic alliance of individual health care professionals including the radiologist, radiology technologist, medical physicist, and pediatrician, creating a powerful force that has changed practice. The Image Gently campaign unifies more than 80 organizations, currently representing more than 800,000 international medical and dental professionals in radiology, pediatrics, physics, and radiology technology. The Image Gently website (http://www.imagegently.org) provides a comprehensive, peer-reviewed resource for a variety of pediatric imaging modalities including CT, digital radiography, nuclear medicine, interventional radiology, fluoroscopy, and dental imaging.

Optimizing CT protocols remains a challenge, particularly when imaging pediatric patients. Many institutions have more than one CT scanner, and many of those institutions have more than one CT vendor in their practice. This necessitates multiple different CT protocols for a similar indication or similar-sized patient. Nevertheless, any given institution's protocols are typically vendor and scanner specific, and as a result, these protocols are not easily transferrable to other institutions. The Image Gently website is an excellent resource for pediatric CT protocols. This resource can serve as a starting point for adult-based radiology practices that image children and wish to develop pediatric specific CT protocols, or for those practices that are seeking general guidance for pediatric CT studies and would like to verify that their existing protocols meet appropriate guidelines.

When a pediatric CT scan is requested, it is important to first consider utilizing alternative imaging modalities such as ultrasound or MRI, which do not require the use of ionizing radiation. However, there should be no hesitation in performing a CT study when it is deemed to be the best imaging test for a given clinical situation. Once the decision to perform a CT is made, it is as important to optimize the CT examination parameters in an effort to minimize dose. Strauss et al provide a nice summary on optimization of CT parameters for pediatric imaging, including specific information on tube current, exposure time, kVp, pitch, and automatic exposure control. Recently the widespread use of iterative reconstruction software has provided further reductions in CT dose, but this new technology also provides another potential level of complexity to protocol generation.

Increased utilization of endoscopy, CT, and MRI has gradually resulted in decreased utilization of fluoroscopy for pediatric chest, gastrointestinal, and genitourinary imaging. However, fluoroscopy remains an important imaging modality for the evaluation of a multitude of pediatric conditions, including neonatal high or low intestinal obstruction, the acutely vomiting infant or child, dynamic large airway imaging, and the evaluation of certain patients with suspected vesicoureteral reflux including patients with a history of febrile urinary tract infection.

In addition to CT dose reduction, national efforts to reduce radiation exposure from medical imaging have included initiatives to reduce unnecessary radiation exposure from fluoroscopic examinations. Despite its virtues, fluoroscopy provides an added challenge for the diagnostic radiologist. This modality is substantially more operator dependent than CT, and doses can vary significantly from patient to patient for similar clinical indications.

When performing a pediatric fluoroscopy study, one should always make an effort to decrease patient dose by minimizing fluoroscopy time, avoiding magnification whenever possible, maximizing collimation, utilizing pulsed fluoroscopy and last image hold, and minimizing the distance between the patient and the image intensifier. These principles are highlighted in the Image Gently Pause and Pulse campaign.

ROLE OF THE CHILD LIFE SPECIALIST AND THE IMPORTANCE OF RELATIONSHIP BUILDING IN PEDIATRIC RADIOLOGY

Certified child life specialists (CLSs) are essential to adequately meet the needs of patients and families entering the pediatric radiology department. For many children, if not most, the radiology department can be a stressful and intimidating environment. Imaging involves machines that may be perceived as loud and frightening, as well as potentially uncomfortable positioning and procedures that may cause discomfort. Radiology is often the first encounter for patients in the medical setting, but likely will not be the last. It is therefore essential to involve CLSs to help create a positive experience and assist children and families in coping with anxiety related to radiologic studies.

Certified CLSs are trained professionals who work with children and families to assist them with the challenges of hospitalization, illness, and disability. They are found throughout the pediatric health care setting. CLSs have a strong background in human growth and development. This specialized training enables them to normalize the hospital environment for children and prepare them for medical experiences, taking into account the age, developmental stage, and unique needs of each patient. As advocates of family-centered care and vital members of the multidisciplinary health care team, CLSs work in partnership with all practitioners to meet the emotional, developmental, and cultural needs of each child and family. CLSs also serve as a resource for other hospital staff members and are active in providing formal and informal education around age-appropriate practices and successful relationship-building skills.

As a clinician working in the pediatric medical setting, it is important to remember that a child's age is not always indicative of the child's developmental stage. Many factors such as acute pathology, chronic illness, a prolonged hospital stay, and even parenting style can affect a child's developmental level. Despite

this, there are universal approaches to interacting with children that are effective across the board. These include making eye contact, addressing fears, being present with children and their families, and clearly communicating your role as part of the health care team. When working to establish a relationship with a patient, it is important to be observant and tuned in to a child's expression and posture. Is the child avoiding eye contact? Is the child clinging to his or her caregiver? Is the child fidgety or biting his or her nails? It is critical to take cues from the patient and tailor your approach accordingly. Information about a child's past experience(s) in the medical setting and coping style should be elicited from a caregiver if possible. Demonstrating an honest interest in the child and individualizing care will go a long way, enhancing the child's ability to cope and facilitating completion of the study or procedure at hand.

It is important to be mindful of age-appropriate techniques in facilitating cooperation with pediatric patients. Infants often respond best when a caregiver is close by and a comfort item is provided. A pacifier dipped in oral sucrose can be very soothing during procedures that may cause discomfort [Fig. 1.1]. Toddlers can be particularly challenging to image, as they are constantly on the move, learning independence, and often strong-willed. Distraction techniques such as singing songs and blowing bubbles are typically very effective with this age group, affording brief windows of opportunity for study completion [Fig. 1.2]. Preschool-aged children are magical thinkers and may see medical experiences as a form of punishment. For them, providing a rationale for imaging may be helpful. A statement such as "the doctor needs to take a picture to make sure everything is working okay inside your body" may facilitate patient cooperation. School-age children are logical thinkers and usually do best when they know what to expect and are given some control of their situation. In preparation for an MRI, one might say, "This test will take 30 minutes, the length of your favorite TV show. You can help us by keeping your body very still. Can you practice being still like a statue?" This type of dialogue involves the child and gives him or her a role related to imaging. For placement of an intravenous line, one might explain to the child, "First you will feel a tight squeeze around your arm, next it will feel cold and wet while we wash it, then you will feel a quick poke. Can you hold the bandage for me and put it on your arm when we are done?" In this setting, the child knows what to expect, has some control, and understands that there will be a beginning and an end to the procedure. Adolescents often see themselves as invincible, and may delay telling caregivers about medical issues they are experiencing and/or withhold important

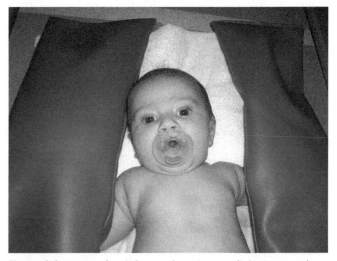

Figure 1.1 Image of an infant undergoing a radiologic procedure. A pacifier has been provided as a comfort item.

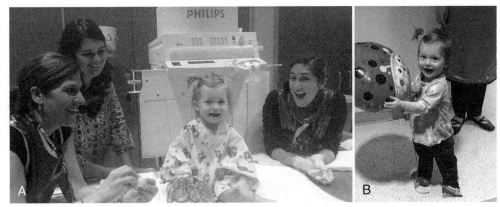

Figure 1.2 Image of a toddler having a voiding cystourethrogram. **A,** A child life specialist (CLS), the patient's mother, and a radiology technologist are with the patient before the procedure begins. The CLS has provided bubbles and toys to be used as distraction techniques during the procedure. **B,** After the procedure, the CLS has rewarded the patient with a balloon.

details. When taking a history before imaging, it is important to speak directly to these older patients and not only to their caregivers. Adolescents should be asked whether they prefer to be alone during imaging or have their caregiver accompany them. Privacy should be considered, particularly when performing an invasive study such as a voiding cystourethrogram (VCUG). If ample staffing is available, it is nice to offer the adolescent patient the option of a male or female practitioner, particularly for these sensitive studies. Options for distraction should be offered. These may include an iPad, a portable DVD player, or even the patient's phone. With all patients and caregivers, medical jargon should be avoided. It is important to remember that terminology that is commonplace to practitioners in the medical setting is often unfamiliar and confusing to others.

Relationship building with parents and other caregivers is equally as important as connecting with pediatric patients. For caregivers to feel confident and secure, trust must be established with the entire imaging team. This can be accomplished by addressing caregivers by name, inquiring about past experiences, allowing ample time for questions, and expressing genuine concern and empathy. Many caregivers present to the radiology department unaware of what will be expected of their child or of them during imaging. This lack of knowledge undoubtedly impacts their comfort level. An open dialogue between the imaging team and the caregiver before a study can clarify expectations for all and allow caregivers to feel empowered and confident. In turn, they are able to be active, supportive participants in the child's medical care. During this discussion, the practitioner should gauge the caregiver's understanding of the imaging study or procedure to be done, clarifying any misconceptions. The practitioner should also clearly define their own role as it pertains to the task at hand. For many radiologic studies, it is appropriate for the caregiver to be present during the examination. If they wish to be, the practitioner should provide concrete examples of how they might be helpful in supporting their child; for example, "Your child will need to lie still for 45 minutes, but you can be right next to her, holding her hand and encouraging her to take deep breaths." As children take their cues from their caregivers and most often respond appropriately, it is imperative to build confidence and empower caregivers to assist in creating a positive imaging environment.

ROLE OF ANESTHESIA AND SEDATION IN PEDIATRIC IMAGING

Anesthesia and sedation for pediatric imaging is an integral part of any pediatric anesthesiologist's role in the hospital

setting. In order to get clear images and complete studies, children must remain motionless for studies that may be rather long in duration. This can be very challenging for younger children, and the imaging environment alone often can be intimidating.

Children between the ages of 3 months and 5 to 6 years typically require sedation or anesthesia for a CT scan, and those between the ages of 3 months and 7 years most often require sedation or anesthesia for an MRI. Infants younger than 3 months can often successfully complete a CT scan or a relatively brief MRI after a "feed and wrap" or while sucking on a pacifier. Because of the duration of the examinations and the noise generated by the magnet, MRI studies require the highest utilization of anesthesia services. Anesthesia is also often required for the completion of nuclear medicine studies.

The concept of requiring general anesthesia or sedation for an imaging study can be very daunting for many parents. As in the operating room, parents may accompany their children into the CT or MR suite for the induction of anesthesia to provide a sense of familiarity and comfort.

The amount and type of anesthesia required varies based on the patient's age, medical condition, and intellectual development. All pediatric patients require a preanesthesia evaluation, similar to that performed for all surgical patients. Some children may need nothing more than an oral anxiolytic such as diazepam (Valium) or midazolam. These medications are associated with minimal cardiorespiratory depression and allow the patient to maintain airway reflexes. Other patients may require intravenous sedation with propofol or ketamine. These agents are administered while maintaining a natural airway in a position that prevents airway obstruction. Sicker children and those needing emergent scans who may not be appropriately NPO often require general anesthesia utilizing intravenous medications or inhalational agents administered via a laryngeal mask airway or endotracheal tube.

From the anesthesiologist's perspective, the administration of anesthesia and sedation in the radiology department poses several unique challenges. The radiology department is often located far from the surgical suite where anesthesia is most often administered and ample personnel and equipment are available. It is critical to have systems in place to keep patients safe in this relatively remote setting. There are standards in place for the administration of anesthesia in nonoperating room areas that must be strictly followed. Sedation protocols and monitoring guidelines exist so that nurses and nonanesthetists can safely care for healthy children with appropriate oversight in specified areas of the radiology department. The MRI suite poses unique challenges for the anesthesiologist because all equipment must be MRI compatible.

Patients must be carefully monitored while under anesthesia or sedation. During an imaging study, this most often means watching the patient through a window with a greater reliance on vital signs than direct observation. Monitoring equipment itself can pose risks to the patient. Tissue burns may occur if any conductive loops exist between the patient and the equipment, and exposed wires may burn the patient's skin.

Children with difficult airways who require anesthesia for imaging studies should be intubated in the controlled setting of the operating room where all necessary personnel and equipment are available before arrival in the radiology suite. In the unfortunate event of a cardiac arrest while a child is in the MRI scanner, the patient should be removed from the magnet and resuscitation should be conducted in an area outside of the scanner where the magnetic field will not interfere with the defibrillator or other ferrous rescue items that may become projectiles.

After anesthesia or sedation for an imaging study, it is important to observe patients in a postanesthesia care unit until they are awake and able to maintain a patent airway. This unit is typically within the radiology department.

With careful planning and close collaboration between pediatric radiologists and anesthesiologists, imaging studies can be successfully completed with anesthesia or sedation while posing minimal risk to pediatric patients.

COMMUNICATING WITH PATIENTS AND PARENTS IN PEDIATRIC RADIOLOGY

A 16-year-old boy with a history of hepatoblastoma, disease free for years, is found on CT to have a new renal lesion. He is sent for a renal ultrasound that demonstrates a solid and vascular lesion. His mother has asked the sonographer what she sees.

A 17-year-old girl presents for a CT scan to evaluate a thigh mass, possibly myositis ossificans. She mentions to the technologist that she is pregnant and planning on a pregnancy termination, but her parents do not know.

A routine abdominal ultrasound performed on a 3-month-old infant at an outpatient "satellite center" demonstrates a large retroperitoneal mass and a liver metastasis. The attending pediatric radiologist, after speaking with the referring pediatrician, must speak to the parents and arrange for them to go to the main hospital center downtown for further care.

A concerned mother asks to speak to the on-call radiology fellow about the radiation dose from a CT scan that is being requested for her 5-year-old son with right lower quadrant pain.

Parents of a 15-month-old girl with a first-time febrile urinary tract infection ask a radiology resident taking the history before a VCUG whether the study really needs to be done.

A radiology nurse meets with the family of an 18-year-old woman who has had debilitating lower urinary tract symptoms. On imaging a mass is noted in the bladder. The diagnosis was revealed to the family while they waited during CT scan. The nurse is waiting with them in the CT waiting room while the logistics are worked out for the patient's disposition.

Each of these narratives provides a snapshot of the challenges that pediatric radiologic practitioners experience when communicating with patients and parents. Some conversations are difficult because of the sheer emotional weight and unexpectedness of the information to be discussed. Other conversations force practitioners to navigate matters of confidentiality. Some may force practitioners to confront the uncomfortable boundaries of their professional roles or knowledge, whether they be technologists, nurses, trainees, or radiologists-in-practice. Other circumstances may require practitioners to communicate sensitive information under conditions that do not provide optimal time or physical space.

Practitioners in pediatric radiology have long prided themselves on their close patient interactions. These difficult conversations entail additional complexity associated with relating to parents and to children of varying developmental stages. Nurses, technologists, and radiologists alike must be able to explain what they are doing and why in terms that children and parents can understand. Further, those who practice in pediatrics must adapt themselves to caring for frightened and sick children who are in pain. They must confront the fact that what they are doing may cause additional pain and other harms in children, sometimes when the benefit is clear and sometimes when the potential benefit seems small or questionable. In all cases, they must remain aware of the best interests of children and be prepared to advocate strongly (but judiciously) when asked to do tests or procedures that seem contrary to the patients' best interests.

Communicating with patients in these circumstances requires a myriad of specific skills. Their application entails a fundamental understanding of the nuances of verbal and nonverbal communication and a facility for recognizing and adjusting to stumbling blocks. Success involves empathy, patience, and an ability to respond reflexively to the moment-to-moment dynamics of the conversation. As with other competencies in radiology, no single avenue exists to acquiring the requisite skills to engage in these conversations on a consistently effective level. Like most areas of radiology, the acquisition of communication skills emerges through a combination of mentorship, observation, and practice. Unlike most other areas of radiology, for which dedicated training curricula form a crucial additional avenue of learning, few training programs provide dedicated curricula for communication skills. Innovative simulation-based communication skills training programs for radiologists have been described. The largest of these demonstrated enhanced comfort among program participants in talking with patients about bad news, radiation risks, and errors. Even for participants of such programs, however, the ability later to implement learned skills is dependent on the supportiveness of the professional cultures in which they practice.

SUGGESTED READINGS

Brenner DJ, Elliston CD, Hall EJ, et al. Estimated risks of radiation-induced fatal cancer from pediatric CT. *AJR Am J Roentgenol.* 2001;176:289-296.

Brenner DJ, Hall EJ. Computed tomography – an increasing source of radiation exposure. *N Engl J Med.* 2007;357:2277-2284.

Brody AS, Frush DP, Huda W, et al. Radiation risk to children from computed tomography. *Pediatrics.* 2007;120:677-682.

Brown C, Chitkara M. Child Life Services, Committee on Hospital Care and Child Life Council. *Pediatrics.* 2014;133:e1471-e1478.

Brown SD. *Communicating Bad News. Case Files: Medical Ethics and Professionalism.* New York, NY: McGraw-Hill Education; 2015:155-163.

Brown SD, Callahan MJ, Browning DM, et al. Radiology trainees' comfort with difficult conversations and attitudes about error disclosure: effect of a communication skills workshop. *J Am Coll Radiol.* 2014;11:781-787.

Carver D, Franceschi A, Thies R. Pediatric imaging. In: Long BW, Rollins JH, Smith BJ, eds. *Merrill's Atlas of Radiographic Positioning and Procedures.* Vol. 3. St. Louis, MO: Elsevier; 2016:99-160.

Debenedectis CM, Gauget J-M, Makris J, et al. Coming Out of the Dark: A Curriculum for Teaching and Evaluating Radiology Resident's Commuinication Skills through Simulation. Annual Meeting of the Radiologic Society of North America; Chicago, IL; 2015.

Donnelly LF, Emery KH, Brody AS, et al. Minimizing radiation dose for pediatric body applications of single-detector helical CT: strategies at a large Children's Hospital. *AJR Am J Roentgenol.* 2001;176:303-306.

Hernanz-Schulman M, Goske MJ, et al. Pause and pulse: ten steps that help manage radiation dose during pediatric fluoroscopy. *AJR Am J Roentgenol.* 2011;197:475-481.

Linton OW, Mettler FA. National conference on dose reduction in CT, with an emphasis on pediatric patients. *AJR Am J Roentgenol.* 2003;181:321-329.

Lown BA, Sasson JP, Hinrichs P. Patients as partners in radiology education: an innovative approach to teaching and assessing patient-centered communication. *Acad Radiol*. 2008;15:425-432.

Luff D, Fernandes S, Soman A, et al. The influence of communication and relational education on radiologists' early posttraining practice. *J Am Coll Radiol*. 2016;13:445-448.

McGee K. The role of a child life specialist in a pediatric radiology department. *Pediatr Radiol*. 2003;33:467-474.

Paterson A, Frush DP, Donnelly LF. Helical CT of the body: are settings adjusted for pediatric patients? *AJR Am J Roentgenol*. 2001;176:297-301.

Pearce MS, Salotti JA, Little MP, et al. Radiation exposure from CT scans in childhood and subsequent risk of leukaemia and brain tumours: a retrospective cohort study. *Lancet*. 2012;380:499-505.

Sandy NS, Nguyen HT, Ziniel SI, et al. Assessment of parental satisfaction in children undergoing voiding cystourethrography without sedation. *J Urol*. 2011;185:658-662.

Slovis TL. Proceedings of the Second ALARA Conference. *Pediatr Radiol*. 2004;34(suppl 3):S159-S248.

Strauss KJ, Goske MJ, Kaste SC, et al. Image Gently: Ten steps you can take to optimize image quality and lower CT dose for pediatric patients. *AJR Am J Roentgenol*. 2010;194:868-873.

Wood J, Collins J, Burnside ES, et al. Patient, faculty, and self-assessment of radiology resident performance: a 360-degree method of measuring professionalism and interpersonal/communication skills. *Acad Radiol*. 2004;11:931-939.

WEB SOURCES

http://www.imagegently.org

http://www.childlife.org

http://www.fda.gov/Radiation-EmittingProducts/RadiationSafety/RadiationDoseReduction/ucm199994.htm

http://www.ncrppublications.org/Reports/160

Chapter 2
Chest Imaging

Patricia Trinidad Chang and Laureen Sena

IMAGING TECHNIQUES AND INDICATIONS

Conventional Radiography

Diagnostic imaging plays an important role in the evaluation of the upper airway and chest in children. Chest radiographs comprise about 40% of all pediatric imaging, in large part because congenital and acquired respiratory disorders are so common.

The most common indication for evaluation of the upper airway is stridor, or noisy breathing caused by airway obstruction. Stridor can be inspiratory, expiratory, or both, and characterization of stridor helps to formulate a practical differential diagnosis and determine the imaging indicated to diagnose the level of obstruction. When stridor is primarily expiratory, the pathology is almost always below the thoracic inlet, and chest radiography with frontal and lateral views is typically performed. When stridor is primarily inspiratory, anteroposterior (AP) and lateral views of the neck soft tissues are performed in addition to chest radiography to evaluate the upper airway. When children have stridor and are suspected to have airway obstruction, they are imaged in a position where they are most comfortable so that symptoms are not exacerbated.

In addition to inspiratory stridor, other indications for upper airway imaging include nasal obstruction, epistaxis, suspected foreign body, evaluation of nasopharyngeal lymphoid tissue, unexplained pulmonary hypertension, hoarseness or abnormal cry, trauma, caustic ingestion, and neck masses. The lateral radiograph of the neck is essential for identifying retained foreign bodies, evaluating for upper airway masses, and diagnosing epiglottitis. An AP view is added for the evaluation for croup or subglottic obstruction.

Indications for chest radiography in children include expiratory stridor, wheezing, tachypnea, chest pain, suspected infectious or inflammatory respiratory illness, trauma, known or suspected heart disease, and evaluation for metastatic or primary tumors. Chest radiography is generally not performed in children for routine hospital admissions or before sedation or anesthesia unless there are concerning symptoms and/or a history of recent respiratory illness.

Obtaining AP or posteroanterior (PA) and lateral views of the chest in children can be challenging, especially when they are younger than 4 years. A variety of immobilization techniques can be used. A pacifier may be helpful to obtain the chest radiograph during quiet inspiration. Supine AP films are usually easiest to obtain, and there is no appreciable difference in magnification between the supine AP and the upright AP or PA view in small children [**Fig. 2.1A**]. At age older than 4 years, PA and lateral views of the chest are performed with the patient standing or sitting upright.

A supplemental view of the chest such as an expiratory image can be helpful to evaluate for and determine the size of a pneumothorax or detect dependent air trapping if there is concern for an aspirated foreign body. Decubitus views are useful to evaluate for layering of a pleural effusion when there is concern for possible loculation. Small amounts of pleural fluid (up to 2 mm thick) can be normal in children.

Ultrasound

Ultrasonography provides valuable diagnostic information to determine the cystic versus solid nature of neck masses and lesions in the superior mediastinum. Ultrasound can be used to distinguish between the normal, homogeneous-appearing thymus and a concerning mediastinal mass [**Fig. 2.1B**]. Cardiac structure and function can be exquisitely assessed by US without the use of ionizing radiation or contrast administration. Echocardiography is primarily performed by pediatric cardiologists. Ultrasound can be used to assess the size and complexity of pleural effusions. It is particularly useful in the setting of complete hemithorax opacification, allowing the detection of pleural fluid associated with collapse or consolidation of an entire lung. Ultrasound can provide an assessment of diaphragmatic excursion during inspiration and expiration in the evaluation for diaphragmatic paresis. Doppler US is useful in the evaluation of intravascular access and the assessment of vessel patency and/ or thrombus formation. Ultrasound has the important benefit of portability, allowing for bedside evaluation of patients who are very ill and/or unable to travel.

Computed Tomography

Modern-day multidetector computed tomography (CT) scanning provides excellent image quality, particularly in the less than cooperative patient. There is a relatively low need for sedation or anesthesia, now used in less than 2% of patients younger than 4 years. The tracheobronchial tree, pulmonary congenital malformations, metastatic and interstitial lung disease, mediastinal pathology, and subpleural and chest wall lesions can now be assessed without breath-holding technique in small children using the rapid scanning techniques of currently available dual-source and volumetric CT scanners. High-resolution computed tomography (HRCT) provides excellent spatial resolution for the depiction of interstitial lung disease. Computed tomography angiography (CTA) has an established role in the evaluation of congenital cardiac anomalies (see Chapter 3) and the assessment of extracardiac thoracic vascular anomalies.

Magnetic Resonance Imaging

Magnetic resonance imaging (MRI) is a useful modality for the evaluation of mediastinal masses. It is particularly useful for demonstrating the extent of posterior mediastinal lesions. MRI and magnetic resonance angiography (MRA) are becoming more widely used in the evaluation of the mediastinal vasculature, congenital cardiac lesions, and anomalies of the great vessels. Both modalities are useful for the assessment and characterization of the vascular supply of congenital bronchopulmonary foregut malformations and vascular lesions of the lung. More recently, rapid MR sequences have allowed improved depiction of the pulmonary interstitium and ventilation and perfusion abnormalities, reducing the cumulative dose from surveillance CT scans. The morphology of congenital cardiac and vascular

6

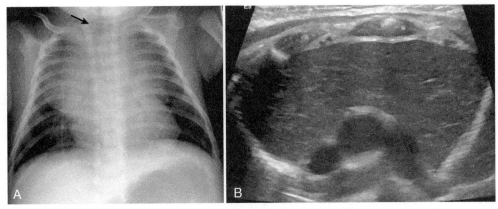

Figure 2.1 **Normal appearance of the chest in a 50-day-old infant. A,** Chest radiograph shows prominence of the superior mediastinum because of size of the thymus at this age. A smooth, undulating contour is noted that conforms to the ribs of the anterior chest wall. The density of the thymus is lower than that of the heart. Note the rightward tracheal buckling (*arrow*) that is often seen on chest radiographs of infants. **B,** Ultrasound of the chest confirms a normal thymus, with homogeneous echotexture and no significant mass effect on the mediastinal vasculature.

lesions and related MRI applications are discussed in detail in Chapter 3.

DEVELOPMENT OF AIRWAY AND LUNGS

Structural Development

In the fourth week of gestation, a ventral diverticulum arises from the developing foregut. This is called the *laryngotracheal tube.* The proximal portion of this develops into the larynx and trachea, and becomes continuous with the pharynx. The distal portion enlarges and divides into three right and two left bronchial buds, which will eventually form the right and left lungs. With continued growth and division, the terminal bronchioles and respiratory bronchioles develop. The process of lung development is complete by 28 weeks' gestation. When the respiratory bronchioles become invested with capillaries, they are called *terminal sacs* or *primitive alveoli.* The primitive alveoli continue to mature until birth. During the last 2 months of prenatal life and up until the age of 8 years, the number of alveoli continues to increase. Growth of the lungs after birth is primarily due to an increase in the number of respiratory bronchioles and alveoli. Alveolar epithelial cells (types I and II) line the terminal sacs. Type II pneumocytes develop by 23 to 24 weeks' gestation and are responsible for pulmonary surfactant production. Respiration is possible at 24 weeks' gestation, when sufficient terminal sacs exist to allow survival of the premature infant with respiratory support in the intensive care unit.

Development of the pulmonary vasculature begins concurrently in the fourth week of gestation. A primitive pulmonary artery arises from the ventral aspect of the right and left sixth aortic arches, extending caudally toward the developing tubular lung bud. This is eventually incorporated into the mesenchymal tissue around the primitive trachea and bronchial buds. A pulmonary artery accompanies each developing bronchial bud. The venous return develops from the mesenchyme and the cardiac wall, and rather than following the bronchial tree, runs between the bronchopulmonary segments and drains to the left atrium.

Tracheal cartilage first begins to differentiate during the fourth week of gestation. Distinct rings of cartilage are present along the trachea and mainstem bronchi by 11 weeks' gestation. The development of cartilage lags behind the branching of the airways; as such, cartilage does not extend into the more peripheral pulmonary bronchi. Any disturbance of this orderly sequence of events may result in a predictable set of developmental aberrations. These are referred to as *bronchopulmonary foregut*

malformations, and they include congenital lobar emphysema, bronchial atresia, and sequestration. These entities are discussed in depth later in this chapter. The submucosal mucous-secreting glands of the bronchi and bronchioles arise from the epithelial cells and migrate into the submucosa. These glands are even slower to develop than the cartilage.

In children, insults (e.g., viruses) to the lungs primarily affect the terminal and respiratory bronchioles. In contrast, in adults such insults primarily affect the interstitium or the airspaces.

Functional Development

Successful lung maturation and function require the completion of both structural development and biochemical development of the surfactant system. Incomplete structural development and/or premature birth before development of the surfactant system will lead to respiratory compromise or insufficiency in the newborn.

Surfactant is a mixture of phospholipids and hydrophobic proteins produced by type II pneumocytes and secreted into the alveolar spaces. The production of surfactant is independent of lung growth. Surfactant decreases the surface tension within alveoli and prevents alveolar collapse during expiration. Surfactant production gradually increases with advancing gestational age, with full maturation by 36 weeks in most fetuses. Therefore birth at any time before 36 weeks' gestation may be associated with respiratory compromise or failure as a result of surfactant deficiency.

In infants, the balance among central airway compliance, peripheral airway resistance, and lung recoil differs compared with that of older children and adults, resulting in different patterns of airflow. Any adverse influences during this period may diminish airway and/or alveolar growth, affecting lung and airway size ultimately attained. Such potentially harmful factors include allergens, viruses, and air pollutants.

Physiologically, the respiratory cycles of a healthy infant are markedly different from those of an infant suffering from peripheral airway disease. Diffuse peripheral airway inflammation is referred to as bronchiolitis. In children with bronchiolitis, the tidal volume of the lungs is small and the residual volume is significantly higher than normal. This leads to air trapping. In severe cases, the degree of air trapping may approach total lung capacity.

On radiographs, hyperinflation is seen in association with thickened (visible) bronchial walls and areas of atelectasis. Peribronchial thickening or "cuffing" is best seen on the lateral radiograph. Other radiographic findings include flattening of the

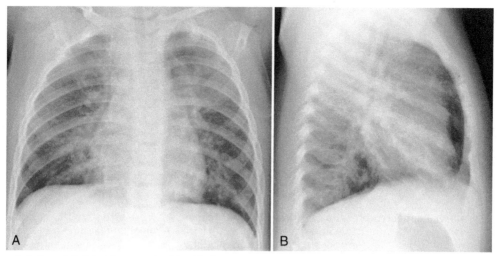

Figure 2.2 Bronchiolitis. Ten-month-old with fever and cough. **A,** Frontal and (**B**) lateral views of the chest demonstrate hyperinflated lungs with perihilar peribronchial cuffing bilaterally. Streaky opacity reflecting atelectasis partially obscures the right heart border on the frontal view and is seen on the lateral view in the region of the right middle lobe. The hemidiaphragms are flattened, and hyperinflated anterior lung causes anterior bowing of the chest wall on the lateral view.

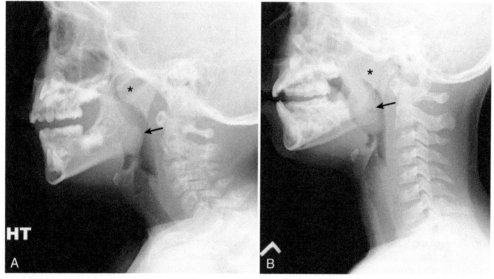

Figure 2.3 Enlargement of the adenoid tissues and tonsils. Lateral views of the neck soft tissues in two different children with recurrent upper respiratory infections and snoring demonstrate enlarged adenoid tissues (*asterisks*) and palatine tonsils (*arrows*).

hemidiaphragms, anterior bowing of the sternum, and a more "horizontal" orientation of the ribs. These radiographic findings reflect the physiologic changes and may vary over time. Atelectasis is relatively frequent in children compared with adults because collateral air circulation through the pores of Kohn and canals of Lambert is less efficient [**Fig. 2.2**].

NORMAL ANATOMY AND VARIANTS

Pharynx

The pharynx is divided into the nasopharynx, oropharynx, and hypopharynx. An important anatomic structure is the Waldeyer ring, composed of the adenoids superiorly, the palatine tonsils laterally, and the lingual tonsils inferiorly. On a lateral radiograph of the neck soft tissues, the retropharyngeal soft tissues extend from the adenoids, which are visible by 3 to 6 months of age, to the origin of the esophagus at the level of C4-C5. Prominent

adenoids become pathologic when they encroach on the nasopharyngeal airway [**Fig. 2.3**]. The palatine tonsils are outlined by air only with marked distention of the hypopharynx. The lingual tonsils are occasionally visible radiographically at the base of the tongue. Measurements of the adenoid tissues and tonsils are notably neither reliable nor useful.

A quantitative assessment of retropharyngeal soft tissue thickness is important. A useful ratio is that of the retropharyngeal soft tissue thickness to the C2 vertebral body width. On a lateral view of the neck obtained in inspiration, this ratio changes from approximately 1.0 until almost 1 year of age to 0.5 by 6 years of age. On average, the retropharyngeal soft tissue width above the level of C4 should not exceed 50% of the vertebral body width [**Fig. 2.4**]. Notably, the retropharyngeal soft tissues may become quite thick on radiographs obtained in expiration or without full neck extension. This can lead to a false-positive diagnosis of retropharyngeal abscess. If an examination is equivocal, a repeat view with full inspiration and neck extension should be obtained.

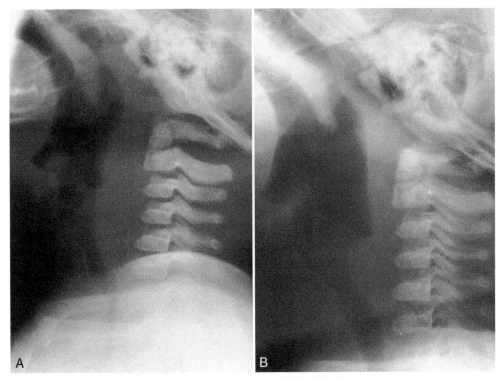

Figure 2.4 A, Lateral radiograph of the neck soft tissues obtained during expiration demonstrates apparent widening of the retropharyngeal soft tissues. **B,** With inspiratory technique, this appearance is no longer seen. The retropharyngeal soft tissue width from C1 to C3 is less than the vertebral body width at these levels.

Larynx

The larynx extends from the base of the tongue to the trachea. It is composed of three major cartilaginous structures—the epiglottis, the thyroid cartilage, and the cricoid cartilage—and three small paired cartilaginous structures—the arytenoid, cuneiform, and corniculate cartilages. A practical anatomic division of the larynx consists of three regions: (1) a supraglottic region containing the epiglottis, aryepiglottic folds, and false vocal cords; (2) a glottic region containing the laryngeal ventricle and the true vocal cords; and (3) a subglottic region extending from the inferior aspect of the true vocal cords to the lower cricoid cartilage. Other anatomic landmarks of the larynx include the hyoid bone, body, and horns, which may be ossified at birth. The horns of the hyoid are oriented in such a way that they "point" to the epiglottis on a conventional lateral radiograph of the neck [**Fig. 2.5**]. Calcification of respiratory cartilage is notably rare in children and is pathologic. It is seen in such conditions as chondrodysplasia punctata and relapsing polychondritis.

Mediastinum

The variable size and shape of the normal mediastinum in children can result in challenges in the interpretation of chest radiographs. Compartmentalization of the mediastinum represents an arbitrary classification to facilitate description of the location of disease and determine pathology. Classically the mediastinum has been divided into a superior portion and an inferior portion by a line drawn from the manubrial sternal junction to the T4-T5 intervertebral disk space. The inferior portion is typically further divided into anterior, middle, and posterior portions by classification systems that vary to some degree. This system is somewhat more difficult to apply to the mediastinum of infants and children.

Using a simplified classification system, the trachea, esophagus, heart, vasculature (including the aorta, superior vena cava

(SVC), inferior vena cava (IVC), and central pulmonary arteries and veins), vagus and phrenic nerves, and lymph nodes comprise the middle mediastinum (M). The thymus occupies much of the anterior mediastinum (A), also referred to as the prevascular space. The posterior mediastinum (P) consists of the structures posterior to a line drawn along the anterior edge of the vertebral bodies, and includes the paraspinal region [**Fig. 2.6**]. This compartmentalization is easily applied to cross-sectional imaging modalities such as CT and MRI [**Fig. 2.7**]. When an anterior or middle mediastinal lesion is suspected on conventional chest radiographs, both CT and MRI are appropriate modalities for further evaluation. When a posterior mediastinal lesion is suspected, MRI is preferred to assess for possible intraspinal extension.

The mediastinum is usually prominent on chest radiographs in children due to the relatively large size of the thymus. The thymus is often visible up to 3 years of age, and may be seen until the age of 8 or 9 years. Maximal thymic size is reached during the first few months of life. The thymus then becomes relatively smaller with further growth of the rest of the body. It has a quadrilateral shape in infancy and gradually becomes triangular-shaped in later childhood and adolescence as it begins to involute. The normal thymus has a soft consistency. It does not compress adjacent structures; instead, it adapts its contour to surround structures of the middle mediastinum. The thymus does not displace the trachea or mediastinal vascular structures.

On chest radiography, the thymus has a similar density to the heart and vascular structures. Thus clear delineation of the borders of these structures may not be possible in the setting of a prominent thymus. Because of its anterior location, the margins of the thymus may be indented by the anterior ribs ("thymic wave" sign) [**Fig. 2.8**]. The right lobe of the thymus can insinuate into the minor fissure, creating a sail-like contour ("thymic sail" sign) [**Fig. 2.8**]. The thymus can change shape during respiration. It can elongate and narrow on inspiration, with

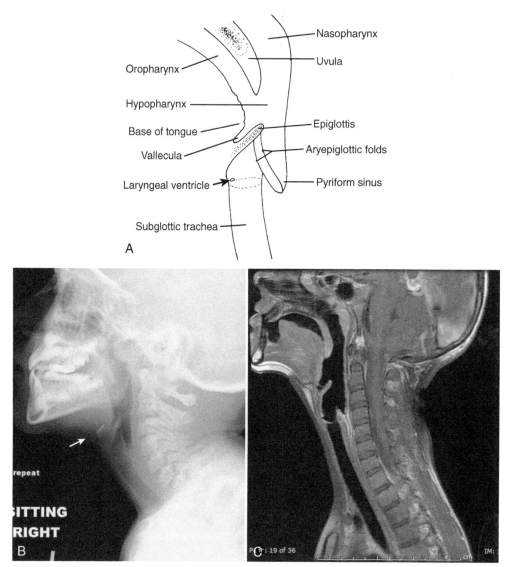

Figure 2.5 A, Diagram depicting the normal anatomy of the upper airway. **B,** Corresponding lateral radiograph of the neck soft tissues and (**C**) sagittal T1-weighted magnetic resonance image. The hyoid bone "points to" the epiglottis on the radiograph (*arrow*).

apparent increase in size on expiration. Occasionally a notch in the mediastinal contour can be seen at the junction of the thymus and the heart. This is called the *cardiothymic incisure.*

The thymus can dramatically decrease in size when a child is under stress. This may occur in the setting of an acute respiratory illness, surgery, steroid treatment, and radiation and/or chemotherapy. The thymus will regenerate when the stress resolves or when therapy is discontinued. Regeneration of the thymus or "thymic rebound" may result in a larger organ than existed before the insult in up to 25% of children. However, in the majority of cases the thymus grows up to 50% of its original size.

The variable appearance of the mediastinum on chest radiographs in children can often be a result of the normal variation in thymic contour. When questions arise, ultrasound is the modality of choice to evaluate for the presence of a normal thymus versus a mediastinal mass [**Fig. 2.9**]. On CT and MRI, normal residual thymic tissue may be visualized until the early teens. It may be seen insinuating between the vessels of the mediastinum. On CT, the thymus appears homogeneous throughout childhood, with attenuation similar to or slightly greater than that of the adjacent chest wall musculature on unenhanced

studies [**Fig. 2.10A**]. On MRI, the thymus is slightly hyperintense to skeletal muscle on T1-weighted images and slightly hypointense to fat on T2-weighted images [**Fig. 2.10B** and **C**].

On chest radiographs, the contour and size of the heart should be evaluated in the context of positioning of the child when the radiograph was obtained. The heart typically appears more prominent when the child is imaged supine as opposed to upright. Regardless of position, the chest radiograph should be obtained with adequate pulmonary inflation. On an expiratory chest radiograph, a misdiagnosis of cardiomediastinal enlargement may be made.

The tracheal air column should be carefully evaluated on both frontal and lateral chest radiographs. On the frontal view, the normal subglottic trachea has a bilaterally symmetric convex appearance, typically described as "shouldering" [**Fig. 2.11**]. As the trachea courses inferiorly into the chest, the diameter should remain uniform to the level of the carina except for a mild, smooth indentation at the level of the aortic arch. The trachea is normally positioned to the right of the midline as it courses by a left aortic arch. When the trachea is positioned in the midline or leftward within the mediastinum, mass effect caused by a right aortic arch or mediastinal mass should be considered.

Careful inspection for associated tracheal narrowing is important to detect, particularly in the setting of stridor. The trachea is relatively more flexible in children younger than 5 years. On expiratory radiographs, the normal trachea may buckle or angle to the side opposite the aortic arch, typically to the right [**Fig. 2.1A**]. This finding is most pronounced in infants. A normal trachea can decrease in diameter up to 50% during expiration, especially in the neonatal period. Collapse of the trachea greater than 50% raises the possibility of tracheomalacia.

Lungs

Chest radiography is most often performed in children for evaluation of the lung parenchyma. Evaluation should begin with an assessment of technique, including patient rotation and the degree of inspiration.

SUPPORT LINES AND TUBES IN INTENSIVE CARE PATIENTS

The evaluation of chest radiographs of neonates in the intensive care unit usually begins with an assessment of support lines and tubes. Incorrect positioning of umbilical venous catheters (UVCs), umbilical arterial catheters (UACs), endotracheal tubes (ETTs), and enteric tubes is important to recognize. Malpositioning of these devices can lead to a prolonged hospital stay, with significant associated morbidity and mortality.

Umbilical venous and arterial catheters enter through the umbilicus, which can be seen as a well-defined, rounded density outlined by air on an abdominal radiograph. Correct positioning of a UVC follows along the expected course of the umbilical vein from the umbilicus into the liver, usually to the right of midline. Blood from the placenta enters the umbilical vein. The umbilical vein then joins the left portal vein, continues to the ductus venosus, then subsequently to the middle or left hepatic vein, the IVC, and the right atrium. Optimal positioning of the UVC is within the suprahepatic IVC just below the right atrium, usually at the level of the right hemidiaphragm. A UVC should take a fairly straight course superiorly to reach the suprahepatic IVC. It should never loop as it courses into the liver [**Fig. 2.12A**]. A UVC may have an abnormal course through the liver parenchyma, terminating in the right or left portal vein. The UVC may also extend into the main portal vein, and subsequently to the superior mesenteric or splenic veins [**Fig. 2.12B**]. Abnormal positioning of the UVC within a portal vein may result in portal

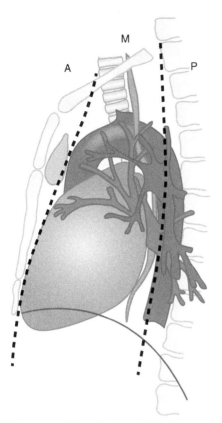

Figure 2.6 Diagram of the chest depicting the anatomic structures within the anterior (*A*), middle (*M*), and posterior (*P*) mediastinal compartments.

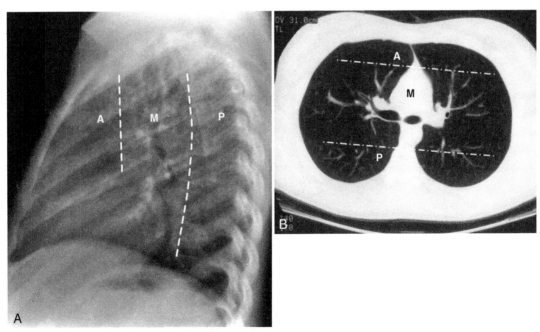

Figure 2.7 Simplified compartmentalization of the mediastinum depicted (**A**) on a lateral chest radiograph and (**B**) on an axial computed tomography image. *A,* anterior; *M,* middle; *P,* posterior.

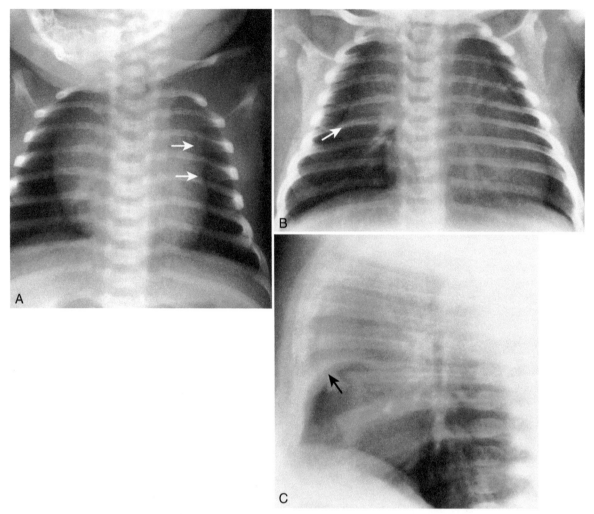

Figure 2.8 Normal variation in the appearance of the thymus on chest radiography in infants. A, The thymus has an undulating contour where it abuts the anterior ribs (*arrows*), creating the "thymic wave" sign. **B** and **C,** The thymus insinuates into the minor fissure, creating the "thymic sail" sign on frontal and lateral views (*arrows*).

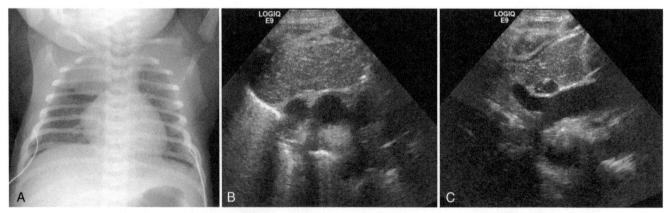

Figure 2.9 Newborn with mild respiratory distress. A, Chest radiograph demonstrates an abnormal, rounded contour to the right side of the mediastinum, raising concern for a mass. **B** and **C,** Subsequent axial and sagittal ultrasound images demonstrate normal, homogeneous-appearing thymus in the location of this finding.

vein thrombosis, liver damage, and even portal vein perforation. If the UVC is advanced too far, it may terminate in the right atrium or extend farther superiorly to enter the SVC. It may cross a patent foramen ovale to terminate in the left atrium. Malpositioning of the UVC within the heart can be associated with arrhythmia or even perforation.

A correctly placed UAC follows the course of one of the paired umbilical arteries through the umbilicus. The umbilical arteries return blood to the placenta from the internal iliac arteries. The UAC takes an inferior course from the umbilicus to enter into one of the umbilical arteries, then turns superiorly to course into the common iliac artery and subsequently into the aorta.

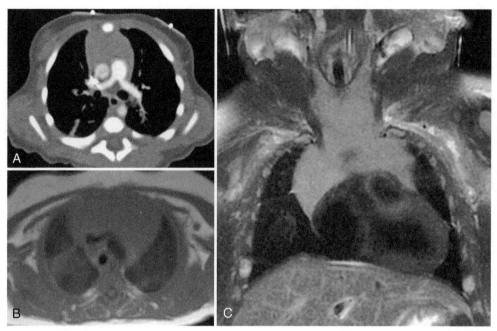

Figure 2.10 Normal thymus on computed tomography (CT) and magnetic resonance (MR) imaging. A, Axial contrast-enhanced CT image shows a normal, homogeneous-appearing thymus in the anterior mediastinum. **B,** Axial T1 and (**C**) coronal T2 MR images of the same patient show the normal thymus in the anterior mediastinum, extending into the lower neck.

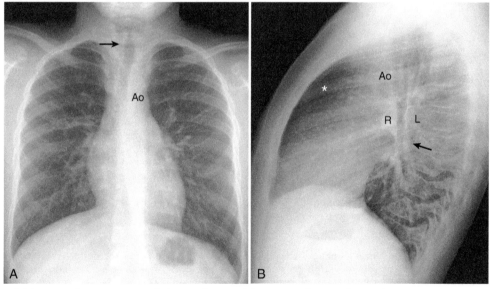

Figure 2.11 Normal appearance of the trachea and lungs on chest radiography. A, On the frontal view, there is normal shouldering of the subglottic trachea (*arrow*). The trachea courses inferiorly with a fairly uniform diameter to the level of the carina apart from a mild, smooth indentation at the level of the aortic arch (*Ao*). The lungs are symmetrically inflated, with normal arborization of the vasculature. The hemidiaphragms are domed, not flattened. The normal heart size is less than 50% the transverse dimension of the chest. **B,** On the lateral view, the trachea is of uniform diameter to the level of the aortic arch, with the exception of a mild, smooth impression from the aortic arch anteriorly (*Ao*). The hemidiaphragms are domed. The heart occupies less than 50% of the anteroposterior dimension of the chest and should not fill the retrosternal clear space (*asterisk*). The bronchus intermedius (*arrow*) courses posterior to the right pulmonary artery (*R*), and the arch of the left pulmonary artery (*L*) projects posterior to the carina.

The UAC ideally terminates within the aorta superior to the origin of the celiac artery and well below the branches from the thoracic aortic arch. This is generally between the T6 and T10 vertebral bodies. This is commonly referred to as a "high" UAC. A "low" UAC is positioned with the tip below the renal arteries or the level of the L3 vertebral body. This positioning is acceptable but may be associated with more complications. A malpositioned UAC may loop in the region of the aorta [**Fig. 2.12**] or take an aberrant course into a branch of the abdominal aorta.

Percutaneously inserted central catheters (PICC) are now being used for long-term access in neonates to avoid the higher

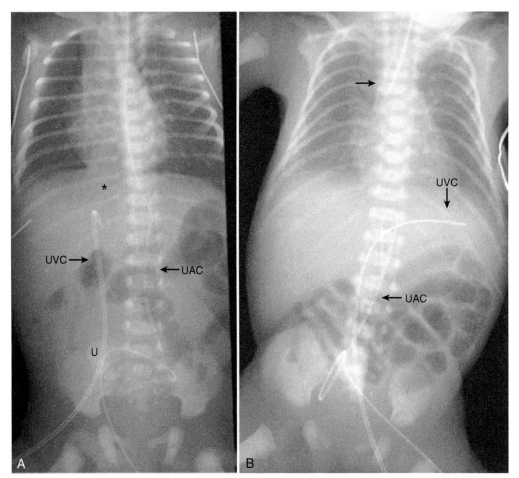

Figure 2.12 Malpositioned support tubes and lines. A, Frontal radiograph of the chest and abdomen of a premature infant shows an abnormally high termination of the endotracheal tube (ETT) in the cervical trachea (*arrow*) and malpositioned umbilical lines. The umbilical venous catheter (*UVC*) takes a normal straight course superiorly from the umbilicus (*U*), but the tip takes a sharp turn inferiorly at the level of the liver rather than continuing superiorly to a normal termination at the level of the cavo-atrial junction (*asterisk*). The umbilical arterial catheter (*UAC*) courses inferiorly from the umbilicus to enter into the left iliac artery, then extends superiorly into the aorta where it loops back on itself and courses inferiorly. A UAC should continue superiorly to terminate between T6 and T10. **B,** Frontal radiograph of the chest and abdomen of another premature infant shows an abnormally low position of the ETT in the right main stem bronchus (*arrow*). The UVC extends superiorly from the umbilicus, then takes an abrupt turn leftward as it courses from the umbilical vein into the left portal vein. The UAC courses inferiorly from the umbilicus to enter the right iliac artery, and loops back on itself within the abdominal aorta, similar to patient in (**A**).

complication rates associated with umbilical catheters. The tip of a PICC inserted from an upper extremity peripheral vein should terminate in the SVC, whereas a PICC inserted from a lower extremity approach should terminate in the IVC inferior to the right atrium.

An ETT should be positioned in the intrathoracic trachea above the level of the carina. High positioning of the ETT within the cervical trachea carries a risk for accidental extubation. Low positioning within a mainstem bronchus may cause hyperinflation of the ipsilateral lung and collapse of the contralateral lung.

Extracorporeal membrane oxygenation (ECMO) provides support to neonates with severe respiratory distress related to conditions such as congenital diaphragmatic hernia (CDH), meconium aspiration, and primary pulmonary hypertension. Venous blood is diverted to an extracorporeal membrane for oxygenation, then returned to the patient via the arterial circulation for combined pulmonary and cardiac support. This is referred to as venoarterial (VA) ECMO. Blood can be returned to the venous circulation alone when only pulmonary support is needed. This is referred to as venovenous (VV) ECMO.

VA ECMO involves separate venous and arterial cannulas, whereas VV ECMO can be performed with a single double-lumen venous cannula [**Fig. 2.13**]. The arterial cannula is often placed via the right common carotid artery, with the tip terminating in the brachiocephalic artery. It can also be placed in the femoral artery. The venous cannula is most often placed via the internal jugular vein, with the tip terminating in the right atrium. Bedside echocardiography is now routinely used for the initial evaluation of cannula placement. Subsequently, follow-up chest radiographs are used to document stability of positioning.

UPPER AIRWAY

Supraglottic Abnormalities

Laryngomalacia

Congenital laryngomalacia is the most common cause of stridor in the newborn. It is characterized by an infolding of the aryepiglottic folds during inspiration, leading to collapse and obstruction of the airway. Infants typically present with inspiratory

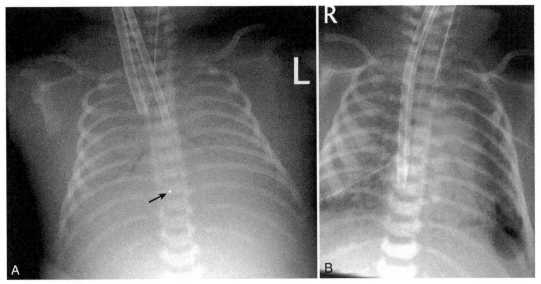

Figure 2.13 **Extracorporeal membrane oxygen (ECMO) catheters. A,** In this infant on venoarterial (VA) ECMO, the radiopaque tip associated with the venous catheter is properly positioned within the right atrium (*arrow*), and the arterial catheter terminates in good position at the aortic arch. **B,** In a different infant on venovenous (VV) ECMO, the single catheter terminates appropriately in the right atrium.

stridor that worsens with feeding, excitement, agitation, crying, and supine positioning.

The diagnosis is usually made by laryngoscopy, although airway fluoroscopy may first be performed to establish the diagnosis. On imaging, downward and posterior displacement of the epiglottis and anterior buckling of the aryepiglottic folds can be seen.

Symptoms are usually self-limiting, with resolution by 12 to 18 months of age. At this point, the arytenoid tissues strengthen and become more firmly attached to the underlying cartilage. Before resolution, serious complications such as airway obstruction and sudden death can occur.

Acute Epiglottitis

Acute epiglottitis is a life-threatening condition caused by infection and inflammation of the epiglottis and aryepiglottic folds, potentially leading to acute airway obstruction. The peak incidence of epiglottitis is between 3 and 6 years of age; however, this entity can also occur in adults. Historically, the most common causative agent was *Haemophilus influenzae* type B (HIB). Since the widespread administration of the HIB vaccine, infection with group A β-hemolytic *streptococcus* has become more frequent. Routine administration of the HIB vaccine in infancy has led to a dramatic decrease in the incidence of epiglottitis in young children. It is now more commonly diagnosed in the older pediatric population.

The clinical presentation can be striking. The affected child assumes a bold upright position, with the head held forward in respiratory distress. In severely affected patients, immediate treatment of acute epiglottitis involves intubation with direct laryngoscopy to secure the airway.

If imaging is obtained, a lateral radiograph of the neck soft tissues should be performed. The patient should be kept in an upright position, and there should be minimal to no manipulation of the neck. The classic radiographic findings of epiglottitis are marked enlargement and edema of the epiglottis and aryepiglottic folds, well-profiled on a lateral view of the neck with the characteristic "thumbprint sign" [**Fig. 2.14**]. The hypopharynx may be overdistended. Subglottic edema, as seen in croup, will also be present in about 25% of patients with epiglottitis.

In addition to airway management, patients with epiglottitis require antimicrobial therapy. The role of steroids is controversial. They may reduce airway inflammation, resulting in improved airway patency.

Glottic Abnormalities
Laryngeal Atresia

Laryngeal atresia is a rare anomaly. It may be characterized by agenesis of the glottis, agenesis of the larynx, or both. The pathogenesis involves maldevelopment of the sixth branchial arch, resulting in failure of the larynx and trachea to recanalize. This entity may occur in isolation or as part of a number of syndromes. It can be associated with tracheoesophageal fistula (TEF), esophageal atresia (EA), urinary tract abnormalities, and limb anomalies.

Prenatal ultrasound may show signs of congenital high airway obstruction syndrome. These include dilated airways distal to the obstruction, bilaterally enlarged and echogenic lungs, and diaphragmatic flattening and/or inversion. Associated fetal ascites, hydrops fetalis, and polyhydramnios may be seen. Fetal MRI can assist in the prenatal diagnosis of this entity and provide a more accurate evaluation of the level of obstruction [**Fig. 2.15**].

Patients typically present with asphyxia at the time of birth, which may require an emergent tracheotomy soon after delivery. If laryngeal atresia is detected in utero, an ex utero intrapartum treatment (EXIT) procedure with tracheotomy can be performed, which may be lifesaving.

Subglottic Abnormalities
Congenital Subglottic Stenosis

Subglottic stenosis is the third most common cause of congenital stridor in the neonate behind laryngomalacia and vocal cord paralysis. It involves narrowing of the subglottic lumen caused by incomplete recanalization during embryogenesis. There are two types of congenital subglottic stenosis: membranous and cartilaginous. Patients with congenital subglottic stenosis may be asymptomatic until an upper respiratory infection causes further narrowing and compromise of the airway. The affected patient may present with stridor and a barking cough. With

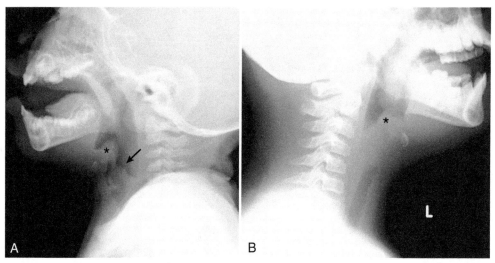

Figure 2.14 Epiglottitis. A, Fourteen-month-old with fever, mouth breathing, and choking while eating. Lateral radiograph of the neck soft tissues shows abnormal thickening of the epiglottis (*asterisk*) and aryepiglottic folds (*arrow*). This patient did well after receiving antibiotic therapy. **B,** Eight-year-old previously immunized with the *Haemophilus influenzae* type B vaccine presenting with fever and worsening sore throat, cough, and noisy breathing, with increased secretions. Lateral radiograph shows severe thickening of the epiglottis (*asterisk*) and aryepiglottic folds, with soft tissue density completely occluding the subglottic airway. This patient required emergent intubation for airway protection and did well after a course of intravenous antibiotics.

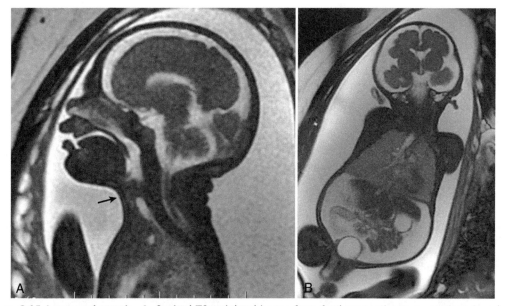

Figure 2.15 Laryngeal atresia. A, Sagittal T2-weighted image from fetal magnetic resonance imaging shows abnormal soft tissue (*arrow*) in the airway, resulting in discontinuity between the hypopharynx and the subglottic trachea. **B,** Coronal T2-weighted image shows a distended trachea, enlarged lungs with scalloped margins, inversion of the hemidiaphragms, and a large volume of intraabdominal ascites.

severe disease, patients present with dyspnea and marked chest retractions.

Although subglottic narrowing may be appreciated on AP and lateral radiographs, congenital subglottic stenosis is a clinical endoscopic diagnosis. CT and MRI can aid in the assessment of the precise location and length of the stenosis. These modalities are also useful for evaluation of the airway distal to the level of narrowing [**Fig. 2.16**].

The management of congenital subglottic stenosis involves supportive care in times of airway compromise. Ultimately surgical reconstruction is needed to provide the patient with an adequate airway for normal activity without the need for tracheostomy.

Croup

Croup, also known as acute laryngotracheobronchitis, is a self-limited viral inflammatory disease of the upper airway. It is caused by parainfluenza or respiratory syncytial virus, and results in symmetric subglottic edema. It is the most common cause of upper respiratory distress in infants and young children, with a peak incidence between 3 and 6 months of age. Acute clinical symptoms include a barky cough, inspiratory stridor, and hoarseness. Symptoms may be preceded by a prodrome of low-grade fever, mild cough, and rhinorrhea.

Imaging is not routinely indicated because the diagnosis is often made clinically. Radiographs are sometimes obtained to exclude more serious causes of stridor such as epiglottitis, a

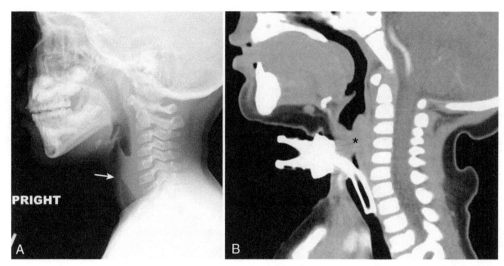

Figure 2.16 Subglottic stenosis. A, Lateral soft tissue neck radiograph of a 10-month-old with stridor and a barking cough. There is severe focal narrowing of the subglottic airway (*arrow*). This patient was successfully treated with antibiotics and steroids. **B,** Sagittal computed tomography (CT) image of a 6-month-old with severe subglottic stenosis (*asterisk*) requiring tracheostomy. CT was performed to assess the distal airway, which was normal.

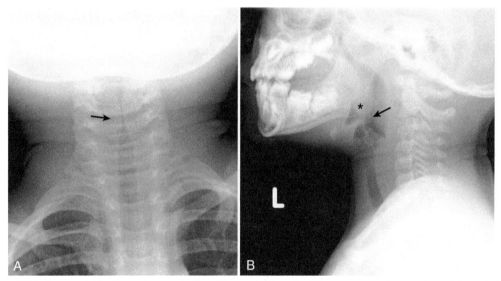

Figure 2.17 Croup. A, On the anteroposterior radiograph, there is diffuse segmental narrowing of the subglottic trachea and loss of the normal tracheal shouldering creating the "steeple sign" (*arrow*). **B,** The lateral view shows distension of the hypopharynx and a normal-appearing epiglottis (*arrow*) that is overlapped by prominent tonsillar tissue (*asterisk*) extending into the hypopharynx.

retained foreign body, or a neck mass. On frontal radiographs, subglottic edema is visualized as loss of the normal shouldering (lateral convexities) of the subglottic trachea, creating a "steeple sign" [**Fig. 2.17**]. Lateral radiographs of the upper airway demonstrate a normal epiglottis with narrowing of the subglottic region. Overdistention of the hypopharynx can be seen on both views.

Croup usually has a self-limited course and resolves within a few days. Therefore supportive care is often sufficient. Oral or inhaled corticosteroids may be administered to decrease the severity of symptoms and potentially avoid hospital admission. Epinephrine nebulizer treatments may be helpful in some cases. Intubation is necessary when disease is severe. In children with atypical, prolonged, or recurrent symptoms refractory to medical therapy, bronchoscopy may be helpful for further evaluation.

Bacterial Tracheitis

Bacterial tracheitis is a bacterial infection of the trachea, with common causative agents including *Staphylococcus aureus, Streptococcus pneumoniae,* and *Haemophilus influenzae.* This infection is associated with a purulent exudate that can cause acute, life-threatening obstruction of the upper airway in rare circumstances. Preschool and early school-aged children are most frequently affected. The clinical features of bacterial tracheitis are similar to those of viral croup and epiglottitis. Children initially present with sore throat, rhinorrhea, cough, and fever, which may escalate to severe upper airway obstruction, high fever, and toxicity.

On a lateral view of the neck soft tissues, linear soft tissue filling defects may be seen along the airway. Irregular plaques along the anterior wall of the trachea may also be seen. This is known as the "candle-dripping sign" [**Fig. 2.18**]. On an AP

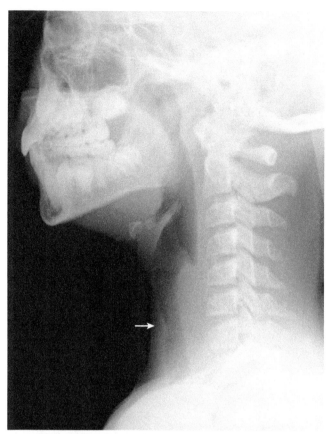

Figure 2.18 Bacterial tracheitis. Lateral radiograph of the neck in a 10-year-old with severe throat pain and hoarseness shows irregularity of the anterior wall of the trachea with mild luminal narrowing (*arrow*). Direct laryngoscopy revealed extensive pus and secretions below the vocal cords.

radiograph of the neck, narrowing of the subglottic airway may be visualized. Notably, concomitant pneumonia can be seen on chest radiographs in approximately half of patients. The most definitive way to diagnose bacterial tracheitis is via direct visualization with bronchoscopy.

Because bacterial tracheitis can result in airway obstruction leading to respiratory failure, treatment is aggressive. Broad-spectrum intravenous antibiotics are initiated as soon as the clinical diagnosis of bacterial tracheitis has been made. If membranes are visualized within the trachea, rigid bronchoscopy can be performed for "stripping" of the airway.

Retropharyngeal Cellulitis/Abscess

Retropharyngeal cellulitis/abscess is a potentially life-threatening infection involving the retropharyngeal space. Retropharyngeal infection can be secondary to pharyngeal trauma from a penetrating foreign body, endoscopy, an intubation attempt, or a dental procedure. It may also occur in association with infectious pharyngitis, vertebral body osteomyelitis, and petrositis. Retropharyngeal infections can range from cellulitis to a mature abscess. The most common causative organisms are *S. aureus, H. influenzae,* and *Streptococcus.* This infection occurs most commonly between the ages of 2 and 4 years.

Children with retropharyngeal abscess generally appear very ill, presenting with sore throat, dysphagia, poor oral intake, dehydration, fever, chills, and an elevated white blood cell count and erythrocyte sedimentation rate. The affected patient may appear toxic, with marked neck pain and limited range

of motion. Airway compromise may be seen at initial presentation.

Imaging evaluation includes lateral radiographs of the neck soft tissues and/or CT scan of the neck with intravenous contrast administration. On lateral radiographs, there may be widening of the retropharyngeal soft tissues with anterior displacement of the airway [**Fig. 2.19A**]. As indicated previously, the normal thickness of the retropharyngeal soft tissues from C1-C4 should be about equal to half of the vertebral body width in children. Rarely, gas may be seen in the retropharyngeal soft tissues in the setting of an abscess.

Contrast-enhanced CT scan is ideal to assess the craniocaudal extent of disease. The retropharyngeal space may be distended by a rim-enhancing fluid collection [**Fig. 2.19B** and **C**]. Sepsis may develop, with septic emboli to the lungs [**Fig. 2.19D**]. Vascular complications including jugular vein thrombosis or thrombophlebitis can be seen in the setting of Lemierre syndrome [**Fig. 2.19E** and **F**]. Narrowing of the internal carotid artery may develop, or rarely, an internal carotid artery pseudoaneurysm and/or rupture may occur.

Traditionally, management of a retropharyngeal abscess has involved surgical drainage. This is evolving, and some cases are now managed with antibiotics alone. This is particularly true for small collections.

Other Causes of Upper Airway Disease

Tonsillar Enlargement/Adenoidal Hypertrophy

Enlargement of the tonsils and adenoids in children may be related to normal development of the immune system. It is usually asymptomatic. However, when there is excessive adeno-tonsillar enlargement associated with sore throat and/or recurrent ear or sinus infections, the affected child may experience difficulty breathing or swallowing. Tonsillar inflammation is typically bilateral and can affect children and young adults. Obstructive sleep apnea may also result from adenotonsillar hypertrophy.

A lateral radiograph of the neck soft tissues can be obtained to evaluate size of the tonsils and adenoids [**Fig. 2.3**]. In the case of tonsillar inflammation with persistent symptoms, a contrast-enhanced CT scan is useful to distinguish between acute tonsillitis and tonsillar/peritonsillar abscess. This distinction is important because these symptoms may progress to lockjaw (trismus) refractory to antibiotic treatment without appropriate management. In the setting of tonsillitis, CT shows bilateral tonsillar enlargement with variable attenuation and a striated pattern of parenchymal enhancement [**Fig. 2.20**].

MR sleep studies are useful to detect both anatomic and dynamic motion abnormalities in children with obstructive sleep apnea related to tonsillar enlargement. These studies include a combination of static T1-weighted imaging and both static and dynamic cine T2-weighted imaging.

Excision of the tonsils and adenoids is indicated in the setting of obstruction and in cases of recurrent acute or chronic tonsillitis.

Foreign Body

Foreign bodies lodged in the larynx can lead to significant morbidity and mortality in children. The majority of patients who present are younger than 4 years, and peanuts are the most common offending agent. Children who ingest or aspirate foreign bodies may have a delayed presentation of acute respiratory distress, days or even months after the aspiration event. This is particularly true if the foreign body aspiration goes unwitnessed. Typically there is a suggestive history marked by an acute episode of paroxysmal cough and stridor. Other common symptoms include cyanosis, choking, and dyspnea.

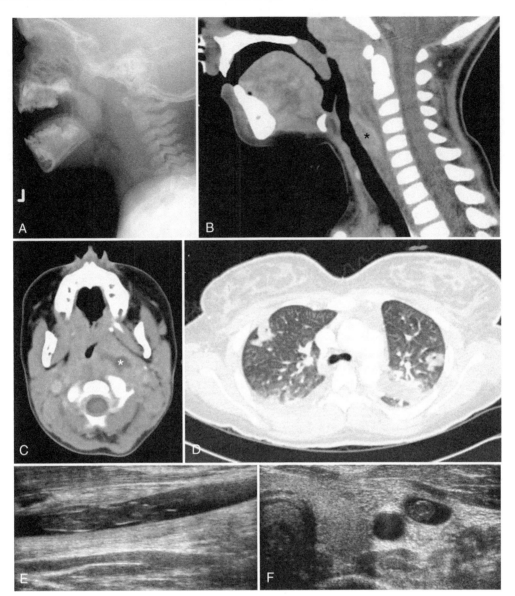

Figure 2.19 Retropharyngeal abscess. A, Lateral radiograph of a 3-year-old with fever and pharyngitis shows prevertebral soft tissue swelling, which measures greater than the anteroposterior diameter of the cervical vertebral bodies. **B,** Corresponding sagittal and (**C**) axial computed tomography (CT) images with contrast administration show heterogeneous thickening and enhancement of the retropharyngeal soft tissues, with a developing fluid collection (*asterisk*) consistent with a retropharyngeal abscess. **D,** Sixteen-year-old with retropharyngeal abscess (not shown) and sepsis. Axial CT image shows multiple peripheral cavitary pulmonary nodules reflecting septic emboli. **E,** Sagittal and (**F**) tranverse images of the neck performed for right-sided pain show a nonocclusive thrombus within the right jugular vein consistent with Lemierre syndrome.

Radiologic evaluation should begin with frontal and lateral views of the neck and chest, which can be helpful in localizing radiopaque foreign bodies such as coins, batteries, lead, mineral fragments, and some pills [**Fig. 2.21**]. Coin ingestion is very common in children. Most coins cause no harm and pass through the gastrointestinal (GI) tract in a few days. However, if a coin becomes impacted at the thoracic inlet or enters the airway, interventional therapy is warranted. Disk (button) batteries are also commonly ingested by children [**Fig. 2.21D**]. These batteries contain a variety of caustic and corrosive agents. Perforation and systemic toxicity related to heavy metal poisoning may occur if their containers are compromised.

In a child with upper respiratory symptoms and suspected foreign body ingestion, radiographic findings may be normal in about one third of cases. When a radiopaque foreign body is not seen, an indirect sign of airway obstruction is differential hyperinflation of the affected lung related to air trapping. This can be diagnosed with expiratory radiographs, or alternatively bilateral decubitus views for young children who cannot hold their breath on command [**Fig. 2.22**]. Other indirect radiographic findings of a foreign body aspiration include regional hyperinflation of a lung lobe and peripheral opacities reflecting atelectasis or consolidation distal to the site of obstruction.

Pharyngeal and laryngeal foreign bodies can lead to airway obstruction and respiratory distress at the time of aspiration. Thus once a foreign body has been identified, flexible or rigid bronchoscopy is indicated to retrieve the aspirated object.

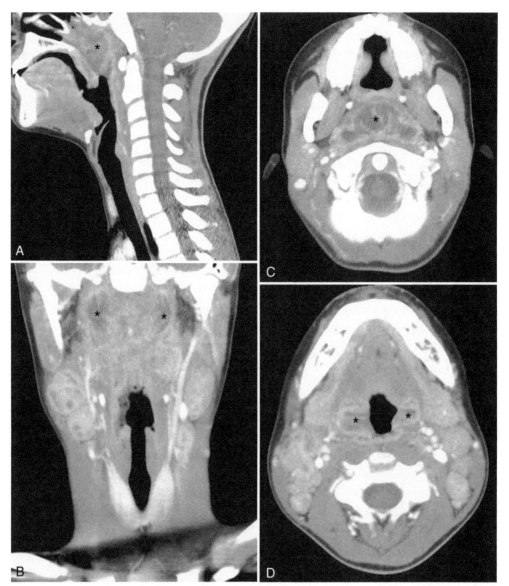

Figure 2.20 Diffuse adenoiditis and tonsillitis in an 11-year-old with exudative pharyngitis refractory to standard antibiotic therapy. A and **B,** Sagittal and coronal computed tomography (CT) images of the neck show enlargement and heterogeneous enhancement of the adenoids (*asterisks*). **C** and **D,** Axial CT images through the pharynx show enlarged, heterogeneously enhancing tonsils (*asterisks*), with narrowing of the oro-pharyngeal and nasopharyngeal airways. The patient also has suppurative adenitis, with marked enlargement of multiple cervical lymph nodes. Cultures were positive for tularemia (Francisella tularensis), which can be associated with tick and deer fly bites.

Neoplasms

Subglottic Hemangioma. Subglottic hemangioma is a rare, benign vascular neoplasm characterized by a proliferative phase of rapid growth during the first 6 to 18 months of life followed by spontaneous involution. Patients are typically symptomatic by 6 months of age due to progressive airway narrowing during the proliferative phase. Symptoms resolve after involution. Presenting symptoms include hoarseness and an abnormal cry. In about 50% of cases, associated cutaneous hemangiomas are seen. Subglottic hemangiomas can be seen as a component of the PHACES syndrome (*p*osterior fossa brain malformations, *h*emangiomas, *a*rterial anomalies, *c*ardiac defects, *e*ye abnormalities, *s*ternal clefts and *s*upraumbilical raphe).

Inspiratory AP and lateral radiographs of the neck demonstrate asymmetric subglottic tracheal narrowing [**Fig. 2.23**]. The modalities of choice for complete assessment of a clinically

suspected subglottic hemangioma are contrast-enhanced CT and MRI. Cross-sectional studies will show an enhancing submucosal mass that may be circumferential, bilateral, or unilateral, with posterolateral positioning most common [**Fig. 2.23**]. Definitive diagnosis is made with direct laryngoscopy or bronchoscopy.

Management varies depending on severity of symptoms. Patients without respiratory or feeding difficulties may be managed conservatively. Symptomatic patients can be treated with systemic and intralesional corticosteroids, CO_2 laser therapy, a trial of interferon, vincristine, or propranolol, or direct excision.

Laryngeal Papilloma. Laryngeal papilloma is the most common benign neoplasm of the larynx in children. In the majority of cases, multiple papillomas are seen in the trachea. Because of the high recurrence rate, this entity is also called

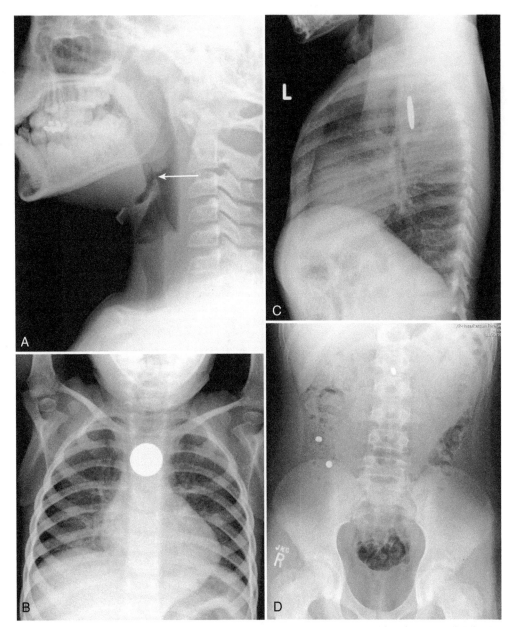

Figure 2.21 **Foreign body ingestions. A,** Lateral neck radiograph of a 9-year-old with pain and difficulty swallowing shows a thin, linear density in the hypopharynx that projects over the epiglottis (*arrow*). A fishbone was subsequently removed. **B** and **C,** Two-year-old with history of a coin ingestion 3 days before presentation. The patient was initially asymptomatic, then developed progressive dysphagia. Frontal and lateral radiographs of the chest show a coin lodged in the proximal esophagus at the level of the aortic arch. Surrounding soft tissue swelling is noted. **D,** Abdominal radiograph shows disc-shaped metallic densities in the region of the large bowel, consistent with button battery ingestion.

recurrent respiratory papillomatosis (RRP). About half of affected patients have a maternal history of condyloma acuminatum. This condition is most often caused by the human papilloma virus types 6 and 11 and is characterized by the proliferation of benign squamous papillomas throughout the aerodigestive tract. Although it is benign, RRP can have an aggressive clinical course in children. It can be fatal because of its tendency to recur and spread throughout the aerodigestive tract.

Children usually present around age 2 or 3 years with worsening hoarseness and stridor. Less commonly, patients can present with chronic cough, recurrent pneumonia, failure to thrive, dyspnea, dysphagia, or acute respiratory distress associated with an upper respiratory tract infection.

RRP can be seen as an irregular filling defect in the glottis on lateral radiographs of the neck soft tissues [**Fig. 2.24**]. Chest radiographs are often normal, particularly if lesions are confined to the larynx. With extension into the subglottic region and seeding of the respiratory tract, pulmonary nodules may develop. Nodules may be solid or cavitary. When papillomas result in airway obstruction, atelectasis, bronchiectasis, and mucous plugging can be seen. On CT, thin-walled cysts with adjacent nodules are visualized. Diagnosis is confirmed with direct laryngoscopy and biopsy.

Laser ablation of laryngeal or airway lesions can be performed for debulking. Repeated procedures may be needed because of the frequency of recurrence of these tumors. Interferon and

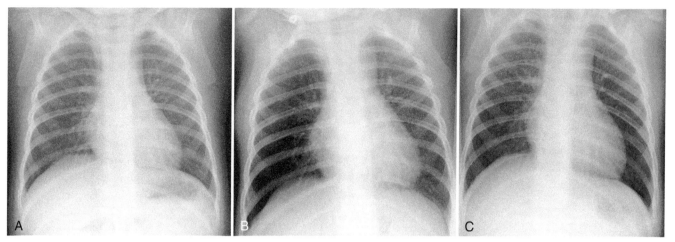

Figure 2.22 Suspected foreign body aspiration in a 13-month-old with stridor. A, Frontal radiograph of the chest demonstrates symmetric inflation of the lungs. **B,** Left-side-down decubitus radiograph shows normal dependent hypoinflation of the left lung. **C,** Right-side-down decubitus radiograph shows relative hyperinflation of the right lung. A walnut was removed from the right main stem bronchus at bronchoscopy.

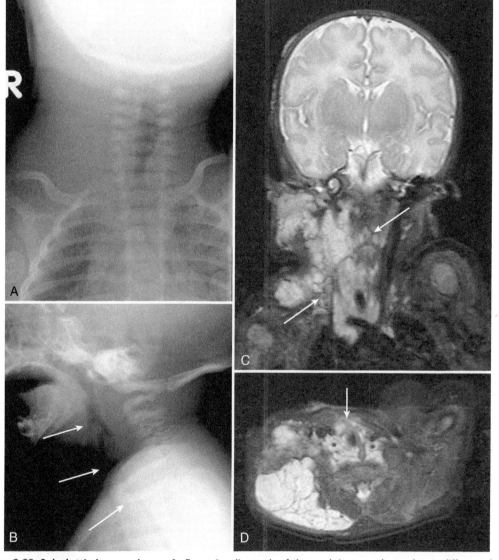

Figure 2.23 Subglottic hemangioma. A, Frontal radiograph of the neck in a newborn shows diffuse enlargement of the soft tissues of the right neck. **B,** Lateral view shows thickened retropharyngeal soft tissues, with displacement and narrowing of the pharynx and trachea (*arrows*). **C** and **D,** Coronal and axial T2-weighted magnetic resonance images show a high signal lobulated mass in the right posterior neck. This extends into the mediastinum, surrounds vascular structures, and narrows the trachea (*arrows*).

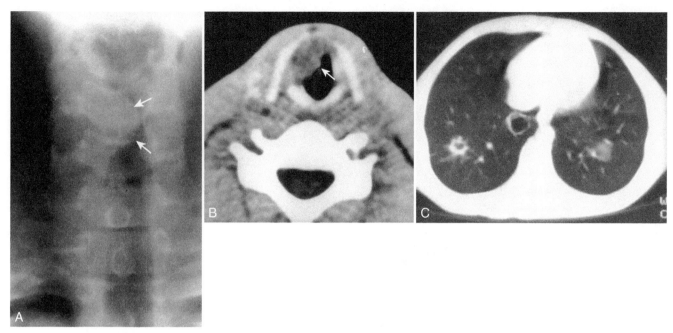

Figure 2.24 Laryngeal papillomatosis. A and **B,** Anteroposterior radiograph and axial computed tomography (CT) image of the neck show an eccentrically positioned soft tissue mass (*arrows*) encroaching on the tracheal air column from the right. **C,** Axial CT image through the lungs demonstrates seeding of the respiratory tract with the development of cavitary pulmonary nodules.

antiviral agents may slow growth but are not curative. There is a small risk for malignant degeneration into squamous cell carcinoma.

LOWER AIRWAY

Tracheobronchomalacia

Tracheobronchomalacia (TBM) is characterized by abnormal collapse of the airway in expiration. It results from abnormal, weakened cartilaginous support of the airway and/or the membranous portion of the posterior tracheal wall. It may be congenital (primary) or acquired (secondary), and it most commonly occurs in young infants in the first year of life because of tracheal flaccidity. Primary TBM results from incomplete development of the tracheal cartilage, and it can involve the entire length of the airway. Secondary TBM may be related to a history of infection, prior surgery, extrinsic compression from cardiovascular structures, or neck and mediastinal tumors. TBM related to tracheal underdevelopment or inflammation is often seen in children with EA and TEF. Children with TBM characteristically present with expiratory wheezing that increases with crying or feeding, cough, stridor, and/or recurrent respiratory infections.

In complex or severe cases of secondary TBM, dedicated expiratory-phase CT imaging can be performed to detect excessive (>50%) collapsibility of the trachea and bronchi, diagnostic of this condition [**Fig. 2.25**]. The most common findings during dynamic expiration are tracheal collapse and crescentic bowing of the posterior membranous trachea. In older patients, a cine CT can be combined with a coughing maneuver. This is the most sensitive method for eliciting tracheal collapse.

For children with mild-to-moderate TBM, conservative management is preferred because symptoms often resolve by 1 to 2 years of age with maturation and strengthening of the tracheal cartilage. For children with more severe symptoms, more aggressive treatment options may be needed. These can include continuous positive airway pressure (CPAP), tracheostomy placement, stent placement, or surgical intervention.

Tracheoesophageal Fistula

TEF results from incomplete or abnormal division of the developing trachea from the ventral foregut during embryogenesis. There are five major anatomic variations of esophageal atresia-tracheoesophageal fistula (EA-TEF) [**Fig. 2.26**]. The level of the fistula varies, but it is most commonly near the carina. There is an increased incidence of TEF in children with Down syndrome. It is also seen with increased incidence in children with VACTERL (*v*ertebral anomalies, *a*nal atresia, *c*ardiac abnormalities, *T*EF and/or *E*A, *r*enal agenesis and dysplasia, and *l*imb defects).

Infants with most forms of EA-TEF present shortly after birth. The exception is the H-type TEF, which may go undiagnosed until late childhood. Symptoms typically include coughing, gagging, cyanosis, vomiting, copious oral secretions, and/or respiratory distress.

Imaging findings depend on the type of EA-TEF. The diagnosis may be suggested on prenatal ultrasound as early as 24 weeks' gestation. Polyhydramnios, absence of a fluid-filled stomach, a small abdomen, lower-than-expected fetal weight, and a fluid-filled, distended esophageal pouch may be seen. Fetal MRI can be obtained to confirm the diagnosis. Postnatally, EA is suggested by the presence of an air-filled, distended upper esophageal pouch on chest radiographs. Clinically, failure to pass a nasogastric tube occurs, with coiling of the tube in the esophageal pouch [**Fig. 2.27**].

Initial postnatal intervention is aimed at minimizing the risk for aspiration pneumonia. Surgical repair consists of closing the fistula, with primary anastomosis of the proximal and distal ends of the esophagus if there is a short-segment atresia. When there is a long-segment atresia or EA without a TEF (type 2), a colonic interposition may be performed. This procedure has varied success rates.

Long-gap EA has also been managed successfully with growth induction via the Foker procedure. In this procedure, sutures are applied to the proximal and distal ends of the esophagus, with a tag on each end. The sutures are externalized and attached to traction devices outside the patient's body. With the patient paralyzed, increasing traction is applied over time, creating

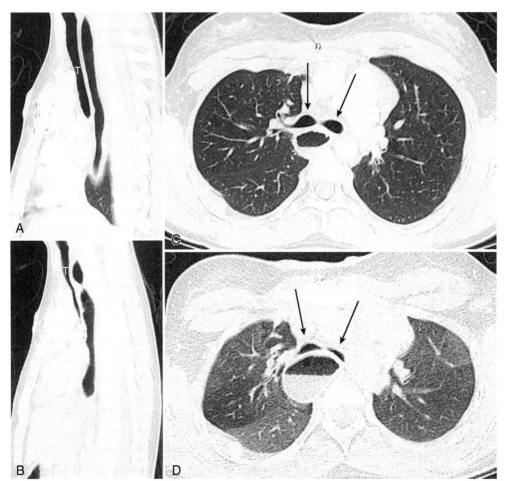

Figure 2.25 Tracheobronchomalacia. A and **C,** Inspiratory and (**B** and **D**) expiratory sagittal and axial computed tomography images show diffuse narrowing of the trachea (*T*) and mainstem bronchi (*arrows*) on expiration in a patient with persistent respiratory symptoms after repair of esophageal atresia. On axial images, the esophagus is dilated with an air–fluid level.

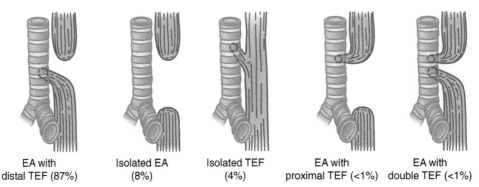

| EA with distal TEF (87%) | Isolated EA (8%) | Isolated TEF (4%) | EA with proximal TEF (<1%) | EA with double TEF (<1%) |

Figure 2.26 Types of esophageal atresia (EA)/tracheoesophageal fistula (TEF). *Type 1* is most common and is characterized by an atresia of the proximal esophagus associated with a fistula from the distal esophagus to the trachea. *Type 2* is EA without a TEF. *Type 3* is a TEF without EA, also referred to as an H-type fistula. Types 4 and 5 are rare. *Type 4* is characterized by EA and a fistula between the proximal esophagus and the trachea. In *type 5,* there is EA with two fistulas extending from both the proximal and the distal segments of the esophagus to the trachea.

stress and leading to natural tissue growth. When growth is determined to be adequate, the proximal and distal ends of the esophagus are connected with a primary anastomosis. After EA-TEF repair, an esophagram is often performed to assess for surgical complications such as anastomotic leak or stricture, recurrent TEF, or esophageal dysmotility.

Asthma

Asthma is characterized by acute, subacute, or chronic paroxysmal airway inflammation caused by hyperreactivity. It is at least partially reversible. It primarily involves the medium-sized and small bronchi, which are thickened due to edema, hyperplasia of the bronchial wall smooth muscle, and an increase in the size

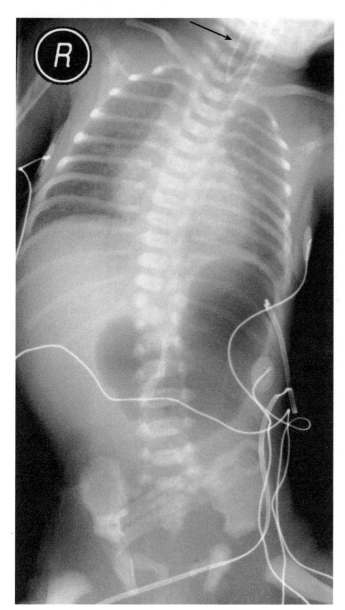

Figure 2.27 Esophageal atresia and duodenal atresia. Intubated newborn with an enteric tube coiled in the proximal esophagus (*arrow*). This tube could not be passed distally because of esophageal atresia. The stomach and proximal duodenum are distended with air, with the remainder of the abdomen appearing gasless. This is the characteristic "double bubble" sign of duodenal atresia (discussed in detail in Chapter 4).

of the airway mucosal glands. Airway hypersensitivity can be related to a number of factors, including viral illnesses, allergens, exercise, medications, and environmental conditions. Symptoms include wheeze, cough, chest tightness, and shortness of breath. Approximately 50% of children suffering from reactive airways disease develop symptoms before the age of 2 years, with 80% to 90% diagnosed by 5 years of age.

Chest radiographs may demonstrate pulmonary hyperinflation, with peribronchial thickening and areas of segmental atelectasis, similar to the findings seen in bronchiolitis [**Fig. 2.2**]. However, the chest radiograph of a child with an asthma exacerbation is most often normal. Radiographs are important as part of the initial diagnostic workup to exclude complications of asthma, which may include pneumomediastinum and pneumothorax. CT can be performed to diagnose associated conditions that may occur, such as allergic bronchopulmonary aspergillosis. In this condition, CT demonstrates central multifocal bronchiectasis with areas of mucoid impaction ("finger-in-glove" appearance), centrilobular nodules, mosaic perfusion caused by air trapping, areas of consolidation and ground-glass opacification, and atelectasis related to bronchial obstruction [**Fig. 2.28**].

With appropriate management of asthma, prognosis is usually excellent. Treatment includes avoidance of known triggers and exacerbating factors, inhaled beta-agonists for bronchospasm, corticosteroids, and inhaled mast cell stabilizers.

Rings and Slings

Vascular rings and pulmonary artery sling are congenital anomalies of the great vessels that can cause stridor in infancy and childhood. They are caused by abnormal development of the embryonic aortic arches. A vascular ring completely encircles the trachea and/or esophagus. A pulmonary artery sling encircles the trachea only.

The embryonic development of the normal aortic arch system was first described by Edwards in 1948. Paired right and left dorsal aortae arising from the truncus arteriosus are present by approximately 21 days gestational age. They are connected by six primitive aortic arches that correspond to the six branchial arches. Early on in development, the first, second, and fifth primitive aortic arches regress. The third arches become the carotid arteries, and the left sixth arch becomes the ductus arteriosus. The right sixth arch will normally regress. The fourth arch forms the proximal portion of the subclavian artery on the right and the major transverse aortic arch segment on the left. The paired dorsal aortae and six primitive arches undergo a structured process that results in a left aortic arch with the normal branching order (the innominate artery followed by the left common carotid and subclavian arteries) and a descending thoracic aorta to the left of the spine. Atresia of segments that should normally persist or persistence of segments that should

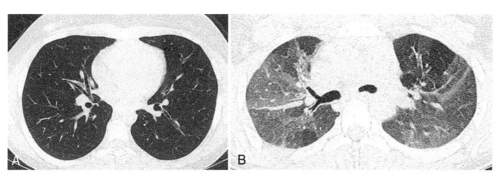

Figure 2.28 Allergic bronchopulmonary aspergillosis in a patient with asthma. A, Axial computed tomography (CT) image on inspiration shows central bronchial dilation related to chronic inflammation. **B,** Axial CT image on expiration shows peripheral subsegmental regions of hyperinflation consistent with air trapping in the setting of small airways inflammation.

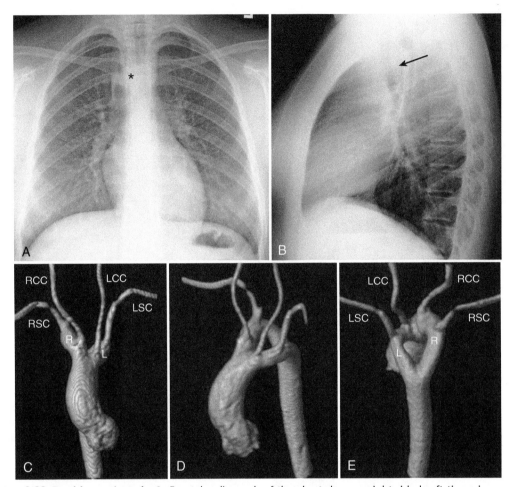

Figure 2.29 **Double aortic arch. A,** Frontal radiograph of the chest shows a right-sided soft tissue impression (*asterisk*) on the trachea, which is deviated leftward. **B,** On the lateral view, the trachea is bowed anteriorly (*arrow*). **C** through **E,** Volume-rendered images from a CT angiogram. **C,** An anterior projection. **D,** A leftward projection. **E,** A posterior projection. Images show a double aortic arch, with a larger and higher right arch (*R*) in comparison with the left arch (*L*). The arches encircle the trachea and esophagus (not shown) and join posteriorly. Note that the right common carotid (*RCC*) and right subclavian (*RSC*) arteries arise from the right arch, and the left common carotid (*LCC*) and left subclavian (*LSC*) arteries arise separately from the right and left arches, respectively.

normally regress can result in complete encircling of the trachea, which may lead to compressive airway obstruction.

In the setting of a vascular ring, there may be displacement or compression of the tracheal air column. This can be detected on radiographs of the neck and chest. When extrinsic compression of the esophagus is detected on a barium swallow or upper GI series, follow-up CTA or MRA of the chest is warranted to delineate the vasculature causing compression of the esophagus and possibly also the airway. Cross-sectional studies provide valuable information necessary to guide surgical management.

In general, respiratory symptoms predominate in the initial presentation of patients with a vascular ring or sling. Stridor is present in almost all cases and is more pronounced with feeding or activity. The three most important vascular causes of stridor are double aortic arch, right aortic arch with aberrant left subclavian artery, and pulmonary sling. Vascular rings may present with dysphagia when there is relatively more compression of the esophagus than the trachea, although this is much less common.

Double Aortic Arch

The most common symptomatic vascular ring is a double aortic arch. This results from persistence of both the right and the left dorsal aortae arising from the ascending aorta. The right and left aortic arches pass to either side of the trachea and esophagus,

and join posteriorly to form a single descending thoracic aorta. The right arch is larger than the left in about 75% of cases and is typically also more superior in position.

On a frontal view of the chest, the right aortic arch may cause deviation of the trachea toward the smaller left aortic arch. On a lateral view, anterior bowing of the trachea may be seen [**Fig. 2.29A** and **B**]. A double aortic arch should be suspected if there is posterior and bilateral extrinsic compression of the esophagus on a barium esophagram or upper GI series. More precise delineation of arch morphology and the degree of tracheal compression requires preoperative planning with an MRA or CTA [**Fig. 2.29C** through **E**]. These cross-sectional studies will show the double arch encircling both the trachea and the esophagus. Right versus left arch dominance can be determined, and any existing coarctation or narrowing in either arch can be identified. The nondominant or narrowed arch and the ligament of the ductus arteriosus are surgically ligated and divided to relieve the compression of the airway.

Right Aortic Arch With Aberrant Left Subclavian Artery

The second most common vascular ring is a right aortic arch with an aberrant left subclavian artery and a left ductal ligament. Ten percent of patients have associated intracardiac defects. The

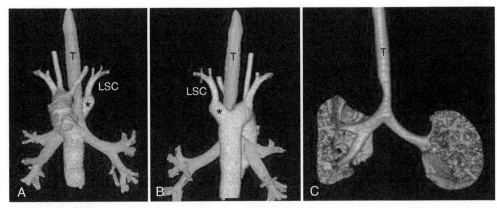

Figure 2.30 Right aortic arch with aberrant left subclavian artery. A, Anterior and **(B)** posterior volume-rendered images from a computed tomography angiogram with the trachea (*T*) added show the aortic arch passing to the right of the trachea. The left subclavian (*LSC*) artery arises as the last branch from the arch and is dilated proximally consistent with a diverticulum of Kommerell (*asterisk*). The presence of a diverticulum of Kommerell indicates that there is a left ductal ligament that needs to be ligated and divided at surgery to release the vascular ring encircling the trachea. **C,** Volume-rendered image of the airway shows an extrinsic impression on and narrowing of the trachea in the setting of a right aortic arch.

aortic arch ascends anterior to the tracheal bifurcation, arches over the right mainstem bronchus, and descends posterior to the esophagus and the trachea. The left subclavian artery originates off the descending aorta, with the ductal ligament coursing from the base of the left subclavian artery to the left pulmonary artery (LPA) [**Fig. 2.30**].

With this entity, there is dilation of the origin of the aberrant subclavian artery, termed the diverticulum of Kommerell. This occurs as a result of in utero ductal blood flow from the LPA to the left subclavian artery to the aorta. When present, this finding indicates that the ductal ligament that needs to be divided to release the ring is on the left side of the mediastinum. When there is no diverticulum of Kommerell in the setting of a right aortic arch, the ductal ligament is on the right, and a complete vascular ring is not present.

On a frontal chest radiograph, a right aortic arch will produce a leftward impression on or leftward deviation of the trachea, which will be more midline in position than usual. Both the lateral chest radiograph and the lateral esophagram can show anterior bowing of the trachea and/or esophagus as they course anterior to the diverticulum of Kommerell. Findings may be very similar to those seen with a double aortic arch. Cross-sectional imaging with CTA or MRA is imperative for definitive diagnosis and preoperative planning [**Fig. 2.30**].

Right Aortic Arch With Mirror Image Branching

A right aortic arch with mirror image branching occurs because of persistence of the right dorsal aorta instead of the left dorsal aorta. It is essentially the mirror image of a left aortic arch with a normal branching pattern. In greater than 90% of cases, it is seen in association with intracardiac defects. These include tetralogy of Fallot (~25%), truncus arteriosus (~25%), and double outlet right ventricle (20%).

A right aortic arch with mirror image branching will not create a vascular ring encircling the trachea provided the ductal ligament is on the right between the proximal descending aorta and the right pulmonary artery (RPA), and the descending aorta descends along the right side of the spine. A complete vascular ring occurs when there is a right aortic arch and the ductal ligament extends between the upper descending aorta and the LPA. This is referred to as a circumflex aortic arch. The ligament pulls or tethers the descending aorta leftward. The deviated aorta descends along the left side of the spine and may cause posterior compression of the trachea [**Fig. 2.31**].

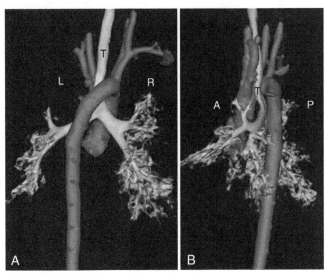

Figure 2.31 Circumflex aortic arch. A, Posterior and **(B)** leftward projections from a volume-rendered computed tomography angiogram with the airway included show a right aortic arch that courses to the right of the trachea (*T*), then descends posterior to the trachea on the left side. Note the significant narrowing of the distal trachea in the anteroposterior plane. *A*, Anterior; *L*, left; *P*, posterior; *R*, right.

Left Aortic Arch With Aberrant Right Subclavian Artery

Left aortic arch with aberrant right subclavian artery is the most common anomaly involving the aortic arch branching pattern. It is usually asymptomatic. The aberrant right subclavian artery courses posterior to the esophagus, and the ductal ligament extends between the aortic isthmus and the LPA. Thus a complete vascular ring is not present. In rare cases, the right subclavian artery will exert extrinsic compression as it courses posterior to the esophagus. This may lead to swallowing difficulty, referred to as dysphagia lusoria.

Pulmonary Sling

A pulmonary sling is defined as an anomalous LPA arising from the RPA, forming a sling that courses between the trachea and

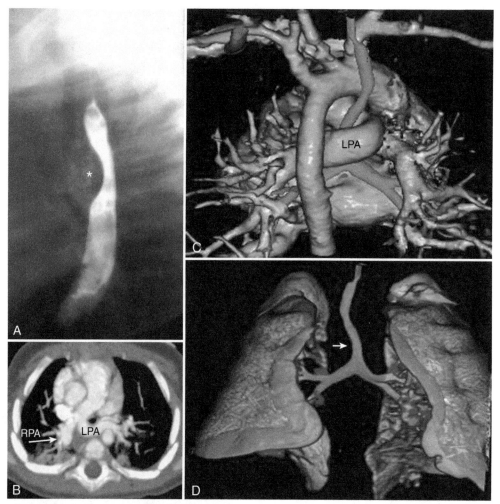

Figure 2.32 **Pulmonary artery sling. A,** Lateral view from a barium swallow shows a mass-like soft tissue density between the trachea and esophagus (*asterisk*). **B,** Axial maximum intensity projection image from a computed tomography angiography (CTA) shows the left pulmonary artery (*LPA*) arising from the right pulmonary artery (*RPA*) (*arrow*) and coursing leftward posterior to the trachea. **C,** Posterior projection image from a volume-rendered CTA with the trachea included shows the LPA coursing posteriorly. **D,** Volume-rendered image of the airway shows an impression on the trachea (*arrow*) due to the rightward bifurcation of the pulmonary arteries and a horizontal or T-shaped configuration of the carina that may be seen in association with an LPA sling.

esophagus. This is the only type of vascular ring in which the abnormal vessel courses between the trachea and esophagus. Approximately half of patients have severe tracheobronchial anomalies, such as tracheomalacia, stenosis, webs, abnormal branching patterns, and/or complete cartilaginous tracheal rings that can result in long-segment tracheal stenosis. The association of pulmonary artery sling with segmental tracheal stenosis related to the presence of complete cartilaginous rings is known as the "ring-sling complex." This anomaly is associated with intracardiac defects in 10% to 20% of children, with atrial and ventricular septal defects most commonly seen.

The anomalous LPA arises from the RPA, and subsequently courses around the right mainstem bronchus. This creates a "sling" that can cause extrinsic compression of the bronchus and resultant hyperinflation of the right lung [**Fig. 2.32**]. On a lateral chest radiograph, anterior bowing of the trachea and posterior deviation of the esophagus may be seen. This classic appearance is well-demonstrated on a lateral esophagram. Preoperative CTA is performed to evaluate the morphology of the pulmonary arteries, determine their relationship to the airway, and delineate the extent of tracheal and/or bronchial compression or intrinsic stenosis.

CHEST

Congenital

Bronchopulmonary Foregut Malformations

The bronchopulmonary foregut malformations are a spectrum of developmental pulmonary anomalies resulting from the abnormal formation of the foregut and tracheobronchial tree during the fourth through seventh weeks of gestation. They include congenital pulmonary airway malformation (CPAM), congenital lobar hyperinflation (CLH), pulmonary sequestration, bronchial atresia, and bronchogenic cyst. Hybrid lesions are seen in more than 50% of pathologic specimens, and most often consist of CPAM and extralobar sequestration (ELS). Distinguishing these entities by imaging is not always possible.

The clinical presentation of bronchopulmonary foregut malformations depends on the size of the lesion, the presence of mass effect on the airway, adjacent lung, and mediastinal structures, and/or any existing superimposed infection. Children with CPAM, ELS, and CLH typically present in infancy with respiratory distress. Those with bronchogenic cyst, intralobar sequestration (ILS), and bronchial atresia often present later, usually with

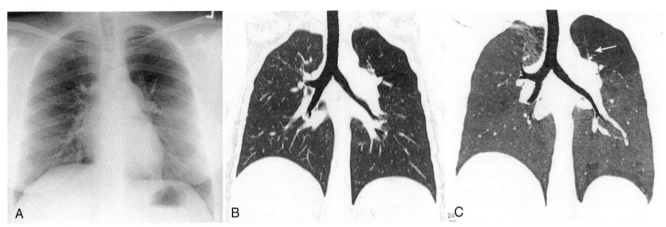

Figure 2.33 **Bronchial atresia. A,** Chest radiograph and (**B**) coronal computed tomography image in a 16-year-old demonstrate hyperinflation of the apical segment of the left upper lobe. **C,** Coronal minimum intensity projection image shows that the origin of the left upper lobe bronchus is absent. A tubular, blind-ended, air-filled structure (*arrow*) is seen, consistent with an atretic bronchus.

recurrent upper respiratory infections. They may also be asymptomatic.

Bronchial Atresia. Bronchial atresia is congenital atresia of a lobar, segmental, or subsegmental bronchus resulting in a blind-ended, atretic proximal bronchus with histologically normal distal architecture. A segmental bronchus is most frequently involved. It is most common in the left upper lobe, followed by the right upper, right middle, and lower lobes. The precise cause of this entity is not known, but it may be secondary to a vascular insult leading to stenosis or atresia of the involved segment. Bronchial atresia typically coexists with bronchopulmonary sequestration, and it is found in the majority of CPAM lesions.

On prenatal imaging, the involved portion of lung will be hyperexpanded. Increased echogenicity is noted on ultrasound, with T2 hyperintensity on fetal MRI. Sometimes a perihilar, tubular, mucous-filled bronchocele/mucocele can be seen on prenatal ultrasound or MRI. On postnatal CT scan, a tubular or rounded opacity reflecting a mucous plug is seen in a dilated central bronchus. This has a "finger-in-glove" appearance. Surrounding hyperlucency and diminished vascularity are characteristically seen [**Fig. 2.33**].

Treatment varies based on clinical symptoms. Surgical resection is usually reserved for symptomatic patients with recurrent infections.

Bronchogenic Cyst. A bronchogenic cyst is the most common of the foregut duplication cysts. It is a congenital malformation of the bronchial tree resulting from abnormal embryogenesis of the airway. It is typically a unilocular, fluid-filled, thin-walled mass. This entity is most commonly encountered in the mediastinum near the carina and within the lower lobes of the pulmonary parenchyma. Intrapulmonary bronchogenic cysts do not communicate with the bronchial tree, and thus are typically not air filled unless there is superimposed infection. They are often detected incidentally unless there is symptomatic compression of the airway or secondary infection of the lesion.

Imaging reveals an oval or round mass with cystic attenuation on CT and characteristic T2 hyperintensity on MRI [**Fig. 2.34**]. There is no internal contrast enhancement of the uncomplicated bronchogenic cyst on CT or MRI. If there is superimposed infection, an air–fluid level, thick, enhancing wall, and surrounding inflammatory changes can be seen.

Treatment is somewhat controversial. If the affected patient is symptomatic and/or growth is demonstrated over time, surgi-

cal resection is indicated. Aspiration can be performed in symptomatic patients who are not surgical candidates.

Congenital Lobar Hyperinflation. CLH, formerly known as congenital lobar emphysema, is caused by intrinsic or extrinsic bronchial narrowing with resultant air trapping, but without associated destruction of lung parenchyma. The left upper lobe is affected most frequently (50%), followed by the right middle lobe (30%), right upper lobe (20%), and lower lobes.

CLH is often indistinguishable from other congenital lung anomalies, particularly bronchial atresia. Similar prenatal imaging features are seen with these two entities. Both appear as an echogenic lesion on ultrasound and a T2 hyperintense lesion on MRI. Cysts are not typically seen, but rather associated with CPAM (to be described). Postnatally, CLH appears as a hyperlucent, hyperexpanded lobe with attenuated pulmonary vasculature, compression of adjacent lobes, and shift of the mediastinum away from the lesion [**Fig. 2.35**].

Surgical lobectomy is the treatment of choice for symptomatic patients. Those with mild or no symptoms can be managed expectantly.

Congenital Pulmonary Airway Malformation. CPAM (historically known as congenital cystic adenomatoid malformation) is a hamartomatous malformation resulting from abnormal proliferation of terminal bronchioles that maintain communication with the bronchial tree. The original classification system by Stocker is based on the size of the cysts that comprise the lesion and is used in clinical practice. In this system, a type I lesion consists of one or more cysts larger than 2 cm, a type II lesion contains multiple thin-walled cysts, and a type III lesion is solid appearing or microcystic. Pathologically, there are five types of CPAM with both cystic and solid pulmonary tissue and disorganized bronchi. It is important to note that the prognosis of CPAM depends more on the size of the lesion than on its classification.

Prenatally, CPAMs are classified based on cyst size. Lesions are evaluated for the presence of microcysts (<5 mm) or macrocysts (≥5 mm) on fetal ultrasound and MRI. The appearance of CPAMs is varied. A multilocular or unilocular cystic mass [**Fig. 2.36**] or solid mass may be seen. A lesion may have no well-defined lobar predilection. A type I CPAM can present as a large cyst in the periphery of the lung and may be radiographically indistinguishable from a predominantly cystic type 1 pleuropulmonary blastoma.

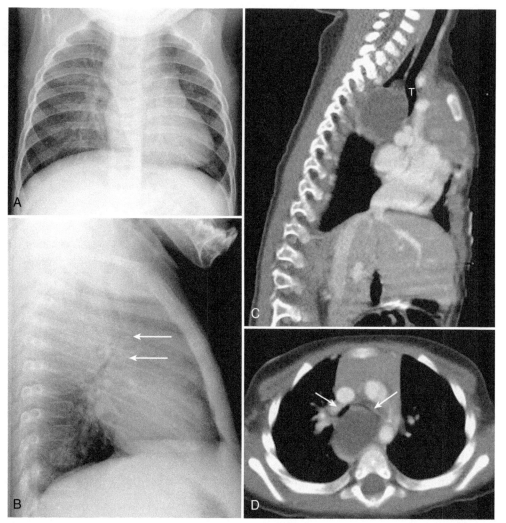

Figure 2.34 Bronchogenic/enteric duplication cyst causing airway compression in a 9-month-old with noisy breathing since birth. A, Frontal chest radiograph demonstrating abnormal increased density within the mediastinum. **B,** On the lateral view, this density projects posteriorly and causes significant anterior displacement and narrowing of the trachea and mainstem bronchi (*arrows*). **C,** Sagittal and (**D**) axial contrast-enhanced CT images show a thin-walled, fluid-filled structure within the posterior mediastinum consistent with a duplication cyst. There is anterior displacement of the trachea (*T*) and the mainstem bronchi (*arrows*). At surgery, the cyst was noted to be attached to both the trachea and the esophagus. It was initially aspirated and marsupialized, but subsequently required surgical resection because of recurrent symptoms from fluid reaccumulation.

Prenatal diagnosis of congenital lung lesions is associated with earlier surgical resection before the development of superimposed infection. This has allowed for more precise histopathologic diagnosis, and it is now known that a congenital lung lesion may be composed of bronchial atresia, CPAM, and/or sequestration simultaneously. Therefore CTA is usually performed before surgery when CPAM is suspected to evaluate for the presence of a hybrid lesion with a concomitant sequestration component. If present, an associated feeding artery from the thoracic or abdominal aorta will be demonstrated. In its purest form, a CPAM is supplied by a pulmonary artery and has venous drainage into the pulmonary veins.

Symptomatic CPAMs are typically resected by lobectomy. Asymptomatic lesions detected postnatally are generally also surgically removed because of the risk for coexistent or subsequent development of pleuropulmonary blastoma or rhabdomyosarcoma within a lesion. Notably, a prenatally detected CPAM will occasionally demonstrate spontaneous involution on early postnatal follow-up imaging.

Sequestration. A bronchopulmonary sequestration is a congenital malformation of the lower respiratory tract that consists of nonfunctioning lung tissue lacking normal communication with the tracheobronchial tree. This lesion usually receives arterial blood supply from the thoracic aorta. Sometimes it may be supplied by branches of the celiac, splenic, intercostal, or subclavian arteries. Venous drainage is primarily via the pulmonary veins into the left atrium, but abnormal connections to the vena cava, azygos vein, or right atrium may also occur.

A sequestration can be intralobar (75%) or extralobar (25%). An ILS is typically embedded within a normal lobe, and therefore not invested by pleura. The majority of ILSs are located in the posterior segment of the left lower lobe. Patients usually present in adolescence or adulthood with recurrent episodes of pneumonia.

An ELS develops as an accessory lung invested within its own pleura. An aberrant systemic vascular supply is present. Venous drainage can be variable and may involve the azygos or hemiazygos veins, the subclavian and intercostal veins, or the portal

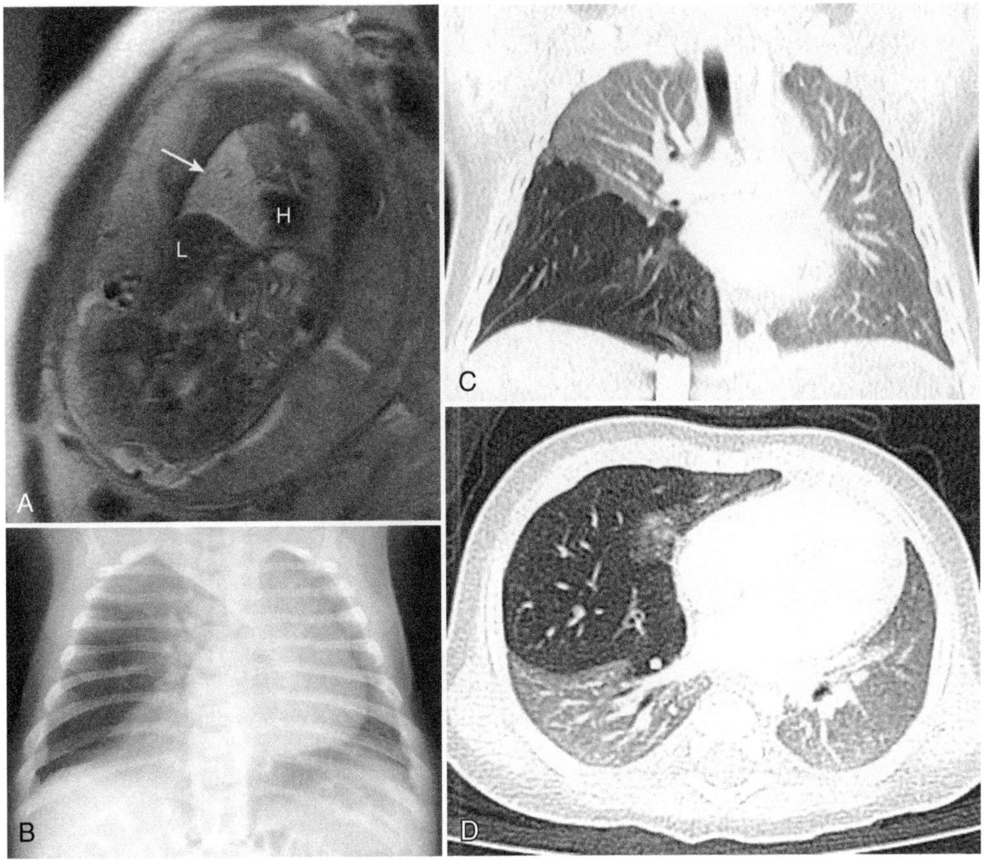

Figure 2.35 **Congenital lobar hyperinflation diagnosed prenatally. A,** Coronal single-shot T2-weighted fetal magnetic resonance image shows abnormal increased signal and mass-like enlargement of a portion of the right lung (*arrow*). *H,* heart; *L,* liver. **B,** Postnatal chest radiograph shows hyperinflation of the right middle lobe. There is mass effect, with displacement of the heart and mediastinum leftward and compressive atelectasis of the right upper and lower lobes. **C,** Coronal and (**D**) axial computed tomography images confirm abnormal hyperinflation of the right middle lobe. This lesion was surgically resected.

venous system. Venous drainage to the pulmonary veins may also be seen. ELS can present as a left subdiaphragmatic or retroperitoneal mass. Patients with ELS usually present in infancy with respiratory compromise. Congenital anomalies are seen in association with ELS with some frequency. These include CDH, CPAM, pulmonary hypoplasia, congenital heart disease, abnormal communications with the GI tract, and vertebral anomalies. Coexistence with CDH is most common. A hybrid lesion consisting of a sequestration and a type II CPAM may be seen.

Imaging features of sequestration overlap with those of CPAM and bronchial atresia, particularly because it is now known that these entities may occur together as hybrid lesions. All may be seen as echogenic lesions on ultrasound, and T2 hyperintense lesions on MRI. On chest radiographs, sequestration appears as a focal opacity with consolidation and/or cysts [**Fig. 2.37**]. On CT, a homogenous or heterogenous solid mass is seen, sometimes with internal cystic components. CTA and MRA are important to detect the anomalous systemic arterial supply to the lesion before surgical resection. When it occurs together with bronchial atresia, an ILS may present as a region of localized emphysema that receives abnormal systemic arterial supply without an associated parenchymal opacity or mass [**Fig. 2.38**].

ILS carries a high risk for associated complications, including recurrent infections, pneumothorax, hemorrhage, and respiratory compromise. Thus lobectomy is the preferred method of treatment. Intrathoracic ELS is typically resected because of the risk for superimposed infection. There is some controversy regarding the management of extrathoracic or intraabdominal ELS. Expectant management of these lesions is often appropriate because they frequently undergo spontaneous involution.

Pulmonary Agenesis/Aplasia/Hypoplasia

There are three main types of pulmonary developmental anomalies: (1) pulmonary agenesis, which refers to the complete absence of a lung or lobe and its bronchi; (2) pulmonary aplasia, which refers to the presence of rudimentary lobar bronchi in the absence of lung tissue; and (3) pulmonary hypoplasia, which refers to an underdeveloped lobe that contains both bronchi and alveoli. Patients with these pulmonary developmental anomalies may be asymptomatic or may present with varying degrees of respiratory distress. There may also be associated congenital malformations involving the heart and vasculature, GI tract, genitourinary tract, or skeletal system. Mass effect from displaced intraabdominal structures into the chest through a CDH in utero often results in hypoplasia of the ipsilateral lung.

Pulmonary agenesis is a rare lesion in which there is a single lung with displacement of the heart and mediastinum to the side of agenesis. A small, radiopaque hemithorax is seen on chest radiographs [**Fig. 2.39**]. The left side is affected more frequently than the right. Right-sided agenesis is notably associated with a much worse prognosis because of greater anatomic distortion of the airway and great vessels, as well as associated TBM and recurrent infections. Postnatally, CT imaging with 2D and 3D

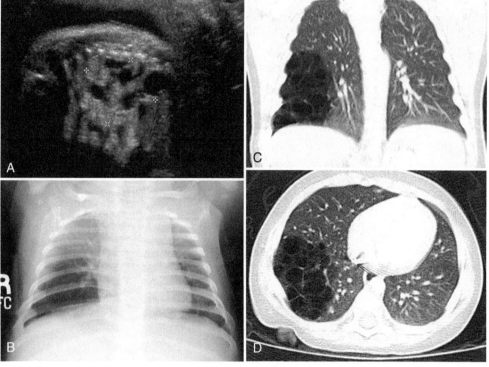

Figure 2.36 **Congenital pulmonary airway malformation (CPAM) detected prenatally. A,** Image from a fetal ultrasound image shows a mixed cystic and solid mass in the right lower lung. **B,** A follow-up chest radiograph at 6 months of age shows a lucent lesion in the right lower lobe. **C,** Coronal and (**D**) axial images from a subsequent computed tomography (CT) scan confirm a multiloculated lucent lesion composed of multiple thin-walled air cysts. No systemic arterial supply was detected on CT angiography. Although this infant remained asymptomatic, the right lower lobe was resected because of the large size of the lesion. A type II CPAM was diagnosed at histopathology.

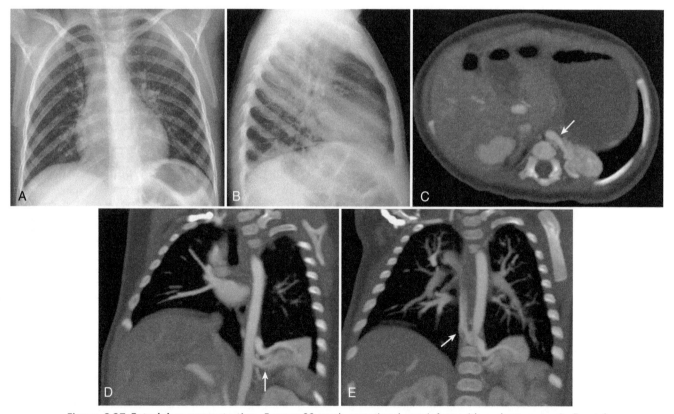

Figure 2.37 **Extralobar sequestration.** Former 33-week gestational age infant with a chest mass. **A,** Frontal and (**B**) lateral radiographs of the chest show a wedge-shaped soft tissue mass in the posteromedial aspect of the left lower lobe. **C** and **D,** Subsequent computed tomography angiography (CTA) in axial oblique and coronal planes demonstrates an enhancing mass with well-defined margins with a large feeding artery from the aorta (*arrow*). **E,** Coronal oblique CTA image shows venous drainage to the azygos vein (*arrow*).

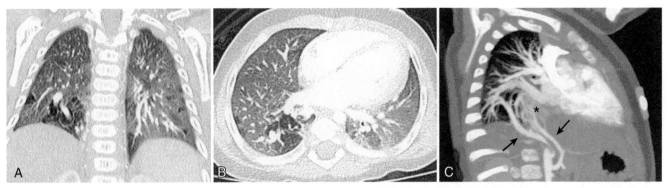

Figure 2.38 Intralobar sequestration associated with bronchial atresia (hybrid lesion). A, Coronal and **(B)** axial computed tomography (CT) images in lung windows show abnormal hyperinflation of the postero-medial aspect of the right lower lobe with abnormal vascular arborization. **C,** Oblique coronal CT angiography image shows an adjacent enhancing mass *(asterisk)*. The entire hybrid lesion is supplied by systemic collateral vessels from the abdominal aorta *(arrows)*.

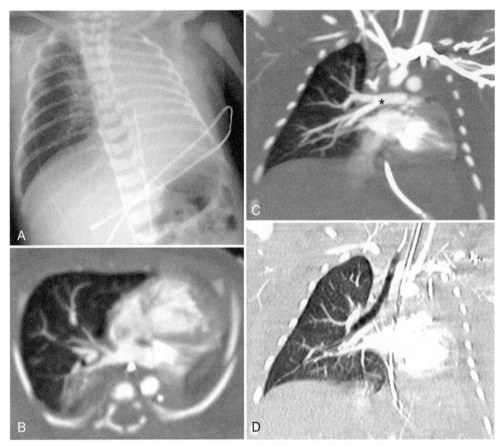

Figure 2.39 Left lung agenesis. A, Frontal chest radiograph shows a small left hemithorax, large right hemi-thorax, and shift of the heart and mediastinal structures into the left chest. **B,** Axial and **(C)** coronal CTA images show the heart displaced into the left chest and a large right pulmonary artery *(asterisk)*. **D,** Coronal CT image in lung windows shows a large but otherwise normal-appearing right lung. No mediastinal left pulmonary artery or left lung tissue was identified, consistent with left lung agenesis.

multiplanar reformats is useful to distinguish among pulmonary agenesis, aplasia, and hypoplasia. MRA is performed to delineate the mediastinal vascular anatomy.

An in utero karyotype should be considered if pulmonary agenesis, aplasia, or hypoplasia is detected, particularly when multiple other anomalies are present. If pulmonary agenesis is detected prenatally, the fetus should be followed for the development of hydrops. Prognosis depends on the degree of

pulmonary development and the presence and severity of other associated congenital anomalies.

Congenital Diaphragmatic Hernia

CDH results from failure of fusion of one of the pleuroperitoneal canals at about 8 weeks' gestation. This results in a diaphragmatic defect through which abdominal contents may herniate.

The most common type of CDH is a Bochdalek hernia, which occurs posteriorly and typically to the left. A hernia may contain stomach, intestine, liver, and/or spleen. CDH can be associated with additional anatomic malformations including neural tube defects. It may also be seen in association with syndromes such as Turner syndrome and other chromosomal anomalies including trisomy 21. Mortality is predominantly due to pulmonary hypoplasia, which results from mass effect on the developing lung. Neonates are typically hypoxic, with persistent fetal circulation (PFC) from pulmonary hypoplasia and resulting pulmonary hypertension.

On radiographs, bubbly lucencies may be seen in the chest reflecting herniated loops of bowel. The heart and mediastinum will be shifted to the contralateral side. Cardiomediastinal shift can alter the expected course of the support lines and tubes, including enteric catheters and umbilical lines [**Fig. 2.40**]. After CDH is detected on prenatal ultrasound, fetal MRI is helpful to

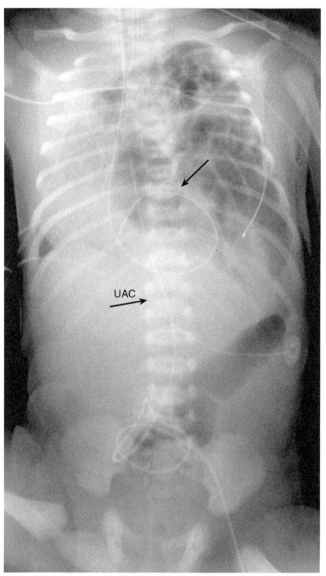

Figure 2.40 Left-sided congenital diaphragmatic hernia. Supine radiograph of the chest and abdomen in a newborn with respiratory distress shows gas-filled loops of bowel filling the left hemithorax, with displacement of the heart and mediastinal structures into the right chest. The enteric tube is coiled in the stomach, which is displaced into the chest (*arrow*). The umbilical arterial catheter (*UAC*) (*arrow*) is positioned in the aorta, which is shifted into the right chest.

assess the hernia and evaluate for secondary pulmonary hypoplasia. This can aid in management decisions regarding the anticipated level of respiratory support needed at the time of delivery. The presence of liver within a hernia is associated with a relatively worse prognosis.

Surgical repair is the definitive treatment. Patients with severe respiratory failure often require support from ECMO.

Hypogenetic Lung or Congenital Venolobar Syndrome

Pulmonary hypoplasia is most often an incidental and clinically insignificant anomaly. An exception is when it is seen with the hypogenetic lung syndrome, also known as congenital venolobar syndrome. This syndrome consists of hypoplasia or aplasia of the lung, persistent systemic arterial supply to the lung from the thoracic or abdominal aorta, anomalous pulmonary venous drainage from one or more lobes of the lung, absence or small size of the pulmonary artery, and occasional vertebral body and rib anomalies. Hypogenetic lung can also be associated with other congenital pulmonary anomalies such as a bronchogenic cyst, horseshoe lung [**Fig. 2.41**], congenital heart disease (most commonly atrial septal defect), and genitourinary tract anomalies. Affected patients may have a varied clinical presentation depending on the degree of pulmonary hypoplasia, the presence and extent of left-to-right shunting leading to pulmonary overcirculation, and the presence of associated congenital malformations.

Scimitar syndrome consists of hypoplasia or aplasia of one or more lobes of the right lung, partial anomalous pulmonary venous connection (PAPVC) below the diaphragm, absence or small size of the pulmonary artery, and occasional vertebral body and rib anomalies. The anomalous pulmonary venous connection is most often right pulmonary venous drainage into the IVC. The name of the syndrome is derived from the appearance of the associated anomalous vein, which resembles a curved Turkish sword or scimitar. Young infants often present with signs and symptoms of congestive heart failure related to right heart volume overload and pulmonary hypertension. In older children, recurrent infections in the right lung base can occur.

Chest radiographs may show the anomalous vein draining medially and inferiorly into the IVC in proximity to the right hemidiaphragm, often in the shape of a scimitar [**Fig. 2.42**]. Echocardiography is indicated to determine the number, location, and course of the pulmonary veins, as well as the direction of blood flow and any potential site of obstruction. CT and MRI with 2D and 3D imaging are used to precisely delineate the cardiac and venous morphology.

If a patient with PAPVC is symptomatic from pulmonary overcirculation and shunting is greater than 2:1, surgical repair may be indicated. The anomalous vein is reconnected to the left atrium, with or without baffling of the common right pulmonary vein into the left atrium. Embolization of the systemic collateral arterial supply may also be performed.

Pulmonary Arteriovenous Malformation

A pulmonary arteriovenous malformation may be single or multiple in 40% of cases. The remaining 60% occur in patients with hereditary hemorrhagic telangiectasia (Osler-Weber-Rendu disease). Affected children may present with cyanosis, dyspnea, hemoptysis, clubbing, and polycythemia. Arteriovenous malformations are most often subpleural in location and are best managed by coil embolization [**Fig. 2.43**].

Inflammatory

Infections

Bacterial Pneumonia. Bacterial infection in the lungs presents as alveolar consolidation in a lobar and segmental

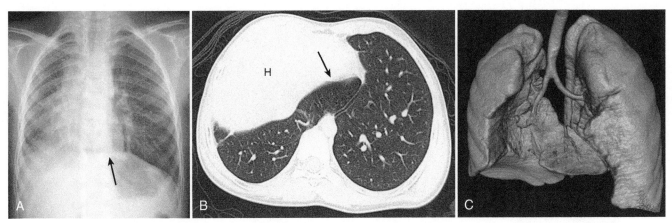

Figure 2.41 Horseshoe lung. A, Frontal chest radiograph in a 4-year-old with recurrent pneumonia demonstrates a small right hemithorax and hypoplastic right lung, with shift of the heart and mediastinal structures into the right chest. Subtle lucency is noted along the margin of the heart (*arrow*), reflecting lung tissue crossing the midline. **B,** Axial computed tomography image shows an abnormal segment of lung (*arrow*) crossing posterior to the heart (*H*) and connecting the right and left lungs. **C,** Volume-rendered image of the lungs with the heart removed shows right and left lung connecting inferiorly across the midline, consistent with a horseshoe lung.

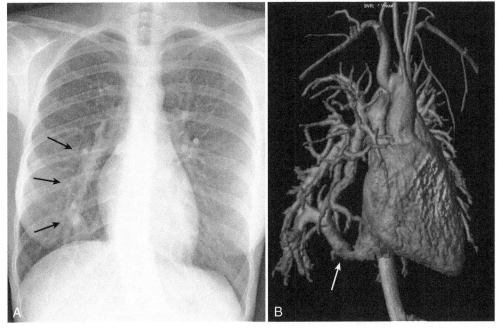

Figure 2.42 Scimitar vein, or partial anomalous pulmonary venous connection to the inferior vena cava (IVC). A, Frontal chest radiograph in a 17-year-old with dyspnea on exertion shows an abnormal vascular structure (*arrows*) extending from the right pulmonary hilum to the right cardiophrenic angle, consistent with a scimitar vein. **B,** Volume-rendered image from a magnetic resonance angiogram shows the abnormal pulmonary venous connection to the IVC (*arrow*), resulting in a left-to-right shunt and volume loading of the right heart.

distribution. Pleural effusions may also be present. The most common causative agents are *S. pneumoniae, H. influenzae,* and *S. aureus.* Staphylococcal pneumonia occurs most commonly in early infancy, *H. influenzae* pneumonia most often between 6 and 12 months of age, and pneumococcus typically between 1 and 3 years of age. Clinically, these infections may be indistinguishable. Children with bacterial pneumonia present with cough, chest pain, and fevers that are often high. Pneumonia most often occurs after a viral upper respiratory infection.

Staphylococcal and *H. influenzae* pneumonia may be complicated by the development of an empyema. Pneumatoceles develop in 50% of patients with staphylococcal infection and are often multiple. They are thought to be a form of pulmonary

interstitial emphysema (PIE) and local emphysema caused by airway obstruction with a subsequent check-valve mechanism. They usually resolve completely in about 6 weeks [**Fig. 2.44**]. Pneumatoceles are less frequently seen in the setting of streptococcal pneumonia.

Imaging is usually not particularly helpful in determining the causative organism in pneumonia. Consolidation is usually lobar, and air bronchograms may be seen. Radiographic abnormality typically resolves in 2 to 3 weeks.

In children younger than 8 years, a staphylococcal or pneumococcal pneumonia can sometimes appear sphere-shaped with indistinct edges. This is referred to as "round pneumonia" [**Fig. 2.45**]. Such a rounded lesion may mimic a mass or a

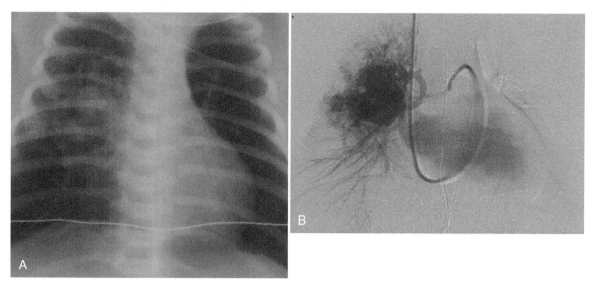

Figure 2.43 Pulmonary arteriovenous malformation (AVM). A, Frontal chest radiograph in a child with hemoptysis demonstrates a patchy opacity in the right upper lobe. **B,** The patient underwent conventional angiography and was diagnosed with a pulmonary AVM that was treated with coil embolization.

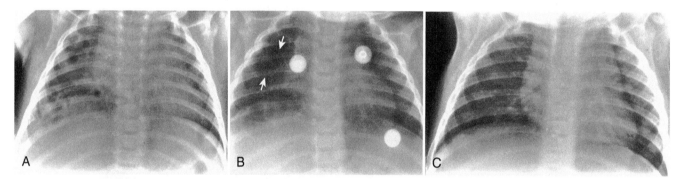

Figure 2.44 Staphylococcal pneumonia. A, Frontal chest radiograph in an infant demonstrates diffuse, patchy alveolar infiltrates. **B,** One week after diagnosis, a pneumatocele has formed in the right upper lobe (*arrows*). **C,** Six weeks after diagnosis, the lungs have cleared.

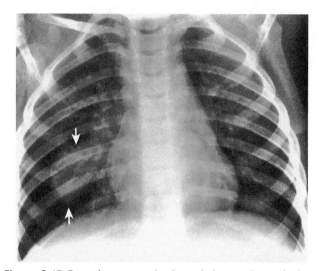

Figure 2.45 Round pneumonia. Frontal chest radiograph demonstrating a well-circumscribed, rounded opacity in the right mid to lower lung (*arrows*) in a 3-year-old with pneumococcal infection. The focal area of consolidation cleared on radiographs obtained 2 weeks after diagnosis.

metastatic lesion. The round shape is thought to be due to the centrifugal spread of bacteria through the pores of Kohn and the canals of Lambert within the pulmonary interstitium. Round pneumonia typically resolves completely after appropriate antimicrobial therapy.

CT scan is not routinely performed for uncomplicated pneumonia in children. Ultrasound evaluation of a parapneumonic effusion may be helpful to evaluate for complexity and also to distinguish a loculated effusion from adjacent consolidated lung. Notably, both exudative effusions (empyema) and transudative effusions may appear complex on ultrasound. A contrast-enhanced CT scan can be performed to distinguish these entities. An enhancing rim surrounds complex pleural fluid in the setting of an empyema.

Pertussis Pneumonia. Pertussis pneumonia most commonly affects children younger than 5 years and is seen more frequently in girls. It is caused by *Bordetella pertussis*. Chest radiographs reveal streaky perihilar infiltrates, with hilar adenopathy that is most often unilateral. This characteristic pattern of infiltrate is sometimes referred to as a "shaggy heart" appearance [**Fig. 2.46**]. Because of the widespread use of the pertussis vaccine in the United States, the incidence of this disease has decreased by more than 80% from the prevaccine era. Pertussis remains a major health problem among children in developing countries.

Mycoplasma Pneumoniae. *Mycoplasma pneumoniae* is a ubiquitous agent that causes epidemics of respiratory infection, primarily in older school-aged children and adolescents. It is the most common cause of pneumonia in children older than 5 years. Of those infected, 50% have tracheobronchitis, 30% have pneumonia, 10% have pharyngitis, and 10% have otitis media. With mycoplasma pneumonia, clinical symptoms are less severe than those seen with true bacterial pneumonias. Chest radiographs may reveal segmental, subsegmental, or reticulonodular interstitial infiltrates. Lobar involvement may be seen, predominantly affecting the lower lobes [**Fig. 2.47**]. Effusions occur in about 20% of patients. Treatment is supportive, and recovery is often relatively slow.

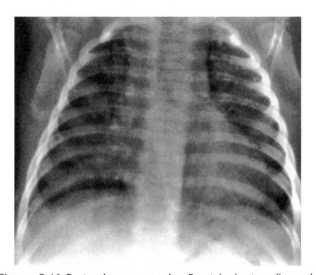

Figure 2.46 **Pertussis pneumonia.** Frontal chest radiograph demonstrates the perihilar interstitial infiltrates resulting in the "shaggy heart" appearance sometimes seen with pertussis and C. *trachomatis* infections.

Mycobacterial Infection. Primary tuberculosis (TB) caused by *Mycobacterium tuberculosis* initially affects the lungs but may spread throughout the body. Almost all cases in the infant and young child begin after exposure through inhalation. An exudative opacity first develops. Subsequently, hypersensitivity develops over 3 to 8 weeks, and hilar and mediastinal lymph nodes become enlarged. In the lung parenchyma, calcification, caseation, and parenchymal scarring may develop.

Radiographically, the constellation of local lymphatic and nodal involvement with parenchymal scarring is referred to as the primary complex of Ranke. With the development of resistance, postprimary TB occurs. This manifests as consolidation of an entire segment or lobe, ipsilateral lymph node enlargement, pleural effusions, and pulmonary cavitation [**Fig. 2.48**]. Seeding of organisms through the lymphatics and the venous system may occur, resulting in miliary (secondary) TB within 6 months [**Fig. 2.49**]. Tiny, 2- to 3-mm pulmonary nodules are characteristic, and widespread dissemination of disease may be seen.

Viral Causative Agents. Airspace disease, whether segmental or lobar, is most likely to be bacterial in origin. In contradistinction, airways disease is more likely to be viral in origin. In children younger than 2 years, infection with respiratory syncytial virus, parainfluenza (types 1, 2, and 3), influenza, and adenovirus leads to inflammation, edema, surface cell necrosis, and increased mucous production in the terminal and respiratory bronchioles. The alveoli are spared. Radiographs show hyperinflation, peribronchial thickening ("cuffing"), and scattered areas of atelectasis ("disordered aeration"). On sequential radiographs, shifting atelectasis may be seen. The lung apices are typically spared. Pleural effusions and complications such as empyema are rare. Resolution may take up to 2 weeks. In children older than 2 years, the radiographic appearance of viral infection is very similar to that of reactive airways disease. Children who experience repeated episodes of bronchiolitis may be evaluated for underlying cystic fibrosis.

Other Infections. Pulmonary mycotic infections are relatively rare in children except in endemic areas. Histoplasmosis is endemic in the central United States, whereas coccidiomycosis

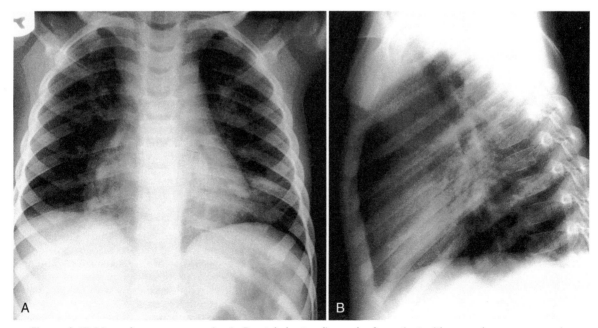

Figure 2.47 **Mycoplasma pneumonia. A,** Frontal chest radiograph of a patient with mycoplasma pneumonia. Subsegmental atelectasis is present in the right lower lobe and lingula. **B,** Corresponding lateral chest radiograph demonstrates hyperinflation, with flattening of the hemidiaphragms and an increased retrosternal clear space.

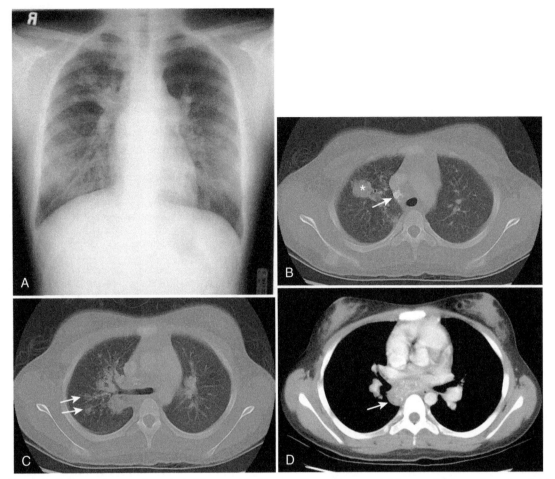

Figure 2.48 *Post primary tuberculosis.* 13-year-old-girl presenting with recurrent fevers, night sweats, and weight loss following treatment for primary TB with isoniazid 2 years prior. **A,** Frontal radiograph of the chest shows perihilar interstitial thickening, enlargement of the right hilar structures, and patchy nodular opacities in the right upper lobe. **B,** Axial CT image shows a dominant nodular opacity in the anterior segment of the right upper lobe (*asterisk*), consistent with a tuberculoma. Calcified lymphadenopathy is noted in the right paratracheal space (*arrow*). **C,** Axial CT image shows centrilobular opacities surrounding the right hilum with smaller nodules in the periphery reflecting endobronchial spread of disease (*arrows*). **D,** Axial CT image in mediastinal windows shows heterogeneous, low density subcarinal adenopathy with distention of the azygoesophageal recess (*arrow*). The patient had repeated exposures to family members with active TB since the time of initial treatment. Sputum culture was positive for mycobacterium tuberculosis, and the patient was treated with multidrug therapy.

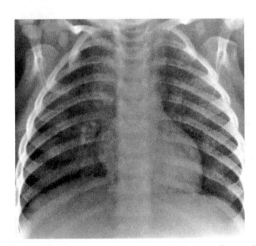

Figure 2.49 Miliary tuberculosis. Frontal chest radiograph demonstrates multiple miliary pulmonary nodules. Right hilar and mediastinal lymphadenopathy are also seen.

is endemic in the southwestern United States. Radiographic findings are often lacking. Findings similar to those seen in primary TB may be noted, with characteristic hilar and mediastinal adenopathy and miliary granulomas in the pulmonary interstitium. With histoplasmosis, late calcification of parenchymal lesions and lymph nodes is common.

Opportunistic pulmonary infections occur in pediatric patients with underlying immunodeficiency. These may be seen in the setting of AIDS, after chemotherapy for leukemia/lymphoma, or after transplant surgery. Relatively more common causative agents include *Pneumocystis carinii* pneumonia, varicella, and certain fungi.

Infection with *P. carinii* occurs in debilitated or otherwise immunocompromised children. It is seen most commonly in those undergoing treatment for leukemia or lymphoma, and is the most common opportunistic pulmonary infection in children with AIDS. Affected patients present with cough, tachypnea, and malaise. The infection is often fatal. Early in the course of disease, chest radiographs may mimic those in children with viral respiratory infections. Subsequently, there is progression from a reticulonodular interstitial process to diffuse alveolar consolidation predominantly affecting the pulmonary hila and lung bases. Lung

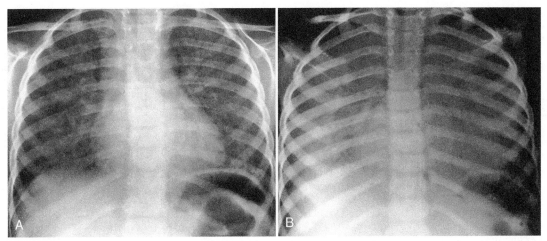

Figure 2.50 Pneumocystis carinii pneumonia. A, Frontal chest radiograph in a patient with *Pneumocystis carinii* infection demonstrates bilateral diffuse reticular infiltrates. **B,** This may progress to diffuse consolidation.

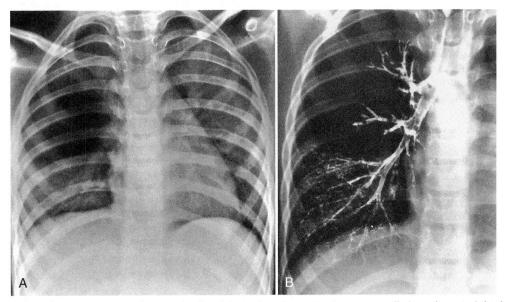

Figure 2.51 Swyer-James syndrome. A, Frontal chest radiograph shows a small, hyperlucent right lung. **B,** Bronchography confirms obliteration of lung tissue in the right upper and middle lobes.

volumes are normal to low, and pleural effusions may occur [**Fig. 2.50**]. Hilar adenopathy is uncommon. Lung biopsy is necessary to confirm the diagnosis.

Chickenpox (varicella) is a highly contagious viral disease of childhood with low mortality in otherwise healthy children. Mortality is higher in immunocompromised children and adults. Children present with cough, fever, and a vesicular rash, generally accompanied by mild constitutional symptoms. Airspace disease may be seen in immunocompromised patients (1% of all cases). Chickenpox may be complicated in relatively older children. Radiographs can demonstrate nodular infiltrates that may progress to large, segmental areas of patchy consolidation, predominantly involving the lung bases and perihilar regions. Total clearing is virtually guaranteed, although punctate parenchymal calcifications may be evident within 2 years after the acute illness and may persist through life.

Aspergillosis is one of the more common sporadic infections that affect children with conditions such as asthma, cystic fibrosis, and chronic granulomatous disease of childhood with some frequency. Aspergillus causes a hypersensitivity reaction. Infection is very common in neutropenic immunocompromised patients and is considered invasive. Superinfection in a preexisting cavitary lesion, or a "mycetoma," is rare in children.

Angioinvasive *Aspergillus* infection is the first variant of disease. Radiographs are characterized by focal consolidation with a surrounding ground glass opacity, or a "halo" sign. In later stages of disease, an "air crescent" sign can be seen, with a focal collection of air surrounding a necrotic mass in the area of consolidation.

Hypersensitivity or allergic aspergillosis may mimic the imaging findings of bronchiolitis. It can also be characterized by mucous plugging, with the "finger-in-glove" sign. Bronchial dilatation may be demonstrated on CT [**Fig. 2.28**], prompting early intervention with steroids to prevent bronchiectasis and irreversible damage to the airways.

Swyer-James Syndrome. Swyer-James syndrome is a manifestation of childhood bronchiolitis obliterans. It is thought to be due to a preceding viral pneumonitis. This entity is characterized by a decrease in the number and size of the airways and pulmonary vessels.

On chest radiographs, a small, hyperlucent lung with diminished vascular markings is often seen. HRCT demonstrates air trapping in the affected lung, small central and peripheral pulmonary arteries, bronchiectasis, and bronchial wall thickening [**Fig. 2.51**].

The differential diagnosis of a unilateral hyperlucent lung includes an endobronchial foreign body, pneumothorax, congenital lobar emphysema, hypoplasia of the lung or pulmonary artery, compensatory hyperinflation, and post–radiation therapy–related change.

Cystic Lung Disease

Cystic Fibrosis. Cystic fibrosis (CF) is the most common lethal genetic disease in Caucasians of Northern European descent. It is an inherited autosomal recessive disorder of exocrine gland function. The lungs, pancreas, liver, and intestine are most commonly affected. This disease is due to mutations in the *CFTR* gene on chromosome 7q31.2. Mutations lead to abnormal transport of chloride and sodium across epithelial membranes, and thick, viscous secretions result. More than 1000 mutations in the *CFTR* gene have been discovered. Thus there is variable phenotypic expression of disease. The clinical spectrum of disease includes recurrent pulmonary infections, chronic sinusitis with nasal polyps, chronic obstruction of the intestinal and biliary systems, pancreatic dysfunction, and infertility.

Pulmonary involvement ranges from repeated episodes of bronchiolitis in infants to chronic cough and recurrent respiratory infections in older children to chronic pulmonary disease in adolescents and young adults. When respiratory insufficiency and progressive pulmonary arterial hypertension develop, death usually occurs by the fourth decade. This is primarily due to complications such as pulmonary hemorrhage.

Chest radiographs may be normal early on, or findings may be indistinguishable from those seen in the setting of bronchiolitis in infants and children. The lungs are often hyperinflated. Progressive mucous plugging of bronchi with superimposed infection leads to bronchial wall thickening, mucoid impaction, and diffuse, often saccular bronchiectasis. Bronchiectasis initially involves the central hilar bronchi, with subsequent peripheral progression. Bronchial dilation occurs throughout the lungs, although it tends to be most pronounced in the upper lobes, lingula, and right middle lobe. Chronic volume loss, cicatricial atelectasis, and scarring ultimately develop [**Fig. 2.52**]. Prominence of the hilar soft tissues may be seen on chest radiographs because of reactive nodal enlargement related to recurrent bouts of infection. This is most often seen in the earlier stages of CF and is often related to recurrent infections with *Pseudomonas aeruginosa* and *S. aureus*. In later stages of disease, enlarged pulmonary arteries in the setting of pulmonary arterial hypertension may also contribute to prominence of the hilar soft tissues.

Complications of CF include pneumothorax, pulmonary hypertension with cor pulmonale, and pulmonary hemorrhage. Pulmonary hemorrhage results from the erosion of hypertrophied bronchial arteries into adjacent bronchi. Bronchial arteries enlarge as a result of chronic lung inflammation.

Supportive care and early implementation of treatment for infections can dramatically increase life expectancy. Treatment includes prolonged antibiotic regimens, oral and inhaled corticosteroids, nutritional support with feeding tube placement and pancreatic enzyme supplementation, and lung transplantation.

Primary Ciliary Dyskinesia. Primary ciliary dyskinesia, also known as immotile cilia syndrome, is an autosomal recessive disorder characterized by a congenital abnormality in ciliary structure. Ciliary immotility is seen due to a deficiency of the dynein arms of the cilia lining the respiratory tract, middle ear, fallopian tubes, and seminiferous tubules, and within the flagella of sperm. Affected patients may suffer from chronic pulmonary and sinus disease, infertility, and deafness. The earliest clinical manifestations of disease are typically chronic sinusitis and chronic otitis media, which may lead to conductive hearing loss and subsequent language delay.

Imaging findings are similar to those seen in patients with cystic fibrosis. Hyperinflation, bronchial wall thickening, and bronchiectasis are seen, with bronchiectasis most pronounced in the lingula, right middle lobe, and lower lobes. There is mucous plugging within dilated airways, centrilobular nodules and tree-in-bud opacities are seen, and air trapping is noted. The triad of situs inversus, sinusitis and/or nasal polyposis, and bronchiectasis raises the possibility of Kartagener syndrome, a subset of primary ciliary dyskinesia [**Fig. 2.53**]. Chronic pulmonary disease, together with a history of infertility or deafness, confirms the diagnosis.

The natural progression of primary ciliary dyskinesia is relatively slow compared with that of cystic fibrosis. Management involves rigorous pulmonary physiotherapy, early treatment of infections, and immunization for common pathogens.

Neoplasms/Mass-Like Lesions

Mediastinal Masses

Mediastinal masses are the most common thoracic masses in children [**Box 2.1**]. The lesions listed in boldface in **Box 2.1** comprise the majority of all masses encountered. Approximately 30% develop before the age of 12 years. About 30% occur in the anterior compartment, 30% in the middle compartment, and 40% in the posterior compartment.

Anterior

Disorders of the Thymus. As previously noted, enlargement of the thymus can mimic a pathologic mediastinal mass on chest radiography in infants. Follow-up imaging with ultrasound, CT, or MRI may be performed for further evaluation in this setting. Pathologic conditions that can be associated with diffuse thymic enlargement include hyperthyroidism, Addison disease, and infiltrative disorders such as lymphoma, leukemia, and Langerhans cell histiocytosis (LCH). Rebound thymic enlargement or thymic hyperplasia can be observed on serial follow-up imaging of patients who have received steroids, chemotherapy, or radiation treatment. The thymus is often small or hypoplastic in premature infants because of stress. Thymic aplasia (DiGeorge

---

BOX 2.1   Mediastinal Masses

ANTERIOR

Thymus: normal, rebound hypertrophy, thymic cyst, thymoma
Teratoma (three layers), dermoid (two layers)
Lymphoma
Ectopic thyroid

MIDDLE

Inflammatory lymph nodes, **lymphoma**
Foregut abnormalities (bronchopulmonary foregut malformations)
Prominent pulmonary vessels, aortic dilatation or aneurysm
Pericardial abnormalities

POSTERIOR

Neurogenic tumors: ganglioneuroma, ganglioneuroblastoma, neuroblastoma
Congenital lesions: sequestration, bronchogenic or neurenteric cyst

SUPERIOR

Lymphatic malformation or cystic hygroma
Bronchogenic cyst
Neurogenic tumors
Rare vascular lesions

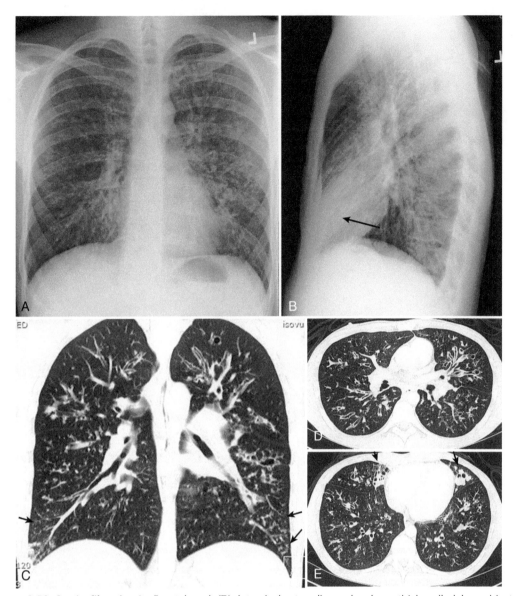

Figure 2.52 Cystic fibrosis. A, Frontal and (**B**) lateral chest radiographs show thick-walled bronchiectasis extending from the hila into the lungs. The right and left heart margins are indistinct. There is bronchiectasis with surrounding opacity anteriorly on the lateral view (*arrow*), consistent with cicatricial atelectasis in the right middle lobe and lingula. **C,** Coronal computed tomography (CT) image in lung windows again shows thick-walled bronchiectasis. Scattered interstitial opacities with a tree-in-bud configuration are seen, most notably in the lateral lower lobes (*arrows*). This appearance reflects inflammatory change. **D** and **E,** Axial CT images show extensive bronchiectasis with dilated, mucous-filled bronchi and cicatricial volume loss in the right middle lobe and lingula (*arrows*).

syndrome) is seen in infants born with little or no thymic tissue (or parathyroid glands) because of maldevelopment of the third and fourth pharyngeal pouches during the 6th to 12th weeks of gestational life. Congenital cardiac anomalies associated with DiGeorge syndrome include tetralogy of Fallot, truncus arteriosus, transposition of the great vessels, ventricular septal defect, and absence of the pulmonary valve.

A thymic cyst is a rare lesion resulting from congenital persistence of the thymopharyngeal tract. Patients are usually asymptomatic and are diagnosed incidentally. A thymic cyst may manifest as a unilocular or multilocular cystic mass with no intrinsic enhancement on postcontrast imaging [**Fig. 2.54**]. MRI can be performed to exclude the presence of mural nodules that may suggest a cystic neoplasm rather than a benign lesion.

A thymoma is the most common primary malignant tumor of the thymus. It arises from medullary thymic epithelium. When thymomas occur in children, they are often diagnosed in the setting of a paraneoplastic syndrome such as myasthenia gravis, red cell aplasia, or hypogammaglobulinemia. Pathologically, thymomas are subdivided into invasive and noninvasive subtypes. Thymomas are typically slow growing and present with nonspecific symptoms such as cough and chest pain.

Chest radiography typically shows a nonspecific appearing anterior mediastinal mass [**Fig. 2.55A** and **B**]. Thymomas may be mildly heterogeneous in attenuation on CT and signal intensity on MRI [**Fig. 2.55C** through **F**]. There can be displacement and/or compression of adjacent mediastinal structures. More aggressive forms of thymoma may demonstrate calcification on CT, or evidence of cystic degeneration or necrosis on CT and MRI after contrast administration. Thymic carcinoma is rare in children. This lesion typically appears more heterogeneous on cross-sectional imaging, sometimes with adjacent lymphadenopathy and distant metastasis. A less favorable prognosis is associated.

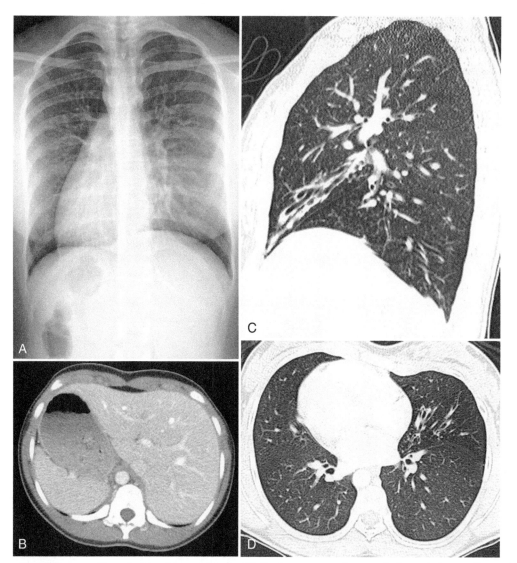

Figure 2.53 Primary ciliary dyskinesia associated with Kartagener syndrome. A, Frontal chest radiograph in a patient with chronic sinusitis shows situs inversus totalis, with dextrocardia and a right-sided stomach. **B,** Axial computed tomography (CT) image of the upper abdomen shows a right-sided stomach and a left-sided liver. **C,** Sagittal and (**D**) axial CT images of the lungs show thick-walled bronchiectasis extending into the morphologic right middle lobe on the left.

Lymphoma. Lymphoma is the third most common neoplasm of childhood after leukemia and central nervous system tumors. It is the most common mass encountered in the anterior mediastinum, and it accounts for 25% of mediastinal masses overall. In about 30% of patients with lymphoma, bilateral mediastinal lymphadenopathy is seen. Similar findings occur in about 50% of children with acute lymphocytic leukemia, giving rise to the "leukemia/lymphoma syndrome" [**Fig. 2.56**].

Lymphoma is classified into Hodgkin and non-Hodgkin subtypes. *Non-Hodgkin lymphoma* (NHL) comprises more than half of lymphomas in children, and more than 70% of patients have disseminated disease at the time of presentation. This disease usually manifests in an insidious fashion, with few specific symptoms. There are four major types of NHL. Type I usually occurs in a supradiaphragmatic location, whereas types II and III are usually subdiaphragmatic. Type IV can occur anywhere but is rare in the mediastinum. Mediastinal NHL is often of T-cell origin, whereas abdominal NHL is often of B-cell origin. NHL manifests primarily as extranodal disease. Overall, the most common site of primary disease is within the ileocecal bowel, followed by the

mediastinum. NHL spreads hematogenously, and a mediastinal mass is encountered in about half of affected patients.

Burkitt lymphoma is the most frequent subtype of NHL in children. It is the most rapidly growing tumor in the pediatric population. Children typically present with extranodal involvement, most often in the abdomen. Common presenting symptoms include abdominal pain, a palpable mass, nausea and vomiting, intestinal obstruction caused by bowel compression or intussusception, and acute appendicitis. Three forms have been described: (1) endemic Burkitt lymphoma, which is linked to Epstein-Barr virus (EBV); (2) sporadic Burkitt lymphoma, for which the cause is unknown; and (3) immunodeficiency-associated Burkitt lymphoma, which occurs in patients with HIV and congenital or posttransplant immunosuppression.

Posttransplant lymphoproliferative disorder (PTLD) represents a heterogeneous group of lymphoproliferative diseases that can occur as a complication of solid-organ and bone marrow transplantation. The incidence of PTLD is much higher in children than it is in the adult population. Most cases of PTLD in children are associated with EBV infection. Any organ system

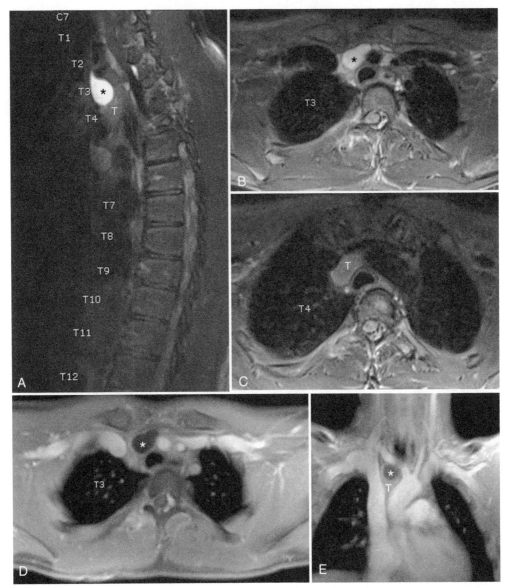

Figure 2.54 Thymic cyst. A, Sagittal T2-weighted magnetic resonance imaging (MRI) of the spine performed for back pain shows an incidental, well-defined cystic structure with a homogeneous appearance (*asterisk*) in the anterior mediastinum at the superior aspect of the thymus (*T*). **B,** Follow-up MRI of the chest shows a bilobed structure with increased T2 signal (*asterisk*) at the level of the aortic arch branches. **C,** Just inferior to this at the level of the aortic arch, a region of lower signal soft tissue is seen in the right paratracheal space. This reflects residual thymus (*T*). **D,** Axial and (**E**) coronal fast gradient recalled echo images after contrast administration show no enhancement of the cystic structure (*asterisk*), with enhancement of normal surrounding thymic tissue (*T*). This confirms a diagnosis of thymic cyst.

can be affected by PTLD, but the GI system and the liver are most commonly involved with extranodal disease. Immunosuppression reduction is the mainstay of therapy. Acyclovir may be used to treat EBV infection.

About 10% of cases of *Hodgkin lymphoma* occur in the pediatric age group. The site of origin is almost invariably nodal, and disease spreads by direct extension [**Fig. 2.57**]. Most patients initially present with a mediastinal mass, although some present with hilar adenopathy. Cervical lymphadenopathy is almost always seen in conjunction with mediastinal involvement. In the abdomen, paraaortic and celiac nodes are much more commonly involved than mesenteric lymph nodes. In contradistinction to NHL, the initial clinical presentation of Hodgkin disease is anything but insidious. Fatigue, malaise, night sweats, and lymphadenopathy are frequently seen.

A critical prognostic factor is the presence or absence of bone marrow involvement. Lack of bone marrow disease is associated with a better prognosis. Staging is extremely important in guiding therapy. CT and MRI are the modalities of choice for diagnostic workup, with scintigraphy (gallium-67 citrate) and positron emission tomography useful in the assessment of response to therapy. Treatment centers around chemotherapy.

Germ Cell Tumors. Germ cell tumors are derived from primordial germ cells and include teratoma, seminoma, and nonseminomatous germ cell tumor (NSGCT). These tumors most often occur in the gonads, but when extragonadal in location, the most common site of disease is the anterior mediastinum.

The most common type of mediastinal germ cell tumor is a mature teratoma. This tumor is usually a complex cystic lesion

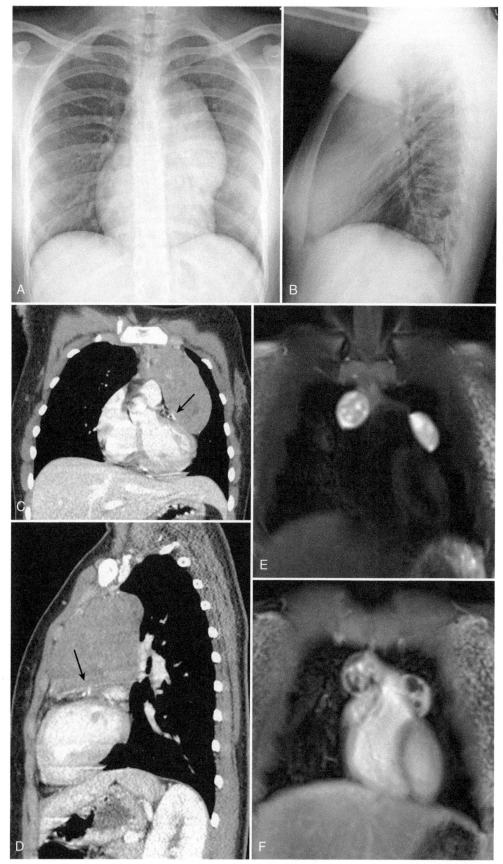

Figure 2.55 Thymoma in a teenager with cough and chest pain. A, Frontal radiograph of the chest shows a dense, lobulated soft tissue mass enlarging the left mediastinal border. **B,** This mass is anteriorly positioned on the lateral radiograph. **C,** Coronal and (**D**) sagittal computed tomography images show a mildly heterogenous mass with some peripheral calcification along its inferior margin (*arrows*). A thymoma was diagnosed after surgical resection. **E,** Coronal T2 with fat saturation and (**F**) T1 gradient recalled echo postcontrast magnetic resonance images in another teenager with a pathology-proven, bilobed thymoma. Well-defined, oval-shaped masses are seen on the right and left sides of the anterior mediastinum. These demonstrate similar heterogeneous increased T2 signal and enhancement.

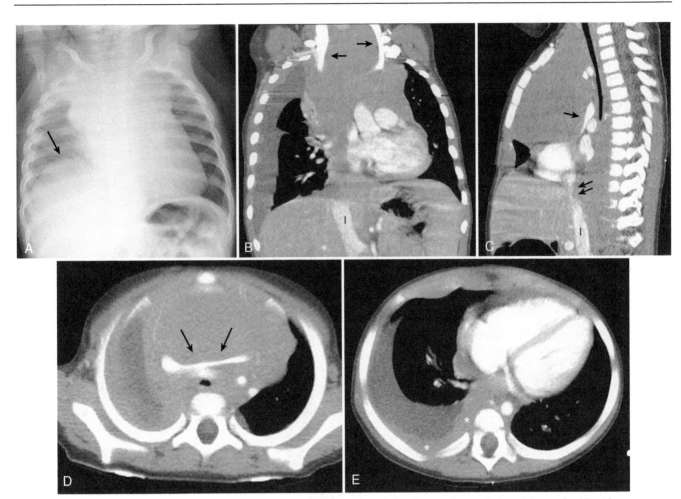

Figure 2.56 Leukemia/lymphoma syndrome. A, Frontal upright chest radiograph in a 19-month-old with cough and wheeze being treated for asthma shows a large, dense mediastinal mass on either side of the trachea. The right lung is hypoinflated and surrounded by pleural fluid, with apparent elevation of the right hemidiaphragm (*arrow*). **B,** Coronal and (**C**) sagittal contrast-enhanced computed tomography (CT) images show a large, homogeneously enhancing anterior mediastinal mass. This extends superiorly into the anterior neck causing lateral, inferior, and posterior displacement of vascular structures (*arrows*). The trachea is diffusely small in caliber in the anteroposterior plane. The right lung is surrounded by a large pleural effusion. The pleural effusion had a significant subpulmonic component on the upright chest radiograph and extends superiorly and laterally on the CT with the patient positioned supine. The mediastinal mass extends inferiorly along the right heart border, then into the retroperitoneum adjacent to the inferior vena cava (*I*), which is narrowed (*double arrows*). **D** and **E,** Axial CT images show the mediastinal mass causing posterior compression of the innominate vein (*arrows,* **D**). Abnormal, thick, enhancing pleura is noted surrounding the large pleural effusion, consistent with tumor (*asterisks*). This is a very characteristic finding of T-cell lymphoblastic leukemia.

containing a combination of soft tissue elements, fat, and calcium [**Fig. 2.58**]. It is typically asymptomatic and discovered incidentally. A malignant teratoma is much less common than its benign counterpart. This tumor is most often seen in adolescent males and presents as a large, symptomatic mass [**Fig. 2.59**]. It most commonly occurs in the sacrococcygeal region, with only 10% encountered in the mediastinum.

Seminomas are the most common primary malignant mediastinal germ cell tumor and are typically seen in adolescents and young adult males. These tumors are usually large, bulky, homogeneous soft tissue masses that are well-marginated with a lobulated contour. They often straddle the midline and cause mass effect on adjacent structures.

NSGCTs include embryonal carcinoma, endodermal sinus tumor, choriocarcinoma, and mixed germ cell tumors. Most patients with a NSGCT are symptomatic, often presenting with distant metastases. On imaging, these tumors are heterogeneous with areas of hemorrhage and necrosis [**Fig. 2.60**].

Middle. The differential diagnosis of a middle mediastinal mass includes lymph node enlargement, hiatal hernia, bronchopulmonary foregut malformations, and vascular anomalies. In the assessment of lymphadenopathy, neoplastic entities such as lymphoma and leukemia are a common consideration. Infectious entities are also common and include granulomatous diseases such as TB, histoplasmosis, and sarcoidosis, and opportunistic infections such as *P. carinii* in immunocompromised patients.

Foregut duplication cysts may communicate with the GI tract (enteric), the airways (bronchogenic), or the spinal canal (neurenteric). Depending on their communication, they may be solid or air-filled, or may contain an air–fluid level. They are more common on the right than on the left and are often related to the carina. Symptoms can result if there is significant compression on the airways or esophagus [**Fig. 2.34**].

Several vascular anomalies may also appear as a mediastinal mass. These include vascular rings, pulmonary artery sling, a

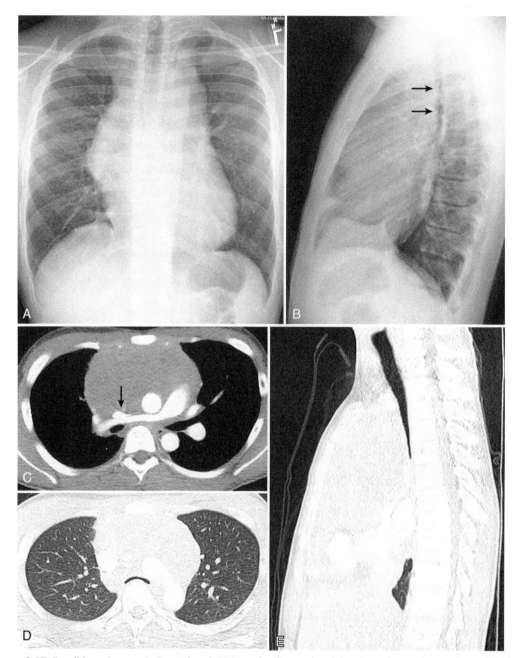

Figure 2.57 B-cell lymphoma. A, Frontal and (**B**) lateral radiographs of the chest show a large, dense, lobulated mass in the anterior mediastinum in a 17-year-old with fever, cough, and night sweats. Note that the trachea has a decreased caliber in the anteroposterior plane as it courses inferiorly (*arrows*). **C,** Axial contrast-enhanced computed tomography (CT) image shows the large mass with posterior displacement and compression of the superior vena cava (*arrow*). **D,** Axial and (**E**) sagittal CT images in lung windows confirm significant narrowing of the trachea and carina.

cervical aortic arch, and enlarged pulmonary arteries in the setting of pulmonary hypertension. Intravenous contrast should always be administered for cross-sectional studies performed in the workup of a middle mediastinal mass.

Posterior. Posterior mediastinal masses account for 40% of all mediastinal masses encountered in children. About 90% are either neuroblastoma, ganglioneuroblastoma, or ganglioneuroma. Neuroblastoma is the most common, and the most aggressive of the three with the least favorable prognosis. This is followed by ganglioneuroblastoma, a more highly differentiated tumor with a better prognosis. Ganglioneuroma is the least common of these tumors. This occurs in older children and is

considered to be a benign lesion with an excellent prognosis. Enlarging posterior mediastinal masses can cause pressure erosion on and displacement of the vertebrae and ribs and can extend into the spinal canal resulting in cord compression [**Fig. 2.61**]. If a posterior mediastinal mass extends anteriorly, it may cause significant mass effect on mediastinal structures leading to respiratory symptoms [**Fig. 2.62**].

Neurenteric cysts are a type of foregut duplication cyst resulting from failure of complete separation of the notochord from the foregut. The majority occur in the posterior mediastinum. Approximately two-thirds of patients present with symptoms of respiratory compromise. If the cyst extends into or communicates with the spinal canal, neurologic symptoms such as

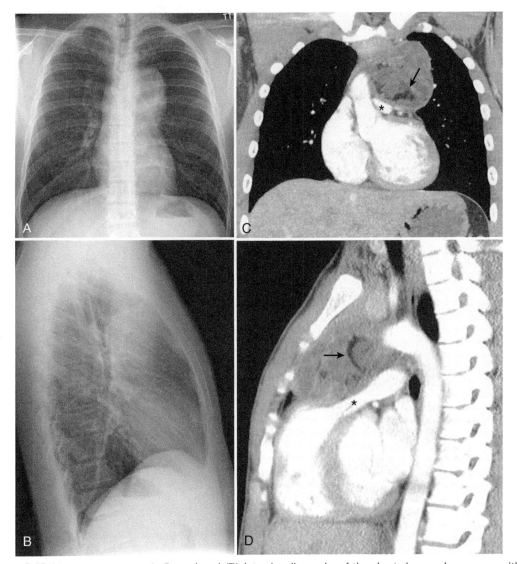

Figure 2.58 Mature teratoma. A, Frontal and (**B**) lateral radiographs of the chest show a dense mass within the left side of the anterior mediastinum. **C,** Coronal and (**D**) sagittal contrast-enhanced CT images show a heterogeneous anterior mediastinal mass causing significant mass effect with narrowing of the main pulmonary artery (*asterisks*). The mass has lobulated regions of fluid density similar to the attenuation of fluid in the stomach and also multiple areas of fat density (*arrows*).

abnormal gait, back pain, and motor or sensory deficits may be present. These lesions may be associated with additional anomalies of the vertebral column, which can vary from spina bifida to hemivertebrae, block vertebrae, and clefts.

Primary Lung Tumors

Primary lung tumors are rare in children. The vast majority of solid parenchymal lung lesions represent inflammatory, infectious, and reactive processes. The most common benign neoplasms of the pediatric lung are inflammatory myofibroblastic tumor and hamartoma, and the most common primary malignant lesions are carcinoid tumor and pleuropulmonary blastoma.

Inflammatory Myofibroblastic Tumor. The inflammatory myofibroblastic tumor has multiple synonyms, including plasma cell granuloma, inflammatory pseudotumor, and histiocytoma as it is composed of varying numbers of histiocytes, lymphocytes, plasma cells, and spindle cells histologically. It can present as a solitary pulmonary nodule or multiple peripheral

nodules. About 25% of lesions are calcified. This tumor may remain stable in appearance over time. When a lesion involves the mediastinum or contains calcification, the imaging appearance may be similar to neuroblastoma, germ cell tumor, or metastatic osteosarcoma. The prognosis is excellent following surgical excision.

Hamartoma. A pulmonary hamartoma is a benign neoplasm that contains normal lung elements (fat, epithelial tissue, fibrous tissue, and cartilage) arranged in an abnormal, disorganized fashion. It is the most common benign pulmonary neoplasm in children. This is a slow-growing lesion that may be variable in size. The majority of lesions are located in the peripheral parenchyma, with less than 10% found in an endobronchial location. Patients are most often asymptomatic, and these lesions are typically found incidentally.

Chest radiographs are nonspecific, demonstrating a solitary pulmonary nodule or mass that may contain calcifications [**Fig. 2.63**]. CT is superior in the detection of intralesional fat and calcification, which are virtually diagnostic. Lesions typically demonstrate a smooth or lobular contour.

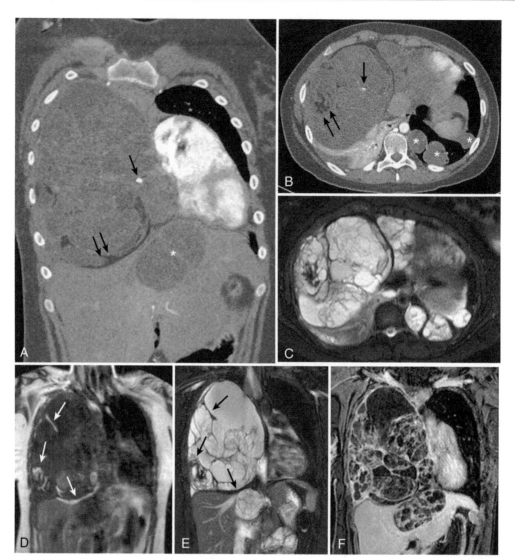

Figure 2.59 Immature teratoma with metastasis. A, Coronal and (**B**) axial contrast-enhanced computed tomography (CT) images of the chest show a large, heterogeneous, predominately low-density mass filling the right hemithorax and displacing the heart leftward. The mass has punctate calcifications (*arrows*) as well as areas of low attenuation consistent with fat (*double arrows*). Metastatic tumor is present in the liver (**A,** *asterisk*) and left lower lobe (**B,** *asterisks*). **C,** Axial T2-weighted magnetic resonance image with fat saturation shows that the lesion and its metastases are composed of multiloculated cysts. **D,** Coronal T1, (**E**) coronal T2 with fat saturation, and (**F**) coronal T1 post contrast with fat saturation images again show the multiloculated cystic character of the mass, with low signal intensity on the T1-weighted image, increased signal on the T2-weighted image, and only rim and septal enhancement after contrast administration. Note the fatty portions of the mass demonstrate high signal intensity on T1-weighted images (**D,** *arrows*), with decreased signal with fat saturation (**E,** *arrows*).

Malignant transformation is rare. Most patients with small peripheral lesions can be carefully monitored. In atypical cases with a symptomatic patient and/or a rapidly enlarging lesion, surgical resection is recommended.

Carcinoid Tumor. Carcinoid tumor is a rare neuroendocrine neoplasm that arises in the bronchial and bronchiolar epithelium. It is the most common primary pulmonary malignancy in children. The majority of tumors arise centrally in the main, lobar, or segmental bronchi. Clinical presentation varies based on location. Patients with central lesions typically present with symptoms related to bronchial obstruction. Chest radiographs may demonstrate a lobar consolidation that does not completely resolve after antibiotic treatment [**Fig. 2.64**]. About half of patients present with hemoptysis because of the

high vascularity of these lesions. Peripheral lesions are generally asymptomatic.

On imaging, a central carcinoid tumor is seen as a well-defined, round or ovoid hilar or perihilar mass. Marked homogeneous enhancement is often seen with contrast administration because of the high vascularity of these lesions. Eccentric calcifications are common, particularly in central lesions.

Prognosis depends on the histologic features of the lesion. Typical carcinoid tumors have a favorable outcome, whereas atypical carcinoids have a worse prognosis. Treatment involves complete surgical excision.

Pleuropulmonary Blastoma. Pleuropulmonary blastoma is a rare malignant embryonal mesenchymal tumor of the lung and pleura. It is the most common pulmonary malignancy of early

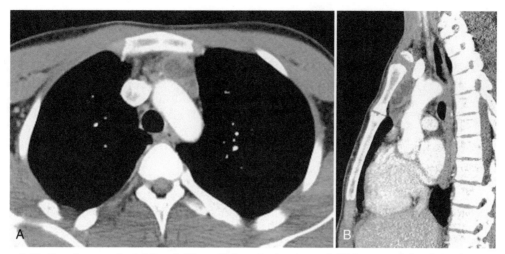

Figure 2.60 Germinoma. A, Axial and (**B**) sagittal contrast-enhanced CT images of the chest show a small, multilobulated cystic mass with peripheral enhancement in the anterior mediastinum. The patient initially presented with a paraneoplastic syndrome consisting of encephalitis, altered mental status, fatigue, and headaches. A germinoma was diagnosed at pathology after surgical resection.

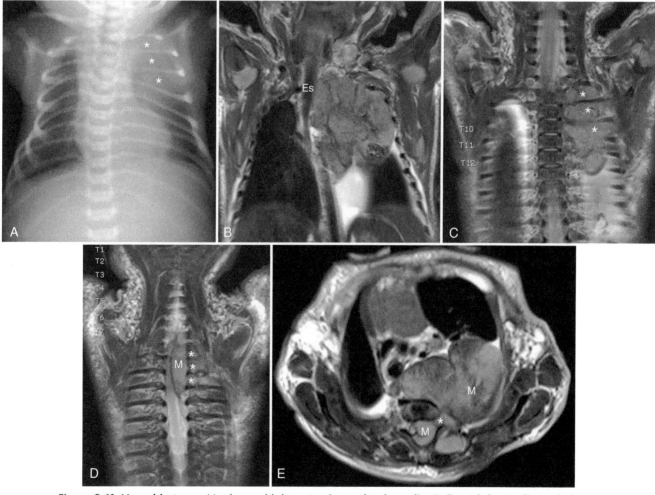

Figure 2.61 Neuroblastoma. Newborn with hypertension and tachycardia. **A,** Frontal chest radiograph shows a hazy opacity in the left upper lobe associated with abnormal widening of the intercostal distances between the left posterior upper ribs (*asterisks*), which are thinned. **B** and **C,** Coronal T2-weighted magnetic resonance images show a heterogeneous posterior mediastinal mass displacing the esophagus (**B**) (*Es*) rightward and extending into the widened intercostal spaces (**C,** *asterisks*). **D,** Coronal and (**E**) axial T2-weighted images with attention to the spine show the mass (*M*) centered in the left paraspinal space, extending through widened neural foramina (*asterisks*) and into the spinal canal, with resultant compression of the spinal cord.

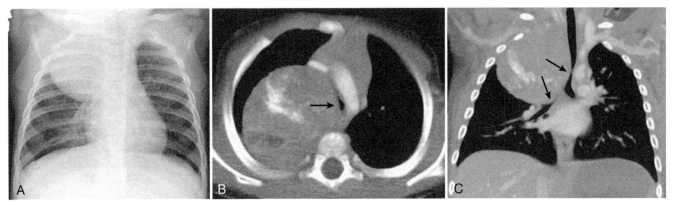

Figure 2.62 Neuroblastoma. Nine-month-old with noisy breathing and wheezing. **A,** Frontal chest radiograph shows a dense mass in the right upper hemithorax causing leftward displacement and narrowing of the trachea. **B,** Axial and (**C**) coronal contrast-enhanced computed tomography images show a partially calcified mass in the right paraspinal area extending into the mediastinum and causing significant mass effect on and compression of the trachea and right mainstem bronchus (*arrows*).

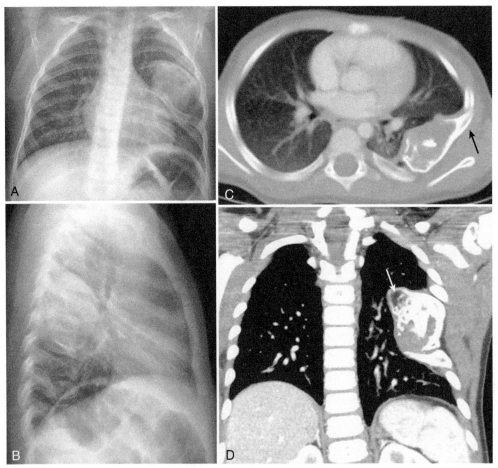

Figure 2.63 Pulmonary mesenchymal hamartoma. A, Frontal and (**B**) lateral chest radiographs show a large, dense lesion with suggestion of internal calcification in the posterior aspect of the left hemithorax. The surrounding ribs are splayed and distorted. **C,** Axial and (**D**) coronal contrast-enhanced CT images show a partially calcified lesion containing a low-density area reflecting fat (**D,** *arrow*) and involving the adjacent ribs (**C,** *arrow*).

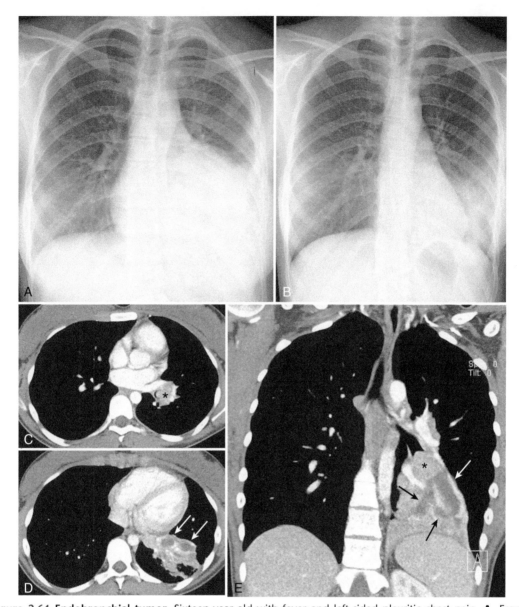

Figure 2.64 Endobronchial tumor. Sixteen-year-old with fever and left-sided pleuritic chest pain. **A,** Frontal chest radiograph demonstrates a dense left lower lobe opacity. The patient was initially diagnosed with pneumonia and a parapneumonic effusion. She was treated with antibiotics and drainage of the effusion, and symptoms improved. **B,** Three months later she presented with cough. Frontal radiograph of the chest shows an improved but persistent left lower lobe opacity. **C** and **D,** Axial and (**E**) coronal contrast-enhanced computed tomography images show a soft tissue mass completely obstructing the left lower lobe bronchus (**C** and **E,** *asterisks*). There are multiple low-density tubular areas within consolidated left lower lobe (**D** and **E,** *arrows*), consistent with dilated, fluid-filled bronchi. This is referred to as "drowned lung" associated with an obstructing endobronchial tumor. The left lower lobe bronchus and parenchyma were surgically resected, and a carcinoid tumor was diagnosed at pathology.

childhood, with the majority of affected patients younger than 6 years. Patients commonly present with nonspecific respiratory distress, signs of respiratory tract infection, or spontaneous pneumothoraces.

Pleuropulmonary blastoma is typically peripheral in location, adjacent to or involving the visceral pleura [**Fig. 2.65**]. It is classified into three subtypes: type 1, predominately macrocystic; type 2, mixed cystic and solid; and type 3, predominately solid. An associated pleural effusion or pneumothorax may be seen. Metastases can occur to the central nervous system and skeletal system, particularly with type 2 and 3 lesions.

Treatment involves surgical excision followed by chemotherapy.

Metastatic Lung Lesions

Metastatic disease to the lungs is far more common than primary pulmonary neoplasms in the pediatric population. Metastases related to Wilms tumor are most common, followed by those related to osteosarcoma and Ewing sarcoma. Osteosarcoma metastasis may be ossified and associated with pneumothoraces [**Fig. 2.66**]. Pulmonary metastasis often occurs hematogenously via the pulmonary arterial system, but may also occur via the lymphatics, the airways, or direct invasion.

Unique Chest Problems in the Neonate

See **Table 2.1**.

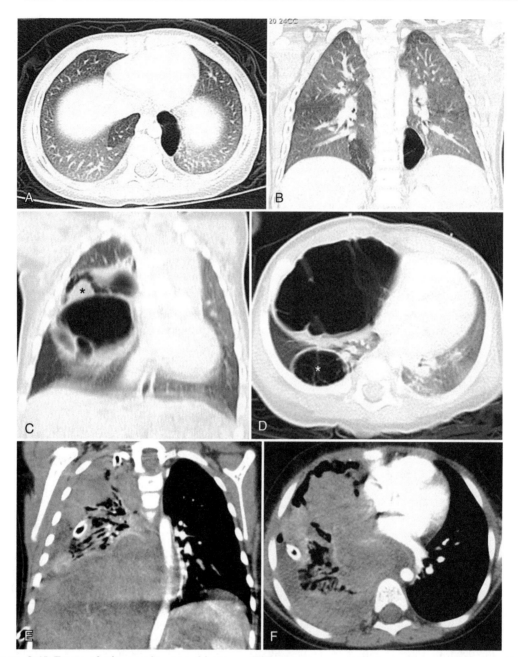

Figure 2.65 Types of pleuropulmonary blastoma (PPB) proven on pathology after surgical resection. **A,** Axial and (**B**) coronal computed tomography (CT) images show a single air-filled cavity with a thin central septation in the posteromedial segment of the left lower lobe, consistent with type I PPB. **C,** Coronal and (**D**) axial CT images in another patient show a complex, thick-walled, air-containing lesion in the right lung that has a soft tissue component (**C**, *asterisk*) and is multiloculated with numerous septations, consistent with type II PPB. A satellite lesion is shown posteriorly (**D**, *asterisk*). **E,** Coronal and (**F**) axial contrast-enhanced CT images in a third patient show an enhancing, lobulated soft tissue mass completely surrounding the collapsed right lung, consistent with type III PPB.

Infant Respiratory Distress Syndrome

Also referred to as surfactant deficiency disease and hyaline membrane disease (HMD), infant respiratory distress syndrome (IRDS) is the most common cause of respiratory distress in the neonatal period. It almost always occurs in premature infants, although term infants of diabetic mothers and infants delivered via cesarean section are occasionally affected. This entity is characterized by pulmonary hypoinflation related to generalized air sac atelectasis. In the premature infant, type I pneumocytes cover approximately 95% of the surface area of the air sacs,

whereas type II pneumocytes cover only 5%. Type II pneumocytes contain osmophilic lamellar inclusion bodies responsible for the synthesis and storage of the lipoprotein surfactant. Pulmonary surfactant lowers the surface tension in the air sacs, increases pulmonary compliance, and decreases the work of breathing. The ability of air sacs to remain distended is part of the "driving force" that prevents the development of pulmonary edema (Starling forces). Surfactant synthesis begins at 24 to 28 weeks' gestation and gradually increases throughout the remainder of fetal life to reach normal levels at birth. Lack of surfactant results in poor lung compliance and the accumulation of

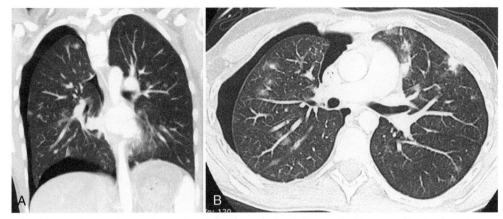

Figure 2.66 Metastatic osteosarcoma. A, Coronal and (**B**) axial computed tomography images show numerous nodular opacities throughout both lungs and a pneumothorax on the right. Metastases to the lungs from sarcomas can involve the pleural surface leading to pneumothorax.

TABLE 2-1   Neonatal Lung Disease

	Infant Respiratory Distress Syndrome	Transient Tachypnea of the Newborn	Meconium Aspiration	Neonatal Pneumonia
Patient history	Premature	Term Cesarean section	Postterm Meconium-stained fluid below vocal cords	Premature rupture of membranes
Time course from birth	Within hours	24–48 hours	12–24 hours	Onset <6 hours
Lung volumes	Decreased	Increased	Increased	Increased
Radiographic features	Diffuse granular opacity	Interstitial edema	Asymmetric coarse interstitial opacity	Perihilar streaky opacities
Pleural effusions	No	Yes	No	Maybe
Complications	Pneumothorax PDA PIE	None	Persistent fetal circulation	Sepsis
Possible therapy	Surfactant		ECMO	ECMO

ECMO, extracorporeal membrane oxygenation; PDA, patent ductus arteriosus; PIE, pulmonary interstitial emphysema.

damaged or desquamated cells, exudative necrosis, and mucus (protein seepage) in the alveolar sacs. This lining of debris stains like hyaline cartilage under the microscope; hence the term *hyaline membrane disease.*

The amniotic fluid lecithin-to-sphingomyelin ratio is used prenatally to predict the probability of development of IRDS in the infant. In the fetus lacking surfactant, this ratio will be decreased. Clinically, infants with IRDS are identified in the first few hours of life. Respiratory distress beginning *after* 8 hours of life is not typically related to surfactant deficiency.

Conventional radiographs show low lung volumes with a bell-shaped thorax, the characteristic "ground-glass" (finely granular) parenchymal opacity, and poor definition of the pulmonary vessels [**Fig. 2.67**]. Air bronchograms are often present and may extend to the periphery of the lungs. A pleural effusion is seldom present. A pneumothorax or pneumomomediastinum at presentation portends a poor prognosis. Hypoinflation may also be seen in infants with neonatal pneumonia, pulmonary hemorrhage, and pulmonary edema. Hyperinflation in a nonventilated infant virtually excludes IRDS as a diagnosis.

To prevent the development of acidosis and hypoxemia in a child with IRDS, the diseased lungs must be ventilated and oxygenated to maintain open terminal air sacs and appropriate arterial blood gas levels. Positive-pressure ventilation (positive end-expiratory pressure [PEEP], CPAP) or oscillating jet

ventilatory support is instituted after placement of an ETT. The "classic" surfactant-deficient, hypoinflated lungs often become relatively hyperinflated with this intervention.

In addition to supportive therapy with oxygen and diuretics, exogenous surfactant is often administered to increase pulmonary compliance and improve gas exchange. Its use has been shown to reduce mortality. Clinical improvement is sometimes evident after a single dose. The effect of surfactant administration on the appearance of the chest radiograph is somewhat variable, although the parenchyma may clear with treatment [**Fig. 2.68**].

After the initial presentation of disease, many of the imaging findings of IRDS reflect complications of ventilatory therapy. These include air leaks, patent ductus arteriosus, and chronic lung disease. Overdistention of the air sacs in poorly compliant lungs may lead to alveolar rupture, with subsequent air leak into the pulmonary interstitium. This is referred to as pulmonary interstitial emphysema (PIE). PIE may develop as early as the first 24 hours of life. This early-onset disease carries a poor prognosis. This entity more typically develops on day 2 or 3 of life. It is characterized by peripheral streaks or bubbles of air in the interstitium, presumably located in the lymphatics. It may be unilateral or bilateral.

Air may migrate centrally resulting in a pneumomediastinum, or peripherally with rupture into the pleural space and a resultant pneumothorax. Because infants are imaged supine and air

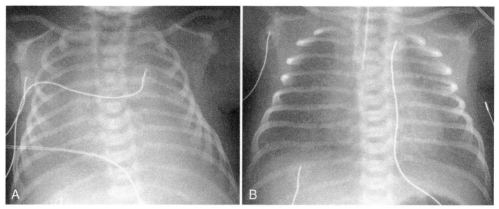

Figure 2.67 Infant respiratory distress syndrome. A, Initial chest radiograph in a premature newborn with respiratory distress shows hypoinflated lungs with diffuse hazy granular opacity. **B,** After intubation and surfactant administration, there is improved aeration of the lungs, although granular opacity persists.

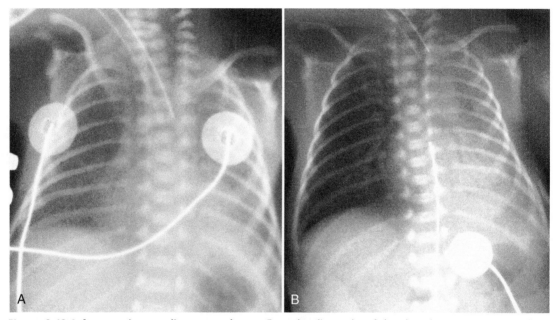

Figure 2.68 Infant respiratory distress syndrome. Frontal radiographs of the chest in a premature newborn with respiratory distress. **A,** Radiograph performed after intubation but before surfactant administration shows low lung volumes and granular pulmonary opacities, left greater than right. **B,** Radiograph obtained 24 hours after surfactant administration shows significantly improved aeration of the right lung in particular, presumably because of the preferential delivery of surfactant into the right mainstem bronchus.

rises to the highest point of the thorax, pneumothoraces are seen in a paramediastinal location and at the lung bases. This creates a "sharp mediastinum" sign [**Fig. 2.69**]. Mediastinal air may also dissect into the neck. One can distinguish a pneumomediastinum from a pneumopericardium by recalling that pericardial air can rise only as high as the pericardial reflections at the level of the pulmonary arteries and tracks around the inferior aspect of the heart. Extraalveolar air collections may also be seen adjacent to the inferior pulmonary ligament [**Fig. 2.69D**].

In premature infants, the ductus arteriosus may remain patent or even reopen because of persistent increased intrapulmonary pressure. This usually becomes clinically evident at about 5 to 7 days of life. The increased interstitial markings related to congestive failure in the setting of PFC may complicate radiographic findings. The clinical picture may not be clear until a series of radiographs has been completed and evaluated over time.

After 28 days of ventilatory support and the related insults to the pulmonary parenchyma, interstitial fibrosis may develop. This occurs in approximately 10% of premature infants. Fibrosis is often accompanied by exudative necrosis, and a "honeycomb" appearance to the lungs may be seen on chest radiographs. This phase of the disease process is referred to as *bronchopulmonary dysplasia* (BPD) [**Fig. 2.70**].

Prolonged exposure to high oxygen concentration is known to result in injury to the lungs at the cellular level. In the past, when a premature newborn received such an exposure for greater than 150 continuous hours under high pressure (CPAP, PEEP), BPD was diagnosed. The definition of BPD has evolved. In the setting of chronic oxygen exposure and respiratory support, there is initial destruction of the type I alveolar epithelium. This is accompanied by mucosal necrosis, peribronchial edema, and hemorrhage. Over time, interstitial fibrosis and cyst-like emphysematous changes develop, and increased lung

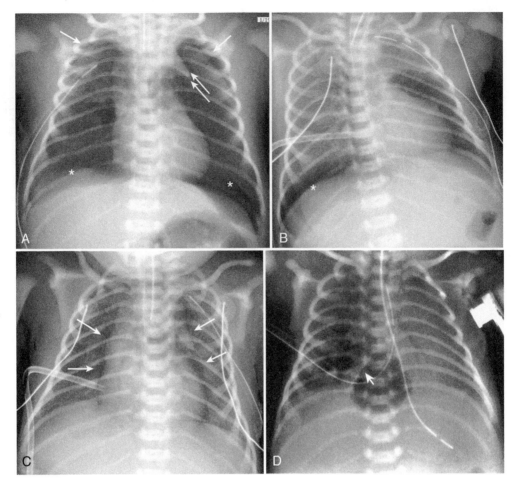

Figure 2.69 Characteristic appearances of pneumothoraces in a supine newborn with respiratory distress. **A,** Initial chest radiograph after intubation and right chest tube placement shows bilateral pneumothoraces primarily located inferior to the lung bases (*asterisks*), with relatively small biapical components (*arrows*). An anteromedial pneumothorax is present on the left, lifting and outlining the thymus (*double arrows*). **B,** After new chest tubes are placed, persistent but improved pneumothoraces outline the sulcus of the hemidiaphragms, best seen on the right (*asterisk*). **C,** After repositioning of both chest tubes, bilateral pneumothoraces have significantly improved, with only small components sharply outlining the cardiomediastinal surfaces (*arrows*). **D,** In a different patient, pneumothorax outlines the inferior pulmonary ligament (*arrow*).

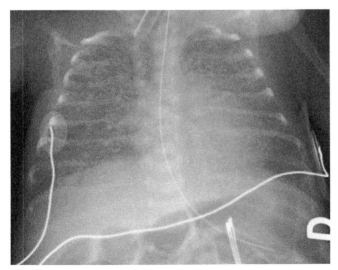

Figure 2.70 Bronchopulmonary dysplasia (BPD). A former severely premature newborn now 44 days old remains intubated, with diffuse coarse interstitial opacities bilaterally.

volumes result. By 4 weeks (28 days) of age, these changes are considered chronic. In the presence of oxygen dependency and respiratory symptoms, they constitute the syndrome of BPD as it is currently defined.

The radiographic appearance of BPD has historically been classified into four stages according to pathologic changes that develop as disease progresses. This classification scheme nicely reflects the sequence of insults caused by the treatment of immature lungs. The radiographic findings of HMD typically appear by day three. By day seven, interstitial edema develops because of capillary leak. Diuretics and surfactant administration may rapidly clear these initial radiographic findings. Thus later stages of disease are seldom seen today. The classification system is useful for following the radiographic changes that occur as BPD develops. The stages are as follows:

- *Stage I* is present at birth. The classic "ground-glass" granularity is seen.
- *Stage II* develops between 4 and 10 days of age. There is increased pulmonary parenchymal density related to exudative necrosis.
- *Stage III* develops between 10 and 20 days of age. It is characterized by a "honeycomb" appearance to the lungs caused

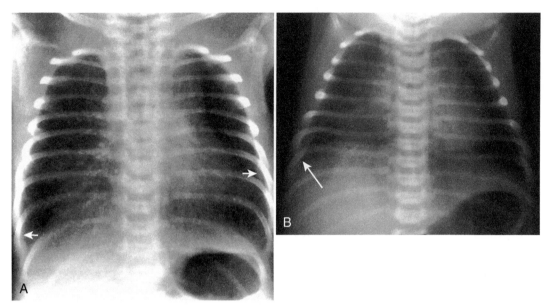

Figure 2.71 Transient tachypnea of the newborn (TTN). A and **B,** Frontal radiographs of the chest in full-term newborn infants with respiratory distress. Characteristic hyperinflation and interstitial prominence are demonstrated. Small pleural effusions (*arrows*) are also seen. All findings cleared within 24 to 48 hours in both patients.

by overdistention of the alveoli and terminal air sacs in the setting of a dysplastic interstitium.

• *Stage IV* develops after 1 month of age. There are fibrotic changes and scattered cystic emphysematous changes. This stage is associated with a mortality rate between 40% and 50%.

If an infant survives, the appearance of chest radiographs may improve and even progress to normal by 3 to 5 years of age (10% of patients with BPD). Unfortunately, pulmonary function parameters remain abnormal, with restrictive changes evident as late as the teenage years. Children with a history of BPD have an overall increased incidence of lower respiratory tract infections.

Wilson-Mikity syndrome is a rare condition seen in premature infants. Respiratory symptoms do not develop until 2 to 4 weeks after birth. Some consider this disease to be a form of pre-HMD that does not require early ventilatory support. Others doubt the existence of this entity. Chest radiographs are usually normal at birth, with the typical changes of BPD developing in subsequent weeks.

Retained Fetal Lung Fluid/Transient Tachypnea of the Newborn

The fetal lung is filled with fluid that contributes to the amniotic fluid. During delivery, part of this fetal lung fluid is expelled from the airways as the baby passes through the birth canal, part is coughed or suctioned out, and part is resorbed by the lymphatics and the pulmonary veins. Impairment or delay of this process leads to difficulty breathing, with respiratory distress in the newborn infant. Delivery by cesarean section, prolonged labor, maternal anesthesia or diabetes, and a precipitous delivery may all contribute to the development of transient tachypnea of the newborn (TTN).

This condition affects about 5% of all term infants. There is an equal sex distribution. The typical infant with retained fetal lung fluid presents with tachypnea during the first 6 hours of life. Symptoms peak at 1 day of age and normalize by 48 hours. Mild cyanosis, retractions, and grunting can occur.

Conventional chest radiographs may show interstitial edema, fluid within the fissures, small pleural effusions, and a mildly enlarged cardiothymic silhouette [**Fig. 2.71**]. The lungs are

most often hyperinflated. Retained fluid begins to clear at 12 hours and should be completely resolved by 48 hours with normalization of the chest radiograph. Differential diagnostic considerations include cyanotic congenital heart disease with congestive heart failure, pneumonia, meconium aspiration, and hypervolemia or PFC.

Meconium Aspiration Syndrome

Approximately 10% of all term deliveries are complicated by meconium staining of the amniotic fluid. Aspiration of this meconium-containing fluid occurs in about half of these deliveries and may result in the presence of meconium below the level of the vocal cords. In 50% of cases, clinical symptoms develop. Meconium aspiration syndrome is related to perinatal stress (hypoxia, prolonged labor), with a vagal response presumably triggering intrauterine evacuation of meconium by the fetus. Concomitant fetal gasping related to distress facilitates aspiration.

Aspirated meconium particles may cause bronchial obstruction and air trapping (check-valve mechanism), as well as a chemical pneumonitis. Secondary infection may occur. Hypoxia and vasospasm result, increasing the risk for pulmonary hypertension and PFC.

Conventional chest radiographs typically show bilateral, asymmetric areas of hyperinflation and atelectasis [**Fig. 2.72**]. Hyperinflation is related to the check-valve mechanism of meconium aspiration, and atelectasis results from the irritative effect of meconium on the bronchial tree. Pneumothorax or pneumomediastinum is seen in about 25% of patients.

Treatment is supportive and consists of antibiotics and oxygen. ECMO is sometimes indicated in severe cases when oxygenation is difficult to maintain. High-frequency jet flow ventilation may be helpful in the setting of pneumonitis. Because intrapulmonary pressure remains high, meconium aspiration is often complicated by PFC.

Neonatal Pneumonia

Neonatal pneumonia may be acquired in utero or perinatally. Predisposing factors include prolonged labor, premature rupture of membranes, placental infection, and ascending infection from

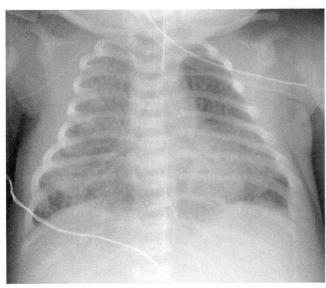

Figure 2.72 **Meconium aspiration syndrome.** A full-term infant with respiratory distress is intubated. The lungs are hyperinflated, and hazy, streaky opacities are seen throughout the right lung and in the left lower lobe.

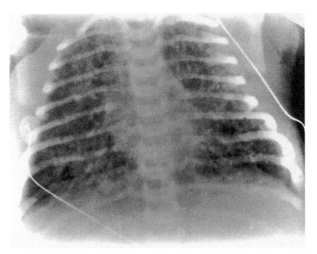

Figure 2.73 **Neonatal pneumonia.** Frontal chest radiograph in an infant with respiratory distress shows bilateral diffuse coarse interstitial infiltrates, which may occasionally become nodular.

the perineum. The most common causative organism is group B β-hemolytic streptococcus, most often acquired in the birth canal. Other common causative agents include *Pseudomonas, Enterobacter, Staphylococcus,* and *Klebsiella.* Clinically, patients present with respiratory distress. Metabolic acidosis may be present and may progress to shock.

The radiologic appearance of neonatal pneumonia is often identical to that seen with TTN or early HMD. A bilateral, patchy interstitial infiltrate is common [**Fig. 2.73**]. An associated effusion is often present. An empyema may develop and suggests infection with *Staphylococcus* or *Klebsiella.*

Left untreated, morbidity and mortality rates related to pneumonia are high. Thus early confirmation of the diagnosis and the prompt institution of appropriate antibiotics are critical.

Persistent Fetal Circulation

PFC is defined as persistent right-to-left shunting after birth. There is no clear cause. Normally, the ductus arteriosus

functionally closes by 15 hours of life, although anatomic closure may take days to weeks. Increased sensitivity to intrauterine hypoxia, altered fetal pulmonary flow, and arterial muscle derangement have been implicated. This entity may also simply be a transitional phenomenon like TTN. If this is the case, time and maturation should allow the normal circulation to predominate as the high intrapulmonary pressure diminishes. Any of the neonatal pulmonary abnormalities previously discussed may be associated with PFC, presumably secondary to increased pulmonary vascular resistance. There are no specific imaging findings.

Interstitial Lung Disease
Idiopathic Pulmonary Hemosiderosis

Idiopathic pulmonary hemosiderosis (IPH) is a rare disorder that most often occurs in children younger than 7 years. It is seen with equal frequency in boys and girls. It is characterized by the triad of hemoptysis, iron deficiency anemia, and recurrent episodes of diffuse alveolar hemorrhage of unknown cause.

Radiographs typically show areas of airspace consolidation or ground-glass opacification, often with a perihilar and lower lobe predominance. On CT, nodules and patchy areas of ground-glass attenuation can be seen in the subacute phase, with more diffuse, confluent areas of ground-glass attenuation in the setting of an exacerbation. On T2-weighted MRI, decreased signal is noted in the lung parenchyma.

The differential diagnosis of pulmonary hemosiderosis in childhood includes Goodpasture syndrome, Heiner syndrome, and pulmonary hemosiderosis in association with cardiac or pancreatic involvement. IPH can be seen in association with celiac disease, known as Lane-Hamilton syndrome.

Diagnosis is confirmed with sputum iron stains or lung biopsy. Although this disease is usually lethal, intensive iron therapy and transfusions to correct anemia can prolong survival.

Pulmonary Alveolar Proteinosis

Pulmonary alveolar proteinosis (PAP) is a rare disease that is characterized by the intraalveolar accumulation of surfactant lipids and proteins, impairing gas exchange and resulting in progressive respiratory insufficiency. Two forms of this disease occur in the pediatric population: congenital alveolar proteinosis and a later-onset form that is generally less severe. When the disease presents before the age of 1 year, there is an association with thymic alymphoplasia. Children may present with diarrhea, vomiting, failure to thrive, and cyanosis more commonly than respiratory symptoms. Growth retardation is also common.

Radiographs demonstrate bilateral, symmetric, perihilar airspace consolidation in a bat-wing distribution [**Fig. 2.74A**]. On CT, a "crazy paving" pattern of opacification is seen, with smooth interlobular septal thickening on a background of patchy or geometric ground-glass opacification [**Fig. 2.74B**]. This is a highly characteristic feature, although not pathognomonic for PAP. Pulmonary consolidation or pulmonary fibrosis may be evident later in the course of disease.

Diagnosis is made with bronchoalveolar lavage (BAL). BAL has also been widely used as a form of treatment. Although it has been associated with long-term survival in adults, its role in children is less clear.

Vasculitis and Collagen Vascular Diseases

Pediatric patients with pulmonary vasculitis typically present in their teen years. Granulomatosis with polyangiitis (GPA), formerly known as Wegener disease, is the most common of the pulmonary vasculitides seen in children. This disease typically

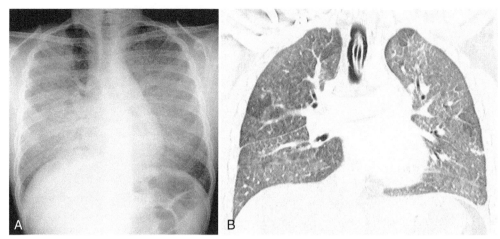

Figure 2.74 Pulmonary alveolar proteinosis (PAP). A, Frontal chest radiograph in a teenager with chronic asthma and recurrent infections shows diffuse hazy interstitial thickening throughout the lungs. **B,** Coronal CT image demonstrates interstitial thickening and diffuse ground-glass opacity. Bronchoalveolar lavage demonstrated characteristic lipid-laden macrophages within the aspirated fluid, and a diagnosis of PAP was confirmed on open lung biopsy.

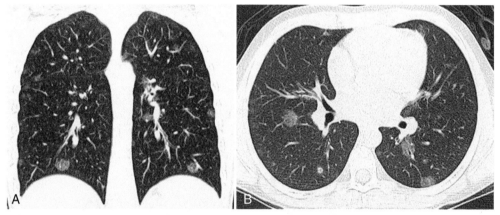

Figure 2.75 Granulomatosis with polyangiitis (GPA). Ten-year-old with anemia, hematuria, and proteinuria associated with glomerulonephritis and antineutrophilic cytoplasmic antibodies detected in the blood. **A,** Coronal and (**B**) axial computed tomography images show rounded, nodular areas of ground-glass opacity of varying size scattered throughout the lung parenchyma, typical of GPA-associated vasculitis.

presents with necrotizing granulomatous lesions in both the upper and lower respiratory tract [**Fig. 2.75**], in addition to glomerulonephritis. GPA is associated with antineutrophilic cytoplasmic antibodies.

Collagen vascular diseases (CVDs) seen in the pediatric population include juvenile arthritis, dermatomyositis, scleroderma, systemic lupus erythematosus (SLE), and mixed connective tissue disease. Pulmonary interstitial disease may be seen in children with these conditions. Pulmonary involvement is seen most frequently in scleroderma and is associated with significant morbidity and mortality. Most CVD has an autoimmune mechanism.

Pulmonary hemorrhage and glomerulonephritis can occur with both the vasculitides and CVDs, most commonly GPA and SLE. In patients with diffuse alveolar hemorrhage, evolving changes are noted on CT scan over time. A crazy paving pattern is often initially seen, with eventual interstitial fibrosis in the setting of recurrent episodes of pulmonary hemorrhage. Advanced stages of CVD may show honeycombing. Pulmonary arterial hypertension may develop in advanced lung disease, particularly in patients with scleroderma.

Treatment for vasculitides and CVDs is aimed at immune suppression with corticosteroids and chemotherapeutic agents.

Langerhans Cell Histiocytosis

LCH is the most common cause of acquired cystic lung disease in children. LCH is a condition caused by uncontrolled monoclonal proliferation of a group of histiocytes known as Langerhans cells, leading to the formation of destructive granulomas. Patients usually present between 1 and 3 years of age, most commonly with osseous lesions. Prognosis is based on the extent of disease. A single site of involvement is associated with a relatively better prognosis than multifocal disease. Involvement of the liver, spleen, lungs, and/or bone marrow is associated with a less favorable prognosis and requires more aggressive treatment. Patients with pulmonary LCH may present with tachypnea, dyspnea, and wheezing. In slightly greater than one quarter of patients, pulmonary LCH can lead to end-stage lung disease.

Initial chest radiographs in patients with pulmonary LCH may be normal, or a reticulonodular pattern of disease with an upper lobe predominance may be seen. HRCT findings of LCH include small pulmonary nodules in a centrilobular, peribronchial, or peribronchiolar distribution. Cysts of varying wall thickness can be seen, with a honeycomb pattern of architectural distortion that evolves with disease progression [**Fig. 2.76**]. Mediastinal and hilar adenopathy are rare in children with pulmonary LCH.

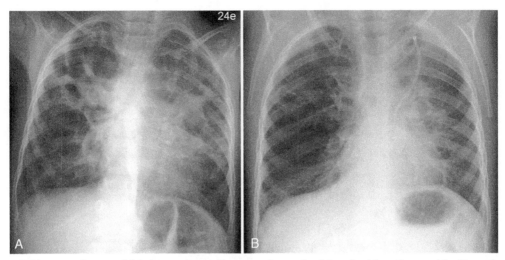

Figure 2.76 **Langerhans cell histiocytosis. A,** Frontal radiograph of the chest in a 3-year-old with worsening respiratory symptoms shows severe parenchymal lung disease, with the majority of both lungs replaced by numerous bullae of varying sizes. **B,** Follow-up chest radiograph 6 months later after treatment with an experimental chemotherapy protocol shows significant improvement of the left lung, with persistent extensive bullous disease involving the right lung.

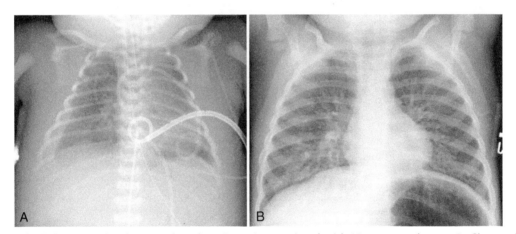

Figure 2.77 **Congenital pulmonary lymphangiectasia associated with Noonan syndrome. A,** Chest radiograph in an intubated newborn with hydrops fetalis shows diffuse interstitial thickening throughout the lungs, a right pleural effusion, and extensive body wall edema. Two pigtail catheters are in place after drainage of left pleural and pericardial effusions. **B,** Chest radiograph in a 2-year-old requiring supplemental oxygen shows hyperinflated lungs with diffuse patchy interstitial opacity.

Treatment of pulmonary LCH depends on the extent of disease. The first line of treatment is usually corticosteroids, vinblastine, or both, with duration of therapy determined by response.

Congenital Pulmonary Lymphangiectasia. Congenital pulmonary lymphangiectasia is a rare anomaly characterized by dilated lymphatic channels without lymphatic proliferation. It is seen almost exclusively in infancy and early childhood. In utero, embryologic lymphatic channels diminish in size to their expected neonatal caliber during weeks 6 to 20 of gestation. This process may be altered by pulmonary venous obstruction or anomalous development of the lymphatic system. About one-third of cases occur in association with congenital cardiac defects that cause pulmonary venous obstruction, such as total anomalous pulmonary venous connection and hypoplastic left heart syndrome.

Antenatal ultrasound may show hydrops fetalis. Chest radiographs can mimic the findings seen in TTN. Alternatively, a nodular pattern of parenchymal opacification may be seen, accompanied by pleural effusions. Similar findings are demonstrated on CT, with perihilar infiltrates and air bronchograms, interstitial and interlobular septal thickening, and pleural effusions [**Fig. 2.77**]. Lymphoscintigraphy can be performed to assess for abnormal radiotracer accumulation in the lungs and an asymmetric appearance of the lymphatic channels.

Treatment is generally supportive, with aggressive neonatal respiratory therapy. Historically, patients with congenital pulmonary lymphangiectasia have generally had poor clinical outcomes. In recent years with more advanced neonatal intensive care capabilities, symptoms associated with this disease have improved over time. This is particularly true for patients with isolated disease.

Neuroendocrine Cell Hyperplasia of Infancy. Neuroendocrine cell hyperplasia of infancy (NEHI) is a type of childhood interstitial lung disease that typically presents before the age of

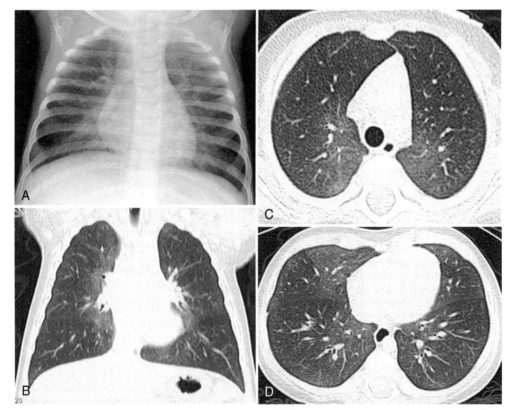

Figure 2.78 Neuroendocrine cell hyperplasia of infancy (NEHI). A, Frontal chest radiograph and (**B**) coronal and (**C** and **D**) axial computed tomography images of the chest in a 6-month-old with tachypnea and hypoxia show hyperinflated lungs with hazy perihilar alveolar opacities. The right middle lobe and lingula are involved in a pattern consistent with NEHI.

2 years with tachypnea, retractions, and hypoxia. Unlike other childhood interstitial lung diseases, NEHI is not responsive to steroid therapy. Thus it is important to be able to differentiate this entity from others to avoid the unnecessary side effects of steroids.

NEHI has a characteristic HRCT appearance. Air trapping is evident, with a mosaic attenuation pattern demonstrated. At least four lung lobes are affected, with geographic ground-glass opacities typically most conspicuous in the right middle lobe and lingula [**Fig. 2.78**]. Because the appearance of this disease is often so characteristic by imaging, biopsy may not be necessary provided clinical history, pulmonary function tests, and imaging findings are typical. Treatment is supportive with supplemental oxygen, which most patients require for many years.

SUGGESTED READINGS

Agrons GA, et al. From the archives of the AFIP: lung disease in premature neonates: radiologic-pathologic correlation. *Radiographics*. 2005;25:1047-1073.

Aukland SM, et al. High-resolution CT of the chest in children and young adults who were born prematurely: findings in a population-based study. *AJR Am J Roentgenol*. 2006;187:1012-1018.

Barlev DM, Nagourney BA, Saintonge R. Traumatic retropharyngeal emphysema as a cause for severe respiratory distress in a newborn. *Pediatr Radiol*. 2003;33:429-432.

Barnacle AM, Smith LC, Hiorns MP. The role of imaging during extracorporeal membrane oxygenation in pediatric respiratory failure. *AJR Am J Roentgenol*. 2006;186:58-66.

Bauman NM, Smith RJ. Recurrent respiratory papillomatosis. *Pediatr Clin North Am*. 1996;43:1385-1401.

Berdon WE. Rings, slings, and other things: vascular compression of the infant trachea updated from the midcentury to the millennium—the legacy of Robert E. Gross, MD, and Edward B. D. Neuhauser, MD. *Radiology*. 2000;216:624-632.

Bove T, et al. Tracheobronchial compression of vascular origin. Review of experience in infants and children. *J Cardiovasc Surg (Torino)*. 2001;42:663-666.

Brody AS. Imaging considerations: interstitial lung disease in children. *Radiol Clin North Am*. 2005;43:391-403.

Brody AS, et al. Computed tomography in the evaluation of cystic fibrosis lung disease. *Am J Respir Crit Care Med*. 2005;172:1246-1252.

Calvert JK, et al. Outcome of antenatally suspected congenital cystic adenomatoid malformation of the lung: 10 years' experience 1991-2001. *Arch Dis Child Fetal Neonatal Ed*. 2006;91:F26-F28.

Castellote A, et al. Cervicothoracic lesions in infants and children. *Radiographics*. 1999;19:583-600.

Chung CJ, et al. Children with congenital pulmonary lymphangiectasia: after infancy. *AJR Am J Roentgenol*. 1999;173:1583-1588.

Cleveland RH. A radiologic update on medical diseases of the newborn chest. *Pediatr Radiol*. 1995;25:631-637.

Cooper M, et al. Congenital subglottic hemangioma: frequency of symmetric subglottic narrowing on frontal radiographs of the neck. *AJR Am J Roentgenol*. 1992;159:1269-1271.

Curtis JM, et al. Endobronchial tumours in childhood. *Eur J Radiol*. 1998;29:11-20.

Donnelly LF, et al. CT findings and temporal course of persistent pulmonary interstitial emphysema in neonates: a multiinstitutional study. *AJR Am J Roentgenol*. 2003;180:1129-1133.

Donnelly LF, Frush DP. Localized radiolucent chest lesions in neonates: causes and differentiation. *AJR Am J Roentgenol*. 1999;172:1651-1658.

Donnelly LF, Frush DP. Langerhans' cell histiocytosis showing low-attenuation mediastinal mass and cystic lung disease. *AJR Am J Roentgenol*. 2000;174:877-878.

Donnelly LF, Jones BV, Strife JL. Imaging of pediatric tongue abnormalities. *AJR Am J Roentgenol*. 2000;175:489-493.

Eggli KD, Newman B. Nodules, masses, and pseudomasses in the pediatric lung. *Radiol Clin North Am*. 1993;31:651-666.

Ghaye B, et al. Congenital bronchial abnormalities revisited. *Radiographics*. 2001;21:105-119.

Helbich TH, et al. Evolution of CT findings in patients with cystic fibrosis. *AJR Am J Roentgenol*. 1999;173:81-88.

Herman M, Michalkova K, Kopriva F. High-resolution CT in the assessment of bronchiectasis in children. *Pediatr Radiol*. 1993;23:376-379.

Johnson AM, Hubbard AM. Congenital anomalies of the fetal/neonatal chest. *Semin Roentgenol*. 2004;39:197-214.

Kang DW, et al. Diffusion weighted magnetic resonance imaging in Neuro-Behcet's disease. *J Neurol Neurosurg Psychiatry*. 2001;70:412-413.

Kao SC, et al. Ultrafast CT of laryngeal and tracheobronchial obstruction in symptomatic postoperative infants with esophageal atresia and tracheoesophageal fistula. *AJR Am J Roentgenol.* 1990;154:345-350.

Kawashima A, et al. CT of posterior mediastinal masses. *Radiographics.* 1991;11:1045-1067.

Kim WS, et al. Congenital cystic adenomatoid malformation of the lung: CT-pathologic correlation. *AJR Am J Roentgenol.* 1997;168:47-53.

Klein MD. Congenital diaphragmatic hernia: an introduction. *Semin Pediatr Surg.* 1996;5:213-215.

Koplewitz BZ, et al. CT of hemangiomas of the upper airways in children. *AJR Am J Roentgenol.* 2005;184:663-670.

Kornreich L, et al. Bronchiectasis in children: assessment by CT. *Pediatr Radiol.* 1993;23:120-123.

Kramer SS, et al. Pulmonary manifestations of juvenile laryngotracheal papillomatosis. *AJR Am J Roentgenol.* 1985;144:687-694.

Kuhn JP, Brody AS. High-resolution CT of pediatric lung disease. *Radiol Clin North Am.* 2002;40:89-110.

Kuhn JP, Fletcher BD, DeLemos RA. Roentgen findings in transient tachypnea of the newborn. *Radiology.* 1969;92:751-757.

Kuint J, et al. Laryngeal obstruction caused by lingual thyroglossal duct cyst presenting at birth. *Am J Perinatol.* 1997;14:353-356.

Langston C. New concepts in the pathology of congenital lung malformations. *Semin Pediatr Surg.* 2003;12:17-37.

Leonidas JC, et al. Radiographic findings in early onset neonatal group b streptococcal septicemia. *Pediatrics.* 1977;59(suppl 6 Pt 2):1006-1011.

Liptak GS, et al. Decline of pediatric admissions with Haemophilus influenzae type b in New York State, 1982 through 1993: relation to immunizations. *J Pediatr.* 1997;130:923-930.

Long FR. High-resolution CT of the lungs in infants and young children. *J Thorac Imaging.* 2001;16:251-258.

Long FR, et al. Comparison of quiet breathing and controlled ventilation in the high-resolution CT assessment of airway disease in infants with cystic fibrosis. *Pediatr Radiol.* 2005;35:1075-1080.

Long FR, Williams RS, Castile RG. Structural airway abnormalities in infants and young children with cystic fibrosis. *J Pediatr.* 2004;144:154-161.

Lopez de Lacalle JM, et al. Congenital epulis: prenatal diagnosis by ultrasound. *Pediatr Radiol.* 2001;31:453-454.

McAdams HP, et al. Bronchogenic cyst: imaging features with clinical and histopathologic correlation. *Radiology.* 2000;217:441-446.

Meuwly JY, et al. Multimodality imaging evaluation of the pediatric neck: techniques and spectrum of findings. *Radiographics.* 2005;25:931-948.

Meyer JS, Nicotra JJ. Tumors of the pediatric chest. *Semin Roentgenol.* 1998;33:187-198.

Miller E, et al. Role of 18F-FDG PET/CT in staging and follow-up of lymphoma in pediatric and young adult patients. *J Comput Assist Tomogr.* 2006;30:689-694.

Moeller KH, Rosado-de-Christenson ML, Templeton PA. Mediastinal mature teratoma: imaging features. *AJR Am J Roentgenol.* 1997;169:985-990.

Newman B. Congenital bronchopulmonary foregut malformations: concepts and controversies. *Pediatr Radiol.* 2006;36:773-791.

Newman B, et al. Congenital surfactant protein B deficiency—emphasis on imaging. *Pediatr Radiol.* 2001;31:327-331.

Nickoloff EL, et al. Pediatric high KV/filtered airway radiographs: comparison of CR and film-screen systems. *Pediatr Radiol.* 2002;32:476-484.

Olutoye OO, et al. Prenatal diagnosis and management of congenital lobar emphysema. *J Pediatr Surg.* 2000;35:792-795.

Orazi C, et al. Pleuropulmonary blastoma, a distinctive neoplasm of childhood: report of three cases. *Pediatr Radiol.* 2007;37:337-344.

Owens C. Radiology of diffuse interstitial pulmonary disease in children. *Eur Radiol.* 2004;14(suppl 4):L2-L12.

Panicek DM, et al. The continuum of pulmonary developmental anomalies. *Radiographics.* 1987;7:747-772.

Paterson A. Imaging evaluation of congenital lung abnormalities in infants and children. *Radiol Clin North Am.* 2005;43:303-323.

Rencken I, Patton WL, Brasch RC. Airway obstruction in pediatric patients. From croup to BOOP. *Radiol Clin North Am.* 1998;36:175-187.

Rosado de Christenson ML, et al. Thoracic carcinoids: radiologic-pathologic correlation. *Radiographics.* 1999;19:707-736.

Rosado-de-Christenson ML, Templeton PA, Moran CA. From the archives of the AFIP. Mediastinal germ cell tumors: radiologic and pathologic correlation. *Radiographics.* 1992;12:1013-1030.

Sakurai H. Congenital diaphragmatic hernia in neonates: variations in umbilical catheter and enteric tube position. *Radiology.* 2000;216:112-116.

Shah A, et al. CT in childhood allergic bronchopulmonary aspergillosis. *Pediatr Radiol.* 1992;22:227-228.

Siegel MJ, et al. Normal and abnormal thymus in childhood: MR imaging. *Radiology.* 1989;172:367-371.

Slovis TL, et al. Thoracic neuroblastoma: what is the best imaging modality for evaluating extent of disease? *Pediatr Radiol.* 1997;27:273-275.

Strollo DC, Rosado de Christenson ML, Jett JR. Primary mediastinal tumors. Part 1: tumors of the anterior mediastinum. *Chest.* 1997;112:511-522.

Stroud RH, Friedman NR. An update on inflammatory disorders of the pediatric airway: epiglottitis, croup, and tracheitis. *Am J Otolaryngol.* 2001;22:268-275.

Svedstrom E, Puhakka H, Kero P. How accurate is chest radiography in the diagnosis of tracheobronchial foreign bodies in children? *Pediatr Radiol.* 1989;19:520-522.

Triglia JM, et al. Tracheomalacia associated with compressive cardiovascular anomalies in children. *Pediatr Pulmonol.* 2001;(suppl 23):8-9.

Valletta EA, et al. Tracheoesophageal compression due to congenital vascular anomalies (vascular rings). *Pediatr Pulmonol.* 1997;24:93-105.

Watts FB Jr, Slovis TL. The enlarged epiglottis. *Pediatr Radiol.* 1977;5:133-136.

Wittenborg MH, Gyepes MT, Crocker D. Tracheal dynamics in infants with respiratory distress, stridor, and collapsing trachea. *Radiology.* 1967;88:653-662.

Wood BP, et al. Exogenous lung surfactant: effect on radiographic appearance in premature infants. *Radiology.* 1987;165:11-13.

Zwiebel BR, Austin JH, Grimes MM. Bronchial carcinoid tumors: assessment with CT of location and intratumoral calcification in 31 patients. *Radiology.* 1991;179:483-486.

Chapter 3
Cardiac Imaging

Jamie L. Frost, Rajesh Krishnamurthy, and Laureen Sena

CONGENITAL HEART DISEASE

Congenital heart disease (CHD) occurs in approximately 1% of all live births, or 40,000 births annually in the United States. It remains the leading cause of birth defect–associated death in infancy. Approximately 25% of CHD defects are critical or severe, resulting in symptoms during the first year of life. About 25% of patients with CHD eventually die of their disease, and approximately 25% of CHD-related deaths occur in the first month of life. Survival rates continue to improve. Today 69% to 95% of patients survive to 18 years of age depending on the type of malformation. There is a continually growing population of patients living with corrected CHD, now estimated to be more than 1.5 million individuals in the United States. Patients are living longer due to improved imaging diagnosis as well as medical and surgical treatment. The majority of patients with CHD are diagnosed during fetal assessment or after birth, with echocardiography as the mainstay of initial diagnostic evaluation. Cardiac catheterization has traditionally been the diagnostic gold standard, providing morphologic and functional information including data on pulmonary vascular resistance and oxygen saturation within chambers and vessels. Magnetic resonance imaging (MRI) and computed tomography (CT) now play increasingly important and complementary roles in the delineation of CHD in the preoperative and postoperative periods.

CHD is a complex disease process that occurs during embryologic development of the cardiovascular system. This chapter will review basic cardiac embryology and morphology, and provide an overview of the segmental approach to CHD that is important in understanding and accurately communicating the morphology and physiology of different types of CHD. The classic radiographic findings of CHD that have traditionally been taught to radiologists in training will be reviewed. In addition, this chapter will provide an overview of the anatomy and physiology of common CHDs and emphasize the role of cross-sectional imaging with CT and MRI before and after cardiac surgery.

Embryology

A basic understanding of cardiac embryology is helpful to understand the complex spectrum of abnormalities that may be encountered in CHD. By definition, cardiac embryology reflects the events that occur in the development of the human heart from conception to the eighth week of gestation. The heart, unlike any other organ, must be able to function while it is undergoing embryologic development.

The major events of cardiac development occur between the third and fifth weeks of gestation. The cardiovascular system arises from the mesoderm as the cardiogenic crescent on the 18th day of fetal life. A straight heart tube develops by the 20th day of gestation, and it is at this point that the heart begins to beat. As cells continue to be added to the heart tube, the tube undergoes the looping process. Typically the heart tube loops to the right, which is referred to as D-looping. The heart may also loop to the left, which is referred to as L-looping. The looping of the heart plays a major role in the eventual spatial relationship of the right ventricle (RV) and left ventricle (LV) [**Fig. 3.1**].

Once looping is complete during the fourth week of gestation, circulation through the heart is in series from the right atrium (RA) to the left atrium (LA), then the LV to the RV to the truncus arteriosus, which serves as a common outflow tract to the aorta and main pulmonary artery (MPA). During this time, the embryologic aortic arches are also developing into the great arteries and their major branches, as well as the ductus arteriosus. The process of convergence, which aligns the RA with the developing RV and the aorta with the developing LV, follows ventricular looping. The heart then undergoes septation during the fifth week of fetal life. The interventricular septum grows from apex to base to septate the ventricles, and the formation of the septum primum and secundum separates the LA and RA. The endocardial cushion tissue lining the atrioventricular canal (AVC) then septates the common AV valve into separate tricuspid and mitral valves. At the same time, the common outflow tract from the ventricles, or the truncus arteriosus, septates to separate the ascending aorta and the MPA. The infundibulum, or conus of muscle forming the right ventricular outflow tract beneath the pulmonary valve, together with the swirling blood flowing out of the developing ventricles, causes the left and right ventricular outflow tracts and aorta and pulmonary artery (PA) to appear wrapped around one another when they are normally developed (i.e., not parallel in configuration) [**Fig. 3.2**]. Separation of the right and left heart is nearly complete by the seventh week of fetal life, but does not completely finish until the final closure of the ductus arteriosus and the interatrial septum after birth.

In summary, the major events in cardiac embryology occur between the third and seventh weeks of fetal life, and include the formation of a straight heart tube with common venous inflow to the developing LV and common arterial outflow from the developing RV. This is followed by looping of the tube to the right (D) or to the left (L), differentiation of morphologic chambers with convergence to provide inflow to the RV and outflow to the LV, valve formation, and chamber separation. Abnormal arrest of this process or defects during any stage of development may result in the wide spectrum of CHDs that can be detected at birth.

Identification of Cardiac Chambers and Great Vessels

The first step in the analysis of CHD by cross-sectional imaging is to accurately identify the morphology of the cardiac chambers and vessels. The *RA* is identified as the chamber that receives the insertion of the inferior vena cava (IVC) and coronary sinus, and also by a broad-based triangular appendage with characteristic pectinate muscle morphology extending to the AV junction. The *LA* is identified by a narrow-based, tubular, finger-like appendage. The pulmonary vein insertion is not reliable for identification of the LA, because the pulmonary veins are often partially or totally anomalous. The situs of the atria can be solitus (S), inversus (I), or ambiguous (A) [**Fig. 3.3**].

The *RV* is identified by the following features:
1. A muscular attachment between the free wall and the interventricular septum called the *moderator band*
2. An AV valve that is slightly more apical in position than the AV valve of the LV
3. The presence of an infundibulum (or conus), which creates a muscular outflow tract that separates the tricuspid valve and the semilunar valve arising from the RV [**Fig. 3.4**]

The *LV* is identified by its smooth superior septal surface, which is devoid of any muscular attachments, and by the absence of a conus, so that the mitral valve and the semilunar valve arising from the LV are in fibrous continuity.

The *PA* is recognized as the vessel that supplies branches to the lungs, but not to the body. The *aorta* is identified as the

Types of Conus

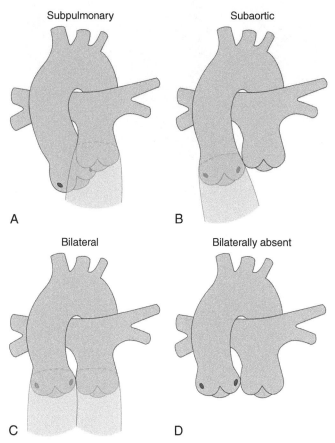

A

B

C

D

Figure 3.2 **Types of conus or infundibulum. A,** The normal heart has a subpulmonary conus as part of the right ventricle (RV), and the left ventricle (LV) normally has no conus when aligned with the aorta. **B,** A subaortic conus occurs when the RV is aligned with the aorta in transposition of the great arteries. **C,** There is both a subaortic and a subpulmonary conus when the RV gives rise to both great arteries, as in double-outlet RV. **D,** Rarely, the conus is entirely absent, as in the setting of double-outlet LV.

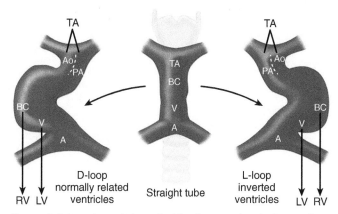

Figure 3.1 **Looping of the primitive heart tube during embryologic development.** Diagram depicting the straight heart tube in the center with a common entrance of the venous system into the common atrium (*A*) that continues to the developing ventricle (*V*), with a single outflow called the *bulbous cordis* (*BC*) that connects to the truncus arteriosus (*TA*). The heart tube can loop to the right (D-looping) to produce normally related ventricles, or to the left (L-looping) to produce inverted ventricles. After looping, there will be further remodeling and septation to create left (LA) and right atria (RA) and left (*LV*) and right ventricles (*RV*), and septation of the TA to the aorta (*Ao*) and pulmonary artery (*PA*).

Types of Visceral and Atrial Situs

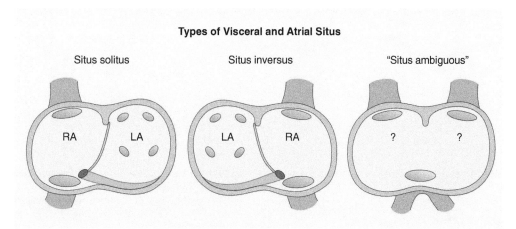

Figure 3.3 **Types of atrial situs.** Diagram depicting the three possibilities for situs of the left (LA) and right atria (RA) as solitus, inversus, or ambiguous. The atrial situs does not always correlate with the visceral situs in the abdomen. Atrial situs ambiguous is associated with a single common atrium because of absence of the interatrial septum and is most often seen in patients with heterotaxy syndrome.

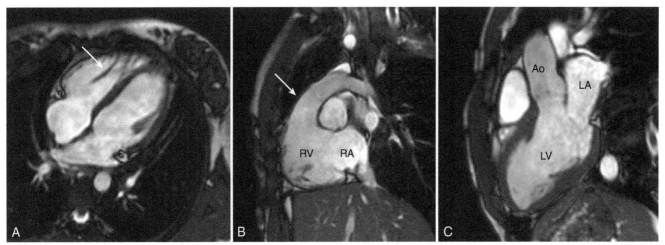

Figure 3.4 Morphologic characteristics of the normal right (RV) and left ventricles (LV). A, Four-chamber steady-state free precession (SSFP) magnetic resonance image shows the moderator band (*arrow*) of a normal RV. The RV is positioned to the right of and anterior to the LV, and the LV has a smooth superior septal surface. **B,** Long-axis sagittal oblique SSFP image through the RV profiles the normal tricuspid and pulmonary valves, which are separated by the conus or infundibulum (*arrow*). **C,** Vertical long-axis SSFP image profiles the normal aortic and mitral valves, which are in fibrous continuity because there is no subaortic conus. *Ao,* Aorta; *LA,* left atrium; *RA,* right atrium.

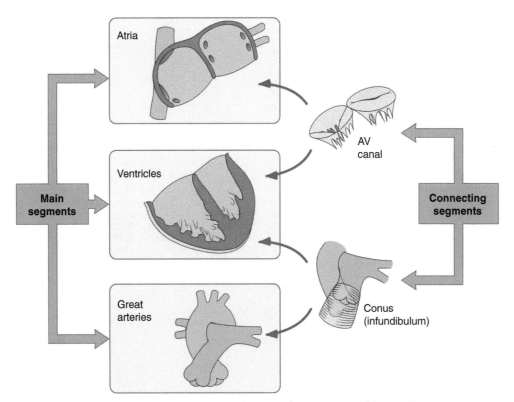

Figure 3.5 **Steps in the segmental approach to congenital heart disease.**

vessel that supplies the coronary arteries and systemic arteries to the body.

Segmental Approach to Heart Disease

Any combination of atrial, ventricular, and great vessel morphology may occur in CHD. One must take a simple, logical, step-by-step approach to understand and describe disease before initiating treatment. The segmental approach to CHD described

by Richard van Praagh **[Fig. 3.5]** involves determination of the following factors:

1. The morphology of the three major cardiac segments: Viscero-atrial situs, ventricular looping, and the relationship of the great arteries
2. How each segment is connected to the adjacent segment: This determination involves analysis of the *AVC*, which connects the atria to the ventricles, and evaluation of the ventriculo-arterial connection, including the *conus* (also

called the *infundibulum*), which connects the ventricles to the great arteries. Potential AV connections are concordant connection (LA to LV and RA to RV), discordant connection (LA to RV and RA to LV), common atrioventricular canal (CAVC), double-inlet LV, unilateral AV valve atresia, straddling AV valve, and overriding AV valve. The options at the level of the conus are normal connection, transposition of the great arteries (TGA), truncus arteriosus, double-outlet right ventricle (DORV), and rarely, double-outlet LV [**Fig. 3.2**]. Description of the conal muscle is important, because this muscle may narrow the outflow tracts and influence subsequent surgical management

3. The presence of associated malformations involving the atrial and ventricular septum or the extracardiac vasculature: Examples include but are not limited to the following: ASD, VSD, partial or total anomalous pulmonary venous connection (TAPVC), bilateral superior vena cava (SVC), and coarctation

4. How segmental combinations and connections, along with the associated malformations, function

As an example, using the segmental approach, a patient would be described as "congenitally corrected" {S,L,L} TGA with pulmonary stenosis and a VSD [**Fig. 3.6**]. Breaking this down to the individual components, there is (1) S-solitus atria, L-looped ventricles, and L-malposed great arteries; (2) a discordant AV connection (LA to RV and RA to LV) and a discordant ventriculo-arterial connection (RV to aorta and LV to PA); (3) pulmonary stenosis and a VSD; and (4) a balanced (physiologically corrected) circulation.

Heterotaxy

Accurate anatomic and physiologic diagnosis of CHD using a structured approach has led to significant improvement in patient outcomes. This method is associated with a more appropriate selection of therapeutic options, whether they be medical, surgical, or both. This is especially true as applied to the patient with complex CHD in the setting of heterotaxy syndrome, or abnormal sidedness of the thoracic and abdominal viscera. With normal development, there is lateralization of the internal thoracic and abdominal organs with respect to the left-right axis, so that the heart is in the left chest with the apex pointing to the left, the stomach and spleen are located in the left upper quadrant, and the liver is located in the right upper quadrant. This is referred to as situs solitus. Situs inversus totalis refers to complete mirror image reversal of the normal position of the thoracic and abdominal viscera and vasculature. Patients with heterotaxy have situs ambiguous or

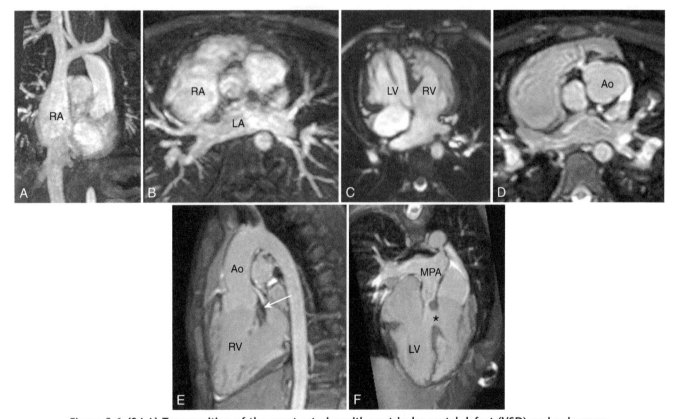

Figure 3.6 {S,L,L} **Transposition of the great arteries with ventricular septal defect (VSD) and pulmonary stenosis, illustrating the steps in the segmental approach to congenital heart disease. A,** Coronal maximum intensity projection (MIP) image from 3D magnetic resonance angiography (MRA) demonstrating the superior and inferior vena cavae connecting to a right-sided right atrium (*RA*). **B,** Axial image at the level of the atria demonstrating the left atrium (*LA*) positioned to the left and receiving the pulmonary veins. **C,** Four-chamber steady-state free precession (SSFP) MR image showing the right ventricle (*RV*) with a trabeculated septum positioned to the left of the left ventricle (*LV*), which has a smooth septal surface. The heart is L-looped. **D,** Axial MIP image from a 3D SSFP showing the aorta (*Ao*) positioned to the left and anterior to the main pulmonary artery (*MPA*), or L-malposed. **E,** Sagittal oblique SSFP image showing the aorta arising from the RV, with a sub-aortic conus (*arrow*) separating the aortic valve from the tricuspid valve. **F,** Coronal oblique SSFP image through the outflow tracts shows the LV aligned with the MPA, narrowing of the subpulmonary outflow tract, and a conoventricular VSD (*asterisk*).

variable lateralization of the thoracic and abdominal viscera and vasculature that does not follow either situs solitus or situs inversus totalis. The exact incidence of heterotaxy is unknown, but it is thought to occur in 1 in 10,000 to 40,000 births, including 3% of all neonates with CHD and 30% who have a cardiac malposition. The prognosis of patients with heterotaxy is primarily based on the severity of the associated cardiovascular malformations.

Heterotaxy encompasses a spectrum of cardiac, vascular, and visceral abnormalities of early embryonic development of the thorax and abdomen that occur in the fifth week of gestation. This spectrum includes abnormalities in septation of the conotruncus, growth of the endocardial cushions, septation between the LA and pulmonary venous plexus, formation of the spleen, rotation of the bowel, and lobation of the lungs. The defining features of heterotaxy therefore include conotruncal anomalies (such as TGA or DORV), endocardial cushion or CAVC defects, anomalous pulmonary and systemic venous connections, symmetry of the atrial appendages with partial or complete absence of the atrial septum, asplenia or polysplenia, malrotation of the bowel, and symmetry of lung lobation (bilateral right- or left-sided morphology).

There is no one feature that is pathognomonic in heterotaxy syndrome. To be able to recognize the numerous different congenital cardiovascular anomalies that may be present, it is helpful to understand that heterotaxy syndrome represents a spectrum between complete bilateral right-sidedness (also called *right isomerism* or *heterotaxy with asplenia*) and bilateral left-sidedness (also called *left isomerism* or *heterotaxy with polysplenia*). Most patients fall somewhere in between these two extremes [**Figs. 3.7** and **3.8**].

Right isomerism or heterotaxy with asplenia is characterized by bilateral right eparterial bronchi and trilobed lungs, absence of a spleen, a midline transverse liver, and a stomach in variable position. Heterotaxy with asplenia may be associated with complex forms of cyanotic heart disease including complete absence of the atrial septum resulting in a common atrium, CAVC, and DORV and/or pulmonary atresia.

Left isomerism or heterotaxy with polysplenia is associated with bilateral left hyparterial bronchi and bilobed lungs, a midline transverse liver, multiple spleens or splenules that can be located on either side of the abdomen, and a stomach in variable position. Heterotaxy with polysplenia may be associated with intracardiac defects similar to those seen in the setting of asplenia, but they tend to be less severe.

Patients with heterotaxy may have numerous different anomalies of the systemic and pulmonary venous connections, including partial or TAPVC and a bilateral SVC. An interrupted IVC at the level of the liver with azygous continuation is more often seen in polysplenia (bilateral left-sidedness), because the IVC is normally a right-sided structure.

Applying the segmental approach to CHD is crucial in the setting of heterotaxy. This method facilitates accurate characterization of complex and variable morphology, and guides decision making in the best approach for management and surgical repair.

Physiologic Subgroups

Chest radiographs play an important role in evaluating the physiology of heart disease and determining palliative therapy at birth by distinguishing between lesions associated with increased pulmonary blood flow (left-to-right shunts and intermixing states with unobstructed pulmonary blood flow), lesions associated with decreased pulmonary blood flow due to right-sided obstruction, and lesions associated with pulmonary venous hypertension due to systemic (left) sided obstruction [**Fig. 3.9**]. Intermixing states are usually due to the presence of a large shunt in lesions associated with a common atrial or single ventricular chamber. Clinically, cyanosis is present due to tremendous mixing of deoxygenated blood with oxygenated blood before it enters into the systemic circulation.

Heterotaxy Syndromes

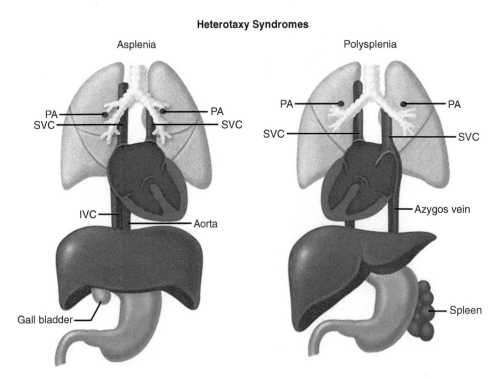

Figure 3.7 Heterotaxy syndrome. Diagram depicting the extremes of bilateral right isomerism (asplenia) versus bilateral left isomerism (polysplenia) of the abdominal viscera and lungs. *IVC*, inferior vena cava; *PA*, pulmonary artery; *SVC*, superior vena cava.

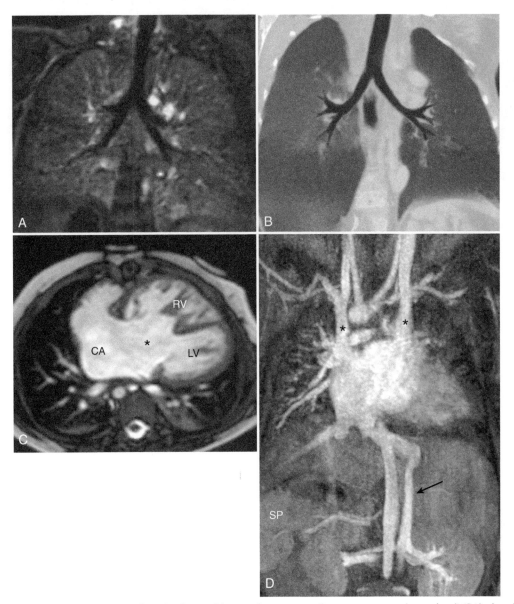

Figure 3.8 Heterotaxy examples. A, Coronal image from magnetic resonance angiography (MRA) showing bilateral right-sided bronchi and minor fissures, and a right-sided stomach in a patient with asplenia. **B,** Coronal computed tomography (CT) image showing bilateral left-sided bronchi in a patient with polysplenia. **C,** Four-chamber steady-state free precession image in a patient with polysplenia showing a balanced common atrio-ventricular canal defect with a common atrium (*CA*) with no interatrial septum and a large inlet ventricular septal defect (*asterisk*). **D,** Coronal maximum intensity projection image from an MRA in the same patient as (**C**) showing a midline liver, a right-sided stomach, and a cluster of splenules (*SP*) in the right upper quadrant. In addition, there are bilateral superior vena cavae (*asterisks*) and an unusual left-sided inferior vena cava (*arrow*) that extends to the right to enter the undersurface of the atria with the hepatic veins. *LV,* left ventricle; *RV,* right ventricle.

With the current diagnostic accuracy of echocardiography for CHD, chest radiography now plays a lesser role in diagnosing the morphology of CHD. In the past, chest radiographs were analyzed together with physiologic information gleaned from clinical examination (murmurs, cyanosis, etc.) to construct a differential diagnosis that would determine the initial treatment needed by the patient at birth. Radiographic classification of CHD may be based on pulmonary blood flow as follows:

I. Increased pulmonary vascularity
  A. Central left-to-right shunts (acyanotic)
    1. Ventricular septal defect (VSD)
    2. Atrial septal defect (ASD)
    3. Atrioventricular septal defect/common atrioventricular canal (CAVC)
    4. Patent ductus arteriosus (PDA)
    5. Less common lesions: partial anomalous pulmonary venous connection (PAPVC), aortopulmonary window, coronary-cameral fistula
  B. Peripheral left-to-right shunts
    1. Vein of Galen malformation
    2. Hepatic hemangioendothelioma
    3. Large extremity arteriovenous malformations
  C. Hyperdynamic states, such as thyrotoxicosis and anemia
  D. Intermixing states without obstruction to pulmonary blood flow (cyanotic)
    1. Transposition of the great arteries (TGA)
    2. Truncus arteriosus
    3. Double outlet right ventricle (DORV)

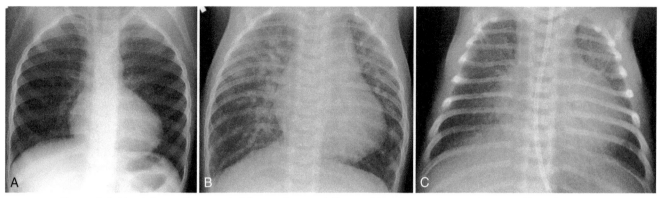

Figure 3.9 **Physiology of congenital heart disease delineated by chest radiography. A,** Mild cardiomegaly with an upturned cardiac apex, a concave main pulmonary artery segment, and symmetric, severely diminished pulmonary blood flow in a 4-year-old with tetralogy of Fallot/pulmonary atresia. **B,** Moderate cardiomegaly and symmetric, increased pulmonary blood flow in a 3-month-old with a large atrial septal defect and ventricular septal defect. **C,** Moderate cardiomegaly with interstitial edema in an 8-day-old with critical aortic stenosis.

4. Single ventricle
5. TAPVC (unobstructed)
II. Decreased pulmonary vascularity
  A. Tetralogy of Fallot (TOF)
  B. Pulmonary atresia with VSD
  C. Intermixing states with obstructed pulmonary blood flow (cyanotic)
    1. TGA with pulmonary stenosis
    2. Truncus arteriosus with pulmonary stenosis
    3. DORV with pulmonary stenosis/atresia
III. Pulmonary venous congestion and edema
  A. Left-sided obstructive lesions
    1. Cor triatriatum
    2. Hypoplastic left heart syndrome (HLHS)
    3. Shone syndrome
    4. Bicuspid aortic valve and aortic stenosis
    5. Aortic coarctation
  B. Hyperdynamic states
  C. Severe left-to-right shunts
IV. Normal pulmonary vascularity
  A. Mild left-sided obstructive lesions
  B. Intermixing states with balanced pulmonary blood flow
  C. Mild right-sided obstruction—pulmonary valve stenosis

Treatment of Congenital Heart Disease

Immediate Palliation

The need for immediate palliative therapy of CHD at birth depends on the patient's clinical and hemodynamic status. The type of palliation is determined by echocardiographic and radiographic findings. For example, in a patient with increased pulmonary vascularity, PA banding to diminish pulmonary blood flow may be considered. In a patient with decreased pulmonary vascularity caused by outflow tract obstruction, pulmonary blood flow can be augmented by surgical relief of the obstruction or placement of a systemic arterial-to-pulmonary arterial shunt such as a modified Blalock-Taussig shunt (BTS) [**Fig. 3.10**]. Older adults with CHD may have had the classic BTS or Waterston or Potts shunts, which are no longer routinely used. Intermixing states are treated in the neonatal period to balance and optimize pulmonary and systemic blood flow. Pulmonary venous hypertension caused by left-sided obstruction is treated through relief of the cause of obstruction.

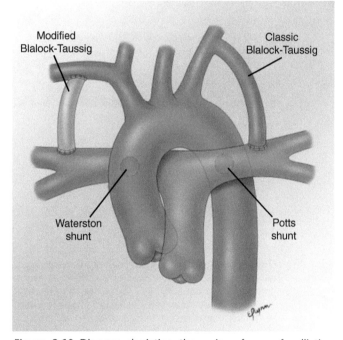

Figure 3.10 Diagram depicting the various forms of palliative shunts used to augment pulmonary blood flow for patients with cyanosis. See section "Named" Pediatric Cardiac Surgical Procedures in the appendix.

Permanent Palliation

After immediate palliation, decisions regarding permanent palliation are based on the number of functioning ventricles and the feasibility of separating deoxygenated and oxygenated blood flows. When there are two well-formed, normal-sized, functioning ventricles in conditions such as TOF, TGA, truncus arteriosus, and some forms of CAVC and DORV that are amenable to a two-ventricle repair, the anatomy is rearranged to restore physiologic venous return and unobstructed systemic and pulmonary arterial outflows.

When there is only one normal-sized, well-functioning RV or LV, this ventricle will be used as the systemic ventricle, and the pulmonary circulation will be palliated by establishing direct

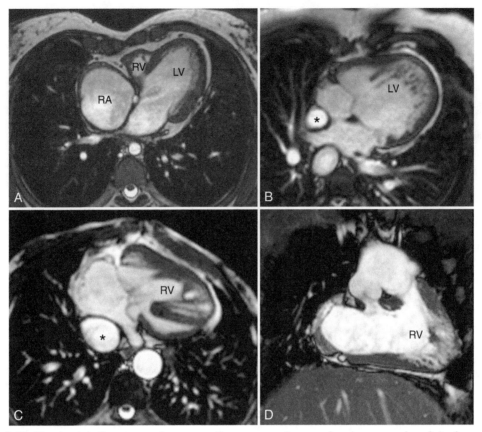

Figure 3.11 **Steady-state free precession magnetic resonance images showing examples of single-ventricle hearts often requiring single-ventricle palliation. A,** Tricuspid atresia. Note the hypoplastic right ventricle (RV) and fat filling the anterior atrioventricular (AV) groove in the expected location of the tricuspid valve. **B,** Double-inlet left ventricle (LV). Both the mitral and the tricuspid valves connect to a single LV. **C,** Unbalanced right dominant AV canal. A single AV valve is aligned with the RV, and a hypoplastic LV is seen posteriorly. **D,** Double-outlet RV. Both the aorta and the main pulmonary artery arise from the RV, and a bilateral conus is seen. *Asterisks* indicate Fontan pathway in cross section. *RA,* right atrium.

connections between the systemic veins and pulmonary arteries or cavopulmonary connections. This is called *single-ventricle repair* [**Fig. 3.11**]. Conditions that can be palliated with single-ventricle repair include unbalanced CAVC, tricuspid atresia, HLHS, double-inlet LV, DORV, and pulmonary atresia with an intact ventricular septum. Occasionally, conditions with two functioning ventricles may end up in the single-ventricle pathway because of an inability to separate the deoxygenated and oxygenated circulations. This may occur with some forms of DORV, straddling AV valves, and crisscross AV valves. A list of named surgical procedures is provided in the appendix to this chapter (see section "Named" Pediatric Cardiac Surgical Procedures).

Indications for Imaging by Computed Tomography and Magnetic Resonance Imaging

In the preoperative period, CT and MRI are used to evaluate CHD when complete characterization of pathology by echocardiography is inadequate due to suboptimal acoustic windows. Evaluation by echocardiography may be suboptimal with abnormalities involving the extracardiac vasculature, such as aortic coarctation, anomalous pulmonary venous connection, systemic venous anomalies, branch PA stenosis, and anomalous coronary artery origin.

In the postoperative period, the goals of imaging change considerably. Information about cardiac function and flow and potential postoperative complications is needed in addition to morphologic assessment. The goals of postoperative imaging are to evaluate ventricular and valvular function, survey the patency of surgically created grafts, conduits, and baffles, and gather information that will aid in the timing of necessary surgical or catheter-based reintervention. Typical indications for postoperative imaging that will help guide subsequent management include the evaluation for recurrent coarctation, the determination of timing of catheter-based or surgical pulmonary valve replacement in repaired TOF, the investigation of the cause of cyanosis after the Fontan operation, the evaluation of the systemic RV after intraatrial repair of TGA, and screening evaluation before staged single-ventricle repair. The role of MRI and CT increases in the postoperative period and in older patients when acoustic windows diminish.

COMMON CONDITIONS

Left-to-Right Shunts

Communications between the systemic and pulmonary circuits that do not result in cyanosis include intracardiac left-to-right shunts and large systemic arteriovenous connections. Common examples of the former are VSD, ASD, AVC defect, and PDA. Less common examples are partial anomalous pulmonary venous connection, aortopulmonary window, and coronary-cameral fistula. Examples of peripheral left-to-right shunts are infantile hepatic hemangioendotheliomas and large systemic arteriovenous malformations such as the vein of Galen malformation in the brain and Parkes-Weber syndrome affecting the extremities.

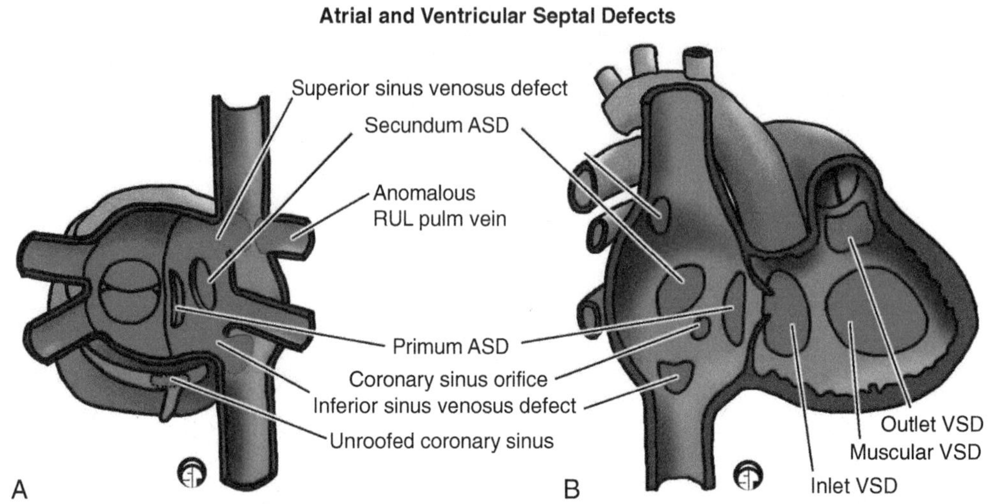

Atrial and Ventricular Septal Defects

Figure 3.12 Diagram illustrating the types of atrial (*ASD*) and ventricular septal defects (*VSD*) as viewed from the (**A**) posterior and (**B**) rightward aspects of the heart. RUL, right upper lobe. (Courtesy of Dr. Andrew Phelps.)

Ventricular Septal Defect

After bicuspid aortic valve, VSD is the second most common congenital intracardiac lesion in children, accounting for 20% to 30% of cases of CHD. Five percent of VSDs are associated with chromosomal abnormalities such as trisomies 13, 18, and 21. Many small VSDs close spontaneously. The classification of VSDs on the basis of location [**Fig. 3.12**] and size is important in deciding whether medical (expectant) or surgical treatment is indicated.

Muscular VSDs are defects in the muscular septum [**Fig. 3.13**]. They may be classified according to their location in the septum (midmuscular, apical muscular). "Swiss cheese septum" describes multiple muscular VSDs.

An *AVC-type VSD* is a defect in the AVC portion of the septum [**Fig. 3.13**]. Also known as an *inlet VSD,* this condition is commonly seen in the setting of heterotaxy.

Several different terms are used for outflow tract VSDs or defects in the interventricular septum associated with the outlet or subaortic or subpulmonary region of the heart. *Conoventricular VSDs* are a form of outlet VSD occurring within or at the junction between the conal septum and the muscular septum. Conoventricular VSDs may be in close proximity to the semilunar valves, and are also referred to as *subarterial VSDs.* Clinically, it is important to evaluate for associated aortic valve prolapse and aortic regurgitation.

The strictest definition of a *membranous VSD* is a defect of only the membranous septum, which would result in a relatively small defect. In day-to-day use, the term *perimembranous* or *paramembranous VSD* usually implies that the defect includes the region of the membranous septum, but also extends into the muscular septum, conal or outflow tract septum, or AVC septum. Outflow tract VSDs can be associated with malalignment, in which the conal septum of the RV outflow tract is displaced. This may create a substrate for outflow tract obstruction. Anterior malalignment of the conal septum often results in the RV outflow obstruction seen in TOF (described later), and posterior malalignment can lead to a VSD with LV outflow tract obstruction and an arch abnormality such as coarctation or complete arch interruption.

A VSD classically presents with a prominent, blowing, pansystolic murmur heard best at the left lower sternal border. Affected patients may have congestive heart failure (CHF), repeated respiratory infections, or failure to thrive. Presentation is usually after the first month of life when pulmonary vascular resistance normalizes and the degree of shunting increases. In an older child, a large, untreated VSD may lead to elevated pulmonary vascular resistance and pulmonary hypertension, which can resolve if the shunt is closed. In rare cases, pulmonary vascular obstructive disease or irreversible pulmonary hypertension can develop, and may even cause reversal of blood flow. This leads to a right-to-left shunt across the septal defect (formerly known as "Eisenmenger physiology"), and eventually to cyanosis. In most cases, corrective surgery is performed before flow reversal across the shunt occurs.

Conventional chest radiograph findings of a left-to-right shunt are usually evident when the ratio of pulmonary to systemic blood flow is greater than 2:1. Pulmonary vascularity is increased, and there is dilatation of the pulmonary arteries and cardiomegaly [**Fig. 3.13**]. A VSD generally results in volume loading of the LA and LV, which may appear prominent on chest radiographs. When pulmonary vascular resistance normalizes after the first month of life, pulmonary blood flow may further increase, resulting in radiographic signs of pulmonary vascular congestion and edema.

Up to 50% of VSDs close spontaneously. Those that do not may be treated with surgical closure of the defect. VSDs that are difficult to reach surgically can be treated with device closure at cardiac catheterization.

Atrial Septal Defect

ASD is the second most common cardiac anomaly in children, accounting for 10% of all cases of CHD. An ASD is the most common intracardiac shunt that persists into adulthood. It is found six to eight times more commonly in females than in males. ASDs are classified according to location in the atrial septum as follows [**Fig. 3.12**]:
- A patent foramen ovale [**Fig. 3.14**] represents defective apposition of the septum secundum and the septum primum, which normally fuse together after birth.
- An ostium secundum (II) ASD [**Fig. 3.14**] is the most common type (60% of cases), and is located in the midseptum in the region of the foramen ovale. It is usually an isolated anomaly.
- An ostium primum (I) ASD (30%) is situated low in the atrial septum and is contiguous with the AV valves. The ostium primum ASD is most commonly seen in the setting of a complete CAVC defect (described later). A *partial AVC defect* refers to a primum ASD associated with a cleft mitral valve.
- A sinus venosus septal defect (5%) does not involve the interatrial septum, but allows LA-to-RA shunting through a defect

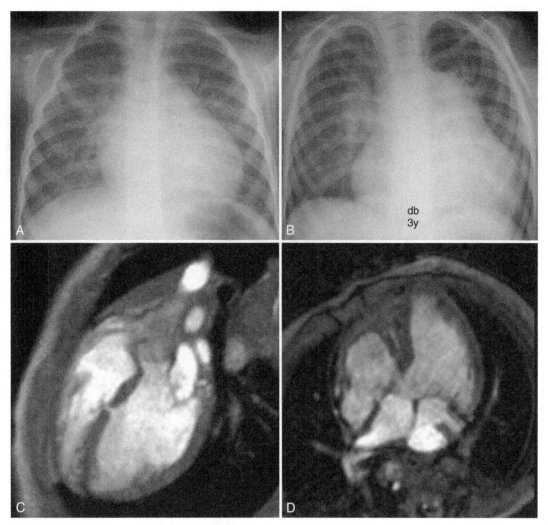

Figure 3.13 Ventricular septal defect (VSD). A, Chest radiograph at birth showing cardiomegaly with increased pulmonary vascularity. **B,** The same patient at 3 years old, with marked enlargement of the main and central branch pulmonary arteries. Note the pruning of the pulmonary arteries as they extend into the periphery of the lungs, consistent with pulmonary artery hypertension. **C,** Long-axis bright blood magnetic resonance (MR) image shows a defect in the mid muscular septum, or a muscular VSD. **D,** Four-chamber MR image of a different patient demonstrates an inlet or atrioventricular (AV) canal type VSD in continuity with the plane of the AV valves.

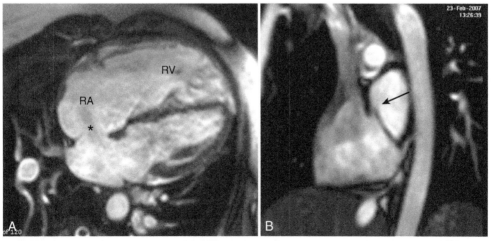

Figure 3.14 Types of atrial septal defects (ASDs). A, Four-chamber steady-state free precession (SSFP) image shows a large secundum ASD (*asterisk*) that is shunting left to right, resulting in dilation of the right atrium (*RA*) and right ventricle (*RV*). **B,** Sagittal oblique SSFP image through the interatrial septum shows the flap of a patent foramen ovale (*arrow*).

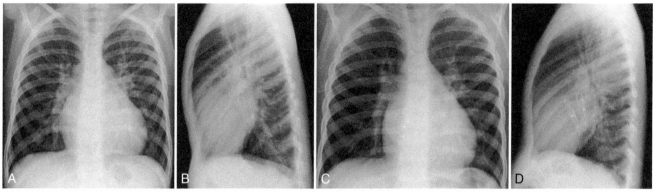

Figure 3.15 Chest radiographs of a 5-year-old with a large atrial septal defect before and after device occlusion. A, There is symmetric enlargement of the central pulmonary arteries on the frontal view. **B,** The right ventricle is enlarged on the lateral view, filling in the retrosternal clear space. **C** and **D,** After catheterization, the discs of an Amplatzer occlusion device are seen across the region of the interatrial septum.

between the posterior wall of the RA (a remnant of the embryonic sinus venosus) and the right-sided pulmonary veins, usually near the entrance of the SVC or IVC. A sinus venosus septal defect is therefore often associated with partial anomalous pulmonary venous drainage and can result in substantial left-to-right shunting.

- A coronary sinus septal defect (also referred to as an unroofed coronary sinus) does not involve the atrial septum proper, but occurs when the common wall separating the coronary sinus from the LA is deficient. A left-sided SVC can appear to connect directly into the LA when present, and the coronary sinus is completely unroofed.
- A common atrium occurs when there are deficiencies of both the septum primum and the septum secundum. It is often associated with heterotaxy syndromes [**Fig. 3.8**]. The interatrial communication can be very large.

Clinically, patients with ASDs are most often asymptomatic. When patients enter adolescence or young adulthood, mild dyspnea may develop, or an asymptomatic, harsh systolic murmur may be heard along the left upper sternal border.

Conventional chest radiographs may be normal in infants with an ASD. Later in childhood, increased pulmonary blood flow and central PA enlargement can be seen. An ASD results in volume loading and dilation of the RA and RV, and their contours can become quite prominent on chest radiographs [**Fig. 3.15**]. LA enlargement does not typically occur because of the immediate decompression of the greater volume of blood from the higher pressure LA to the lower pressure RA during both systole and diastole.

CT or MRI can be used to determine the site and size of the ASD before treatment with surgery or percutaneous device closure. These cross-sectional modalities are also useful to screen for the presence of coexistent anomalous pulmonary venous connection, which can be difficult to assess in larger patients by transthoracic echocardiography.

Cardiac MRI can be performed to quantify ventricular volumes and shunt size (pulmonary-to-systemic flow ratio, otherwise known as the Qp:Qs ratio) by MR flow velocity mapping for simple left-to-right shunts such as VSD, ASD, and PDA, as well as for any form of CHD where an imbalance between pulmonary and systemic blood flow exists. Quantification of ventricular volumes and shunt fraction can aid in decision making as to conservative versus surgical management. Large shunt lesions resulting in significant ventricular dilation and a Qp:Qs greater than 1.5:1 in symptomatic patients will generally require closure [**Fig. 3.16**].

Common Atrioventricular Canal

Endocardial cushion defect and *atrioventricular septal defect* are alternate terms for CAVC. The AV junction fails to develop normally into two distinct AV valves and complete the atrial septum and ventricular septum. *CAVC* therefore refers to a range of defects, from an isolated primum ASD with a cleft mitral valve (partial CAVC), to an isolated inlet VSD (incomplete CAVC), to a common AV valve with both a primum ASD and a VSD (complete CAVC) [**Fig. 3.17**]. The common AV valve may be symmetrically located over both ventricles, resulting in a *balanced CAVC* with both ventricles of approximately equal size. An *unbalanced CAVC* occurs when the AV valve is malaligned, or when there are valve attachments that impede flow to one of the ventricles and result in one ventricle being larger than the other [**Fig. 3.11C**]. About 40% to 50% of patients with CAVC have trisomy 21 (Down syndrome). Complete CAVC defects are often seen in patients with heterotaxy syndrome [**Fig. 3.8**].

Conventional chest radiographs show enlargement on the right side (RA and RV) and increased blood flow within the lungs [**Fig. 3.17**]. In the setting of trisomy 21, skeletal anomalies such as 11 or 13 pairs of ribs or a bifid manubrium sternum may be seen.

Corrective surgery involves patching of the ASD and VSD and separation or resuspension of the valve leaflets.

Patent Ductus Arteriosus

PDA constitutes 8% to 10% of all CHD, occurring in 1 in 3000 term infants. It is more common in girls (2:1) and premature infants (50% of those weighing less than 1500 g). A PDA is defined as a communication between the proximal descending thoracic aorta and the PA caused by persistence of the fetal ductus arteriosus, a remnant of the distal sixth aortic arch. Less commonly, the ductus arteriosus may connect the main or a branch PA to the subclavian or innominate artery [**Fig. 3.18**].

The ductus arteriosus communication normally functionally closes by 48 hours after birth because of an increase in arterial oxygen with ventilation and a decrease in circulating prostaglandins that are metabolized in the lungs. A PDA becomes anatomically closed in 95% of infants by the third month of life. Low oxygen tension in the arterial blood flow and/or elevated fetal prostaglandin levels will inhibit contraction and closure of the ductus.

A PDA is usually asymptomatic. The clinical presentation of a large PDA can range from detection of a machinery-like murmur

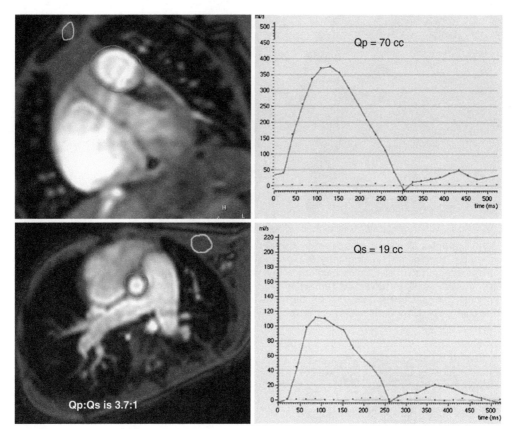

Figure 3.16 Calculation of pulmonary-to-systemic flow ratio on magnetic resonance (MR) imaging. The ratio of pulmonary blood flow (Qp) to systemic blood flow (Qs) can be calculated by MR flow velocity mapping using a phase velocity cine MR imaging sequence. Flow is measured across the main pulmonary artery and ascending aorta. This patient has a large systemic to pulmonary shunt with a Qp:Qs ratio of 3.7:1.

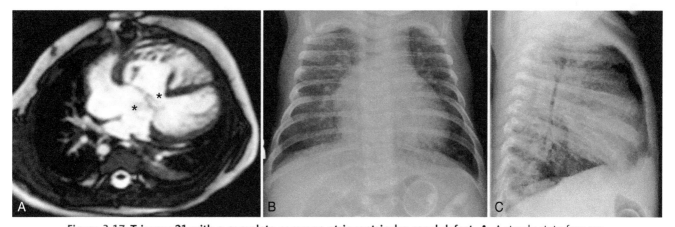

Figure 3.17 Trisomy 21 with a complete common atrioventricular canal defect. A, A steady-state free precession image in the four-chamber plane shows a primum atrial septal defect in direct continuity with the plane of a single atrioventricular valve and an inlet ventricular septal defect (*asterisks*). **B,** Frontal and (**C**) lateral radiographs of the chest show moderate cardiomegaly with a prominent right atrium and symmetrically increased pulmonary blood flow. Eleven pairs of ribs and a hypersegmented sternum are present.

to frank CHF in infancy, depending on the degree of shunting. Surfactant deficiency disease in the premature infant may facilitate persistence of a PDA in 25% of patients. The patent ductus may be treated medically with indomethacin or surgically with placement of a clip.

Conventional chest radiographs in the neonate with a PDA may show cardiomegaly with increased pulmonary vascularity and pulmonary edema. These findings may be difficult to evaluate if concomitant changes of surfactant deficiency or bronchopulmonary dysplasia are present. In the premature infant, interstitial edema (CHF) commonly occurs because there are fewer pulmonary arterioles to accommodate the increased blood flow. The classic patient with a PDA is a premature infant who develops radiographic signs of CHF at approximately 7 to 10 days of life when pulmonary vascular resistance starts to fall.

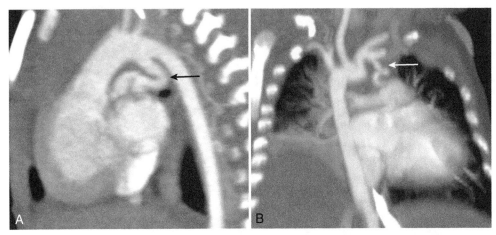

Figure 3.18 Examples of patent ductus arteriosus (PDA). A, Sagittal oblique maximum intensity projection (MIP) computed tomography angiography (CTA) image shows a large PDA (*arrow*) arising from the aortic isthmus and extending to the left pulmonary artery in a patient with pulmonary atresia. **B,** Oblique coronal MIP CTA image shows a small, tortuous PDA (*arrow*) arising from the left proximal subclavian artery and extending to the proximal left pulmonary artery. This patient has tetralogy of Fallot and a right aortic arch with mirror image branching. The left innominate artery arises as the first branch from the transverse arch.

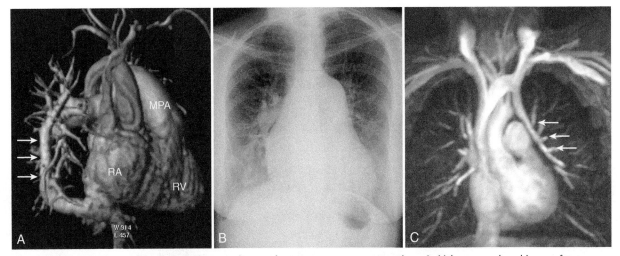

Figure 3.19 Examples of partial anomalous pulmonary venous connection. A, Volume-rendered image from magnetic resonance angiography (MRA) shows a large scimitar vein (*arrows*) draining most of the right lung to the inferior vena cava, resulting in a large left-to-right shunt with enlargement of the right atrium (*RA*), right ventricle (*RV*), and main (*MPA*) and branch pulmonary arteries. **B,** This patient's chest radiograph shows the enlarged heart shifted into the right chest, as the right lung is hypoplastic relative to the left lung. **C,** Coronal maximum intensity projection MRA image showing an anomalous left upper lobe pulmonary vein (*arrows*) draining to the innominate vein.

On imaging, a surgical clip or small closure device may indicate a surgically treated PDA. A closed ductus may also be evident as ligamentum calcification on CT. Partial closure of a ductus that remains open at the aortic end results in a ductus "bump" or ductus diverticulum, an incidental finding. This may occasionally enlarge to form a ductal aneurysm, which usually resolves spontaneously.

Partial Anomalous Pulmonary Venous Connection

In partial anomalous pulmonary venous connection, at least one or more, but not all, of the pulmonary veins return to the systemic veins (SVC, IVC, innominate vein, etc.) or directly to the RA. This results in a left-to-right shunt that causes volume loading of the RV, similar to the pathophysiology of an ASD.

A scimitar vein is defined as a right lower pulmonary vein or the entire pulmonary venous return from the right lung connecting to the IVC at the level of the diaphragm. Scimitar syndrome is characterized by a scimitar vein and right lung hypoplasia, resulting in dextroposition of the heart [**Fig. 3.19**]. This syndrome also can be associated with persistent systemic arterial supply from the abdominal aorta to the right lung.

MRI is helpful to evaluate for the presence of anomalous pulmonary vein(s), delineate their connections, assess for the presence of associated venous obstruction, quantify the degree of left-to-right shunting (Qp:Qs), and evaluate for associated anomalies such as branch PA hypoplasia, systemic arterial supply to the lung, or other developmental lung anomalies such as horseshoe lung or sequestration.

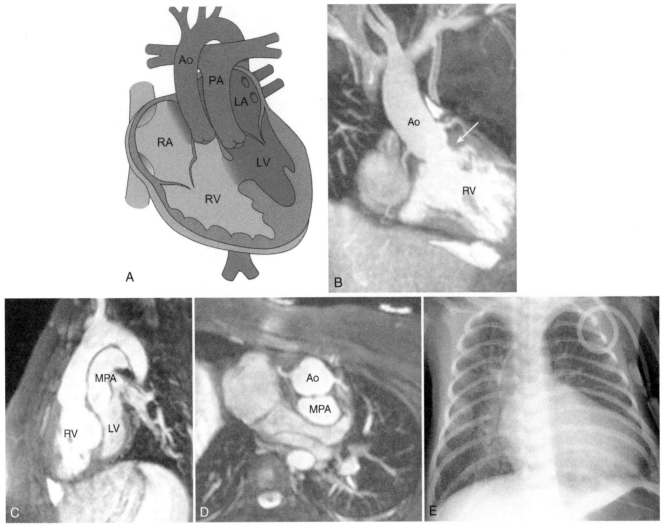

Figure 3.20 D-looped transposition of the great arteries (TGA). A, Diagram of D-TGA, with the main pulmonary artery (*MPA*) arising from the left ventricle (*LV*) and the aorta (*Ao*) arising from the right ventricle (*RV*). The degree of cyanosis is variable and depends on the presence of intracardiac shunts such as an atrial septal defect or a ventricular septal defect (VSD) to get oxygenated blood into the systemic circulation. **B** and **C,** Oblique reformatted images from a 3D steady-state free precession sequence show (**B**) the Ao arising from the anterior RV with a subaortic conus (*arrow*), and (**C**) the MPA arising from the posterior LV. **D,** The Ao and MPA have a parallel "back-to-front" arrangement. **E,** This parallel back-to-front arrangement contributes to the narrow mediastinum and "egg on a string" appearance seen on chest radiography. This patient has a large VSD with increased pulmonary blood flow. *LA,* Left atrium; *PA,* pulmonary artery; *RA,* right atrium.

Intermixing States

Common anomalies associated with intermixing include conotruncal anomalies such as TGA, truncus arteriosus, double outlet right ventricle (DORV), total anomalous pulmonary venous connection (TAPVC), and single ventricle.

Transposition of the Great Arteries

TGA is the most common form of cyanotic CHD (5% of cases). The incidence of dextro-TGA (D-TGA) is 1 in 4000 live births. It is higher in infants of mothers with diabetes, and boys with D-TGA outnumber girls 2.5:1.

In this condition the aorta and MPA originate from the "wrong" ventricle; the aorta arises from the RV, and the PA arises from the LV. This is also referred to as ventriculo-arterial discordance [**Fig. 3.20**]. The atria, AV connections, and ventricles may be normal. Typically the aorta lies anterior and to the right of the MPA (D-malposition). About 50% of infants with TGA have

an intact ventricular septum, 25% have a conoventricular VSD, and 25% have a VSD with pulmonary stenosis. The subaortic conal muscle of the RV can narrow the ventricular outflow tract, decreasing flow of blood to the aorta during development and resulting in coarctation.

With D-TGA, deoxygenated and oxygenated blood is separated into two independent circuits. Deoxygenated blood from the body returns to the RA, flowing through the RV and aorta, then back to the body. Oxygenated blood circulates from the LA and LV to the lungs and back again. This arrangement of two circuits in parallel is incompatible with life unless there is a communication at the level of the atria, ventricles, or ductus arteriosus.

This disorder commonly manifests as cyanosis in the first 24 hours of life. The extent of mixing of deoxygenated and oxygenated blood through an ASD, VSD, or PDA and the amount of pulmonary blood flow contribute to the level of cyanosis a patient may have and a variable appearance that may be seen on chest radiography. Substantial pulmonary blood flow can result in

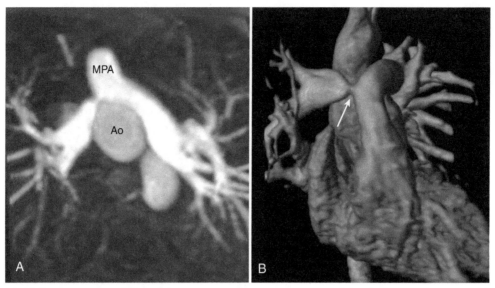

Figure 3.21 Dextro-transposition of the great arteries status post arterial switch operation. A, Axial refor-matted magnetic resonance angiography (MRA) image in a postoperative patient. The main pulmonary artery (MPA) and aorta (*Ao*) have been switched, leading to the very characteristic postoperative appearance with the MPA located anterior to the Ao and the branch PAs draped on either side of the Ao as they extend to the hila. **B,** Note the severe narrowing of the proximal right pulmonary artery (*arrow*) on an anterior volume-rendered image from MRA in the same patient.

cardiomegaly and edema with less significant cyanosis. Dimin-ished pulmonary flow, particularly in the setting of concomitant pulmonary valve stenosis, will result in decreased pulmonary vascularity on chest radiographs and more significant cyanosis. The cardiac silhouette is usually normal in size immediately after birth, but subsequently enlarges if shunting is present for ade-quate venous return and mixing of deoxygenated and oxygen-ated blood. A narrow mediastinal vascular contour is often seen in TGA because of the parallel "back-to-front" arrangement of the aorta and PA, as well as lack of a normal thymic contour caused by "stress." This appearance has often been referred to as an "egg on a string" [**Fig. 3.20**].

Palliative therapy centers on creation of a large ASD by means of balloon atrial septostomy (Rashkind procedure) to improve mixing of venous return and direct more oxygenated blood from the pulmonary veins into the systemic circulation via the RV to the aorta.

The goal of permanent palliation of TGA is to surgically redi-rect blood flow so that the deoxygenated systemic venous return enters the PA and oxygenated pulmonary venous return enters the aorta. There are two ways to accomplish this goal. Blood may be redirected at the atrial level (Mustard or Senning "atrial switch" procedure). Alternatively, a switch of the great arteries may be performed (Jatene "arterial switch" procedure). The arte-rial switch operation is the procedure of choice, and it requires coronary artery transfer and VSD closure. When there is LV outflow tract obstruction, the LV can be baffled to the aorta through the VSD, and a conduit can be placed to connect the RV to the PA. Complications after the arterial switch operation include neo-aortic root dilatation, branch PA stenosis [**Fig. 3.21**], and coronary artery ostial stenosis or kinking. MRI and CT play important roles in noninvasive monitoring for and diagnosis of complications after surgical palliation of TGA.

Congenitally Corrected Transposition of the Great Arteries

Congenitally corrected TGA is not an intermixing state, but it is discussed in this section because of its anatomic similarity

to D-TGA. Congenitally corrected or {S,L,L} TGA occurs when the heart undergoes L-looping instead of D-looping in utero, and there is both AV and ventriculo-arterial discordance [**Fig. 3.22**]. There is normal morphology of the atria, and the ven-tricles are inverted so that the RV is posterior and to the left of the LV (L-looping). The great arteries are transposed, and the aorta is to the left and anterior arising from the RV (L-malposition). When there is a solitus relationship of the atria, the blood flowing through the heart is "physiologically" corrected. The morphologic RV receives pulmonary venous return from the LA, which then exits to the aorta, and the morphologic LV receives systemic venous return from the RA, which then exits to the PA [**Fig. 3.6**]. Coexisting lesions include VSD (in more than 50% of cases), tricuspid valve anomalies (incompetence, atresia, and Ebstein anomaly), left ventricular outflow tract obstruction and/or pulmonary valve stenosis, and conduction system anomalies leading to arrhythmia.

The clinical presentation of patients with physiologically cor-rected levo-TGA (L-TGA) is variable depending on the severity of the associated intracardiac lesions listed earlier. If these lesions are absent or mild, a patient may escape clinical detection for many years, and the condition may be picked up incidentally in adulthood.

Conventional chest radiographs often appear normal but may show an abnormal fullness along the left upper cardiomediasti-nal border where the ascending aorta arises from the left-sided RV [**Fig. 3.22**]. The pulmonary vascularity is often decreased because of the high incidence of associated pulmonary stenosis. Late RV failure is common because the RV is usually not capable of sustaining a systemic workload for an entire life span. MRI plays an important role in the preoperative period in clarifying chamber morphology and connections and in monitoring sys-temic RV function.

A "double-switch" procedure is performed for L-TGA in early childhood at some centers. This consists of both atrial switch and arterial switch operations, with the goal of making the LV the systemic ventricle. Long-term results of this procedure are still unknown.

Congenitally Corrected Transposition

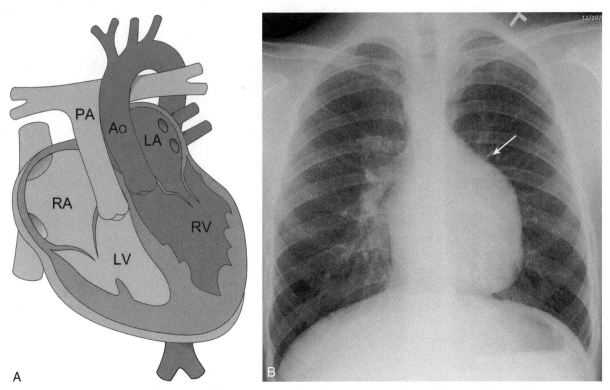

A

B

Figure 3.22 **Congenitally corrected levo-transposition of the great arteries (L-TGA). A,** Diagram illustrating L-TGA with L-looped ventricles and atrioventricular and ventriculo-arterial discordance. The right ventricle (*RV*) is located to the left and posterior to the left ventricle (*LV*), and gives rise to a levoposed ascending aorta (*Ao*). **B,** This results in filling in of the anteroposterior window and a prominent contour of the left superior heart margin on the chest radiograph (*arrow*), which may be mistaken for a dilated left atrial appendage. The Ao ascends from the left, then courses to the right of the trachea, forming a right aortic arch. *LA,* Left atrium; *PA,* pulmonary artery; *RA,* right atrium.

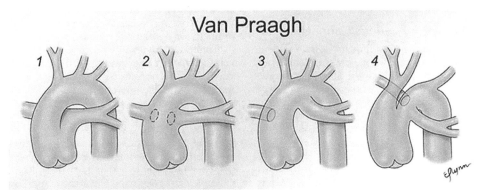

Figure 3.23 **Classification of truncus arteriosus.** Type 1: main pulmonary artery arises from the ascending aorta. Type 2: branch pulmonary arteries arise separately from the ascending aorta. Type 3: one branch pulmonary artery arises from the ascending aorta, the other from a ductlike collateral. Type 4: truncus arteriosus associated with interruption of the aortic arch.

Persistent Truncus Arteriosus

Persistent truncus arteriosus accounts for approximately 1% to 4% of CHD. It is associated with a right aortic arch in 21% to 36% of cases and with an interrupted aortic arch in 11% of cases. About 30% to 35% of patients with persistent truncus arteriosus have a 22q11 deletion (DiGeorge syndrome). Truncus arteriosus is classified according to the origin of the pulmonary arteries and the presence or absence of a VSD and an interrupted aortic arch [**Fig. 3.23**].

Persistent truncus arteriosus is defined as a single artery arising from the base of the heart and giving rise to the coronary, systemic, and pulmonary circulations. It represents a failure of septation of the primitive truncus arteriosus into the aorta and PA. The resultant single trunk arises from a single semilunar valve possessing anywhere from two to six cusps. A VSD is almost always present below the semilunar valve.

Patients with truncus arteriosus present early in infancy with cyanosis, failure to thrive, dyspnea, and CHF. Chest radiographs

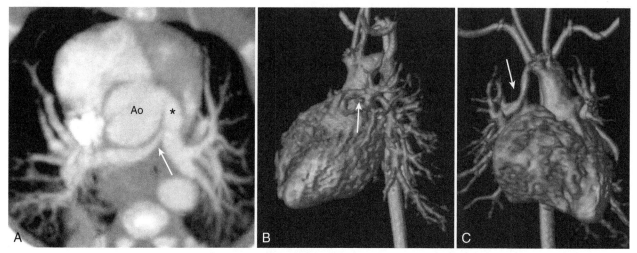

Figure 3.24 Examples of truncus arteriosus. A, Type 1: oblique axial maximum intensity projection computed tomography angiography image shows the main pulmonary artery (*asterisk*) arising from the leftward aspect of the ascending aorta (Ao) and bifurcating. There is stenosis of the proximal right pulmonary artery (RPA) (*arrow*), and the left pulmonary artery (LPA) is of normal caliber. **B** and **C,** Volume-rendered images from magnetic resonance angiography show (**B**) the LPA arising directly from the proximal truncal root (*arrow*), and (**C**) a ductlike collateral vessel from the innominate artery supporting the hilar RPA (*arrow*). (**A,** Courtesy Dr. Beverley Newman.)

typically demonstrate cardiomegaly and increased pulmonary vascularity. Preoperative computed tomography angiography (CTA) or magnetic resonance angiography (MRA) can be helpful in cases in which the PA anatomy cannot be determined by echocardiography [**Fig. 3.24**].

Treatment consists of assigning the truncal valve to the LV, closing the VSD, separating the branch pulmonary arteries from the aorta, and connecting them to the RV with a valved conduit, often an aortic homograft. The conduit will require replacement with somatic growth, and MRI plays an important role in determining the timing of follow-up surgery.

Total Anomalous Pulmonary Venous Connection

TAPVC is present when all of the pulmonary veins connect anomalously to the systemic venous circulation. The four types of TAPVC (supracardiac, intracardiac, infracardiac, and mixed) are named based on the site of drainage of the pulmonary veins into the systemic venous circulation. Supracardiac TAPVC connects above the heart, usually into the left innominate vein, and accounts for 40% of all cases of TAPVC. Intracardiac TAPVC connects to the heart, either via the coronary sinus or directly into the atria, and accounts for 20% of cases. Infracardiac TAPVC connects below the heart, often to the portal or hepatic veins in the abdomen, and accounts for 35% of cases. Mixed TAPVC is the rarest type, accounting for less than 5% of cases. In this condition, the pulmonary veins typically connect to two or more systemic veins (eg, the SVC and the portal vein). All forms of TAPVC have a risk for pulmonary venous obstruction, with a significantly higher incidence with the infracardiac and mixed types [**Fig. 3.25**].

Infants with TAPVC usually present in the first week of life. Because all of the pulmonary venous blood eventually returns to the RA, an intracardiac communication such as an ASD is necessary to bring some oxygenated blood to the left heart and systemic circulation. If there is modestly increased pulmonary blood flow and good admixture of the pulmonary venous blood through an ASD, cyanosis will be mild. With more significant pulmonary venous obstruction, severe cyanosis and pulmonary edema will manifest after birth, and intervention is mandatory to preserve life. In about one third of patients with TAPVC, major

associated conditions occur. These include heterotaxy, D-TGA, and HLHS.

Classically, chest radiographs of patients with obstructed TAPVC show a normal-sized cardiac silhouette with severely congested pulmonary vessels and pulmonary interstitial edema. In patients with TAPVC without obstruction, there is cardiomegaly (dilated RV and RA), an enlarged PA segment, and increased pulmonary blood flow. The classic "snowman" or figure-of-eight cardiomediastinal silhouette is seen in older patients with unobstructed supracardiac TAPVC and good intermixing [**Fig. 3.25**], but not in infants and children. CT and MRA are useful to trace the entire course of the anomalous pulmonary venous system, especially when there is mixed TAPVC, and to evaluate for pulmonary venous obstruction.

Treatment involves rerouting of the anomalous pulmonary veins to the LA and closure of the ASD. Recurrent pulmonary venous obstruction after TAPVC repair is an important indication for MRA and CTA, and carries a poor prognosis.

Right-Sided Obstructive Lesions

The congenital lesions included in this category have a common denominator: right-sided obstruction of varying severity and the presence of a right-to-left shunt that results in cyanosis. Common examples are TOF, tricuspid atresia, and Ebstein anomaly.

Tetralogy of Fallot

TOF is the most common cyanotic CHD in children and adults, accounting for 8% to 10% of cases. The pathologic substrate is anterior, superior, and leftward deviation of the conal septum, resulting in RV outflow tract obstruction, a conoventricular or malalignment VSD, RV hypertrophy, and overriding of the VSD by the aorta [**Fig. 3.26**].

If the RV outflow tract obstruction is mild (one third of cases) and the VSD is large, the infant will not be overtly cyanotic, the so-called pink tet. These patients tend to become more cyanotic as they get older and can display the characteristic "squatting" behavior when they become cyanotic during exercise. Squatting increases systemic venous return to the right heart to drive more blood flow into the lungs and improve oxygenation. At the other

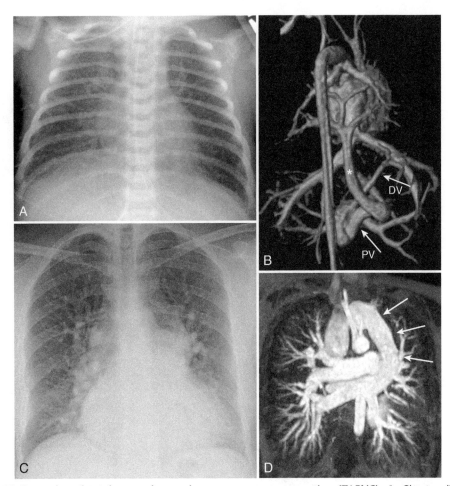

Figure 3.25 Examples of total anomalous pulmonary venous connection (TAPVC). A, Chest radiograph in a cyanotic newborn shows diffuse interstitial edema and a normal heart size. **B,** Posterior volume-rendered image from magnetic resonance angiography (MRA) shows infracardiac TAPVC, with all of the pulmonary veins joining to a pulmonary venous confluence (*asterisk*) and connecting to a dilated portal vein (*PV, arrow*). There is significant pulmonary venous obstruction because the ductus venosus (*DV, arrow*) is closing. **C,** Chest radiograph in an adult shows cardiomegaly with enlarged central pulmonary arteries and a prominent contour of the superior mediastinum. **D,** Oblique coronal maximum intensity projection image from MRA shows the right and left pulmonary veins connecting to a large vertical vein (*arrows*) that continues to a dilated innominate vein. A right superior vena cava is demonstrated. Findings are consistent with supracardiac TAPVC.

end of the spectrum is TOF with pulmonary atresia. In this condition, pulmonary blood flow depends on a PDA or major aortopulmonary collateral arteries (MAPCAs), embryologic vessels that support the lungs and abnormally persist when blood flow through the pulmonary arteries is compromised [**Fig. 3.26**].

TOF can be associated with trisomy 21, tracheoesophageal fistula, and the VACTERL association (*v*ertebral abnormalities, *a*nal atresia, *c*ardiac abnormalities, *t*racheoesophageal fistula and/or *e*sophageal atresia, *r*enal agenesis and dysplasia, and *l*imb defects).

Typical chest radiographic findings in the patient with TOF [**Fig. 3.27**] include (1) decreased pulmonary blood flow (although flow may be normal or even increased in patients with "pink tet"); (2) absence or small size of the pulmonary segment of the left mediastinal contour; and (3) RV hypertrophy, which creates a prominent, upturned cardiac apex. The thymus may be small because of stress atrophy, or absent in patients who have DiGeorge syndrome and TOF. Up to 25% of patients with TOF have a right-sided aortic arch. This constellation of findings creates the classic appearance of the coeur-en-sabot, or boot-shaped heart. Patients with TOF with pulmonary atresia and

MAPCAs may have abnormal arborization of the pulmonary vasculature [**Fig. 3.27**].

The treatment for TOF is surgical correction. Timing of surgery and procedures varies depending on the patient's anatomy and physiology (the severity and level of RV outflow tract obstruction, the size of the pulmonary arteries, the presence of aortopulmonary collaterals, and other associated cardiac defects). In the past, initial palliative procedures for patients with severe pulmonary oligemia included central aortopulmonary shunts like the Potts shunt, Waterston shunt, and BTS as discussed earlier. The current treatment in most surgical centers is total correction in infancy, with closure of the VSD and enlargement of the RV outflow tract and PAs with a synthetic or pericardial patch material. When there is pulmonary valve atresia, a conduit is placed from the RV to the PA, typically an aortic homograft.

With a transannular patch repair, an incision is made through the pulmonary valve annulus, leaving the patient with no functional pulmonary valve and resulting in chronic pulmonary regurgitation. This results in progressive RV volume overload leading to RV systolic and diastolic dysfunction, LV dysfunction,

Tetralogy of Fallot

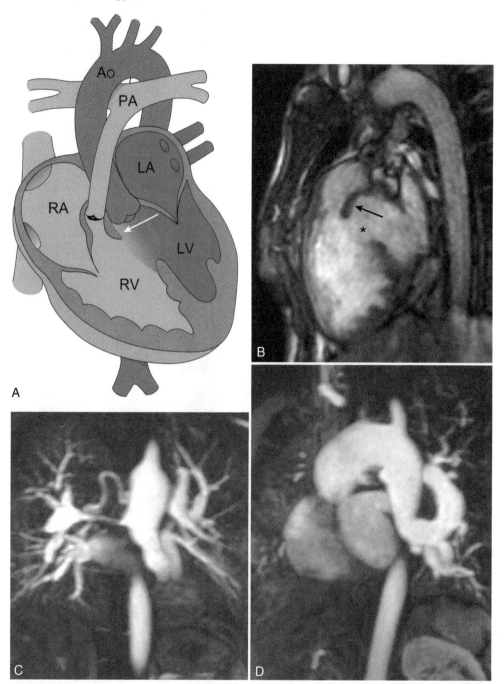

Figure 3.26 Tetralogy of Fallot (TOF). A, Diagram depicting the typical morphology caused by anterior and leftward deviation of the conal septum (*arrow*). This results in right ventricular outflow tract obstruction, a conoventricular or malalignment ventricular septal defect (VSD), right ventricular hypertrophy, and overriding of the VSD by the aorta (*Ao*). Right-to-left shunting of deoxygenated blood across the VSD results in cyanosis. **B,** Sagittal oblique steady-state free precession image through the right ventricular outflow tract shows anterior deviation of the conal septum (*arrow*), resulting in narrowing of the outflow tract and a malalignment VSD (*asterisk*). Maximum intensity projection images from magnetic resonance angiography in (**C**) coronal and (**D**) sagittal planes in a patient with TOF and pulmonary atresia. Major aortopulmonary collateral arteries arise from the descending aorta to support blood flow to the right and left lungs because the mediastinal branch pulmonary arteries are absent. *LA,* Left atrium; *LV,* left ventricle; *PA,* pulmonary artery; *RA,* right atrium; *RV,* right ventricle.

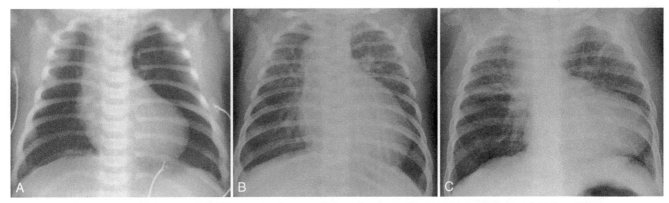

Figure 3.27 Spectrum of findings on chest radiography in patients with tetralogy of Fallot (TOF). **A,** Severely decreased pulmonary blood flow (PBF) associated with severe right ventricular outflow tract obstruction. **B,** Normal to increased PBF caused by mild right ventricular outflow tract obstruction. **C,** Abnormal arborization of vessels with a region of decreased PBF in the right lower lobe in a patient with TOF, pulmonary atresia, and aortopulmonary collaterals. All of these patients have a right aortic arch, concave main pulmonary artery segment, and upturned cardiac apex typical of TOF.

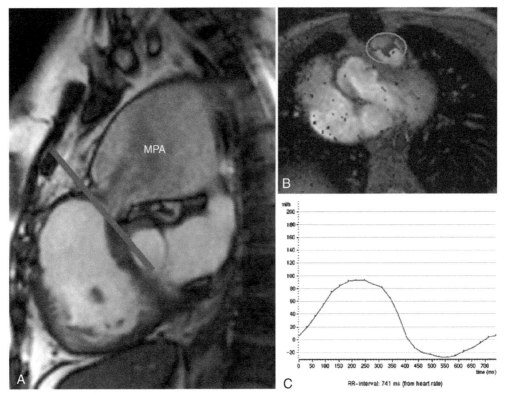

Figure 3.28 Postoperative magnetic resonance imaging (MRI) evaluation of tetralogy of Fallot. A, Recurrent right ventricular outflow tract (RVOT) obstruction with poststenotic dilatation of the main pulmonary artery (MPA) demonstrated on a bright blood image. Flow-velocity mapping was performed across the RVOT in a plane marked by the *solid gray bar,* yielding a cross-sectional image of the RVOT as shown in **B**. A region of interest is drawn around the RVOT on the phase image to quantify the volume of forward flow and regurgitant flow within the RVOT, yielding a pulmonary regurgitant fraction of approximately 35%, as shown in **C**.

and arrhythmias, requiring many patients to have pulmonary valve replacement in adulthood. The current surgical approach is to avoid the transannular patch repair if there is mild RV outflow tract obstruction, but this type of repair may still be needed when there is severe outflow tract obstruction.

MRI plays an important role in the postoperative setting to monitor RV size and function and determine the optimal timing of pulmonary valve replacement. Patients with homografts often require RV to PA conduit replacement or transcatheter

pulmonary valve replacement within the conduit. MRI and CTA are helpful in screening such patients for stenosis and determining the optimal time for surgery [**Fig. 3.28**].

Tricuspid Atresia

Tricuspid atresia is complete absence of the tricuspid valve with no direct communication between the RA and RV [**Fig. 3.11A**]. The RV is typically hypoplastic. The degree of hypoplasia varies

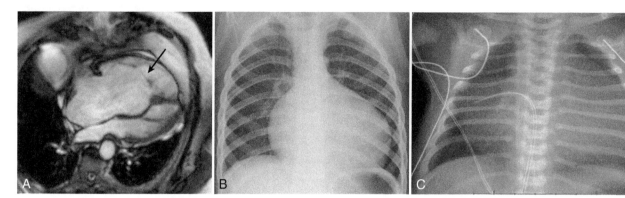

Figure 3.29 Ebstein anomaly of the tricuspid valve. A, Four-chamber steady-state free precession magnetic resonance image shows apical displacement of the septal leaflet of the tricuspid valve, resulting in partial "atrialization" of the right ventricle. Note the sail-like anterior leaflet (*arrow*). **B,** Chest radiograph in a 3-year-old with severe Ebstein anomaly shows cardiomegaly with small hilar branch pulmonary arteries and decreased peripheral pulmonary blood flow. **C,** Large, box-shaped heart caused by a severely enlarged right atrium in a patient with Ebstein anomaly.

with the presence and size of associated VSDs. Infants with an atretic tricuspid valve are cyanotic at birth and require an obligatory ASD or VSD to survive. The "RV" in tricuspid atresia lacks an inflow portion and may consist only of the infundibulum or outlet chamber. Absence of the tricuspid valve is accompanied by pulmonary stenosis (or more rarely, pulmonary atresia) in more than 50% of cases, and TGA in 30% of cases. The associated VSD may become restrictive over time, producing subpulmonary or subaortic stenosis.

Radiographs of the chest in a patient with tricuspid atresia show normal or decreased pulmonary flow and a "rounded" cardiac apex caused by the RA enlargement. The RA contour is prominent, there may be a concave PA segment, and the aorta may be on the right side in 15% of children with tricuspid atresia.

The goal of initial palliation is to maintain pulmonary flow. This may be accomplished with prostaglandin therapy to maintain the PDA and surgical creation of a modified BTS. Permanent palliation is accomplished by a single-ventricle repair or Fontan procedure. The survival rate is about 70% at 5 years.

Ebstein Anomaly

Ebstein anomaly is uncommon, constituting less than 1% of all cases of CHD. It is an abnormality in the formation of the tricuspid valve, resulting in apical displacement of the annular attachments of the septal and inferior leaflets [**Fig. 3.29**]. The anterior leaflet is usually attached at the normal position of the annulus, but it is dysplastic and sail-like. The malformed leaflets do not coapt normally, resulting in significant tricuspid regurgitation. A portion of the RV becomes "atrialized" with a thin myocardium.

When Ebstein anomaly results in severe tricuspid regurgitation and an ASD is present, blood shunts from right to left leading to severe cyanosis at birth or within the first month of life. Patients with mild Ebstein anomaly may be diagnosed in later adolescence or even adulthood.

Radiographic findings depend on the extent of dilatation of the right side of the heart. The cardiac silhouette may appear "box-shaped," or may resemble the appearance seen in the setting of a pericardial effusion [**Fig. 3.29**]. The central pulmonary arteries may be small, and overall pulmonary vascularity may be diminished. This is due to a combination of tricuspid regurgitation and right-to-left shunting at the atrial level.

Treatment of the newborn with severe Ebstein anomaly may be palliative, consisting of extracorporeal membrane oxygenation until pulmonary vascular resistance decreases and

pulmonary blood flow improves. The prognosis is variable; there is a 50% neonatal mortality rate in the first month of life for severe forms of Ebstein anomaly.

The differential diagnosis for the imaging findings of Ebstein anomaly includes tricuspid insufficiency associated with the even more rare condition of Uhl anomaly. The latter consists of focal or complete absence of RV myocardium, resulting in a thin-walled, poorly functioning RV.

Left-Sided Obstructive Lesions

The most important left-sided obstructive lesions are (from distal to proximal) coarctation, congenital aortic stenosis, Shone syndrome, HLHS, and cor triatriatum.

Coarctation of the Aorta

There are two types of coarctation, the discrete or focal form, which involves the aortic isthmus, and the diffuse form, which involves a longer segment of the aorta including the transverse arch [**Fig. 3.30**]. Discrete coarctation is thought to occur from constriction and fibrosis of ductal tissue extending from the ductus arteriosus into the wall of the aortic isthmus, resulting in focal narrowing distal to the origin of the left subclavian artery. Discrete coarctation accounts for about 5% of all congenital heart lesions. Males are affected twice as often as females. The diffuse form is frequently associated with other obstructive lesions of the left ventricular outflow tract, such as bicuspid aortic valve, aortic stenosis, Shone syndrome, and HLHS.

The presentation of the patient and timing of surgery depend on the severity of coarctation. Most children with discrete coarctation of the aorta are asymptomatic and are identified incidentally because of hypertension. Patients with more diffuse narrowing of the aortic arch tend to present with CHF in the neonatal period when the ductus arteriosus closes.

The chest radiograph may show LV enlargement, particularly on the lateral view, as well as poststenotic dilatation of the proximal descending aorta. Occasionally, the contour of the proximal descending thoracic aorta will demonstrate a "figure-of-three" sign, formed by the combination of prestenotic and poststenotic bulging of the aorta around the narrowing at the isthmus [**Fig. 3.30**]. The "reverse three," or "E" sign, is the mirror image of these findings that can be seen on an esophageal contrast study (no longer performed for diagnosis today). Rib notching may be seen in the setting of coarctation, although it is

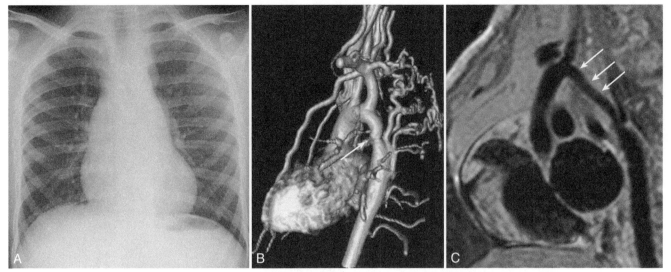

Figure 3.30 Aortic coarctation. A, Chest radiograph in a patient with coarctation showing the classic "3 sign" created by prestenotic and poststenotic dilation of the aorta around the narrowed isthmus. **B,** Volume-rendered image from magnetic resonance angiography showing discrete or focal narrowing of the aortic isthmus (*arrow*) with abundant collateral flow to the descending thoracic aorta. **C,** Sagittal oblique black blood magnetic resonance image shows long-segment diffuse hypoplasia and elongation of the transverse aortic arch and isthmus (*arrows*).

notably rarely observed in children younger than 8 years. It is typically seen along the inferior margins of the fourth through eighth ribs, and represents pressure erosion by enlarged, hypertrophied intercostal arteries serving as collaterals to the lower body distal to the arch obstruction. It is usually a bilateral finding unless there is an aberrant right subclavian artery, in which case there is no notching on the right side.

In young infants with coarctation, echocardiography can fully characterize the degree of arch obstruction, provide a pressure gradient measurement across the coarctation, and detect associated LV hypertrophy with hyperdynamic systolic function. Reduction in LV systolic function with CHF in infancy is an ominous sign associated with severe coarctation.

When echocardiography windows become limited in older children and adolescents, the best noninvasive measure of the anatomic extent and severity of coarctation and the presence of collaterals is obtained with MRA or CTA. When the utility of echocardiography decreases, velocity encoded cine MRI of the descending aorta can be used to assess for blunted flow distal to the coarctation, and the peak velocity across the coarctation can be used to calculate a pressure gradient across the stenosis using the modified Bernoulli equation.

Surgical treatment of coarctation of the aorta involves excision of the coarctation segment followed by direct end-to-end or end-to-side anastomosis. More severe, diffuse coarctation may require patch augmentation. The subclavian flap repair is not favored as an option because of possible vertebral artery steal and compromise to upper extremity circulation postoperatively [**Fig. 3.31**]. MRA and/or CTA are used in the postoperative setting to assess for recurrent coarctation or aneurysm formation at the repair site.

Congenital Aortic Stenosis

Aortic valve abnormalities constitute the most common form of CHD overall. Valvular aortic stenosis is most commonly seen, with a dysplastic, thickened, and frequently bicuspid aortic valve (70%) [**Fig. 3.32**]. Obstruction of the left ventricular outflow tract can also be subvalvular and/or supravalvular. Subvalvular aortic stenosis may be fixed and discrete, caused by a fibromuscular ring or membrane, or may be dynamic and diffuse, sometimes referred to as tunnel-type stenosis. Subvalvular obstruction may also result from septal hypertrophy in the setting of hypertrophic obstructive cardiomyopathy.

Supravalvular stenosis may be sporadic or familial, or may be related to Williams syndrome (elfin facies, mental retardation, and neonatal hypercalcemia). Patients with Williams syndrome can have a characteristic hourglass deformity of the ascending aorta caused by a fibrotic constriction of the sinotubular junction [**Fig. 3.33**], as well as stenosis of the branch pulmonary, renal, and coronary arteries. The obstructive nature of these aortic valve abnormalities eventually results in pressure overload of the LV.

Patient age at presentation is inversely related to the severity of the obstruction. The clinical spectrum ranges from CHF in the newborn period due to critical stenosis to an asymptomatic murmur in older children and adolescents. Valvular stenosis tends to be progressive with age, and it is characterized by a harsh systolic murmur at the right upper sternal border.

Conventional chest radiographs may also vary in appearance, from cardiomegaly with edema in newborns with critical aortic stenosis to a normal heart size in older children. The ascending aorta may be border forming along the right side of the mediastinum because of poststenotic dilatation [**Fig. 3.32**]. MRI can help delineate the location, extent, and nature of obstruction, especially in the setting of subvalvular or supravalvular stenosis.

Newborns with critical valvular stenosis are initially treated with balloon dilatation. If this is unsuccessful, a surgical aortic valve commissurotomy is performed. Additional surgical approaches to subvalvular and supravalvular stenoses include

- *Konno procedure:* For subvalvular aortic stenosis, the aortic annulus and LV outflow tract are enlarged by excising a portion of the ventricular septum and inserting a patch, followed by replacement of the aortic valve with a mechanical or homograft valve.
- *Ross procedure:* For aortic valvular insufficiency and/or stenosis, the aortic root is removed, the pulmonary root is "transplanted" (autografted) to the aortic position, the coronary arteries are reimplanted into the pulmonary or neo-aortic root,

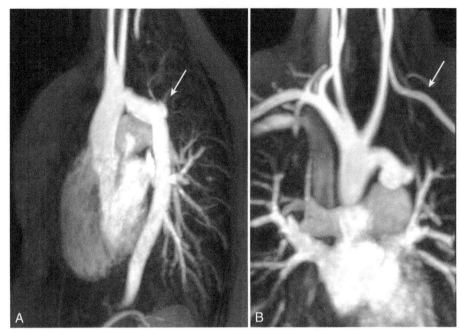

Figure 3.31 Subclavian artery steal after subclavian artery flap repair for coarctation. A, Sagittal oblique maximum intensity projection (MIP) image from magnetic resonance angiography shows an elongated transverse arch with a focal bulge in the contour of the isthmus (*arrow*), consistent with a small aneurysm after coarctation repair. There is no evidence for recurrent stenosis. **B,** Coronal oblique MIP image shows the right innominate and left common carotid arteries arising from the proximal transverse aortic arch. The left proximal subclavian artery is not visualized because it has been used for the coarctation repair. The left distal subclavian artery (*arrow*) is reconstituted from the left vertebral artery.

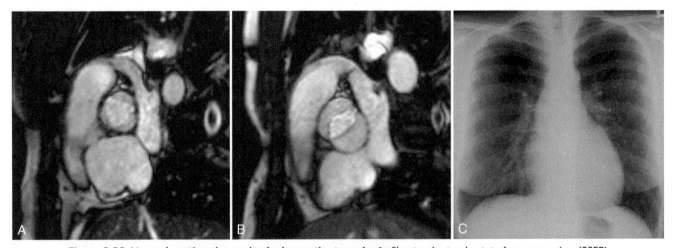

Figure 3.32 Normal aortic valve and valvular aortic stenosis. A, Short-axis steady-state free precession (SSFP) white blood image through the aortic root shows a normal trileaflet aortic valve with a triangular opening during systole. **B,** Short-axis SSFP white blood image shows a typical bicuspid aortic valve with a fish-mouth opening during systole. This valve has a good-sized orifice without significant stenosis. **C,** Chest radiograph of a patient with significant valvular aortic stenosis shows poststenotic dilation of the ascending aorta, creating an accentuated border along the right side of the mediastinum.

and an aortic homograft is used as a conduit to connect the RV to the MPA.

Hypoplastic Left Heart Syndrome

HLHS, a relatively common cause of CHF in the neonate, manifests at birth and represents a spectrum of severe forms of left heart obstruction that are insufficient to sustain the systemic circulation. The major components of HLHS are hypoplasia or atresia of the aortic and mitral valves and varying degrees of hypoplasia of the LA, LV, and ascending aorta and aortic arch [**Fig. 3.34**]. There is an obligatory left-to-right shunt, most often at the atrial level. Chest radiographs show globular cardiomegaly with congestive changes in the lungs within 24 hours of birth.

The initial palliative surgery for HLHS is the stage I Norwood procedure, which includes several steps. The MPA is ligated and divided, and the ascending aorta is reconstructed using the

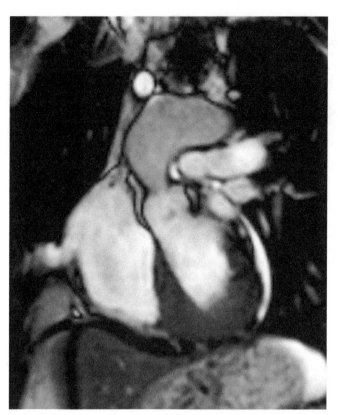

Figure 3.33 **Supravalvular aortic stenosis.** Coronal oblique long-axis steady-state free precession image through the left ventricular outflow tract shows discrete narrowing and wall thickening of the sinotubular junction between the aortic root and ascending aorta in a patient with Williams syndrome.

pulmonary valve as the neo-aortic valve and enlarged with patch augmentation. Thus the RV becomes the systemic ventricle (Damus-Kaye-Stansel procedure). An atrial septectomy is performed so that pulmonary venous blood will return to the RA and RV. A BTS or a small RV to PA conduit is placed to provide pulmonary blood flow. The end result of the stage I Norwood operation is that the RV supports both the systemic and the pulmonary circulations. The stage II procedure includes creation of the superior cavopulmonary shunt (bidirectional Glenn) connecting the SVC directly to the branch PAs and take down of the BTS. Stage III involves creation of a total cavopulmonary shunt (Fontan procedure, in which the IVC blood is directly connected to the PA), so that the entire systemic venous system will return passively to the lungs without a ventricular pump [**Fig. 3.35**].

The usual role of MRI in patients with HLHS is to clarify the status of the aortic arch before the stage I Norwood procedure and to determine the status of the branch pulmonary arteries, pulmonary veins, and systemic veins before the stage II and III procedures. This imaging modality is also helpful to monitor ventricular function, screen for thrombosis, and determine the cause of cyanosis after the stage III or Fontan procedure.

Shone Syndrome

Shone syndrome is a complex of four potentially obstructive anomalies of the left heart: supramitral ring, parachute mitral valve with a single papillary muscle of the LV [**Fig. 3.36**], subaortic stenosis, and coarctation of the aorta. All four findings are not always present. In the neonatal period, an important decision must be made regarding surgical palliation. Patients with Shone syndrome may undergo two-ventricle palliation, or alternatively single-ventricle palliation similar to patients with HLHS. MRI can accurately quantify LV volume and function, and also

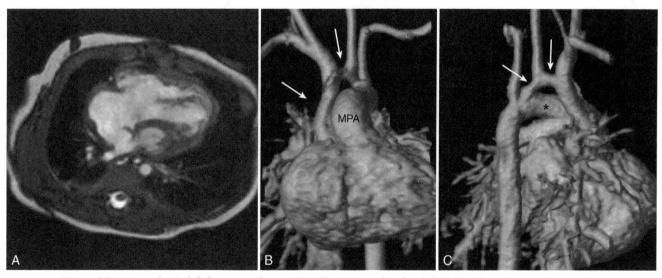

Figure 3.34 **Hypoplastic left heart syndrome (HLHS). A,** Four-chamber bright blood steady-state free precession image shows severe hypoplasia of the left ventricle and an apex-forming right ventricle (RV). A large atrial septa defect is present, allowing the pulmonary venous return to enter the right atrium to the RV and main pulmonary artery (*MPA*). A patent ductus arteriosus (PDA) is mandatory to bring oxygenated blood from the MPA to the aorta for systemic perfusion. Volume-rendered magnetic resonance angiography images in (**B**) anterior and (**C**) rightward projections from another patient with HLHS show a diffusely hypoplastic ascending aorta and transverse arch (*arrows*). The MPA is dilated, and a large PDA is present (*asterisk*) to deliver oxygenated blood from the RV to the aorta for the systemic circulation.

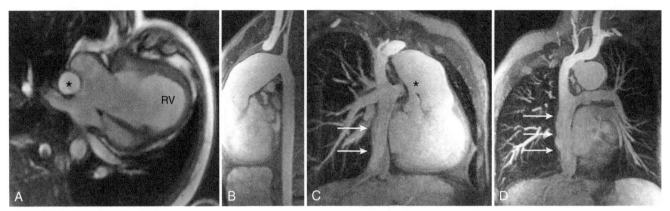

Figure 3.35 Hypoplastic left heart syndrome status post single-ventricle palliation. A, A four-chamber steady-state free precession image shows the hypoplastic left ventricle posterior to the dominant, apex-forming right ventricle (*RV*). The Fontan pathway is in cross section (*asterisk*). **B,** Sagittal oblique reformatted image from magnetic resonance angiography (MRA) shows the reconstructed aortic arch. The RV supports the reconstructed aortic arch to the body, and the native ascending aorta and coronary arteries via the Damus-Kaye Stansel anastomosis between the native ascending aorta and the main pulmonary artery. **C,** This is shown in a coronal oblique reformatted MRA image (*asterisk*). The extracardiac Fontan pathway (*arrows*) connects the inferior vena cava to (**C**) the right pulmonary artery (RPA) and (**D**) the left pulmonary artery (LPA). There is also a superior cavopulmonary anastomosis between the right superior vena cava and the RPA so that all of the systemic venous return is routed directly to the branch pulmonary arteries.

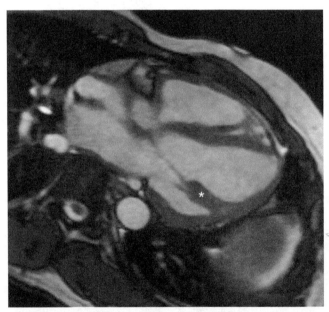

Figure 3.36 Parachute mitral valve. A four-chamber steady-state free precession image shows a form of congenital mitral stenosis referred to as a parachute mitral valve. All of the chordal attachments from both of the mitral valve leaflets connect to a single papillary muscle (*asterisk*), narrowing the opening of the mitral valve into the left ventricle.

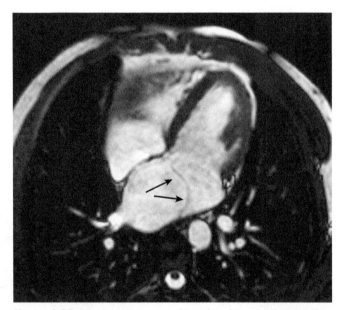

Figure 3.37 Cor triatriatum. A four-chamber steady-state free precession image shows a membrane (*arrows*) dividing the left atrium into two chambers. The membrane has a very small opening, which creates significant obstruction to pulmonary venous blood flow.

quantify the amount of blood flow across the mitral and aortic valves to help with surgical decision making.

Cor Triatriatum

Cor triatriatum results from a failure of complete incorporation of the pulmonary veins into the LA. A perforated membrane bisects the LA and impedes blood return from the lungs, resulting in pulmonary venous obstruction. The pathophysiology is similar to that seen in mitral valve stenosis. Radiographs may initially show interstitial edema with a normal-sized heart. When

echocardiography findings are inconclusive, MRI is diagnostic, showing a membrane dividing the LA into two separate chambers [**Fig. 3.37**].

MISCELLANEOUS CONDITIONS

Pericardial Absence and Pericardial Cysts

Pericardial absence is classified as partial or complete, with partial left-sided defects being the most common. A partial pericardial defect on the right side is rare. In one third of cases, there

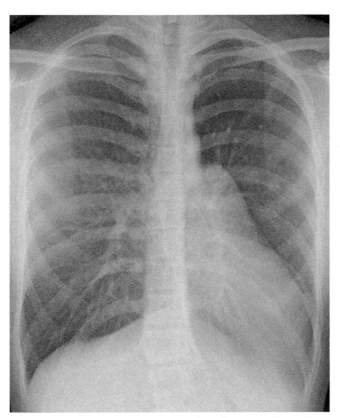

Figure 3.38 Congenital absence of the left pericardium. Chest radiograph of a 17-year-old. The heart is rotated into the left hemithorax. Lung tissue extends between the aortic knob and main pulmonary artery segment.

is an associated intracardiac defect such as a PDA, ASD, or TOF. Pericardial absence may also be seen together with omphalocele, diaphragmatic hernia, and ectopia cordis in the pentalogy of Cantrell.

In the setting of a small, partial pericardial defect, the chest radiograph may show an abnormal protuberance in the region of the LA appendage and MPA. Herniation of these structures through the defect is a rare complication. In the setting of a large left-sided pericardial defect, the heart is rotated away from the sternum creating an unusual cardiomediastinal contour with lung tissue separating the aortic knob and MPA [**Fig. 3.38**]. Large pericardial defects are usually detected incidentally on chest radiography and have no clinical significance.

Pericardial cysts may be true or false. True cysts are located within the pericardial sac, although they have no direct communication with it. False cysts, or diverticula, are protrusions of parietal pericardium, and consequently do communicate directly with the pericardial space. True cysts can occur anywhere on the pericardium but are found most often in the right costophrenic angle [**Fig. 3.39**].

Pericardial cysts are clinically symptomatic in only a small number of cases and are usually diagnosed incidentally. If associated symptoms of dyspnea or chest pain are present, percutaneous aspiration or thoracoscopic resection may be performed.

Kawasaki Disease

Kawasaki disease is a mucocutaneous lymph node syndrome characterized by fever, rash, conjunctivitis, and cervical adenopathy. The peak incidence is between 1 and 3 years of age.

Symptoms are due to a generalized vasculitis, with involvement of the coronary arteries and myocardium being a characteristic feature. Coronary artery vasculitis may be complicated by aneurysm formation and stenoses of the proximal portions of both the left and the right coronary arteries. Rarely myocardial infarction may occur, which is often clinically occult.

Conventional chest radiographic findings are often normal, except for rare instances of cardiac enlargement in severe cases of myocarditis. MRI is preferred for serial follow-up of patients with Kawasaki disease. This modality can accurately detect aneurysms of the coronary and systemic arteries, significant stenoses of the proximal coronary arteries, active vasculitis, and the presence of myocardial damage [**Fig. 3.40**]. Low-dose coronary CTA is performed when significant coronary artery stenosis is detected. It may also be performed before bypass surgery when necessary.

Aspirin and intravenous gamma-globulin administered early in the course of disease are typically quite effective in the prevention of aneurysm formation.

Rheumatic Heart Disease

Rheumatic heart disease is caused by acute rheumatic fever. This is a delayed complication of streptococcal disease, a throat infection with group A beta-hemolytic streptococci. This can result in long-term damage to the heart muscle or heart valves, especially in the setting of repeated, untreated episodes. Myocarditis may result, and involvement of the mitral (85%) and aortic (55%) valves may be seen. Rheumatic heart disease is rare in the western world but is still a common affliction in developing countries. It is the most common cause of acquired valvular insufficiency and/or stenosis.

If mitral stenosis or mitral regurgitation occurs, chest radiographs often show LA enlargement and a prominent LA appendage. An "atrial double density sign" may be seen [**Fig. 3.41**]. If pulmonary venous hypertension develops, there may be signs of congestive failure with interstitial edema and Kerley B lines demonstrated.

In children, treatment with appropriate antibiotics is often sufficient early in the course of the disease. In the setting of established rheumatic heart disease, however, surgery for the affected valves may be required.

APPENDIX

Cardiac Position

Levocardia: Heart in the left chest, apex pointing leftward (normal position)
Mesocardia: Heart in the midline, apex pointing inferiorly
Dextrocardia: Heart in the right chest, apex pointing rightward
Ectopia cordis: Heart partially or completely outside the chest
Dextroposition: Rightward displacement of the heart with apex pointing leftward, as may be seen with a left-sided tension pneumothorax
Dextrorotation: Most commonly, the base of the heart is in the normal position, but the apex has rotated rightward
Dextroversion: A previously used term that has been replaced by *isolated dextrocardia,* which refers to dextrocardia in the setting of situs solitus
Isolated levocardia: Levocardia in the setting of situs inversus; there is a high incidence of CHD with isolated dextrocardia and isolated levocardia

Visceral Situs and Atrial Situs

Situs refers to the position of the unpaired organs (liver, spleen, stomach) as well as the atria. There are three possibilities:

I

'll

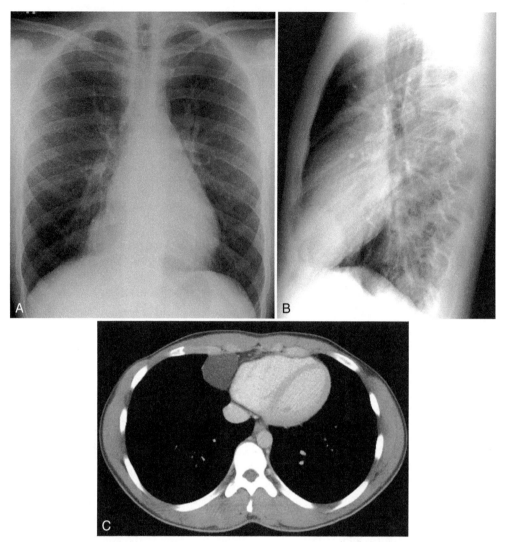

Figure 3.39 Pericardial cyst. A, Frontal radiograph shows a rounded density within the right cardiophrenic angle. **B,** This is seen anteriorly on the lateral view. **C,** Axial computed tomography image with contrast shows a nonenhancing lesion of homogeneous fluid density, consistent with a pericardial cyst.

Situs solitus (S): Usual position; liver on right, spleen on left, RA on right, LA on left

Situs inversus (I): Mirror image of the usual position; liver on left, spleen on right, RA on left, LA on right

Situs ambiguous (A): Neither solitus nor inversus; midline liver, asplenia or polysplenia, common atrium or indeterminate morphologic RA and LA; also referred to as heterotaxy and frequently associated with complex CHD

Classic Radiographic Signs in Congenital Heart Disease

These signs are explained in the text:

Egg on a string: D-TGA
Snowman sign: Supracardiac TAPVC to the left innominate vein
Coeur-en-sabot or boot-shaped heart: TOF
Box-shaped heart: Ebstein anomaly
Scimitar sign: Partial anomalous pulmonary venous connection of the right lung to the IVC
Gooseneck deformity: Elongation of the LV outflow tract in the CAVC

Figure-of-three and reversed-three signs: Coarctation of the aorta

"Named" Pediatric Cardiac Surgical Procedures
Aortopulmonary Shunts

The indication for these procedures is to increase pulmonary blood flow in lesions with inadequate pulmonary blood flow.

BTS: The first palliative surgery for cyanotic heart disease; a classic BTS consists of an end-to-side anastomosis of the subclavian artery to the PA; the modified version consists of interposition (side-to-side) of a polytetrafluoroethylene (PTFE; GORE-TEX) tube graft between the subclavian artery and the PA

Central shunt: PTFE tube graft from the ascending aorta to the PA

Potts shunt: Direct anastomosis of the descending aorta to the left PA

Waterston (Cooley) shunt: Direct anastomosis of the ascending aorta to the right PA

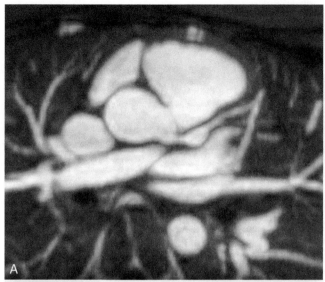

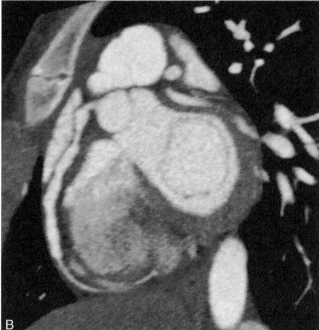

Figure 3.40 Coronary artery aneurysms in two patients with Kawasaki disease. A, Axial maximum intensity projection (MIP) image from a contrast-enhanced 3D gradient recalled echo sequence shows focal enlargement of the origin of the left main coronary artery and a focal aneurysm of the proximal left anterior descending coronary artery. **B,** Oblique MIP image from a coronary computed tomography angiography shows fusiform, long-segment, irregular dilatation of the right coronary artery (Courtesy of Dr. Cynthia Rigsby.)

Procedures for Transposition of the Great Arteries

Blalock-Hanlon atrial septectomy: A closed-heart procedure using clamps to isolate the posterior part of the atrial septum and cut it out; it is rarely used today.

Rashkind balloon atrial septostomy: A catheterization procedure using a stiff balloon pulled across the foramen ovale from the LA to the RA to rip the atrial septum and make a larger ASD.

Arterial switch operation (Jatene procedure): The great arteries are divided and switched so that the aorta is connected to the LV, and the PA is connected to the RV. The coronary arteries

are transferred to the neo-aortic root. The Lecompte maneuver refers to the repositioning of the pulmonary arteries in front of the neo-aorta from their original position behind the aorta.

Atrial switch procedures: Senning and Mustard: Also known as intraatrial baffle procedures; the end physiology of these two operations is the same, but the procedures differ in the use of baffle material and placement. The native atrial septum is removed, and baffles are constructed to redirect the systemic venous return into the mitral valve, LV, and out the PA. The pulmonary venous return is directed into the tricuspid valve, RV, and out the aorta.

Rastelli procedure for TGA with VSD and pulmonary stenosis: "Rastelli" is a term used for any RV to PA conduit, but the original operation was for TGA with a VSD and pulmonary stenosis. The VSD is closed in a way to connect the LV with the aorta, and a conduit is used to connect the RV with the PA.

Single-Ventricle Palliations

Norwood procedure—stage I: Initially devised for HLHS, but also applied to any single-ventricle lesion with systemic outflow obstruction. The first part is the Damus-Kaye-Stansel procedure, in which the ascending aorta is connected to the MPA (thus, the RV is used to pump systemic blood flow). The aortic arch is augmented. A modified BTS is placed to provide pulmonary blood flow, and the atrial septum is excised to ensure free mixing of blood at the atrial level.

Bidirectional Glenn procedure—stage II: This procedure directs the systemic venous return from the upper body directly into the lungs by connecting the SVC to the pulmonary arteries.

Fontan procedure—stage III: The basic concept is to create a pathway for all venous blood to flow directly into the pulmonary arteries without passing through the heart. The *original Fontan* procedure connected the RA appendage to the pulmonary arteries. There was a high incidence of RA dilatation and atrial arrhythmias with this procedure, so the *lateral tunnel Fontan* procedure was developed to utilize only a portion of the atrium as a connection from the IVC to the pulmonary arteries. A fenestration (small hole) is usually left in the patch to provide a "popoff" for venous blood to return to the heart. There is still a high incidence of atrial arrhythmias with this variation, so the *extracardiac conduit Fontan* procedure was developed to involve less suturing in the atrium. A homograft is used to connect the IVC to the PA outside the heart.

Differential Diagnoses

Dilated PA:
- Valvular pulmonary stenosis
- Left-to-right shunts (VSD, ASD, PDA)
- Pulmonary arterial hypertension

Concave PA:
- TOF
- Pulmonary atresia
- TGA

Dilated ascending aorta:
- Aortic valvular stenosis
- Bicuspid aortic valve
- Marfan syndrome
- PDA

Right aortic arch:
- TOF
- PDA
- DORV
- D-TGA
- Tricuspid atresia (rarely)
- Truncus arteriosus

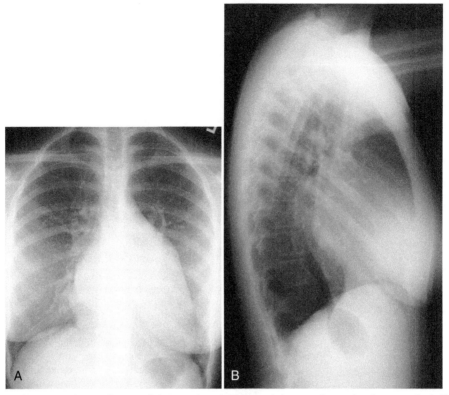

Figure 3.41 Rheumatic heart disease. (A) Frontal and **(B)** lateral chest radiographs show marked dilatation of the left atrium and left atrial appendage. There is downward displacement of the cardiac apex related to left ventricular enlargement in the setting of severe mitral stenosis and regurgitation.

SUGGESTED READINGS

Allen HD, Driscoll DJ, Shaddy RE, et al., eds. *Moss and Adams' Heart Disease in Infants, Children, and Adolescents: Including the Fetus and Young Adults.* 7th ed. Philadelphia, PA: Lippincott Williams & Wilkins; 2008.

Araoz PA, Reddy GP, Higgins CB. Congenital heart disease: morphology and function. In: Higgins CB, de Roos A, eds. *Cardiovascular MRI and MRA.* Philadelphia, PA: Lippincott Williams & Wilkins; 2002:307-338.

Degenhardt K, Singh MK, Epstein JA. New approaches under development: cardiovascular embryology applied to heart disease. *J Clin Invest.* 2013;123:71-74.

Gaca AM, Jaggers JJ, Dudley LT, et al. Repair of congenital heart disease: a primer—part 1. *Radiology.* 2008;247:617-631.

Gaca AM, Jaggers JJ, Dudley LT, et al. Repair of congenital heart disease: a primer—part 2. *Radiology.* 2008;248:44-60.

Helbing WH, Ouhlous M. Cardiac magnetic resonance imaging in children. *Pediatr Radiol.* 2015;45:20-26.

Kellenberger CJ, Yoo SJ, Büchel ER, et al. imaging in neonates and infants with congenital heart disease. *Radiographics.* 2007;27:5-18.

Krishnamurthy R. Pediatric cardiac MRI: anatomy and function. *Pediatr Radiol.* 2008;38:S192-S199.

Krishnamurthy R, Chung T. Pediatric cardiac MRI. In: Lucaya J, Strife JL, eds. *Pediatric Chest Radiology: Chest Imaging in Infants and Children.* 2nd ed rev. Medical Radiology/Diagnostic Imaging. Berlin: Springer-Verlag; 2007.

Krishnamurthy R, Lee EY. Congenital cardiovascular malformations: noninvasive imaging by MRI in neonates. *Magn Reson Imaging Clin N Am.* 2011;20:xviii.

Rhodes JF, Hijazi ZM, Sommer RJ. Pathophysiology of congenital heart disease in the adult. Part II: simple obstructive lesions. *Circulation.* 2008;117:1228-1237.

Sommer RJ, Hijazi ZM, Rhodes JF Jr. Pathophysiology of congenital heart disease in the adult. Part I: Shunt lesions. *Circulation.* 2008;117:1090-1099.

Sommer RJ, Hijazi ZM, Rhodes JF. Pathophysiology of congenital heart disease in the adult. Part III: Complex congenital heart disease. *Circulation.* 2008;117: 1340-1350.

Valsangiacomo Buechel ER, Fogel MA. Congenital cardiac defects and MR-guided planning of surgery. *Magn Reson Imaging Clin N Am.* 2011;19:823-840, viii.

Van Praagh R. Terminology of congenital heart disease: glossary and commentary. *Circulation.* 1977;56:139-143.

Van Praagh R. The segmental approach clarified. *Cardiovasc Intervent Radiol.* 1984;7:320-325.

Chapter 4
Gastrointestinal Imaging

Stephanie DiPerna and Carlo Buonomo

To the radiologist who cares for adults, the exact age of a patient is rarely of great importance. To be sure, one approaches the chest radiograph of a 30-year-old differently from that of an 80-year-old. For the most part, however, we are all equally prey to the afflictions of senescence. For the pediatric radiologist, the situation is entirely different. To offer an interpretation of an image of a child without knowing the precise patient age is often an exercise in futility. This is especially true in the field that is the subject of this chapter: pediatric gastrointestinal (GI) imaging. To give just one example out of many that are possible, there is essentially no overlap in the differential diagnosis of small-bowel obstruction in children who are 1 day, 1 week, 1 month, or 1 year old. As discussed later in this chapter, it is an excellent rule of thumb that in any child between 3 months and 3 years of age, a small-bowel obstruction is due to intussusception until proven otherwise. Intussusception, however, almost *never* occurs in a newborn. In pediatric GI radiology, it is only a slight exaggeration to say that to know the patient's age is to know the patient's diagnosis.

It is for this reason that this chapter, devoted to imaging of the GI tract, is organized by age and not by the perhaps more familiar anatomic or pathologic categories. We believe it is more practical to present the GI radiology of the newborn than to organize a discussion around "developmental anomalies" or "diseases of the colon."

This chapter will focus primarily on conventional radiography and fluoroscopy. The interpretation and, in the case of fluoroscopy, the performance of these studies are sometimes described as dying arts. It is probably true that the radiology resident is often most uncomfortable with these more traditional modalities. It is hoped that this chapter will prove them to be as indispensable as ever.

IMAGING TECHNIQUES

Conventional Radiography

In a child with abdominal complaints, conventional radiographs are most often the recommended initial imaging evaluation. Although the referring clinician may request ultrasound or computed tomography (CT) as the first-line study in a diagnostic workup, radiographs may provide useful information to best tailor cross-sectional imaging to a patient's specific problem.

A two-view study is most often obtained for children with acute abdominal symptoms, with supine and upright projections. In babies and patients who are very ill or uncooperative, a left lateral decubitus view may replace the upright image. An additional prone image can be useful when obstruction cannot be excluded with standard views. Air will rise to the rectum in the prone position when obstruction is not present. A single supine view alone will suffice in certain clinical settings, such as the evaluation for constipation, the search for an ingested foreign body, or the localization of catheter placement.

Normal Bowel Gas Pattern

In the newborn, air is typically present in the stomach at birth. By 6 hours of life, the stomach and the majority of the small bowel are usually filled with air. Air should reach the rectum by 24 hours of age, although this most often occurs much earlier. Loops of gas-filled bowel should be uniformly distributed throughout the abdomen and pelvis in a so-called polygonal pattern [**Fig. 4.1A**].

Abnormal Bowel Gas Patterns

Absence of air in the stomach by 1 hour of life should raise concern for an esophageal obstruction, as may be seen in the setting of esophageal atresia (EA). The presence of a "double-bubble" sign [**Fig. 4.1B**], reflecting distention of the stomach and proximal duodenum, raises concern for an upper GI obstruction. The presence of many dilated bowel loops on a neonatal abdominal radiograph raises concern for a distal bowel obstruction [**Fig. 4.1C**]. Neonatal bowel obstruction will be covered extensively in subsequent sections of this chapter.

Adynamic ileus may be seen in infants and older children. This commonly occurs after surgery and may also be seen in the setting of an acute illness such as gastroenteritis. Radiographs typically show distention of small bowel, with air–fluid levels noted on the upright or decubitus view.

With dynamic ileus, there is an anatomic cause for mechanical obstruction. Relatively common causes beyond the neonatal period include inflammation related to acute appendicitis, intussusception [**Fig. 4.2**], inguinal hernia, postoperative adhesions, and midgut volvulus.

Abdominal Masses

An abdominal or pelvic mass may be first detected on radiographs [**Fig. 4.3**]. An abnormal soft tissue opacity may be seen, or a solid visceral contour may be enlarged, distorted, or ill-defined in the presence of a mass. Associated calcification(s) may be present. Bowel loops may be compressed or significantly displaced by a mass, and a secondary bowel obstruction can be seen.

Pneumoperitoneum

Free air in the abdomen most often results from perforation of a hollow viscus. It is also commonly observed in the postoperative setting. Small amounts of free air may be seen on upright and decubitus views, but may be difficult to detect on a supine view. Large amounts of free air are typically readily identifiable on a supine radiograph [**Fig. 4.4**]. A "Rigler sign" may be seen, with air on both sides of the bowel wall. A "football sign" may also be noted, with free air outlining the falciform ligament.

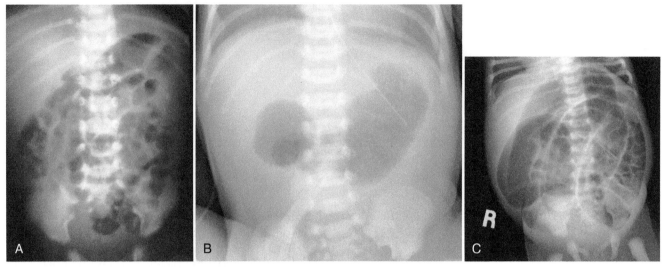

Figure 4.1 **Normal and abnormal neonatal bowel gas patterns. A,** A normal abdominal radiograph shows air evenly distributed throughout nondilated loops of small and large bowel. **B,** An abdominal radiograph demonstrating a dilated stomach and proximal duodenum in a neonate with a high bowel obstruction. **C,** An abdominal radiograph showing many dilated bowel loops in a neonate with a low or distal bowel obstruction.

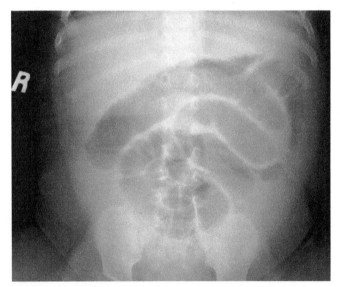

Figure 4.2 **Small-bowel obstruction.** A frontal supine abdominal radiograph demonstrating a small-bowel obstruction in the setting of intussusception.

Ascites

Ascites has many causes in the pediatric population, as in adults. In the neonate, urinary ascites may be seen in the setting of posterior urethral valves, with obstruction of the collecting system and resulting forniceal rupture. Peritonitis may be seen after bowel perforation in the setting of meconium ileus or necrotizing enterocolitis (NEC). Chylous ascites may result from birth trauma and may also be seen in the postoperative setting.

Regardless of cause, ascites appears similar on radiographs. Bowel loops are centralized on the supine view, the hepatic margin may be indistinct, and the properitoneal fat planes may be obliterated by free fluid in the paracolic gutters. Notably, ultrasound and CT are more sensitive modalities for the detection of small amounts of free fluid in the abdomen.

Calcifications

Calcifications are well visualized on abdominal radiographs. Sheetlike calcifications may be present along the peritoneal cavity in a newborn with meconium peritonitis [**Fig. 4.5**], or a meconium pseudocyst may be seen [**Fig. 4.6**]. Calcification of the adrenal gland(s) related to neonatal hemorrhage may be noted. Renal calculi, gallbladder calculi, and appendicoliths are often detected on radiographs. Calcified tumors may be first suggested on radiographs, as indicated earlier.

Fluoroscopy

Contrast Agents

Barium is routinely used in the evaluation of the pediatric GI tract, most commonly for the upper GI series. Barium compounds are less frequently used for evaluation of the lower GI tract. They are relatively thick and tenacious, and often are difficult to evacuate from the colon after a contrast enema. A relative contraindication to the use of barium is suspected bowel perforation. Barium in the peritoneal cavity or retroperitoneum may result in peritonitis, granuloma formation, and adhesions.

Several *water-soluble contrast agents* exist. *Diatrizoate meglumine/sodium (Gastrografin)* is a hyperosmolar water-soluble contrast medium. It is never used in the routine diagnostic evaluation of the upper GI tract. There is a serious risk for pulmonary edema or death with aspiration because aspirated Gastrografin can trigger the release of histamine or histamine-like substances in the lung. Hyperosmolar, hydrophilic contrast agents like Gastrografin also draw fluid into the GI tract lumen and can result in massive and potentially dangerous fluid shifts. This is particularly true in neonates. If ingested from above, marked dilution of hyperosmolar agents occurs as early as the third portion of the duodenum, limiting their diagnostic utility for the remainder of the GI tract. The hyperosmolar quality of these agents may be exploited in the large bowel in certain clinical settings (to be described). Through appropriate dilution of these contrast agents, near isotonicity can be achieved.

Iothalamate meglumine (Cysto-Conray) is less hypertonic than agents like Gastrografin. The relatively low iodine content of this contrast medium limits adequate visualization of detail for upper GI studies. However, Cysto-Conray does provide adequate

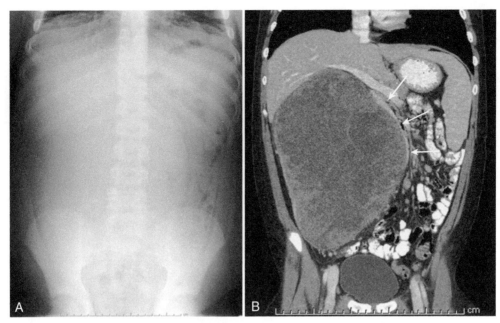

Figure 4.3 Abdominal mass. A, A frontal abdominal radiograph demonstrates a large soft tissue mass occupying much of the right hemiabdomen and central abdomen. Bowel is displaced leftward and compressed. **B,** A coronal reformatted image from a contrast-enhanced computed tomography scan shows a heterogeneous mass arising from the right kidney. A "claw sign" is noted (*arrows*), with the compressed, enhancing renal parenchyma stretched around the mass. This patient was diagnosed with Wilms tumor.

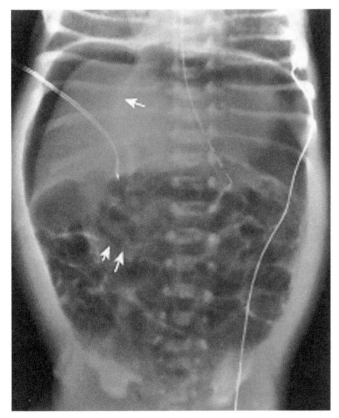

Figure 4.4 Free intraperitoneal air. An anteroposterior supine abdominal radiograph in a baby with necrotizing enterocolitis and free air demonstrates generalized lucency throughout the abdomen. Note that free air outlines the falciform ligament ("football sign") (*arrow*), and air is seen on both sides of the bowel wall ("Rigler sign") (*double arrows*).

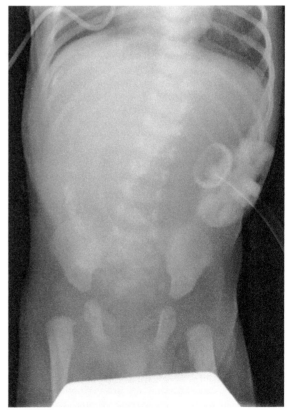

Figure 4.5 Abdominal calcifications. An abdominal radiograph in a baby with meconium peritonitis shows clusters of calcification over the liver, along the right flank, and in the pelvis. The patient has a gastrostomy tube.

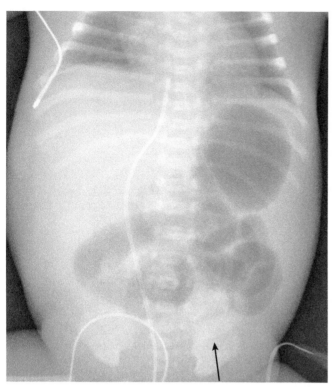

Figure 4.6 Abdominal calcifications. An abdominal radiograph in a baby with meconium peritonitis demonstrates a calcified meconium pseudocyst in the left lower quadrant (*arrow*).

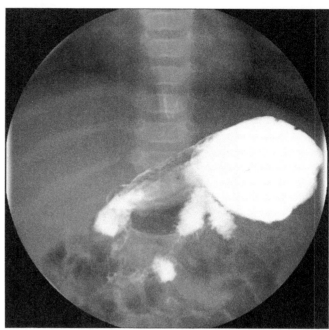

Figure 4.7 An anteroposterior image from a normal upper gastrointestinal series shows the duodenal jejunal junction to the left of a left-sided spinous pedicle and at the level of the duodenal bulb.

visualization of the lower GI tract and is the agent of choice for routine diagnostic contrast enemas.

Water-soluble agents with relatively lower osmolality include *iopamidol (Isovue)*, *ioversol (Optiray)*, and *iohexol (Omnipaque)*. These agents contain sufficient iodine concentration for adequate visualization of the upper GI tract but are low enough in osmolality to prevent clinically significant fluid shifts. They are useful when the anatomic integrity of the GI tract must be evaluated in the sick neonate, as in the setting of NEC. They are also useful in the postoperative setting after bowel anastomosis, when the risk for perforation is relatively high. Notably, use of these agents is best reserved for these and other specific circumstances. They are more costly and often less revealing than more radiopaque barium.

Common Examinations

The *upper GI series* is routinely performed in the pediatric population. Common indications include the assessment for upper GI obstruction in a neonate, malrotation of the bowel with or without midgut volvulus, and anatomic malformations such as tracheoesophageal fistula (TEF). These and other entities will be discussed in detail in later sections of this chapter.

Pediatric patients most often ingest dilute barium alone for an upper GI. The swallowing mechanism is assessed, and evaluation for laryngeal penetration and tracheal aspiration is performed. The contour and motility pattern of the esophagus and the gastroesophageal (GE) junction are evaluated, and the anatomic integrity of the stomach, duodenum, and proximal jejunum is assessed. Most importantly, the location of the duodenojejunal junction (DJJ) is determined to assess for normal rotation and positioning of the GI tract. Normally, the DJJ is positioned to the left of the spine posterior to the stomach at the level of the duodenal bulb [**Fig. 4.7**]. A normal DJJ may be located a bit medial to this overlying a left-sided spinous pedicle, or slightly

lower than the level of the duodenal bulb. The duodenal C-sweep is usually smooth but may demonstrate some degree of undulation or redundancy. These represent variations of normal; the position of the DJJ itself is of paramount importance.

Double-contrast studies are worthwhile for the evaluation of the GI tract mucosa. However, these studies are infrequently indicated in the pediatric population and not typically believed to be high yield. The *contrast enema* is another routine fluoroscopic examination in the pediatric population. This study is most commonly performed to evaluate for low bowel obstruction in the neonate, as may be seen in Hirschsprung disease, small left colon syndrome, meconium ileus, and ileal atresia.

As indicated earlier, water-soluble contrast agents such as iothalamate meglumine (Cysto-Conray) are most appropriate for a diagnostic contrast enema.

The contrast enema is typically performed with a small, straight-tipped catheter inserted low in the rectum so that distal pathology is not missed. Contrast is instilled throughout the large bowel, ideally with reflux to the distal ileum. The caliber and contour of the colon are assessed, and evaluation for areas of narrowing or obstruction is performed.

Occasionally a therapeutic enema may be performed. Indications include the therapeutic contrast enema performed for meconium ileus in the newborn with cystic fibrosis (CF) and distal intestinal obstruction syndrome (DIOS) in the older patient with CF. The contrast agent of choice for these studies is diatrizoate meglumine/sodium (Gastrografin). The high osmolality of Gastrografin causes fluid shifts into the GI tract lumen, with the potential to relieve obstruction related to tenacious meconium or significant stool impaction.

Another commonly performed therapeutic enema in the pediatric population is the air enema for intussusception reduction. This procedure is outlined in detail later in this chapter.

THE NEWBORN

Intestinal Obstruction in the Newborn

Intestinal obstruction is the most common abdominal emergency in the newborn period. Almost all babies with the conditions to be described will present in the first day or two of life. The single exception is malrotation with midgut volvulus. Even with this condition, however, babies will usually develop symptoms within the first month of life.

Neonatal bowel obstruction is usually classified as high or low [**Box 4.1**]. High or proximal obstruction involves the stomach, duodenum, jejunum, and proximal ileum; low or distal obstruction involves the distal ileum and colon. Obviously there is no precise location after which a "high" obstruction becomes "low." By the end of this section, however, it should be clear why such a seemingly vague classification is not only necessary but also extraordinarily useful.

The presentation of both types of obstruction may be identical. Babies can present with vomiting that is often bilious, abdominal distention, delayed or absent passage of meconium, or poor feeding. Fortunately, the distinction between high and low obstruction can almost always be made from a single abdominal radiograph. Air is an excellent contrast medium. Air is swallowed at birth and either passes out the other end of the GI tract or stops at the point of obstruction. Neonates with a high obstruction will have one, two, or a few air-filled dilated bowel loops, and those with a low obstruction will have many [**Fig. 4.1**]. This distinction is critical because virtually all babies with a high obstruction need surgery. Babies with low obstruction initially need a contrast enema. The enema will usually yield a specific diagnosis and, in some cases, may be therapeutic.

Low Intestinal Obstruction

As stated earlier, all newborns with signs and symptoms of intestinal obstruction need an abdominal radiograph. To the request frequently made of the radiologist, "We have a newborn with bilious vomiting and would like an upper GI series to rule out malrotation," the appropriate response is, "Let's start with a plain radiograph. After that, we will decide which study is indicated." If the radiograph demonstrates multiple dilated bowel loops, the baby may have a low or distal obstruction and needs an enema, not an upper GI. The exact level of the obstruction, whether in the distal small bowel or the colon, cannot be determined from the radiograph alone. The contrast enema will be definitive.

BOX 4.1   Differential Diagnosis of Bowel Obstruction in a Neonate

HIGH OBSTRUCTION

Duodenal atresia
Duodenal stenosis
Duodenal web
Annular pancreas
Malrotation with midgut volvulus
Jejunoileal atresia

LOW OBSTRUCTION

Hirschsprung disease
Small left colon/meconium plug syndrome
Colonic atresia
Meconium ileus
Ileal atresia
Anorectal malformation

The enema should be performed with water-soluble contrast material. We use a relatively dilute ionic agent such as that used for cystography. There is no need for more expensive nonionic agents or for barium because we are rarely interested in mucosal detail in newborns. Babies with meconium plug/small left colon syndrome or meconium ileus (discussed later) may actually benefit from a water-soluble enema. Further, in our experience, the use of barium as a diagnostic agent actually *decreases* the chance of subsequent successful therapeutic reduction of meconium ileus. The diagnostic enema should be performed with a small-caliber tube barely inserted into the rectum so that very distal pathology is not missed.

The differential diagnosis of low obstruction is limited [**Box 4.1**]. Three conditions involve the colon: Hirschsprung disease, small left colon/meconium plug syndrome, and colonic atresia. Two conditions involve the distal ileum: meconium ileus and ileal atresia. A radiologist may spend many years in a busy pediatric hospital and see only these conditions.

Anorectal malformations such as imperforate anus may, of course, cause low obstruction, although the diagnosis should be clinically obvious. Preoperative imaging in these patients is usually unnecessary. Anorectal malformations are discussed at the end of this section.

The crucial differential diagnostic finding on the contrast enema is the presence or absence of a microcolon. A microcolon is simply a colon of very small caliber. The entire colon must be small, not just a part of it. The assessment of the colon as "small" or "micro" is necessarily subjective and requires some experience [**Fig. 4.8**]. A microcolon is an unused colon. The caliber of the postnatal colon depends on the amount of succus entericus which reaches it. If little or no succus reaches the colon, it will be of small caliber. If there is a proximal small bowel obstruction such as a duodenal atresia, the colon will be of normal caliber because the small bowel between the atresia and the colon is of sufficient length to produce a normal amount of succus. Thus with rare exceptions, a newborn with a microcolon *must* have a high-grade distal small-bowel obstruction: for all practical purposes, ileal atresia or meconium ileus. There are two exceptions to this rule: total colonic Hirschsprung disease (discussed later) and extreme prematurity. All very premature

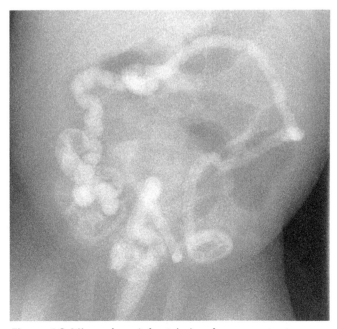

Figure 4.8 Microcolon. A frontal view from a contrast enema shows a colon that is diffusely small in caliber. The baby was diagnosed with meconium ileus.

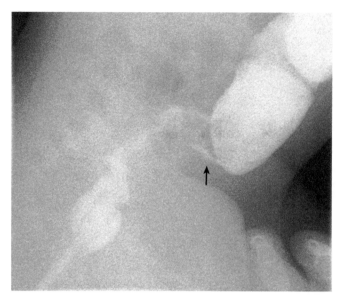

Figure 4.9 Hirschsprung disease. A lateral view from a contrast enema demonstrates a transition zone (*arrow*) from the narrow, aganglionic rectum to the larger, normally innervated sigmoid colon.

infants have microcolons related to underdevelopment. A contrast enema in these tiniest of babies rarely yields any useful information.

Hirschsprung Disease

Hirschsprung disease is the congenital absence of intestinal intramural ganglion cells resulting in failure of colonic relaxation and subsequent bowel obstruction. The aganglionic segment of bowel is continuous, extending proximally from the anus without "skip areas."

Hirschsprung disease affects boys more than girls. It is usually not inherited, except in the relatively rare total colonic or total intestinal varieties. With the exception of trisomy 21, it is not usually associated with other anomalies.

Abdominal radiographs in newborns with Hirschsprung disease will show the typical pattern of low bowel obstruction. As in all newborns with presumed low obstruction, a contrast enema is the next step. The classic finding on the enema is a "transition zone" from nondilated, aganglionic distal bowel to relatively distended, normally innervated proximal bowel [**Fig. 4.9**]. This transition zone will be best demonstrated on the lateral view, particularly in the phase of early filling. In most babies with Hirschsprung disease, the transition zone is gradual rather than abrupt, and thus may be relatively subtle.

The most common zone of transition on a contrast enema is the rectosigmoid colon; this is also the most common histopathologic zone of transition. The correlation between the radiologic and pathologic transition zones is quite good, but far from perfect. Intraoperative biopsy is necessary to document the absence of ganglion cells before proceeding to definitive treatment.

A helpful concept to keep in mind is the so-called rectosigmoid index. On a normal examination, the diameter of the rectum should be greater than the diameter of the sigmoid on all views. Thus the ratio of the diameter of the rectum to that of the sigmoid (the rectosigmoid index) should be greater than 1. In Hirschsprung disease, the index is reversed and the sigmoid is larger than the rectum [**Fig. 4.10**]. Attention to this simple observation will prevent many missed diagnoses of Hirschsprung disease.

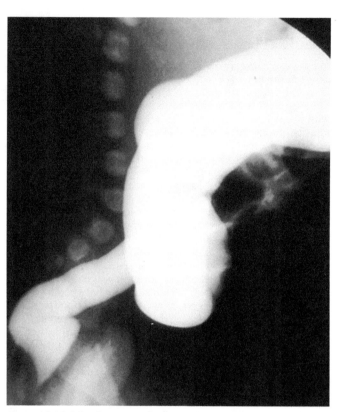

Figure 4.10 Hirschsprung disease. A lateral view from a contrast enema shows an abnormal rectosigmoid index. The diameter of the sigmoid colon is larger than that of the rectum.

An additional fluoroscopic finding in Hirschsprung disease is a "sawtooth" appearance to the rectum related to irregular contractions in the aganglionic segment. Delayed evacuation of contrast material after the enema may also be noted. These findings are much less sensitive and specific than the transition zone. A small percentage of babies may present with clinical and imaging findings of enterocolitis, which may be severe.

In the rare patient with total colonic or total intestinal Hirschsprung disease, the findings on enema are variable and may include a true transition zone, in which the radiologic transition zone corresponds to the pathologic transition zone, a pseudotransition zone in which the radiologic and pathologic transition zones do not correspond, a short colon, or a microcolon.

Infrequently, the enema in a baby with Hirschsprung disease may be normal. Notably, this is the only condition that causes low bowel obstruction in which the enema may be normal. Thus any baby with a low obstruction and a normal enema should be presumed to have Hirschsprung disease until proven otherwise by biopsy.

Meconium Plug/Small Left Colon Syndrome

The cause of meconium plug syndrome, also called small left colon syndrome, is unknown. It is usually attributed to functional immaturity of the colon. There is an increased incidence in babies whose mothers have diabetes or have received magnesium sulfate for eclampsia. However, many affected babies have no identifiable risk factors. They present with low obstruction, but often have less severe symptoms than babies with other causes of bowel obstruction.

The contrast enema will demonstrate a normal-caliber rectum, a small-caliber sigmoid and descending colon, and an abrupt transition zone at the splenic flexure to a relatively distended

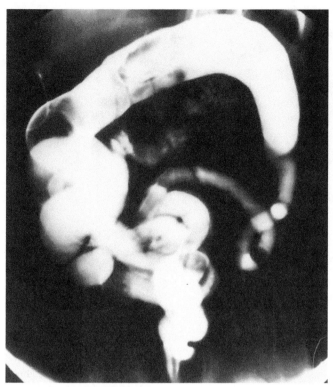

Figure 4.11 Small left colon syndrome. A frontal view from a contrast enema shows a small sigmoid colon and descending colon, with a transition point near the splenic flexure to a dilated transverse and ascending colon. The rectum is notably normal in caliber.

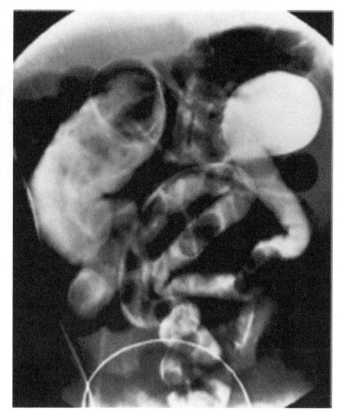

Figure 4.12 Hirschsprung disease. A frontal image from a contrast enema shows that the rectum is of the same caliber as the small left colon. In small left colon syndrome, the rectum is of normal caliber.

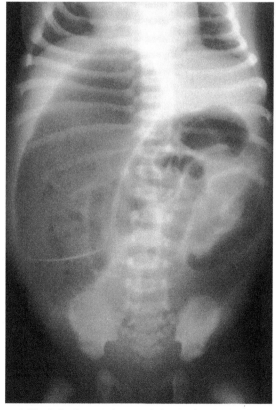

Figure 4.13 Colonic atresia. An abdominal radiograph demonstrates a disproportionally dilated loop of bowel in the right hemiabdomen at the point of obstruction.

transverse colon [**Fig. 4.11**]. It cannot be stressed enough that the radiologist cannot make the diagnosis of meconium plug/small left colon syndrome in the absence of these findings. The rectum should be of normal caliber. If the rectum is as small as the left colon, Hirschsprung disease should be suspected [**Fig. 4.12**]. The transition zone must be at the splenic flexure; a transition zone elsewhere suggests Hirschsprung disease. Meconium "plugs" may or may not be present. The amount of meconium in the colon of a newborn is a finding that is rarely of diagnostic value. It bears repeating that with a microcolon, the entire colon, not just the left colon, is small.

Many babies with functional immaturity will improve after the enema, and may in fact even pass the classic "meconium plug" on the fluoroscopy table. If the baby does not improve, a rectal biopsy should be performed to exclude Hirschsprung disease.

Colonic Atresia

Colonic atresia, like jejunoileal atresia, is caused by a prenatal vascular insult. Notably, newborns with colonic atresia may have additional areas of atresia.

Radiographs show a low bowel obstruction, often with a disproportionately dilated loop of bowel just proximal to the atretic segment [**Fig. 4.13**]. When a radiograph demonstrates such a loop in a baby with obstruction at any level, an atresia should be suspected. Contrast enema shows a microcolon distal to an abrupt transition at the level of the atresia.

Meconium Ileus

Meconium ileus is a bowel obstruction seen almost exclusively in babies with CF. It is caused by inspissation of abnormally viscous meconium in the terminal ileum. The diagnosis is often

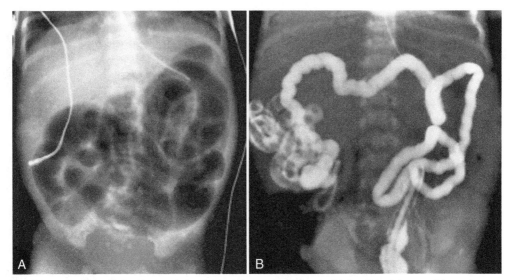

Figure 4.14 Meconium ileus. A, An abdominal radiograph shows multiple dilated loops of bowel suggesting a low obstruction. **B,** A frontal view from a contrast enema demonstrates a microcolon. Meconium pellets are noted in a nondilated terminal ileum, diagnostic of meconium ileus.

made prenatally. The mother of a fetus found to have many dilated bowel loops on prenatal ultrasound may be tested for mutations causing CF. If the diagnosis is not made prenatally, meconium ileus remains in the differential diagnosis in a newborn with a low bowel obstruction. The finding of meconium ileus on enema should prompt an evaluation for CF.

Contrast enema shows a microcolon. As noted earlier, the finding of a microcolon essentially limits the differential diagnosis to either meconium ileus or ileal atresia. The presence of filling defects (pellets of abnormal meconium) impacted in a nondilated terminal ileum with progressive dilatation of the proximal small bowel is diagnostic of meconium ileus [**Fig. 4.14**].

In 30% to 50% of newborns, meconium ileus may be "complicated." In these babies, the massively dilated distal small bowel can twist upon itself, causing a segmental volvulus that may ultimately lead to ischemia and perforation. When perforation occurs, meconium spills into the peritoneal cavity and almost immediately calcifies. Radiographs show evidence of meconium peritonitis, with sheets of calcification around the liver, along the flanks, and in the deep pelvis [**Fig. 4.5**]. Meconium peritonitis may notably occur in conditions other than meconium ileus when bowel perforation has occurred. Infrequently, a mass of dead bowel, fluid, and debris may form a meconium pseudocyst, the rim of which may calcify [**Fig. 4.6**]. In some patients, a gasless abdomen may be seen. Unfortunately, radiographs in babies with complicated meconium ileus may in some cases be indistinguishable from those with uncomplicated meconium ileus.

Once a diagnosis of meconium ileus is made, the radiologist may be asked to perform a therapeutic contrast enema. Even though the technique of hydrostatic reduction with Gastrografin was introduced in 1969, there is still no consensus about the best way to do it. We have found that Gastrografin is more effective than other water-soluble agents. Notably, half-strength Gastrografin works just as well as full strength. Gastrografin is extremely hyperosmolar, and it presumably works by pulling water into the bowel and breaking up inspissated meconium. In our experience, the greatest predictor of failure of the procedure is a prior diagnostic enema with barium. This, as noted earlier, is one of the reasons for performing all diagnostic enemas in newborns with water-soluble contrast material. The goal of the radiologist should be to reflux contrast into the dilated distal small bowel. In babies who are stable and in

whom the procedure appears to be working, several attempts can safely be made.

It cannot be stressed enough that reduction is a procedure that should be performed only by experienced radiologists in a center with experienced neonatologists. Even dilute Gastrografin is extremely hyperosmolar and may cause fluid shifts resulting in severe dehydration, electrolyte abnormalities, and even death. As indicated earlier, repeated attempts should be made only in babies who are clinically stable and in whom some therapeutic progress is being made. A lack of progress with reduction may imply that the baby has complicated meconium ileus. In babies with uncomplicated meconium ileus, the procedure is often successful and perforation is rare.

Ileal Atresia

Ileal atresia may be caused by either ischemic injury from an in utero vascular accident or mechanical obstruction, as may be seen with in utero volvulus related to meconium ileus. Radiographs show a low bowel obstruction, often with a disproportionately dilated loop of bowel. Contrast enema shows a microcolon. Unlike meconium ileus, the point of obstruction is not necessarily in the terminal ileum. If one is lucky enough to reflux beyond the ileocecal valve on contrast enema, the postatretic ileum will be of small caliber to the point of the obstruction [**Fig. 4.15**].

Anorectal Malformation

Anorectal malformation, also commonly though inaccurately called *imperforate anus,* is likely the result of abnormal separation of genitourinary (GU) and hindgut structures in fetal life. This failure of separation results in an atresia of the rectum and a variable persistent communication between the GU and GI systems. This is analogous to the failure of separation of the respiratory and GI systems that results in EA and TEF (to be described).

Classification of the malformation is based on the position of the atretic rectum in relation to the levator sling. Atresias ending above the levator sling are classified as "high," and those ending below it as "low." The lesion may be further classified according to the anatomy of the termination. In most infants with high lesions, the atretic rectum ends in the GU tract. In boys, this is usually in the posterior urethra; in girls, it is typically in the

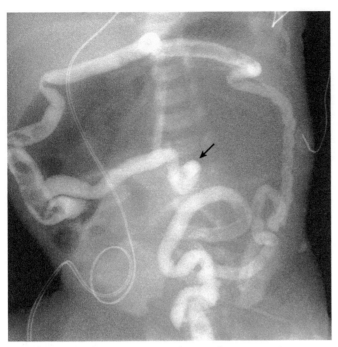

Figure 4.15 Ileal atresia. A frontal image from a contrast enema shows a microcolon with reflux into small-caliber distal ileum to the level of the atresia (*arrow*). Note the dilated, unopacified bowel proximal to the atresia. Meconium is absent from the terminal ileum, excluding a diagnosis of meconium ileus.

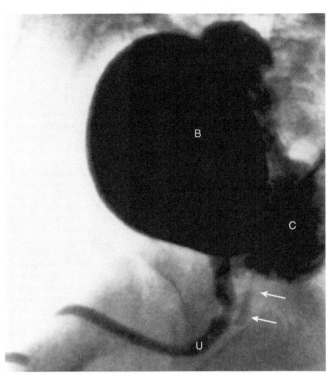

Figure 4.16 Imperforate anus. A lateral view from a contrast study with opacification of both the bladder (*B*) and the colon (*C*) shows communication between the posterior urethra (*U*) and the rectum (*arrows*) in a boy with imperforate anus.

vagina. In low lesions, there is usually a visible perineal orifice which may be stenotic or covered ("true" imperforate anus). There is not usually a communication with the GU tract.

The role of preoperative imaging is limited. Associated anomalies of the kidneys and spine are relatively common, and screening for these anomalies should be performed. After colostomy, the expected fistula to the urethra in boys may be delineated by a contrast study [**Fig. 4.16**]. In girls, the communication is usually clinically obvious. Magnetic resonance imaging (MRI) can clearly define the musculature of the pelvic floor.

High Intestinal Obstruction

Obstruction of the Stomach

Congenital obstruction of the stomach, as may be seen in microgastria or pyloric atresia, is rare. Pyloric stenosis, although an extremely common cause of gastric outlet obstruction in infancy, almost never occurs in newborns younger than 1 week. A newborn with a dilated stomach is much more likely to have an obstruction of the duodenum than of the stomach.

Duodenal Obstruction

The duodenum is the most common site of intestinal atresia. Duodenal atresia is more common than duodenal stenosis or duodenal web. The cause of all three is notably the same: a failure of the solid fetal duodenum to recanalize. About 30% of infants with duodenal obstruction have trisomy 21.

Although duodenal atresia leads to complete duodenal obstruction, duodenal stenosis or web may be associated with partial or complete obstruction. An annular pancreas may be associated with duodenal atresia, stenosis, or web. Annular pancreas is due to a persistence of the embryonic ventral portion of pancreas, which encircles the second portion of the duodenum and contributes to obstruction.

Most infants with duodenal obstruction present with bilious vomiting within hours of birth because the site of obstruction in the setting of duodenal atresia, stenosis, or web is typically just distal to the ampulla of Vater. The diagnosis of duodenal atresia can usually be made from the abdominal radiograph alone. A "double bubble" is seen, reflecting air within a dilated stomach and proximal duodenum [**Fig. 4.17**]. If distal gas is absent, duodenal atresia is the diagnosis. If distal gas is present, the diagnosis is usually duodenal stenosis or web, but importantly may also be malrotation with midgut volvulus (to be described). In all cases, surgery is usually the next step after radiographs, with the specific diagnosis made in the operating room.

There is never a reason to administer contrast from above to a baby with a double bubble and no distal air on radiographs because a complete obstruction is clear. In this setting, air is an excellent contrast medium. In babies with partial obstruction, in contrast, the surgeon may request an upper GI series to differentiate duodenal stenosis or web from midgut volvulus. This distinction is key because duodenal stenosis and web do not require immediate surgery, whereas midgut volvulus is a surgical emergency. Many surgeons also request a contrast enema to exclude additional distal atresia(s).

On the upper GI of an infant with duodenal stenosis, contrast will outline a narrowing in the second portion of the duodenum [**Fig. 4.18**]. If a duodenal web is present, it may appear as a thin, curvilinear filling defect in the lumen of the second portion of the duodenum [**Fig. 4.19**]. Frequently, in babies with stenosis or web, the upper GI will simply demonstrate partial or complete duodenal obstruction. It is critically important to remember that obstruction caused by duodenal atresia, stenosis, or web occurs in the *second* portion of the duodenum. In contrast, obstruction caused by midgut volvulus occurs in the *third* portion.

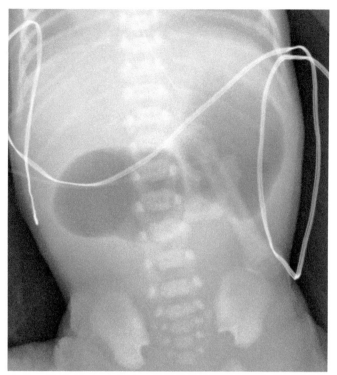

Figure 4.17 Duodenal atresia. An abdominal radiograph demonstrating a "double bubble," with a dilated stomach and proximal duodenum. A lack of distal bowel gas is noted.

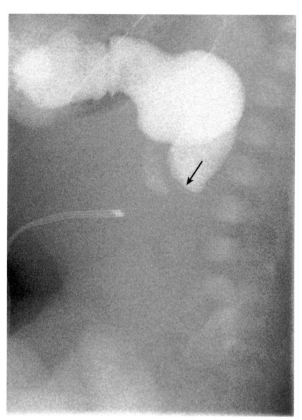

Figure 4.19 Duodenal web. A right lateral decubitus image from an upper gastrointestinal series demonstrates a curvilinear filling defect (*arrow*) in the second portion of the duodenum.

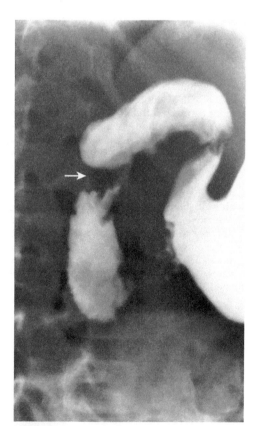

Figure 4.18 Duodenal stenosis. An anteroposterior image from an upper gastrointestinal series shows a focal narrowing (*arrow*) in the second portion of the duodenum.

Malrotation

Malrotation with midgut volvulus is the most important cause of duodenal obstruction, and the only one that is a surgical emergency. During normal fetal development, bowel loops rotate into a position such that the mesentery has a long pedicle extending from the left upper quadrant at the ligament of Treitz to the right lower quadrant at the cecum. If this process is arrested at any point, bowel loops will be malpositioned and consequently abnormally fixed with a shorter mesenteric root [**Fig. 4.20**]. The possibility of twisting around this shorter pedicle then exists. The twisting of abnormally fixed intestines around a short mesentery is referred to as midgut volvulus. The phrase *midgut volvulus* should not be used interchangeably with the more general term *volvulus*, which simply means the twisting of a viscus, hollow or otherwise. Midgut volvulus is a specific surgical and radiologic entity in children with malrotation and abnormal fixation in which the entire midgut twists about the axis of the superior mesenteric artery (SMA). This results first in obstruction of the duodenum (hence the classic symptom of bilious vomiting) and second in obstruction of the mesenteric vessels, ultimately leading to ischemia and bowel necrosis.

Most patients with midgut volvulus present in the first month of life, and often in the first week of life. One may, however, present at any age. Vomiting is almost always present and is often bilious. Babies may be entirely well, or critically ill in cases of vascular occlusion.

Radiographs in patients with midgut volvulus reflect the underlying pathologic anatomy. Patients with an early or intermittent twist will usually have normal radiographs. Even with normal radiographs, all babies with bilious vomiting need an upper GI series. Radiographs in babies with higher degrees of duodenal obstruction may demonstrate gastric outlet

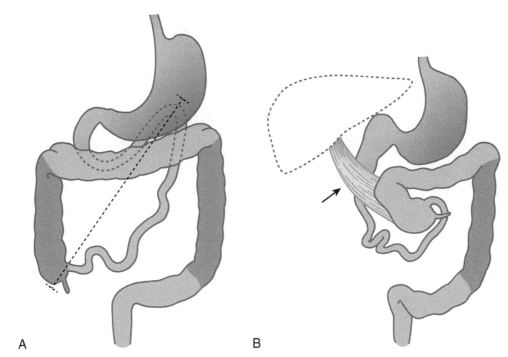

Figure 4.20 Schematic representations of normal fixation (*stippled*) (**A**) and malpositioned intestinal tract (**B**). Note the Ladd bands (*arrow*) extending from the malpositioned cecum to the liver, traversing the duodenum.

obstruction or complete or incomplete duodenal obstruction. In children with ischemia, radiographs may demonstrate an ileus pattern or even a gasless abdomen.

Patients with abnormal mesenteric fixation may have abnormal intraperitoneal fibrous bands called *Ladd bands* [**Fig. 4.20**]. Ladd bands usually extend from the malpositioned cecum across the duodenum and attach to the liver. Bands can entrap and obstruct the duodenum. Any obstruction of the third portion of the duodenum, however, should be considered a midgut volvulus and a surgical emergency; the diagnosis of Ladd bands is the job of the surgeon, not the radiologist.

The upper GI remains the study of choice in patients with suspected malrotation. It is simple, safe, and highly sensitive and specific. Barium is the contrast agent of choice and may be most efficiently introduced via a nasogastric (NG) tube in sick children. Attention must be paid to detail. Views of the DJJ should be obtained in both anteroposterior (AP) and lateral projections, and care must be taken to ensure that on the AP view the patient is absolutely straight on the fluoroscopy table. Malrotation is diagnosed on an upper GI when the DJJ is *not* to the left of a left-sided spinous pedicle and/or at the level of the duodenal bulb [**Fig. 4.21**]. Malposition of the DJJ implies abnormal fixation. If there is a volvulus, passage of contrast will be completely or incompletely obstructed at the third portion of the duodenum in the midline. Rarely, the classic "corkscrew" appearance of a volvulus will be seen [**Fig. 4.22**].

If there is any uncertainty about the position of the DJJ on an upper GI series, contrast should be followed to the cecum. With malrotation, the jejunum is usually found on the right, and the cecum is higher and more midline than normal. However, in 20% of patients with malrotation, the cecum is normally positioned. Therefore the most specific sign of malrotation is the malpositioned DJJ. A point worth mentioning is that in children with distended bowel, the DJJ can be pushed inferiorly, leading to pseudomalrotation.

Recently cross-sectional imaging, particularly ultrasound, has been more frequently used in the evaluation of rotational anomalies. Identifying the position of the SMA and superior mesenteric vein (SMV) on ultrasound can aid in the diagnosis of malrotation.

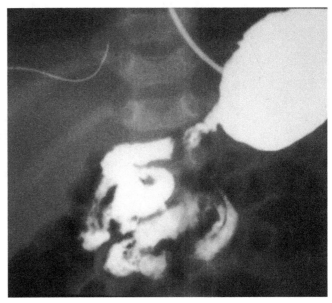

Figure 4.21 Malrotation. An anteroposterior image from an abnormal upper gastrointestinal series shows the duodenojejunal junction in the midline.

Most patients with malrotation have an inverted SMA/SMV relationship, with the SMA on the right and the SMV on the left (the opposite of the normal relationship) [**Fig. 4.23**]. However, in about one-third of patients with malrotation, the SMA/SMV relationship is notably normal.

Jejunal or Proximal Ileal Obstruction

Jejunoileal atresia, unlike duodenal atresia, is caused by an in utero vascular accident. Infants with jejunal or proximal ileal atresia present with bilious vomiting. Radiographs show a few dilated loops of bowel, more than seen in the setting of duodenal

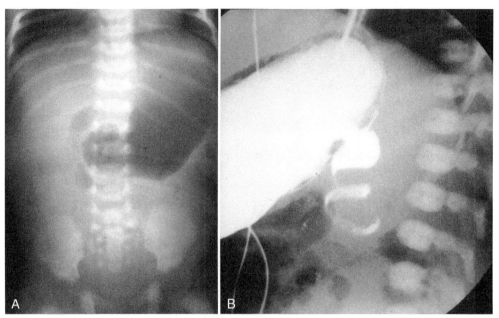

Figure 4.22 **Midgut volvulus. A,** An abdominal radiograph shows a dilated stomach and proximal duodenum. **B,** A lateral view from an upper gastrointestinal series demonstrates the "corkscrew" appearance of a midgut volvulus.

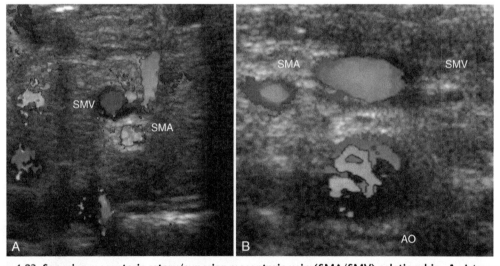

Figure 4.23 **Superior mesenteric artery/superior mesenteric vein (SMA/SMV) relationship. A,** A transverse ultrasound image of the abdomen in a patient with normal bowel rotation shows the SMA on the left and the SMV on the right. **B,** A similarly acquired ultrasound image in a baby with malrotation shows reversal of the SMA/SMV relationship. The SMA is on the right and the SMV is on the left.

obstruction, but less than encountered with a low bowel obstruction. As is the case with atresia in other locations, there may be a disproportionately dilated loop of bowel just proximal to the level of the atresia [**Fig. 4.24**].

Patients suspected to have jejunal or proximal ileal atresia based on symptoms and radiographs can usually proceed directly to surgery. There is no role for contrast studies from above. A contrast enema may be performed in the preoperative setting to evaluate for additional sites of more distal atresia. An enema will show a relatively normal-caliber colon with a proximal jejunal atresia, but a microcolon with a more distal atresia.

Esophageal Atresia and Tracheoesophageal Fistula

EA is a common congenital anomaly. It results when the trachea and esophagus fail to separate normally in fetal life. In most cases, there is an atresia of the esophagus at the junction of its proximal and middle thirds, with a variable persistent communication with the trachea in the form of a TEF. By far the most common type of EA is atresia with a distal fistula, that is, a fistula from the distal (postatretic) esophagus to the trachea, usually around the carina. Other less common types include atresia without a fistula, atresia with a proximal or distal fistula (or both), or fistula without an atresia (H-type fistula) [**Fig. 4.25**]. About half of patients with EA have associated anomalies in the VACTERL spectrum (vertebral, anorectal, cardiac, tracheoesophageal, renal, limb). Of these, cardiac anomalies are the most common.

Today, EA is usually diagnosed prenatally. Polyhydramnios develops in utero because the fetus is unable to swallow amniotic fluid. In babies who are not diagnosed prenatally, EA will present shortly after birth with drooling, cyanosis, coughing and choking, and an inability to pass an NG tube. The postnatal

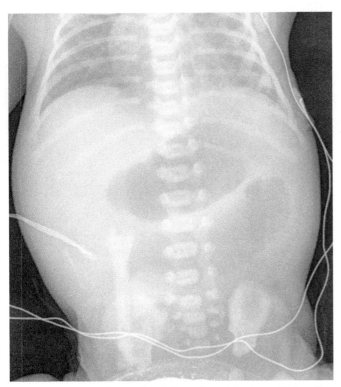

Figure 4.24 Jejunal atresia. A frontal supine abdominal radiograph demonstrates a few dilated loops of bowel, suggesting a jejunal obstruction.

radiologic diagnosis is made on chest radiograph with the finding of an NG tube coiled in the proximal esophageal pouch. The presence of bowel gas suggests there is a distal TEF [**Fig. 4.26**], whereas the absence of bowel gas indicates isolated EA.

Usually chest and abdominal radiographs alone are sufficient for the preoperative evaluation of babies with EA/TEF. Fluoroscopic studies ("pouch-o-grams") are reserved for challenging cases and are rarely requested. Postoperative imaging is of critical importance for the identification of postoperative complications such as anastomotic leaks, strictures, and recurrent fistulae. These studies are generally performed only in specialty centers.

A circumstance worthy of discussion is TEF without EA, the rare "H-type" TEF. Affected patients may present later in childhood with coughing and choking with feeding and recurrent episodes of pneumonia. Importantly, these symptoms are much more commonly related to aspiration or GE reflux, rather than the presence of a relatively rare H-type TEF. In our experience, most H-type fistulae are found during a modified barium swallow (videofluoroscopic swallowing study), which is also the study of choice for suspected swallowing dysfunction and aspiration. A standard barium esophagram with *adequate esophageal distention* will also usually be diagnostic, although not always. The diagnosis does *not* require the injection of contrast through an NG tube in the esophagus. The H-type fistula usually extends cephalad from the anterior wall of the esophagus to the trachea at the level of the thoracic inlet [**Fig. 4.27**].

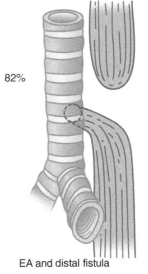
82%
EA and distal fistula

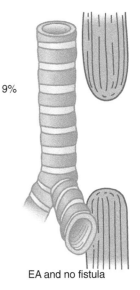
9%
EA and no fistula

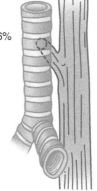
6%
No EA but "H" fistula

2%
EA and 2 fistulas

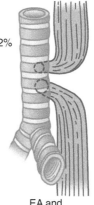
1%
EA and proximal fistula

Figure 4.25 An illustration of the types of esophageal atresia (EA) and tracheoesophageal fistula (TEF). The most common type is EA with a distal TEF; all other types are much less common.

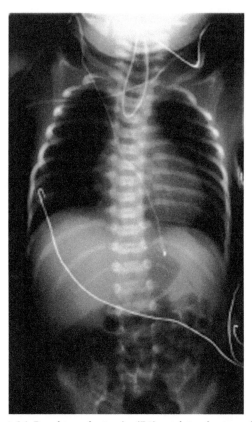

Figure 4.26 Esophageal atresia (EA) and tracheoesophageal fistula (TEF). An anteroposterior radiograph of the chest and abdomen shows a nasogastric tube coiled in the proximal esophageal pouch. There is air within the bowel, indicating the presence of a TEF.

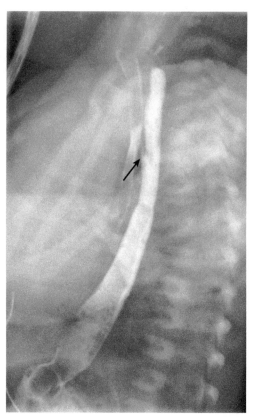

Figure 4.27 H-type tracheoesophageal fistula (TEF). A lateral view from an esophagram shows contrast opacifying the TEF (*arrow*).

Omphalocele and Gastroschisis

Omphalocele and gastroschisis are the most common congenital anomalies of the abdominal wall. The cause of each is quite distinct. Omphalocele is thought to arise from a developmental failure in the closure of the abdominal wall. This results in a midline defect into which any abdominal organ may herniate. The herniated organ(s) are covered by a sac of amnion and peritoneum. The umbilical cord inserts into these membranes at the apex of the omphalocele. The majority of babies with omphalocele have associated anomalies. Chromosomal abnormalities are common, as is heart disease. Omphalocele is also part of the Beckwith-Wiedemann syndrome.

Gastroschisis, in contrast, is probably the consequence of an in utero vascular accident that leads to a defect lateral to the umbilicus. The umbilicus itself is normal. With gastroschisis, it is usually exclusively bowel that herniates through the defect. Herniated bowel is not covered by a membrane and is, therefore, exposed to amniotic fluid. This direct contact in some way damages the bowel and may result in strictures or atresias. Unlike babies with omphalocele, those with gastroschisis typically do not have other congenital anomalies.

Other than screening the baby with omphalocele for associated anomalies, preoperative imaging is rarely obtained for these conditions. Postoperative contrast studies are frequently necessary and useful in children with a history of gastroschisis and abdominal complaints. Children with both conditions obviously and necessarily will have malrotation. Volvulus is rare, however, due to the inevitable adhesions.

Necrotizing Enterocolitis

NEC is the often severe entity that afflicts premature infants in neonatal intensive care units. Only 10% to 15% of cases of NEC occur in term or late preterm infants. In term infants, NEC may be associated with congenital heart disease or with Hirschsprung disease. Most cases of NEC occur in infants younger than 34 weeks gestational age. The age of onset of NEC is inversely proportional to gestational age at birth. Whereas babies born after 34 weeks gestation usually experience development of NEC in the first week or so of life, babies born before 34 weeks of gestation may not present until the second or third week of life.

The causes of NEC are not completely understood. This entity likely results from a complex interaction of multiple factors including microbes, an immature immune system and blood/gut barrier, and milk substrate (often associated with early feeding). The frequent occurrence of spatial and temporal clusters of cases of NEC suggests that microorganisms play a significant part in its pathogenesis. Notably, no specific or consistent microbe has been identified as playing a causative role. Although NEC may affect any part of the GI tract, it most commonly occurs in the distal ileum and right colon. The final common pathology in NEC is hemorrhagic/ischemic necrosis.

The presenting signs and symptoms of NEC are nonspecific: abdominal distention, feeding intolerance, vomiting, and blood in the stool. Multiorgan system failure and shock may rapidly ensue. The mortality rate from NEC may be as high as 40%.

The abdominal radiograph remains the indispensable initial study of choice for babies with suspected NEC. In babies who are more severely ill, a supine radiograph should be accompanied by a horizontal beam radiograph, either a cross-table lateral or left-side-down decubitus image, to evaluate for free air. The advantage of the cross-table lateral view is that it does not require moving the baby. However, free air may be more easily detected on a decubitus view.

The diagnosis of NEC is made based on clinical signs and symptoms as well as radiographic findings. Unfortunately, the radiographic findings may be as nonspecific as the clinical findings, particularly in early or suspected NEC. The most common radiographic finding in babies with NEC is diffuse gaseous distention of the bowel. Notably, most normal babies have more intestinal air than typically seen in older children and particularly in adults. The reasons for this relative abundance of air should not be surprising. Babies suck in air as they feed from the breast or bottle, and are usually unhappy and crying while they are submitting to radiographs. In healthy babies, air should be evenly distributed throughout the abdomen in a so-called polygonal pattern, without areas devoid of gas and without asymmetrically focally dilated loops [**Fig. 4.28**]. In babies who are significantly distended, including babies with NEC, a uniform distribution of bowel gas may be preserved. Most premature babies in the neonatal intensive care unit with diffuse gaseous distension of the bowel do not have NEC. Most simply have intestinal dysmotility, an almost invariable consequence of prematurity. Babies treated with continuous positive airway pressure are also frequently distended. A somewhat more specific sign of early NEC is distension with loss of the normal symmetrical distribution of gas, most likely related to focal inflammation [**Fig. 4.29**]. The persistence of a single dilated loop for hours to days ("fixed loop sign") may be a manifestation of more advanced NEC [**Fig. 4.30**]. Needless to say, even such asymmetrical distension is a nonspecific finding.

In the appropriate clinical setting the presence of intramural gas, or pneumatosis intestinalis, is considered pathognomic of

NEC. The reported incidence of pneumatosis varies widely. It probably occurs in the majority of cases of NEC, although certainly not in all. The amount and distribution of pneumatosis does not necessarily correlate with the clinical severity of NEC. It is probably true, however, that the presence of extensive pneumatosis on the initial radiograph obtained for suspected NEC is an ominous prognostic sign. To further complicate matters, the resolution of pneumatosis does not always imply or accompany an improvement in the patient's clinical condition.

Pneumatosis may involve any portion of the GI tract, but it is most frequently seen in the distal small bowel and the colon. The intramural gas may be submucosal, where it has a "bubbly" or cystic appearance, or subserosal, where it has a linear configuration [**Fig. 4.31**]. Submucosal gas may be confused with stool. In babies who have not been fed, a "bubbly" appearance is most likely due to pneumatosis, although the distinction between intramural air and stool is often more difficult than generally admitted.

Ultrasound may detect small amounts of intramural air that are not evident on plain radiographs. The air is echogenic and may give the bowel wall a speckled appearance. There is generally an indistinct or "dirty" shadow. Ultrasound may be useful when suspicion for NEC is high and radiographs are nonspecific.

The other virtually pathognomonic sign of NEC is portal venous gas. It may be present in up to one third of cases and is usually, although not invariably, associated with advanced disease. On radiographs, it appears as branching lucencies projecting over the liver [**Fig. 4.32**]. Portal venous gas is often transient. Its "disappearance" on an abdominal radiograph does not necessarily imply clinical improvement. As is the case with pneumatosis, portal venous gas may occasionally be more evident on ultrasound, seen as hyperechoic foci within the smaller portal venous branches.

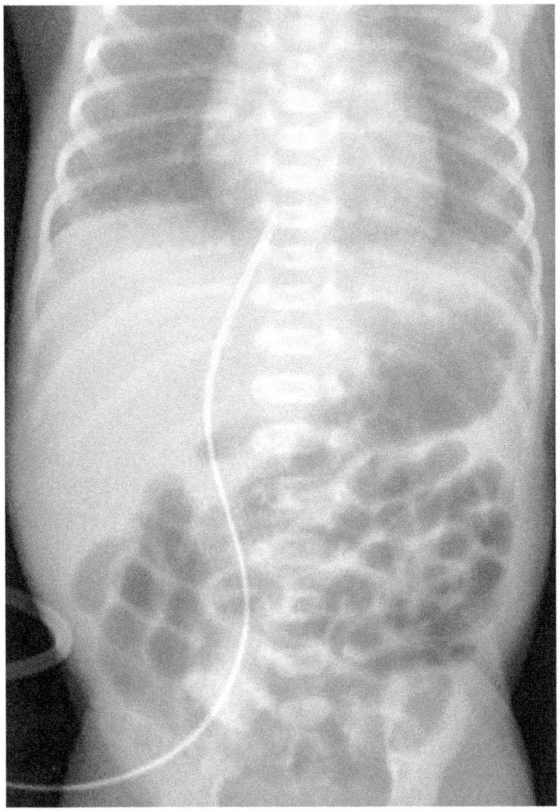

Figure 4.28 Normal bowel gas pattern in a neonate. An abdominal radiograph shows a uniform distribution of air throughout the bowel. An umbilical venous catheter is noted terminating at the inferior vena cava–right atrial junction.

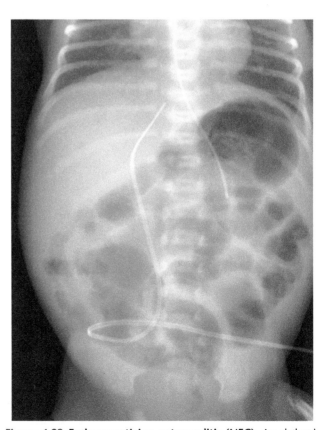

Figure 4.29 Early necrotizing enterocolitis (NEC). An abdominal radiograph shows an asymmetric distribution of bowel gas.

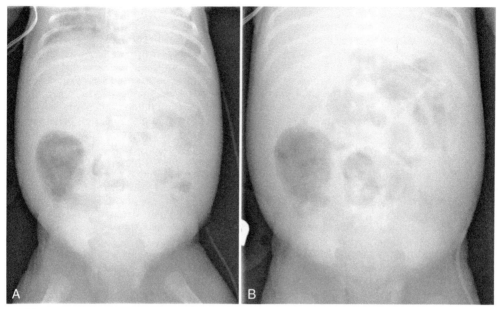

Figure 4.30 Necrotizing enterocolitis (NEC). A, An abdominal radiograph shows an asymmetric bowel gas pattern with a dilated loop of bowel in the right hemiabdomen. **B,** Several days later, this "fixed loop" of dilated bowel remains, appearing unchanged.

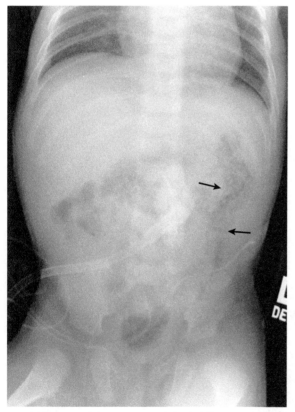

Figure 4.31 Necrotizing enterocolitis (NEC). Pneumatosis. An abdominal radiograph shows "bubbly" lucencies in a linear pattern in the left hemiabdomen (*arrows*), indicating intramural gas.

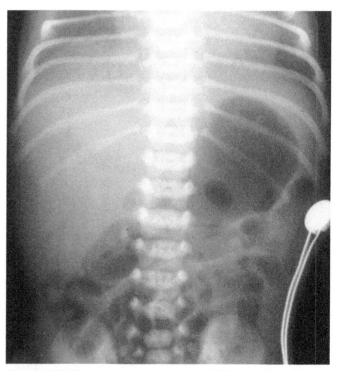

Figure 4.32 Necrotizing enterocolitis (NEC). Portal venous gas. An abdominal radiograph shows branching lucencies over the liver.

The morbidity and mortality of NEC is due to hemorrhagic/ischemic necrosis, which may result in intestinal perforation, sepsis, and shock. The challenge for the neonatologist and the radiologist is to identify babies in whom perforation is imminent and in whom surgery may prevent peritonitis. At the very least,

we hope to identify all babies in whom perforation has occurred. In these cases, surgery is absolutely necessary and potentially lifesaving. Unfortunately, just as the radiographic signs of early NEC are nonspecific, the late signs are also either nonspecific or relatively insensitive. It should be apparent by now that the *N* in NEC is sometimes thought to stand for "nonspecific."

The only universally accepted indication for surgery is free intraperitoneal air. In most settings, horizontal beam radiographs are exquisitely sensitive for the detection of free air. However, only half to three quarters of babies with NEC and perforation

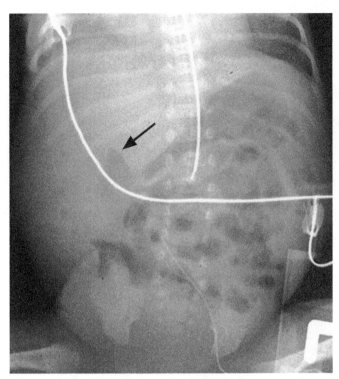

Figure 4.33 Necrotizing enterocolitis (NEC). Free air. A frontal supine abdominal radiograph demonstrates a triangular lucency in the right upper quadrant reflecting air in Morison's pouch (*arrow*) in the setting of perforation.

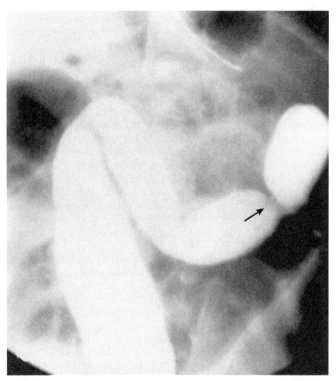

Figure 4.34 Necrotizing enterocolitis (NEC). Stricture. A frontal image from a contrast enema shows a focal narrowing in the descending colon (*arrow*) consistent with a stricture.

will have visible free air, even on lateral decubitus or cross-table lateral radiographs.

It is important to be able to identify free air on a supine radiograph. This may be the only view obtained in infants when there is clinical concern for NEC, but suspicion for perforation is not high. Large amounts of free air are generally easy to see, giving an overall lucency to the abdomen and outlining such structures as the falciform ligament ("football sign") [**Fig. 4.4**]. Smaller amounts of free air may collect in Morison's pouch and present as a triangular lucency in the right upper quadrant on radiographs [**Fig. 4.33**]. It is probably good practice to assume that any air present on a supine radiograph that cannot confidently be localized to a hollow viscus is free air until proven otherwise. Such proof is complicated by the fact that not all "free" air will rise above the liver with left lateral decubitus positioning or collect anteriorly on cross-table lateral radiographs. Air seen on both sides of the bowel wall ("Rigler sign") [**Fig. 4.4**] is notoriously unreliable in small babies with abdominal distension because the multiple air–bowel interfaces may give a misleading impression of intraluminal and extraluminal air.

Other signs sometimes thought to be predictive of perforation or impending perforation are ascites (as seen on ultrasound) or the "fixed loop sign" [**Fig. 4.30**] discussed earlier. Rarely will a surgeon intervene without the definitive presence of free air.

In summary, the most common radiographic finding in early or suspected NEC is diffuse gaseous distention of bowel. This finding is nonspecific and is seen in many premature infants who do not have and will not experience development of NEC. The pathognomic signs of NEC are pneumatosis intestinalis and portal venous gas. The presence of pneumatosis, unless extensive, is not always an indication of advanced disease, and its disappearance does not always imply improvement. Portal venous gas is usually an indicator of severe disease, but it is present in a minority of cases and is often transient. The only specific sign of perforation is free air, but free air is not always

detectable, even on horizontal beam radiographs. Ultrasound is more sensitive for the detection of pneumatosis and portal venous gas, but it remains to be seen whether use of this modality will have any impact on clinical outcomes of babies with NEC.

The most important complications of NEC are intestinal strictures and short gut syndrome. The latter results from extensive bowel resection and is an increasingly common and important problem in babies who survive NEC. Strictures occur in about 20% of babies who have had medical or surgical NEC. Strictures may be found anywhere in the intestine, but most occur in the left colon near the splenic flexure. Patients typically present weeks to months after their episode(s) of NEC with obstruction, which may only be clinically evident with feeding. Babies with suspected strictures related to NEC should undergo a contrast enema [**Fig. 4.34**].

In addition to NEC, extremely premature infants are at risk for isolated intestinal perforation. The perforation occurs in the terminal ileum, and it is not associated with other areas of inflammation. Patients usually present in the first week of life with pneumoperitoneum without signs of systemic disease. This may progress to peritonitis, sepsis, and death in up to 40% of cases. There is an increased incidence in patients who have been treated with indomethacin (Indocin) for patent ductus arteriosus.

THE INFANT AND YOUNG CHILD

Hypertrophic Pyloric Stenosis

In hypertrophic pyloric stenosis (HPS), hyperplasia and hypertrophy of the circular muscle of the pylorus result in thickening and elongation of the pyloric channel. This eventually leads to gastric outlet obstruction. HPS is a very common cause of vomiting in babies who are 2 to 6 weeks old, but only rarely occurs before 1 week or after 3 months of age. HPS is more common in boys than in girls, and there is a strong hereditary predisposition. Its cause is unknown.

Infants with HPS usually present with persistent, forceful, nonbilious vomiting often described as "projectile." Ultrasound is the study of choice in children with suspected HPS. Focused examination of the right upper quadrant is performed using a high-frequency linear transducer. The gallbladder is used as a landmark for the antropyloric region of the stomach. This technique will usually readily demonstrate the hypoechoic thickened muscularis of the pylorus which defines HPS. Muscle thickness of 3 mm or greater as measured on a longitudinal view of the midline of the pylorus is diagnostic of HPS [**Fig. 4.35**]. The elongated pyloric channel is also routinely measured and is generally greater than 16 mm in HPS. Channel length is noted to be less specific than muscle thickness, and the diagnosis should never be made unless the muscle thickness is 3 mm or greater.

Although the diagnosis of HPS is usually straightforward, there are some potential pitfalls. If the stomach is empty, giving the baby a small bottle of sugar water can facilitate visualization of the pylorus. However, if the stomach is overdistended, the pylorus can sometimes be difficult to locate because it may be more posteriorly directed than expected. Changing patient position may help, as may NG tube decompression of the stomach. Transient pylorospasm can mimic a thickened pylorus; although during real-time observation, pyloric channel opening with passage of gastric contents into the duodenum excludes a diagnosis of HPS.

Even though the treatment for HPS is surgery, it is not a surgical emergency. If there is any doubt as to the diagnosis of HPS, an infant with borderline pyloric thickness can be observed clinically and reimaged in a few days.

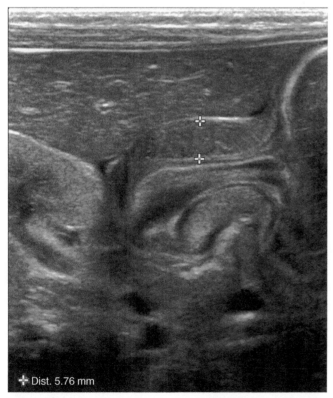

Dist. 5.76 mm

Figure 4.35 Hypertrophic pyloric stenosis (HPS). A longitudinal sonographic image through the pylorus shows abnormal thickening of the pyloric musculature. The calipers measure the muscular wall thickness from the serosa to the mucosa. The pyloric channel is also abnormally elongated.

Intussusception

Intussusception is the invagination of a segment of bowel (the "intussusceptum") into a contiguous distal segment of bowel (the "intussuscipiens"). In children, more than 90% of cases of intussusception are ileocolic [**Fig. 4.36**]. Intussusception leads to bowel obstruction and, if untreated, to ischemia and bowel necrosis.

Intussusception is most common between the ages of 3 months and 3 years, with most cases occurring between 6 months and 1 year of age. It is rare in newborns and affects boys more than girls. Childhood intussusception is usually described as idiopathic, although it has long been thought that the abundant and often hypertrophied lymphoid tissue in the distal small bowel of children may serve as a "lead point" for the intussusception. True pathologic lead points are found in only 10% of cases of childhood intussusception. Pathologic lead points are almost always present in the rare newborn with intussusception, and they become more common with increasing age after about 5 or 6 years. There is obviously no specific age after which a child *must* have a pathologic lead point, but it is probably safe to say that a 5-year-old is much more likely to have an "idiopathic" intussusception and a 10-year-old more likely to have an intussusception due to a pathologic lead point. In younger children, the lead point is usually benign, and most often a Meckel diverticulum. In older children, the lead point is often malignant, usually lymphoma.

The clinical presentation of intussusception may include intermittent episodes of abdominal pain, vomiting, and bloody stools that are often described as resembling currant jelly. Babies with intussusception are frequently lethargic, sometimes alarmingly so.

Intussusception is an emergency and should be treated as such by all involved parties. Surgical consultation is mandatory. It is ultimately the attending surgeon who must decide whether a reduction can be attempted by the radiologist, and who must be ready to operate expeditiously should the attempted reduction fail.

The task of the radiologist is straightforward: to identify *all* children who present with intussusception in a timely manner, and to safely and successfully treat as many of those children as

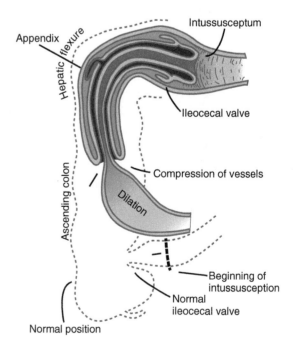

Figure 4.36 Intussusception. A schematic illustration of an ileocolic intussusception.

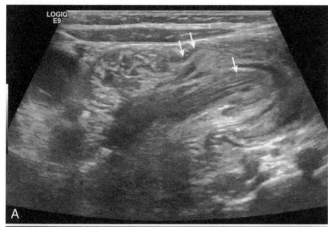

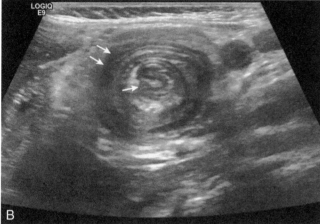

Figure 4.37 Intussusception. A, Longitudinal and (**B**) transverse ultrasound images of an intussusception demonstrate invagination of the intussusceptum (*arrow*) into the intussuscipiens (*double arrow*). The involved loops of bowel are thickened and edematous.

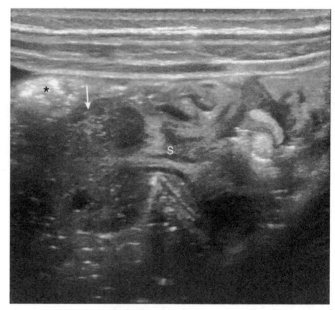

Figure 4.38 Intussusception. Ultrasound shows a polyp (*arrow*) with a stalk (*S*) serving as a pathologic lead point extending into the intussuscipiens (*asterisk*).

possible. The radiologic evaluation of the child with suspected intussusception has traditionally begun with plain radiographs of the abdomen. However, in many centers, ultrasound has more recently become the initial study of choice, and for good reason. Ultrasound is not associated with exposure to ionizing radiation. It is highly sensitive and specific for the diagnosis of intussusception. The invagination of one bowel loop into another is displayed with exquisite clarity [**Fig. 4.37**]. Ultrasound may also demonstrate a pathologic lead point, which may alter the chosen therapeutic approach [**Fig. 4.38**]. Finally, as will be discussed further, some sonographic features of the intussusception may help predict success or failure of reduction.

We continue to obtain plain radiographs of the abdomen in children with suspected intussusception for several reasons. First, although we acknowledge that there is little agreement about the utility of plain radiographs in intussusception, it has been our experience that few patients with intussusception will have normal radiographs. In those patients with abnormal radiographs, the findings are often diagnostic. These patients may proceed to reduction without further diagnostic workup and delay. Second, ultrasound is a highly *operator-dependent* modality. Although the diagnosis of intussusception may be straightforward for a pediatric radiologist or sonographer, it may not be so for the less experienced. Finally, an ultrasound performed to "rule out intussusception" is often quite limited, looking only for the presumed pretest diagnosis. Given these potential limitations, a few targeted ultrasound images may be an insufficient

record of an encounter with a child with an abdominal complaint. Although normal radiographs will obviously not exclude all significant intraabdominal pathology, they may offer some reassurance.

One need not be dogmatic about any of this. A diagnostic approach to intussusception should be tailored to the strengths and weaknesses of individual radiologists, departments, and institutions. Whatever the approach, it is most important to avoid falsely negative evaluations. Accomplishing this goal will sometimes require ultrasound, but it will just as frequently assume the correct interpretation of radiographs. For many reasons, not all children with intussusception will get an ultrasound. In our experience, in most cases in which the diagnosis is missed or delayed, it is because the plain radiograph findings have not been recognized.

Plain radiograph findings can be explained by the pathologic anatomy of the intussusception. As noted previously, in normal abdominal radiographs there is a uniform distribution of air. In children with intussusception, air in the cecum and right colon is replaced by the intussusceptum, usually the distal ileum. Thus in most patients, there will be no air in the cecum and right colon [**Fig. 4.39**]. This is the most sensitive radiographic finding for intussusception. Occasionally small bowel is seen in the right lower quadrant in the expected location of the cecum. This finding is referred to as "lateralization of the ileum," and it increases the specificity of the radiograph substantially [**Fig. 4.40**]. In many cases, the intussusception mass may be seen, with the leading edge outlined by air ("crescent sign"). This further increases the specificity of the radiograph [**Fig. 4.41**]. Up to one quarter of patients with intussusception will present with a small-bowel obstruction [**Fig. 4.2**]. Small-bowel obstruction is obviously not specific for intussusception, but it is probably a good rule of thumb that any child between the ages of 3 months and 3 years with a small-bowel obstruction should be presumed to have an intussusception until proven otherwise.

A radiograph in which the entire cecum is filled with air and stool virtually excludes the presence of an ileocolic intussusception. This strict definition of a normal radiograph must be applied if one is asked to "rule out" intussusception. Care must be taken not to mistake lateralized small bowel for cecum.

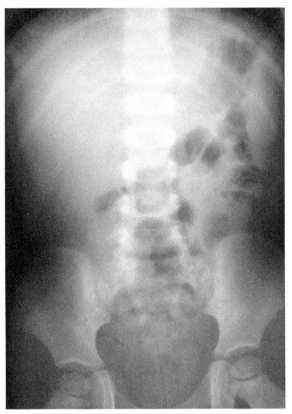

Figure 4.39 Intussusception. A frontal supine abdominal radiograph demonstrates a paucity of bowel gas in the right lower quadrant.

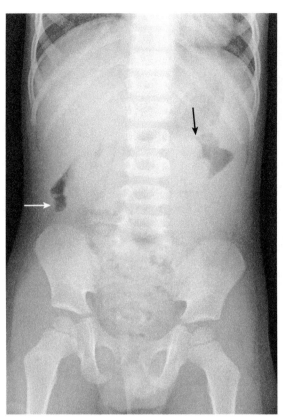

Figure 4.41 Intussusception. A frontal supine abdominal radiograph shows a soft tissue mass (*black arrow*) outlined by bowel gas ("crescent sign") in the left upper quadrant. Also note the lack of bowel gas in the right lower quadrant and "lateralization of the ileum" (*white arrow*).

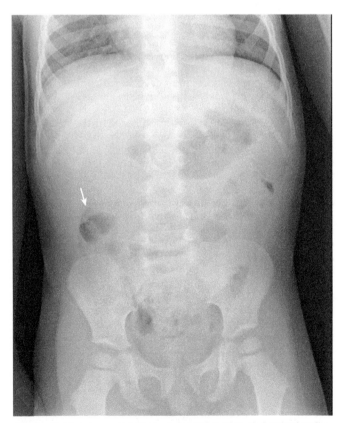

Figure 4.40 Intussusception. A frontal supine abdominal radiograph shows "lateralization of the ileum" (*arrow*).

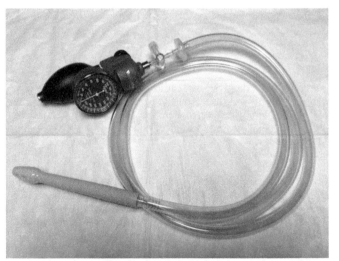

Figure 4.42 Intussusception reduction kit. A photograph of an air reduction device consisting of an aneroid gauge and insufflator attached to plastic tubing with an enema tip.

Once the diagnosis of intussusception has been made, preparation for reduction may begin. For many years, the most widely used method was hydrostatic reduction under fluoroscopic guidance using barium or water-soluble contrast material. The standard of care in most pediatric centers is now air reduction under fluoroscopic guidance. In many parts of the world, hydrostatic reduction with ultrasound guidance is used, but this method is not widely used in the United States. Our discussion will be limited to air reduction.

When the child with intussusception is in the radiology department, he or she is the responsibility of the radiologist. Many children with intussusception are very ill, with dehydration, tachycardia, and even hypotension. A reduction should never be attempted in a child who is hemodynamically unstable. Even with a stable patient, reduction should not begin without adequate personnel present to care for the patient. To be clear, being sick is not a contraindication to reduction. On the contrary, it is the best reason for doing one. No specific guidelines for reduction will be suitable for all institutions and all patients. It is ultimately up to the radiologist to assess the patient and decide how much help may be needed. Inability to reduce an intussusception is not a failure, but attempted reduction without the appropriate level of medical expertise and adequate support may be.

The only universally accepted contraindications to reduction are peritonitis and pneumoperitoneum. Pneumoperitoneum is notably rare in patients with intussusception. Despite this, we routinely obtain horizontal beam radiographs prior to attempted reduction.

Although peritonitis and pneumoperitoneum are the only absolute contraindications, additional clinical and radiographic findings suggest that the chance of successful reduction may be diminished. Among these are longer duration of symptoms, copious rectal bleeding, small-bowel obstruction, and lack of blood flow in the affected bowel on Doppler ultrasound. Sonographic demonstration of peritoneal fluid "trapped" within the intussusception has also been associated with a lower reduction rate. These are not contraindications to reduction; however, the presence of these factors may influence how aggressively reduction is attempted.

Reduction can be attempted in almost all children. After adequate medical support has been established, the procedure should be thoroughly explained to the patient's parents or guardian. It should be made clear that the alternative to reduction is surgery. The small risk for perforation (to be discussed) should be acknowledged. Most importantly, the painful nature of the procedure should be conveyed. Sedation is not routinely used. It adds a layer of delay and potential complication to the procedure. Further, as most pediatric radiologists know, it is during crying and straining (Valsalva maneuver) that reduction is usually achieved. Most parents will understand and accept this rationale.

After appropriate evaluation, explanation, and preparation, air reduction may proceed. Air reduction systems are commercially available and vary little from center to center. The reduction device consists of two parts: a reusable aneroid gauge and insufflator, similar to that of a sphygmomanometer, and a disposable tubing set with an enema tip and filter (to protect the gauge and insufflator) [**Fig. 4.42**]. There are a few important points regarding technique. In the therapeutic reduction of intussusception, one should use the largest tube possible, inserted deeply but safely into the rectum. This is in contradistinction to diagnostic enemas performed for bowel obstruction, when it is critical to use the smallest tube possible barely inserted into the anus. It is essential that an airtight seal be maintained throughout attempted reduction. This is usually accomplished through a combination of sturdy taping and continuous manual compression of the buttocks. Most intussusceptions are reduced at relatively low pressures. The insufflation pressure *should not exceed 120 mm Hg* with the child at rest. When the patient strains or cries, pressures may rise much higher. It is often during this "Valsalva maneuver" that reduction is achieved.

The intussusception is typically encountered near the hepatic flexure, where it is well seen as an intraluminal filling defect [**Fig. 4.43A**]. When the intussusception is reduced, air flows freely into the small bowel. Reflux of air may occur before complete reduction, but this "trickle" of air is usually easy to distinguish from the "rush" of air that occurs with complete reduction [**Fig. 4.43B**]. A tangential beam radiograph should be obtained after reduction to exclude a perforation that was not recognized during the procedure. There is a relatively steep learning curve for air reduction. However, with a little experience, it is fairly straightforward.

Some reductions are very difficult. There are no generally accepted guidelines for termination of the procedure. In our institution, we generally persevere in children who are not extremely ill, who do not have predictors of a lower rate of successful reduction or predictors of perforation (to be discussed), and in whom progress is being made. There are radiologists and surgeons at other institutions who may be more aggressive in their approach.

Reported success rates for air reduction vary widely depending on several factors, including patient population, definition of success, and aggressiveness of approach. The experienced pediatric radiologist should probably aim for an 80% to 90% success

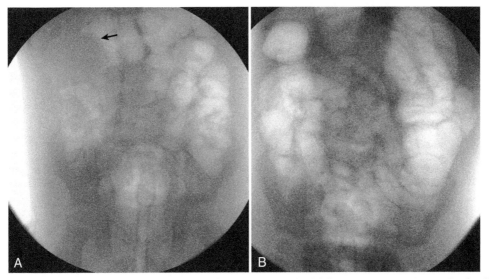

Figure 4.43 Air enema for intussusception reduction. A, An initial fluoroscopic spot image in the frontal projection shows the intussusceptum (*arrow*) near the hepatic flexure. **B,** A postreduction spot image shows interval resolution of the mass with reflux of air to the small bowel.

rate. As noted earlier, less than 10% of childhood intussusceptions are caused by pathologic lead points. Most intussusceptions associated with lead points are notably not reducible. Detection of lead points is the best argument for careful ultrasonography before air enema.

There is about a 10% recurrence rate after air reduction. Recurrence rate is lower after surgical reduction. Most recurrences occur within hours to days of the initial reduction. Recurrences may be multiple. Children with recurrent intussusception are no more likely to have lead points than those with single episodes. Successful reduction is the best proof that there is no lead point.

The most important complication of air reduction is perforation. Some perforations occur in necrotic bowel and are probably unmasked by reduction. Others, however, occur in normal bowel and are presumably due to barotrauma. Reported perforation rates vary widely. Overall, the rate is probably less than 1%. Perforation may be more common in babies who are younger than 6 months and in those with a longer duration of symptoms.

Most babies who sustain a bowel perforation during reduction will do well. Rarely, however, perforation may result in tension pneumoperitoneum. Left untreated, this can lead to diminished venous return and cardiovascular collapse. Tension pneumoperitoneum usually occurs when free air is not recognized during the procedure. If large amounts of free air are recognized and/or clinical deterioration occurs, the abdomen must be immediately decompressed with an 18-gauge needle inserted into the midline of the abdomen above the umbilicus.

Esophageal Foreign Bodies

Children often swallow foreign objects such as coins, buttons, small toys, batteries, and pins. In most cases, the foreign body passes through the GI tract without difficulty. In cases when it does not, it most frequently becomes impacted in the esophagus. In order of decreasing frequency, esophageal foreign bodies lodge at the thoracic inlet, the level of the aortic arch/left mainstem bronchus, and the GE junction.

Most children with an impacted esophageal foreign body are acutely symptomatic. Dysphagia, drooling, gagging, and chest pain are common. In young children with prolonged impaction, the predominant symptoms may be respiratory, possibly with signs of airway obstruction. This is due to inflammation of the trachea, and it may be especially striking when the impaction has resulted in esophageal perforation and mediastinitis.

Most ingested foreign bodies are radiopaque. This includes coins, one of the most commonly swallowed objects. Radiographs are the initial imaging step in a child suspected to have an ingested foreign body. It is important to image the entire GI tract from the mouth to the anus to search for foreign bodies. An AP view of the chest and abdomen and a lateral view of the neck and upper thorax should be performed. Typically, a coin in the esophagus is seen as a round, flat object in the frontal projection and on the edge on the lateral view [**Fig. 4.44**]. The opposite is true for tracheal aspiration, which is less common. Careful attention should be made to discern a disk battery (such as those found in cameras, hearing aids, and watches) from a coin because batteries may cause serious chemical injury to the esophagus. Batteries have a characteristic bilaminar structure, with a step-off at the cathode and anode ends [**Fig. 4.45**].

In the setting of an esophageal foreign body, radiographs are useful to assess for signs of inflammation surrounding the trachea and esophagus. One may see tracheal narrowing or an increased distance between the trachea and the esophagus in the lateral projection.

When radiographs are negative but suspicion for an esophageal foreign body persists, an esophagram may be performed with water-soluble contrast material. A water-soluble esophagram is also useful in cases of difficult foreign body removal to assess for esophageal perforation.

In cases of prolonged esophageal foreign body, CT scan with intravenous and/or oral contrast material may be helpful to look for complications such as mediastinitis or tracheoesophageal or aortoesophageal fistulae.

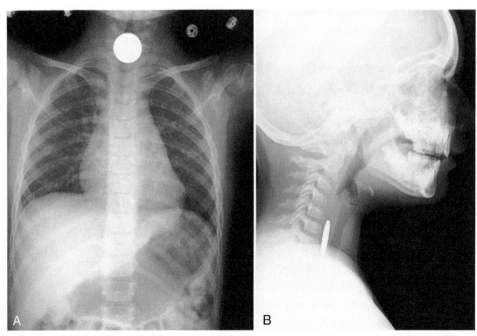

Figure 4.44 Esophageal foreign body. Radiographs demonstrating an impacted coin in the lower cervical esophagus. **A,** This appears as a round, flat object in the frontal projection. **B,** On the lateral view, it is profiled on edge.

Gastric Volvulus

The stomach is normally firmly fixed to surrounding organs by the gastrophrenic, gastrohepatic, gastrocolic, and gastrosplenic ligaments. Volvulus of the stomach is quite unusual. It occurs when fixation is deficient, as may occur in the setting of diaphragmatic hernia, eventration, or asplenia.

Two types of gastric volvulus are possible: organoaxial and mesenteroaxial [**Fig. 4.46**]. Organoaxial volvulus is rare in childhood. In this condition, the stomach rotates on its long axis. The greater curvature of the stomach will lie superiorly and the lesser curvature will lie inferiorly. This is usually a consequence of a hiatal hernia and is typically intrathoracic in location.

In the more common mesenteroaxial volvulus, the stomach rotates on an axis perpendicular to its long axis, from right to left. The gastric antrum passes superiorly and anteriorly to lie near the expected location of the GE junction, and the GE junction is pulled inferiorly. Obstruction may occur at both the pylorus and the GE junction in a closed loop.

Mesenteroaxial volvulus is typically acute. Abdominal pain and retching without vomiting are the classic symptoms. Plain radiographs will show gastric distension, air–fluid level(s), and a "beak" at the obstructed gastric antrum [**Fig. 4.47**]. Treatment is surgical.

Gastrointestinal Duplication and Meckel Diverticulum

A GI duplication is a cystic structure lined with alimentary tract epithelium and attached to adjacent bowel. The duplication cyst and the adjacent bowel share a muscular wall and blood supply. The cyst rarely communicates with the lumen of the attached bowel. The mucosal lining of the duplication may be "ectopic," that is, different from that of the adjacent bowel. The

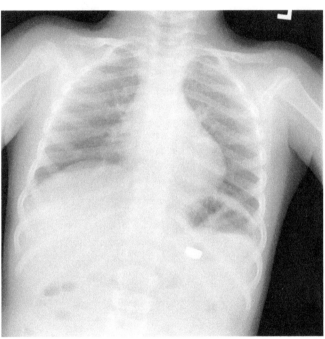

Figure 4.45 **Ingested battery.** Note the bilaminar configuration, which distinguishes the battery from a coin.

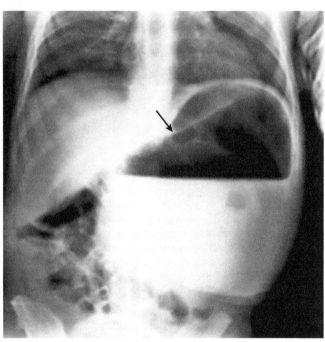

Figure 4.47 **Mesenteroaxial volvulus.** A frontal abdominal radiograph shows a distended stomach with an air–fluid level. The gastric antrum is rotated to the expected position of the gastroesophageal junction. A "beak" is noted at the obstructed antrum (*arrow*).

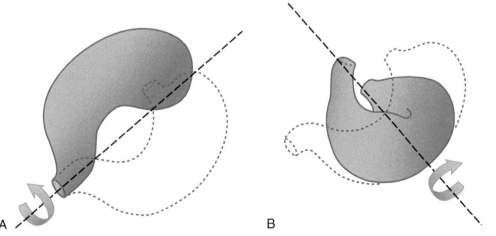

Figure 4.46 **Gastric volvulus.** A schematic illustration of organoaxial volvulus (**A**) and mesenteroaxial volvulus (**B**).

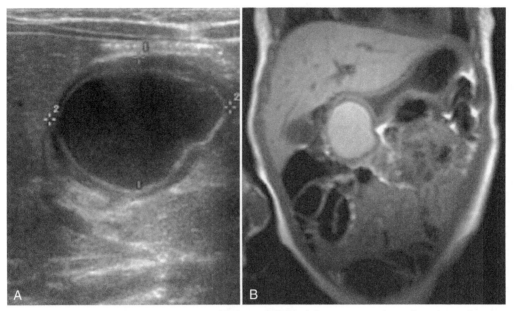

Figure 4.48 Gastric duplication. A, A sonographic image of the right upper quadrant shows a cystic mass with an inner echogenic mucosal layer and an outer hypoechoic muscular layer ("gut signature"). **B,** A coronal T2-weighted magnetic resonance image of the same patient demonstrates the fluid-filled cyst in the right upper quadrant.

most frequently found types of ectopic mucosa are gastric and pancreatic. A duplication is named for the bowel to which it is attached, not for its mucosal lining.

Duplications may be located anywhere along the alimentary tract but are most commonly found in the distal ileum and esophagus. The signs and symptoms of a duplication depend on location. Some are asymptomatic. In the esophagus, a duplication may cause compression of the airway. A small-bowel duplication may lead to obstruction, either by compression of adjacent bowel or by serving as a lead point for intussusception. In any location, a duplication that contains gastric mucosa may ulcerate, leading to hemorrhage and perforation.

The diagnosis of a duplication is usually established by ultrasound, which demonstrates a cystic mass with pathognomonic "gut signature" reflecting an inner layer of echogenic mucosa and an outer layer of hypoechoic muscle [**Fig. 4.48**]. CT and MRI are sometimes useful in the diagnosis of esophageal duplication but are somewhat nonspecific, usually demonstrating a spherical fluid-filled mass adjacent to the esophagus.

Meckel diverticulum and GI duplication share some important clinical and imaging features, although the causes of these entities are distinct. Meckel diverticulum is the most common remnant of the omphalomesenteric duct, the embryonic connection between the ileum and the extraembryonic yolk sac. It is located on the antimesenteric border of the ileum near the ileocecal valve. Like other true diverticula and like duplication, a Meckel diverticulum contains all the layers of the bowel wall. As with a duplication, the mucosa may be ectopic, most frequently gastric. Unlike a duplication, a Meckel diverticulum by definition communicates with normal bowel.

A Meckel diverticulum may cause symptoms in two ways. In infants and young children, a diverticulum may invert from its usual position and serve as a lead point for intussusception (as previously described). Older children may present with GI bleeding related to ectopic gastric mucosa within the diverticulum.

The diagnosis of Meckel diverticulum is most frequently made by ultrasound, often in a child with intussusception. The Meckel diverticulum is seen as a tubular, fluid-filled structure

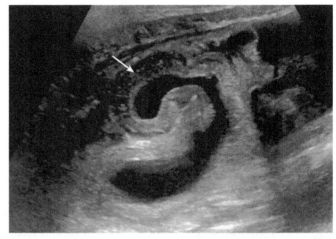

Figure 4.49 Meckel diverticulum. An ultrasound image of the right lower quadrant shows a tubular fluid-filled structure (*arrow*) with a thick wall and characteristic "gut signature."

with gut signature [**Fig. 4.49**]. In children without intussusception, it may be difficult to distinguish a Meckel diverticulum from surrounding normal bowel. Nuclear scintigraphy with technetium-99m (^{99m}Tc) pertechnetate will be positive only if the diverticulum contains gastric mucosa. Gastric mucosa, although present in only one quarter of cases of Meckel diverticulum, is almost always found in children with bleeding.

Gastroesophageal Reflux and Hiatal Hernia

Textbooks of pediatric radiology have traditionally devoted many words to GE reflux. In the 21st century, such an emphasis can hardly be justified. Most pediatric radiologists would agree that imaging has little or no role to play in the diagnosis and management of reflux. Why then devote even a few paragraphs to this subject? Mostly because we are still quite frequently asked to "rule out reflux."

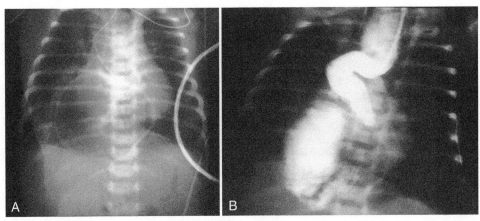

Figure 4.50 Hiatal hernia. A, A frontal radiograph of the chest in a 2-week-old infant shows a large, air-filled structure in the right hemithorax. **B,** A frontal image from an upper gastrointestinal series shows this air-filled structure to be the stomach. The gastroesophageal junction is above the hemidiaphragm, and the esophagus has a kinked configuration.

GE reflux is a common problem in infancy. Some regurgitation of gastric contents is normal in young babies. This is the "spitting up" with which all parents are familiar. When spitting up becomes pathologic, we may see failure to thrive, malnourishment, extreme irritability related to esophagitis, or respiratory disease caused by aspiration of refluxed gastric contents. It goes without saying that we should not be asked to do studies on well children who are "spitters." With regard to the upper GI performed in this setting, we have learned over the years that the younger the child, the more barium administered, and the longer the duration of fluoroscopic observation, the more likely reflux will be seen. The presence or absence of reflux on an upper GI has little correlation with reflux in real life and certainly cannot predict whether reflux is or will become pathologic.

An upper GI is more often requested in children whose reflux has been deemed pathologic to "rule out anatomic abnormalities." Experience has taught us that underlying anatomic abnormalities that might be contributing to presumed reflux, such as incomplete obstruction caused by webs, stenosis, or malrotation, are rarely found. This is also the case with abnormalities that may be the consequence of reflux, such as esophageal strictures.

The anatomic abnormality that is most frequently suspected as the cause of reflux is the hiatal hernia. Small sliding hiatal hernias commonly seen in adults with reflux are distinctly uncommon in early childhood. Very large hiatal hernias may occur in newborns. Their appearance is typical. On chest radiographs, the hernia is seen as a large, air-containing retrocardiac mass that almost invariably extends to the right hemithorax [**Fig. 4.50**]. If contrast is given, the hernia will be noted to be of the sliding type, with the GE junction above the diaphragm. The esophagus is kinked and the stomach is twisted to some degree.

A baby with a large hernia will usually have intractable vomiting. These hernias should not be confused with the relatively common Bochdalek hernia or the more rare Morgagni hernia.

THE OLDER CHILD

Distal Intestinal Obstruction Syndrome

DIOS, formerly (and in our opinion, more accurately and helpfully) known as "meconium ileus equivalent," is a unique type of small-bowel obstruction that occurs in older children and adults with CF. In a manner analogous to meconium ileus in

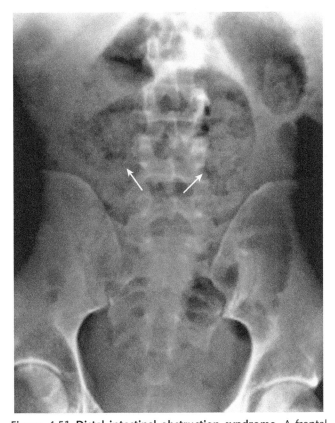

Figure 4.51 Distal intestinal obstruction syndrome. A frontal abdominal radiograph in a patient with cystic fibrosis shows dilated, fecalized small-bowel (*arrows*) and related bowel obstruction.

newborns, obstruction results from inspissation of abnormally viscous stool in the ileum and right colon. There is a clinical and radiographic continuum from constipation, a relatively common problem in CF, to DIOS. In the appropriate clinical setting, the diagnosis is confirmed by radiographs demonstrating a large amount of stool. In more advanced cases, radiographs will demonstrate fecalized small-bowel and frank obstruction [**Fig. 4.51**]. Patients with CF are also at risk for small-bowel obstruction from other causes, including appendicitis and adhesions related to prior surgery. Thus the diagnosis of DIOS should not be

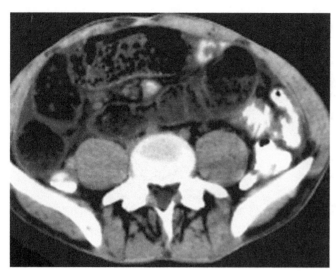

Figure 4.52 Distal intestinal obstruction syndrome. An axial computed tomography image through the abdomen in a patient with cystic fibrosis confirms fecalized small bowel as the source of bowel obstruction.

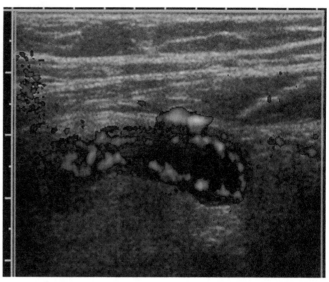

Figure 4.53 Acute appendicitis in a 7-year-old with right lower quadrant pain and fever. A sagittal power Doppler image through the right lower quadrant shows a dilated, fluid-filled appendix with marked mucosal hyperemia.

made unless the radiograph demonstrates constipation and obstruction. When the diagnosis is unclear, CT may be very useful [**Fig. 4.52**].

The initial treatment of DIOS is usually either Gastrografin or a colonic "clean-out" solution by mouth. In refractory cases or in patients who cannot tolerate oral agents, an enema with Gastrografin may be very effective. In DIOS, Gastrografin presumably works just as it does in meconium ileus. In both entities, it is important to reflux contrast material into the terminal ileum.

Appendicitis

Appendicitis affects up to 90,000 children each year in the United States. It is the most common condition requiring intraabdominal surgery in infancy and childhood. Although the peak incidence of childhood appendicitis occurs during adolescence, approximately 10% of cases occur in children 2 to 5 years of age. The typical clinical presentation includes lower abdominal pain with vomiting, fever, and leukocytosis. However, the clinical presentation in young children is often atypical, and delayed diagnosis is common. In addition, the risk for appendiceal perforation at presentation for children younger than 5 years is more than nine times higher than that for older children. A high index of suspicion is the key to early diagnosis in this patient population.

Acute appendicitis occurs in the setting of luminal obstruction, which may be caused by a fecalith, lymphoid hyperplasia, parasitic infestation, or rarely, carcinoid tumor of the appendix. Obstruction results in increased intraluminal pressure, mucosal ischemia, bacterial overgrowth and invasion, and eventual appendiceal perforation.

Sonography is the preferred modality for the initial evaluation of children with suspected appendicitis. A targeted right lower quadrant evaluation is performed with a high-frequency linear transducer using a graded compression technique. Additional imaging of the pelvis through a well-distended urinary bladder using a 5-MHz curved array transducer may be helpful to identify an appendix in the deep pelvis. Evaluation of the right flank from the liver and right kidney to the iliac crest may reveal a retrocecal appendix.

Direct criteria for the diagnosis of appendicitis by ultrasound include the presence of a fluid-filled, distended (≥6 mm in

diameter), noncompressible tubular structure with or without an appendicolith either anterior to the psoas muscle or retrocecal in position. Secondary signs of appendicitis include loculated periappendiceal fluid, hyperechoic periappendiceal fat, and a focal inflammatory mass in the right lower quadrant or deep pelvis. Appendiceal and mesenteric hyperemia on color Doppler sonography is a useful confirmatory finding [**Fig. 4.53**].

Sonography is widely available and is relatively inexpensive and safe. It has a high specificity for the diagnosis of appendicitis in children (approximately 94%). The major drawback of ultrasound is a relatively low sensitivity rate (88%), such that a negative examination does not exclude appendicitis unless a normal appendix is visualized with a high degree of confidence. Visualization rates vary widely in the published literature from a high of 98% to a low of 22%. As such, a negative ultrasound in the presence of ongoing clinical suspicion is not sufficient to exclude the presence of acute appendicitis. CT is often used in patients with persistent clinical signs and symptoms and a negative ultrasound examination. Published sensitivity and specificity values for CT are consistently high (94% and 95%, respectively) in the diagnosis of pediatric acute appendicitis despite a wide range of clinical protocols in use.

The size of a normal appendix on CT can vary widely, sometimes reaching up to 10 mm in diameter. This degree of distention is not uncommon in patients with CF. The normal appendix is often filled with gas or fecal material. The identification of a normal appendix on CT excludes the diagnosis of appendicitis. In the absence of secondary signs of appendiceal inflammation, CT nonvisualization of the appendix also constitutes a negative examination for appendicitis.

When inflamed, the appendix appears as a distended, thick-walled, blind-ended tubular structure with increased contrast enhancement. One or more appendicoliths may be present. Secondary signs of appendicitis are commonly seen, including mesenteric stranding, mesenteric adenopathy, free peritoneal fluid, and cecal wall thickening. With appendiceal perforation, a focal inflammatory phlegmon may form, and the appendix itself may no longer be visible.

Diagnostic imaging plays an important role in the prompt and accurate diagnosis of acute appendicitis in children and in the detection of alternative causes of acute abdominal pain. An effective imaging protocol should include *both* ultrasonography and

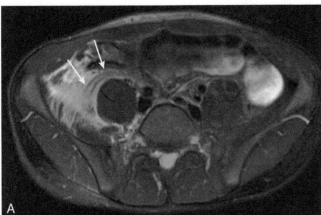

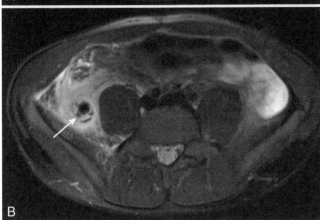

Figure 4.54 Acute appendicitis in a 16-year-old with a 2-day history of abdominal pain. **A,** An axial T2-weighted magnetic resonance image through the pelvis shows a distended, thick-walled appendix (*arrows*) draped over the right psoas muscle. The mid to distal portion of the appendix is somewhat ill-defined. There is considerable surrounding edema and inflammatory change. **B,** Just inferior to this, a large appendicolith (*arrow*) is seen near the appendiceal tip. At surgery, this patient had acute gangrenous appendicitis with focal perforation.

CT. If the ultrasound study is inconclusive or fails to show the appendix, a CT with intravenous contrast material should be performed. Alone or in conjunction with clinical practice guidelines, this sequence of imaging has a high combined sensitivity, specificity, and overall accuracy of at least 94%.

The role of MRI in pediatric appendicitis is evolving. At this time limited MRI with or without contrast administration shows promise as an alternative to CT in suspected appendicitis [**Fig. 4.54**].

SUGGESTED READINGS

Applegate KE, Anderson JM, Klatte EC. Intestinal malrotation in children: a problem-solving approach to the upper gastrointestinal series. *Radiographics*. 2006;26:1485-1500.

Berdon WE, Baker DH, Santulli TV, et al. Microcolon in newborn infants with intestinal obstruction. Its correlation with the level and time of onset of obstruction. *Radiology*. 1968;90:878-885.

Berdon WE, Slovis TL, Campbell JB, et al. Neonatal small left colon syndrome: its relationship to aganglionosis and meconium plug syndrome. *Radiology*. 1977;125:457-462.

Buonomo C. Neonatal gastrointestinal emergencies. *Radiol Clin North Am*. 1997;35:845-864.

Daneman A, Kozlowski K. Large hiatus hernias in infancy and childhood. *Australas Radiol*. 1977;21:133-139.

Daneman A, Navarro O. Intussusception. Part 1: a review of diagnostic approaches. *Pediatr Radiol*. 2003;33:79-85.

Daneman A, Navarro O. Intussusception. Part 2: an update on the evolution of management. *Pediatr Radiol*. 2004;34:97-108, quiz 187.

Epelman M, Daneman A, Navarro OM, et al. Necrotizing enterocolitis: review of state-of-the-art imaging findings with pathologic correlation. *Radiographics*. 2007;27:285-305.

Herliczek TW, Swenson DW, Mayo-Smith WW. Utility of MRI after inconclusive ultrasound in pediatric patients with suspected appendicitis: retrospective review of 60 consecutive patients. *AJR Am J Roentgenol*. 2013;200:969-973.

Maxfield CM, Bartz BH, Shaffer JL. A pattern-based approach to bowel obstruction in the newborn. *Pediatr Radiol*. 2013;43:318-329.

Navarro O, Daneman A. Intussusception. Part 3: diagnosis and management of those with an identifiable or predisposing cause and those that reduce spontaneously. *Pediatr Radiol*. 2004;34:305-312, quiz 369.

Saucier A, Huang EY, Emeremni CA, et al. Prospective evaluation of a clinical pathway for suspected appendicitis. *Pediatrics*. 2014;133:88-95.

Sharma R, Hudak ML. A clinical perspective of necrotizing enterocolitis: past, present, and future. *Clin Perinatol*. 2013;40:27-51.

Strouse PJ. Disorders of intestinal rotation and fixation ("malrotation"). *Pediatr Radiol*. 2004;34:837-851.

Teele RL, Smith EH. Ultrasound in the diagnosis of idiopathic hypertrophic pyloric stenosis. *N Engl J Med*. 1977;296:1149-1150.

Chapter 5

Hepatobiliary, Pancreas, and Spleen Imaging

Erica L. Riedesel and George A. Taylor

LIVER AND BILIARY TREE

Anatomy and Embryology

The liver, gallbladder, and biliary tree originate from endodermal cells that form a diverticulum arising from the duodenal region of the primitive embryonic gut between 4 and 10 weeks' gestation. The larger cranial division (pars hepatica) gives rise to the liver, whereas the smaller, caudal portion (pars cystica) develops into the gallbladder and cystic duct. The intrahepatic and extrahepatic components of the biliary tree develop independently and unite by 12 weeks' gestation. At birth, the liver represents about 5% of total body weight (200 g). Bile secretion commences between 12 and 16 weeks' gestation. Hematopoiesis normally occurs only in the fetal liver and ceases by the age of 6 weeks in healthy infants.

Although the liver is usually located in the right upper quadrant, it may be midline and more symmetric in patients with heterotaxy syndromes [**Fig. 5.1**]. This is seen in approximately 80% of patients with asplenia and about 50% of patients with polysplenia.

The portal venous system supplies between 70% and 80% of the blood supply to the liver. The portal venous branches, hepatic arterial branches, and biliary radicles run parallel to one another in the center of hepatic segments, the so-called portal triad arrangement. Accessory lobes of the liver are rare. Caudal elongation of the right lobe of the liver, known as a Riedel lobe, is a normal variant.

Developmental Anomalies

Biliary Atresia

Jaundice in an infant older than 2 weeks should raise suspicion for underlying liver disease. The clinical differential diagnosis of neonatal jaundice is broad. It may be related to sepsis, hemolysis, infection (cytomegalovirus, hepatitis A and B, rubella), and metabolic abnormalities (α_1-antitrypsin deficiency, cystic fibrosis [CF]). When these causes of jaundice have been excluded, neonatal hepatitis and biliary atresia account for more than two-thirds of the remaining cases of conjugated hyperbilirubinemia in the neonate. It is postulated that neonatal hepatitis and biliary atresia are part of the same clinical spectrum of cholestatic jaundice and hepatomegaly.

Biliary atresia is relatively rare in the United States, with an incidence of 1/10,000 to 20,000 infants. Progressive ductal inflammation leads to fibrosis and obliteration of the extrahepatic bile ducts, with occasional involvement of the intrahepatic bile ducts. Disruption of the biliary system results in chronic cholestasis, which eventually leads to liver fibrosis and biliary cirrhosis. Obliteration of the bile ducts may be present at the time of birth or may occur shortly after birth. Although there are many hypotheses regarding the etiology of this disease, the exact cause remains unknown.

The Kasai system is most commonly used to classify biliary atresia based on location of disease involvement [**Fig. 5.2**]. The diagnosis of biliary atresia requires definitive imaging of the biliary ductal system. Intraoperative cholangiogram is considered the gold standard for evaluation of the biliary tree, and liver biopsy is needed for microscopic evaluation to determine involvement of the intrahepatic bile ducts. These are invasive procedures and not without significant risk in the infant population. Thus evaluation often begins with ultrasound and hepatobiliary scintigraphy to determine which patients should go on to more definitive diagnostic procedures.

Findings on ultrasound include the "triangular cord sign," an abnormal triangular or tubular echogenic band of fibrous tissue in the porta hepatis representing the obliterated common hepatic duct [**Fig. 5.3**]. Because this structure lies immediately adjacent to the portal vessels, it can sometimes appear as a relative thickening of the anterior wall of the right portal vein. On a longitudinal ultrasound image, an anterior wall thickness of greater than 4 mm can be used to define the triangular cord sign.

In 25% of cases of biliary atresia, the gallbladder is absent. If the gallbladder is identified, it is often abnormal. Ultrasound evaluation of the gallbladder before and after feeding can be helpful because the abnormal gallbladder in biliary atresia will not typically demonstrate the expected change in size between the fasting and recently fed states. Ultrasound can also help to identify alternative causes of cholestasis, such as a choledochal cyst or other mass causing biliary obstruction.

Hepatobiliary scintigraphy with ^{99m}Tc-iminodiacetic acid derivatives is often the second diagnostic imaging study used to evaluate biliary atresia. In the normal liver, radiotracer is taken up and excreted by hepatocytes into the biliary tree within 10 to 15 minutes of venous injection. In biliary atresia, the tracer cannot be excreted and remains in the liver parenchyma. A lack of tracer excretion into the small bowel by 24 hours after tracer injection is suggestive of biliary atresia [**Fig. 5.4**]. This finding is notably nonspecific and can be seen in any disorder that results in cholestasis. Poor hepatocellular function, as may be seen in neonatal hepatitis, can also result in delayed biliary excretion. Thus an infant undergoing a hepatobiliary scan is typically pretreated with phenobarbital for 5 days before the examination. This enhances hepatocellular function and decreases the chance of a false-positive result. If an infant has not been pretreated with phenobarbital and there is no tracer excretion into the small bowel at 24 hours, an infusion of ursodiol can be given, with repeat imaging at 48 and 72 hours.

Treatment of biliary atresia is surgical, with the best outcomes seen when surgery is performed before 40 to 60 days of life. The surgery of choice is the Kasai procedure. The abnormal extrahepatic biliary tree is mobilized from the liver, and the cut liver surface is directly anastomosed to a Roux-en-Y loop of small bowel. This allows direct drainage of bile from the liver. After 3 months of age, intrahepatic bile duct involvement and resultant hepatic fibrosis are often severe enough to render the Kasai procedure ineffective. In these patients, and in those who undergo a Kasai procedure with no significant improvement in cholestasis, liver transplant is the only treatment option.

Choledochal Cyst

A choledochal cyst is a localized cystic dilatation of the biliary ductal system. It is postulated that this develops when there is an anomalous junction of the common bile duct and the pancreatic duct, forming a long common channel and allowing for reflux of pancreatic enzymes into the biliary tree. This leads to inflammation and focal duct stenosis, with resultant proximal dilation or outpouching of the bile duct. Choledochal cysts occur four times more commonly in females than in males, and they have a high prevalence among individuals from East Asia.

A choledochal cyst is a rare cause of neonatal cholestatic jaundice; however, when identified in this age group, concomitant biliary atresia should always be ruled out.

In older patients, clinical manifestations of a choledochal cyst include abdominal pain, jaundice, and a palpable right upper quadrant "mass." This complete constellation of clinical findings

is notably seen in less than 60% of patients. Laboratory workup reveals a direct hyperbilirubinemia. Most patients present before the age of 10 years.

Four types of congenital biliary cysts have been described [**Fig. 5.5**]. The most common is type 1 (80%–90% of cases), which is confined to the extrahepatic bile ducts. Type 2 is a diverticulum arising from the common bile duct (2% of cases). Type 3 occurs just proximal to the ampulla of Vater in the distal intraduodenal wall segment of the common bile duct, with extension into the duodenal lumen. Type 4 consists of multiple regions of cystic dilatation of the extrahepatic or intrahepatic biliary tree.

Ultrasound is a useful imaging modality for the evaluation of choledochal cysts. Cysts appear as anechoic structures in the region of the porta hepatis or under the liver, separate from the gallbladder and in direct communication with the biliary tree [**Fig. 5.6**]. Enlargement of the proximal common bile duct or dilation of the intrahepatic ducts can be seen. If a choledochal cyst is suspected, the entire biliary tree should be closely interrogated to identify the extent of disease. With significant cystic dilation of the common bile duct, biliary lithiasis can be seen secondary to bile stasis. Magnetic resonance imaging (MRI) and computed tomography (CT) show findings similar to ultrasound, and can also be used to better define any associated intrahepatic disease. Hepatobiliary scanning may be useful to confirm communication between the cyst and the hepatobiliary tree. However, it yields little additional anatomic information.

Caroli Disease

There are two forms of Caroli disease; both are rare inherited disorders. The most common form is an autosomal dominant disorder characterized by cystic dilatation of the intrahepatic biliary tree with no evidence of biliary obstruction. Patients may present from infancy through young adulthood with clinical symptoms of fever, intermittent abdominal pain, and hepatomegaly. This form of Caroli disease can be complicated by cholangitis, stone formation, and rarely, cholangiocarcinoma.

The second form of the disease is called *Caroli syndrome*. This is a more complex, autosomal recessive condition associated with congenital hepatic fibrosis and autosomal recessive polycystic kidney disease. The genetic basis for the hepatic and renal abnormalities is a series of mutations in the *PKHD1* gene that result in malformed biliary ducts and renal collecting tubules.

Caroli disease has a distinct pattern on cross-sectional imaging, with fusiform or saccular dilation of the intrahepatic bile ducts [**Fig. 5.7**]. Also seen is the classic "central dot sign," which reflects a portal vein radical surrounded by a dilated bile duct. These findings can be seen with sonography, MRI, and CT. In patients with Caroli syndrome, imaging findings consist of hepatomegaly, dilatation of the biliary radicles, and fibrous

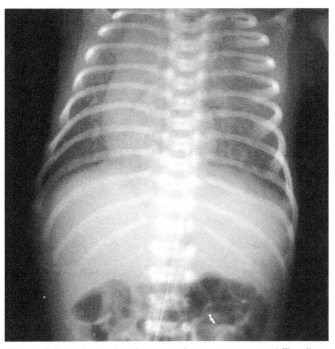

Figure 5.1 Abdominal radiograph demonstrating a midline liver in heterotaxy syndrome.

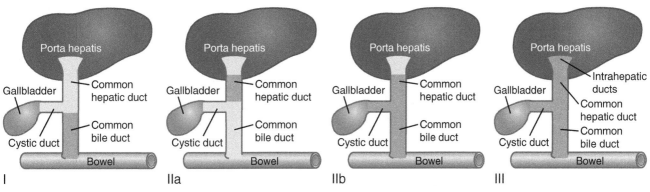

Figure 5.2 Kasai classification of biliary atresia.

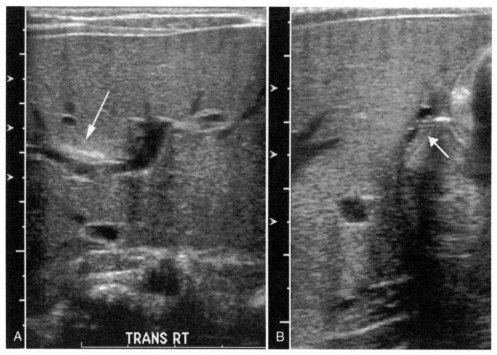

Figure 5.3 Two-month-old with biliary atresia. A, A transverse sonographic image shows a tubular echogenic cord of fibrous tissue anterior to the right portal vein (*arrow*). **B,** A sagittal sonographic image shows a diminutive gallbladder (*arrow*).

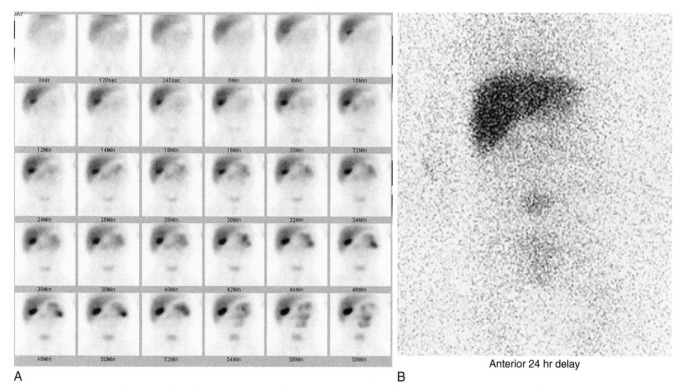

Figure 5.4 Biliary atresia. A, An anterior image from a normal hepatobiliary iminodiacetic acid (HIDA) scan shows sequential excretion of tracer into small bowel. **B,** An anterior image from a hepatobiliary HIDA scan obtained 24 hours after tracer administration in a 3-month-old infant with biliary atresia shows no excretion of tracer into the bowel.

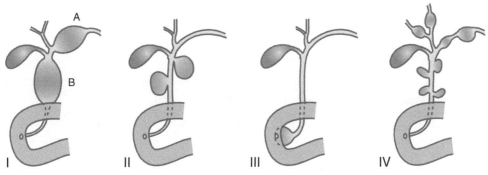

Figure 5.5 Classification of choledochal cysts.

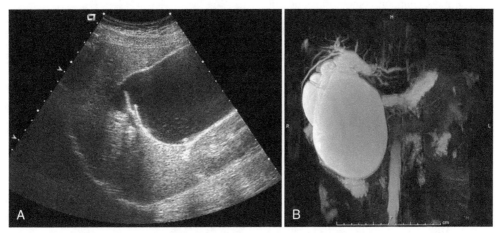

Figure 5.6 Choledochal cyst in a 16-year-old with upper abdominal pain and a palpable mass. A, A sagittal ultrasound image shows cystic dilatation of the common bile duct. **B,** Magnetic resonance cholangiopancreatography confirms a type IV choledochal cyst with dilatation of the central intrahepatic ducts.

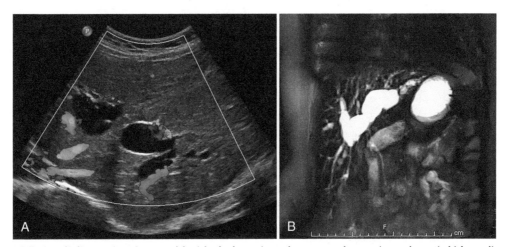

Figure 5.7 Caroli disease in a 9-year-old with cholestasis and autosomal recessive polycystic kidney disease. A, A transverse color Doppler ultrasound image shows saccular dilatation of intrahepatic ducts. **B,** An oblique magnetic resonance cholangiopancreatography image confirms dilatation and beading of the intrahepatic ducts.

replacement of liver parenchyma. Hepatic fibrosis progressively leads to symptomatic portal hypertension.

Antibiotics can be used to treat intercurrent infections, and ursodeoxycholic acid can be administered for stone formation. Endoscopic stent placement and liver transplantation have been used successfully in selected patients.

Acquired Conditions

Cholelithiasis and Choledocholithiasis

Gallstones are a common finding in children. In infants, hepatic immaturity is associated with decreased secretion of bile salts, and immature biliary conjugation pathways contribute to the formation of pigmented stones and bile sludge. Predisposing factors include the use of diuretics (furosemide) in premature infants, the administration of total parenteral nutrition, extended fasting, and an altered enterohepatic circulation, as may be seen in infants with short bowel syndrome. In these clinical settings, stones often resolve spontaneously.

Cholelithiasis is idiopathic in approximately 40% of older children. Hemolytic diseases such as sickle cell disease and thalassemia are responsible for an additional 30% of cases. Other conditions including inflammatory bowel disease affecting the ileum, CF, obesity, and short gut syndrome (after bowel surgery) have also been associated with gallstone formation. With these entities, an interrupted enterohepatic circulation is contributory.

It is important to remember that up to 50% of pediatric patients will be asymptomatic with gallstones. Another large percentage of patients will present with nonspecific, intermittent abdominal pain. The most common complications of gallstones in pediatric patients are acute calculus cholecystitis and acute pancreatitis in the setting of cystic duct or pancreatic duct obstruction.

Although conventional abdominal radiographs may demonstrate up to 50% of gallstones, ultrasound is considered the imaging modality of choice for evaluation, with an accuracy of more than 95% for the detection of cholelithiasis. Luminal debris/sludge, bile concretions, and calculi are all well demonstrated by ultrasound. Dilatation of the common duct is often the only indirect sign of downstream calculi because direct stone visualization may be difficult in the setting of overlying bowel gas.

Even though the appearance of most gallstones on CT is identical to that seen on radiographs, some stones will be isodense to background bile in the gallbladder, and thus can be missed on CT.

Gallstones are seen on MRI as T2 hypointense foci against a background of T2 bright bile in the gallbladder. Stones can also be evaluated with magnetic resonance cholangiopancreatography (MRCP), which will demonstrate filling void(s) in the gallbladder or biliary tree.

In asymptomatic patients, treatment is typically expectant with periodic ultrasound surveillance. Patients who are symptomatic from gallstones should have them removed. Endoscopic retrograde cholangiopancreatography (ERCP) is often the treatment of choice in symptomatic patients without predisposing underlying disease. If ERCP is unsuccessful, laparoscopic cholecystectomy is performed.

Biliary Sludge

Noncalcified biliary debris (sludge) is a common, transient phenomenon resulting from biliary stasis. Predisposing conditions include biliary obstruction, extended fasting, parenteral nutrition, and hemolysis. Although usually asymptomatic, the presence of biliary sludge may be associated with a dramatic but transient rise in conjugated bilirubin. On sonographic evaluation, sludge is moderately echogenic and usually lacks acoustic shadowing. It may be associated with a fluid–debris level or may coalesce into focal echogenic "masses" (tumefactive sludge) [**Fig. 5.8**]. Sludge is typically mobile with changes in patient position.

Biliary sludge does not require specific therapy in most situations. However, frequent sonographic monitoring is useful to document resolution or progression to calculus formation.

Cholecystitis

Acute cholecystitis occurs far less commonly in children than in the adult population. However, mortality rates in young children approach 30% because of associated serious concomitant illness and a high risk for ischemia and perforation. Cholecystitis may be classified as calculous or acalculous based on the presence or

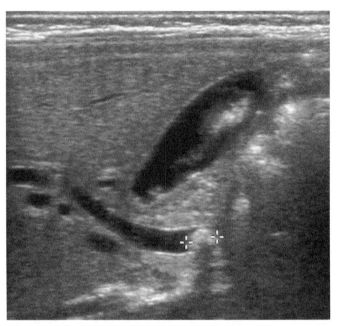

Figure 5.8 Tumefactive bile sludge in a 15-day-old infant with rapidly rising total bilirubin levels. A sagittal ultrasound image shows biliary sludge floating in the gallbladder lumen, with an obstructing sludge ball in a dilated common bile duct (*cursors*).

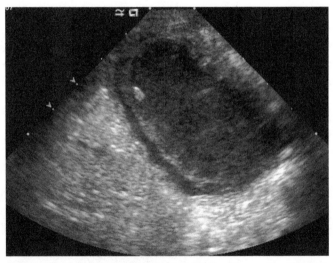

Figure 5.9 Acute acalculous cholecystitis in a 9-month-old infant with urosepsis. A transverse ultrasound image of the gallbladder shows a dilated, debris-filled, thick-walled gallbladder.

absence of obstructing calculi in the bladder neck or cystic duct. The common pathway in both conditions involves distention of the gallbladder, with increased intraluminal pressure and bile stasis. Bile stasis results in chemical injury to the gallbladder mucosa, with progressive edema, ischemia, and necrosis of the gallbladder wall. Perforation may occur in severe cases. Acalculous cholecystitis constitutes more than 50% of cases in infants and young children and has been associated with severe gram-negative bacterial infections, cytomegalovirus, and Epstein-Barr virus [**Fig. 5.9**].

Sonography is the imaging modality of choice to diagnose acute cholecystitis. Ultrasound findings in pediatric patients are similar to those seen in adults. An obstructing biliary stone often can be identified in the gallbladder neck, cystic duct, or common bile duct. A positive sonographic Murphy sign may be helpful

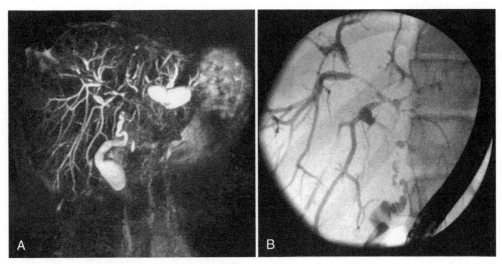

Figure 5.10 Primary sclerosing cholangitis in a 15-year-old with Crohn disease and acute abdominal pain. **A,** Magnetic resonance cholangiopancreatography shows irregular beading of the intrahepatic ducts. **B,** An oblique image from an endoscopic retrograde cholangiopancreatography confirms narrowing and irregular beading of multiple hepatic ducts.

when present, although this finding is not always reliable in the pediatric population. Gallbladder wall thickening (>3 mm) and pericholecystic fluid are important secondary findings. An additional secondary finding is edema involving the adjacent liver parenchyma.

Gallbladder wall thickening should be approached with caution because this finding can be seen in multiple pathologic states. The differential diagnosis of gallbladder wall thickening is broad and includes pseudothickening in the postprandial state, acute or chronic cholecystitis, reactive change secondary to acute hepatitis, edema in the setting of congestive heart failure, and edema related to third-spacing in hypoalbuminemia.

Findings of acute cholecystitis on CT and MRI are similar to those seen with ultrasound. MRI may be more sensitive for the detection of inflammation within the gallbladder wall and in the liver and mesentery surrounding the gallbladder. Evaluation of the biliary tree with MRCP can demonstrate an impacted stone in the gallbladder neck or cystic duct. Although frequently used in the past, CT is not currently recommended for this clinical indication in pediatric patients because of the associated radiation exposure.

Hepatobiliary scanning is not commonly used in the pediatric population for the diagnosis of biliary obstruction. It is typically reserved for cases with high clinical suspicion and equivocal findings on ultrasound. The most common positive scintigraphic finding in pediatric acute cholecystitis is lack of visualization of the gallbladder by 40 minutes after tracer administration.

Medical treatment consists of supportive measures, intravenous antibiotics, and occasional percutaneous cholecystotomy before definitive surgery.

Hydrops of the Gallbladder

Gallbladder hydrops is characterized by marked distension of the gallbladder without evidence of secondary inflammation. It occurs in the setting of transient, self-limiting acalculous obstruction of bile flow. On imaging, the hydropic gallbladder is often longer than the adjacent right kidney but maintains normal wall thickness with no appreciable hyperemia or pericholecystic fluid. Both gallbladder hydrops and acute acalculous cholecystitis may occur in Kawasaki disease, presumably because of direct vascular compromise to the gallbladder.

Cholangitis

Ascending cholangitis may be caused by a number of conditions, including calculi, parasitic infestation, immunodeficiency syndromes, and biliary obstruction caused by neoplasms. It may also occur as a complication of surgical (Kasai) repair of biliary atresia. Sclerosing cholangitis is typically an autoimmune disease. More than 80% of patients with primary sclerosing cholangitis (PSC) have concomitant inflammatory bowel disease, and about one-third of patients have associated autoimmune hepatitis. Other diseases associated with sclerosing cholangitis in children include Langerhans cell histiocytosis and CF. Patients typically present in the second decade of life with jaundice, hepatomegaly, and abdominal pain.

Dilatation and irregular wall thickening of the common bile duct and large intrahepatic ducts are seen on ultrasound, CT, and MRI. At sonography, hyperechoic portal triads, a thickened gallbladder wall, and calculi are also demonstrated in patients with PSC. Abnormal contrast enhancement of the biliary duct walls may be seen on contrast-enhanced CT. In many pediatric institutions, MRI with MRCP is the preferred imaging modality in patients with suspected PSC. This technique well demonstrates focal areas of hepatic parenchymal signal abnormality and a beaded appearance of the common bile duct and large intrahepatic ducts [**Fig. 5.10**]. In older children, MRCP has a reported sensitivity greater than 85% and a specificity greater than 90% for the detection of PSC.

Treatment with ursodeoxycholic acid alone or in combination with immunosuppressive therapy may temporarily contain disease activity. However, up to one-third of patients with PSC will eventually go on to require liver transplantation.

Hepatic Parenchymal Disorders

Hepatic Infections

Viral Hepatitis. Viral hepatitis is the most common diffuse infection of the liver in otherwise healthy children. In the newborn, cytomegalovirus and hepatitis B virus are the most common causative agents associated with chronic inflammatory change, fibrosis, and eventual cirrhosis. In older children, viral hepatitis is most commonly caused by the hepatitis A, B, and C viruses, although cytomegalovirus, herpes simplex virus, varicella zoster virus, and Epstein-Barr virus can all result in hepatic inflammation.

The diagnosis of viral hepatitis is made clinically and on the basis of laboratory data. The clinical presentation of viral hepatitis varies with the pathogen. Hepatitis A presents with a flu-like illness and fever, and is sometimes associated with jaundice. In children, the disease is typically self-limited and may be clinically inapparent. Both hepatitis B and C cause acute disease, which may progress to chronic hepatitis and possibly the development of cirrhosis and hepatocellular carcinoma (HCC).

If imaging is performed during the early stages of illness, the liver is usually normal in appearance. As the disease progresses, there may be hepatomegaly, and the liver parenchyma may appear somewhat echogenic and heterogeneous on ultrasound. In severe acute hepatitis, there is diffusely decreased parenchymal echogenicity with relative increased echogenicity of the portal triads, resulting in the classic "starry-sky" appearance. Other findings on ultrasound include enlargement of lymph nodes in the porta hepatis and reactive inflammatory change involving the gallbladder, including gallbladder wall thickening and pericholecystic fluid. CT may show mild hepatomegaly, heterogeneous liver parenchyma, decreased periportal attenuation, and gallbladder wall thickening. On MRI, there may be periportal hyperintensity on T2-weighted sequences. Unfortunately, the imaging findings of acute hepatitis are nonspecific and require appropriate clinical correlation.

In some children, viral hepatitis may result in fulminant hepatic failure, characterized by severe impairment of hepatic function with necrosis of hepatocytes in the absence of preexisting liver disease. Necrotic areas contract in size and may have internal hemorrhage or inflammatory cell infiltration.

Pyogenic Abscess. Pyogenic abscesses are typically polymicrobial, with the most common agents being gram-negative aerobic and anaerobic organisms such as *Escherichia coli* and *Klebsiella* and gram-positive organisms such as *Staphylococcus aureus* and *Streptococcus pneumoniae*.

The most common route of entry is via the portal venous system in the setting of an intraabdominal infection such as appendicitis or colitis. Abscesses are typically solitary and most commonly seen in the right hepatic lobe. In the very early stages of infection, a cluster of microabscesses may be seen that eventually coalesce into a larger confluent pyogenic abscess cavity. Bacteria may also enter the liver through the hepatic arterial system in the setting of sepsis, resulting in multifocal peripheral abscesses. Biliary entry is also possible after ERCP or biliary surgery. Resultant abscesses are more centrally located or along the path of the intrahepatic biliary tree. Superinfection of necrotic tissue can occur after hepatic trauma.

On cross-sectional imaging, the appearance of pyogenic abscesses may range from a single, well-defined, homogeneous lesion to poorly defined, heterogeneous regions of distorted hepatic parenchyma [**Fig. 5.11**]. Internal septations and debris can be seen when abscesses are large. There is often increased surrounding vascularity on color Doppler sonography and peripheral enhancement on CT and MRI. All abscesses lack blood flow centrally. Internal gas can be seen in infection with gas-forming organisms. A thin surrounding rim of hepatic edema may be noted.

Treatment of a pyogenic hepatic abscess varies based on size. Smaller abscesses (<3 cm) are typically treated with intravenous antibiotic therapy. Larger collections usually warrant percutaneous aspiration and catheter drainage. Surgical drainage is performed when catheter drainage fails or treatment of an underlying cause of the abscess is required.

Fungal Infection. Hepatic fungal infection occurs frequently in the setting of disseminated fungal disease in immunocompromised patients. In pediatrics, this includes patients on

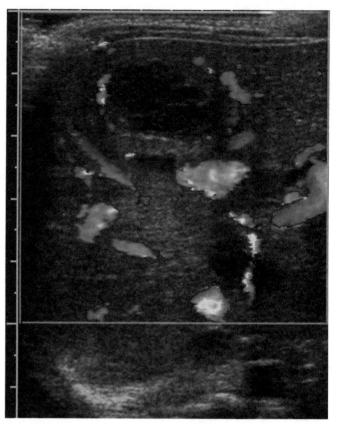

Figure 5.11 *E. coli* abscess in a 3-week-old with sepsis. A transverse color Doppler ultrasound image through the right hepatic lobe shows a complex, septated cystic lesion with intense peripheral vascularity and no blood flow centrally.

chemotherapy and those who are status post bone marrow or solid organ transplant. The most common causative organism is *Candida albicans*, which typically presents with microabscesses involving multiple organs including the liver, spleen, and occasionally the kidneys. Other less common causative organisms include *Aspergillus*, *Coccidioides*, *Cryptococcus*, and *Histoplasma*. Colonization of the gastrointestinal (GI) tract is the preliminary path of dissemination of *Candida*, with the presence of mucositis in immunocompromised patients facilitating spread of the organism.

Notably, the diagnosis of hepatic fungal disease is limited on all imaging modalities when the patient is neutropenic and unable to mount a sufficient immune response. In these patients, it is important to consider repeat imaging after recovery of the neutrophil count, especially if clinical suspicion is high and the patient is not responding to conventional antibiotic therapy.

Four sonographic patterns of hepatic candidiasis have been described, representing the different stages of hepatic infection. The "wheel-within-a-wheel" and "bull's-eye" or "target" appearances are commonly seen during the active phase of infection. The most common pattern seen later in the course of disease is diffuse, tiny (<4 mm), uniformly hypoechoic foci throughout the liver, reflecting the formation of small microabscesses [**Fig. 5.12**]. Punctate echogenic foci generally indicate healing or healed fungal infection.

Findings on noncontrast CT include multiple foci of low attenuation of varying size, generally between 2 and 20 mm. Microabscesses usually enhance centrally, although peripheral enhancement may occur.

As with ultrasound, the imaging appearance of hepatic fungal disease on MRI varies with the phase of infection and stage of treatment [**Fig. 5.12**]. Several authors suggest that MRI is

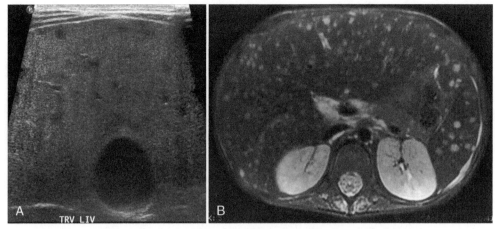

Figure 5.12 **Hepatic *Candida* microabscesses in a 5-year-old with leukemia with fever and neutropenia.** **A,** A transverse ultrasound image through the liver shows multiple hypoechoic nodules. **B,** An axial T2-weighted magnetic resonance image shows innumerable T2 bright lesions throughout the liver and spleen.

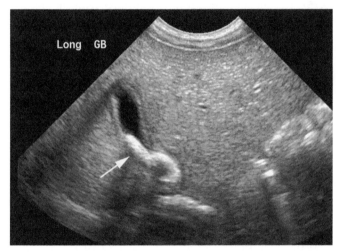

Figure 5.13 Ascariasis of the biliary tree in a 2-year-old with recurrent right upper quadrant pain and jaundice. A transverse ultrasound image at the level of the gallbladder shows a linear echogenic worm in the cystic duct (*arrow*).

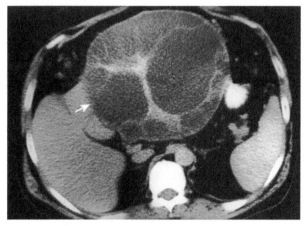

Figure 5.14 An axial computed tomography image shows a liver abscess (*arrow*) in a child with *Echinococcus* infection. A large, complex cystic lesion is seen, with multiple daughter cysts noted.

superior to CT for the identification of hepatosplenic fungal disease, with a reported sensitivity of 100% and specificity of 96%. Thus many institutions now use limited MRI protocols consisting of fast-acquisition T2-weighted sequences rather than CT for rapid imaging assessment for fungal disease in pediatric patients. More extensive MRI protocols are used to follow disease change after the implementation of treatment.

Parasitic Infections. Although rare in developed countries, parasitic disease is estimated to affect almost 1 billion people worldwide. The three most common infections—ascariasis, echinococcosis, and amebiasis—are endemic in many parts of the world.

Ascariasis is a parasitic infection that is prevalent in tropical and subtropical regions of the world. It occurs when the parasite eggs are inadvertently ingested. Eggs develop into larvae in the bowel and subsequently develop into long, thin, pencil-shaped worms that penetrate through the intestinal wall, enter the portal venous system, and eventually travel to the liver. Clinical symptoms depend on the stage of infection. Biliary obstruction can occur, resulting in dilation of the intrahepatic bile ducts on ultrasound. Occasionally, worms can be identified within the bile ducts or the portal vasculature [**Fig. 5.13**].

Echinococcal, or hydatid disease, is somewhat more common. It is endemic in regions of South America, the Middle East, and the Mediterranean. After ingestion of eggs from contaminated soil or water, the protective covering of echinococcal eggs is broken down by gastric acid, and larvae pass through the mucosa into the portal venous system. Larvae then become lodged in the liver and slowly grow into hydatid cysts. Daughter cysts, a pathognomonic finding, form from brood capsules along the periphery of an endocyst [**Fig. 5.14**]. As they enlarge, echinococcal cysts are prone to rupture. In a "contained rupture," the endocyst membrane pulls away from the pericyst, resulting in a "floating" internal membrane. If rupture is not contained, cystic contents can spill into the peritoneal cavity and result in seeding of the peritoneum.

Definitive treatment of an echinococcal cyst requires removal of the entire cyst and its contents. Primary surgical removal is often not attempted because of concern for cyst rupture and peritoneal spillage. Initial treatment typically consists of percutaneous drainage in conjunction with antiparasitic therapy with albendazole. This is subsequently followed by complete surgical excision.

An amebic abscess may have a variable imaging appearance. Features are often similar to those of a pyogenic abscess. Both

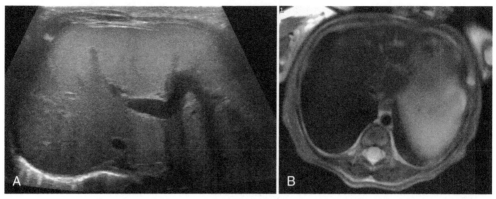

Figure 5.15 Primary hemochromatosis in a 6-week-old infant with cholestasis and hepatitis. A, A transverse ultrasound image of the liver shows hepatomegaly and diffusely increased hepatic echogenicity. **B,** An axial T2-weighted magnetic resonance image with fat saturation shows markedly decreased hepatic signal caused by iron deposition.

pyogenic and amebic abscesses are more common in the right hepatic lobe and are often peripheral in location near the liver capsule. Treatment of an amebic abscess is medical. Metronidazole is typically administered, with a rapid response most often observed within 24 to 72 hours.

Hepatic Steatosis

Hepatic steatosis is caused by excessive accumulation of triglycerides within hepatocytes. It is the most common cause of chronic liver disease in pediatric patients. The pathologic diagnosis of hepatic steatosis is made when more than 5% of the total liver weight is replaced by fat. Adolescents are affected more often than younger children, with a higher prevalence in boys than girls. Obesity and associated insulin resistance are the most common risk factors for hepatic steatosis. The overall incidence of disease is increasing in the United States with the increase in pediatric obesity. Fatty infiltration of the liver may be focal or diffuse. When focal, fatty deposition classically occurs along the falciform ligament and the gallbladder fossa. Areas of focal fat deposition demonstrate well-defined margins.

Metabolic Diseases

Several hereditary metabolic diseases may cause liver damage with liver failure or cirrhosis, with or without associated injury to other tissues. These include hemochromatosis, tyrosinemia type I, α1-antitrypsin deficiency, CF, and glycogen storage disease (type I). Although individually rare, together they account for approximately 10% of liver transplants in children.

Hemochromatosis/Iron Deposition. Iron overload can occur by three basic mechanisms, including excess intestinal absorption, repeated blood transfusions, or inborn errors of metabolism. As systemic iron concentration overwhelms the capacity of ferritin to bind to and store iron, unbound iron accumulates in the cytoplasm of cells in the liver, spleen, pancreas, and bone marrow, resulting in cellular damage. A neonatal form of hereditary hemochromatosis known as neonatal iron storage disease exists, with the onset of liver disease in utero. Illness is usually evident within hours of birth, with features of fulminant hepatic failure.

Parenchymal alterations on both ultrasound and CT are considered nonspecific and nondiagnostic. MRI is the most useful noninvasive diagnostic tool for the identification of hepatic iron overload. As iron concentration in the hepatic parenchyma increases, signal intensity on T2 and gradient echo sequences decreases, leading to the appearance of a "black" liver [**Fig.

5.15**]. Treatment of primary disease involves frequent phlebotomy, whereas treatment of secondary disease involves iron chelation therapy.

Tyrosinemia Type I. Tyrosinemia type I is a rare disorder caused by a defect in the enzyme fumarylacetoacetate hydrolase. This defect leads to the accumulation of caustic metabolites in the liver and results in damage to DNA and a predisposition to the development of HCC. Patients may present with acute liver failure, chronic liver disease, or acute neurologic decompensation. In up to 42% of patients, clinical manifestations develop within the first year of life. Nephromegaly is frequently present. This entity should be considered when cirrhosis presents in early infancy. Treatment with 2-[2-nitro-4-(trifluoromethyl)benzoyl] cyclohexane-1,3-dione (NTBC) can be effective if started early. NTBC blocks the formation of caustic alkylating metabolites in the liver.

Glycogen Storage Disease. Glycogen storage disease type I (von Gierke disease) is an autosomal recessive condition that results from a defect of the enzyme glucose-6-phosphatase, with resultant accumulation of glycogen in the liver, kidneys, and intestines. This disease may manifest in infancy with hypoglycemia, hepatomegaly, and nephromegaly. Hepatic adenomas and HCC have been described.

Ultrasound and CT most commonly show hepatomegaly and heterogeneous hepatic architecture. Nodules rarely occur and may appear hyperdense or hypodense on CT.

Hepatic Neoplasms

Primary hepatic tumors are relatively uncommon, accounting for 0.5% to 2% of all pediatric neoplasms. As in the adult population, the most common neoplasm involving the liver is metastatic disease, usually from neuroblastoma, Wilms tumor, or lymphoma. Malignant lesions account for approximately two-thirds of all primary liver tumors in children. A focused differential diagnosis for a liver tumor can be generated based on the age of the patient, serum tumor markers such as α-fetoprotein, and imaging characteristics.

Benign Lesions

Hemangioma. Hemangioma is the most common hepatic mass presenting within the first 6 months of life, with nearly 50% of cases manifesting by the age of 1 month. Girls are affected more often than boys. This is a benign vascular tumor consisting of proliferation of endothelium-lined vascular spaces.

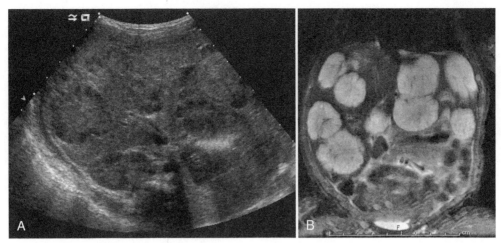

Figure 5.16 Congenital hepatic hemangiomas in a 12-day-old infant with congestive heart failure. A, A transverse ultrasound image through the liver shows multiple nodules with a peripheral hypoechoic rim representing dilated blood vessels. **B,** An axial fast spin echo inversion recovery magnetic resonance image shows multiple hyperintense hemangiomas throughout the liver.

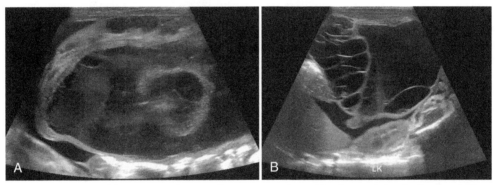

Figure 5.17 Mesenchymal hamartoma in a newborn presenting with a large abdominal mass. A, Transverse and **(B)** sagittal ultrasound images through the inferior aspect of the liver show a multiseptated cystic mass arising from the liver edge, with internal echogenic debris. Treatment is typically surgical resection.

Concomitant cutaneous hemangiomas occur in up to 50% of affected individuals. Hemangiomas are classified as infantile or congenital. The infantile form typically begins to grow after birth and slowly involutes after the second year of life. Congenital hemangiomas are present at birth and further subclassified as rapidly involuting congenital hemangiomas that regress within the first 14 months of life and noninvoluting congenital hemangiomas, which follow a clinical course similar to that seen with the infantile form.

Most hemangiomas present as a painless upper abdominal mass. However, serious clinical complications may occur. High-output congestive heart failure may be seen with high-flow lesions. This may be exacerbated by hypothyroidism caused by high levels of tumor-produced iodothyronine deiodinase. Occasionally, the Kasabach-Merritt syndrome of intratumoral consumptive coagulopathy may be seen. α-Fetoprotein levels are rarely elevated with this tumor.

The imaging appearance of hepatic hemangiomas may be quite variable. Multifocal lesions are typically small and relatively uniform in appearance. Large focal lesions are often heterogeneous, with areas of hemorrhage, infarction, and dystrophic calcification. Diffuse lesions result in marked enlargement of the liver, with replacement by large, vascular masses [**Fig. 5.16**]. Hepatic arteries and veins are commonly enlarged, with prominent feeding and draining vessels within and surrounding the tumor(s). With bolus injection of contrast material and serial CT or MRI at the level of a lesion, early centripetal

enhancement with delayed central enhancement over time will be observed.

Medical therapy using propranolol with or without concurrent steroids is highly effective in the management of hepatic hemangiomas. Additional supportive measures to treat congestive failure and hypothyroidism may be indicated.

Mesenchymal Hamartoma. Mesenchymal hamartoma is the second most common benign hepatic tumor in young children after hemangioma. The median patient age at presentation is 11 months, with the majority of children presenting before age 2 years. There is a slight male preponderance. There are no specific laboratory markers for mesenchymal hamartoma. Serum α-fetoprotein levels are typically within normal range for age and are useful in distinguishing this tumor from hepatoblastoma.

A mesenchymal hamartoma is a solitary, multicystic, septated mass. Cysts vary in size and are filled with gelatinous or clear fluid. Rarely, the tumor may be solid or pedunculated. In 75% of cases, the mass arises in the right hepatic lobe. Histologically, a mesenchymal hamartoma consists of a mixture of mesenchyme, bile ducts, hepatocytes, and inflammatory and hematopoietic cells.

The imaging appearance depends on the predominance of cysts or stroma (mesenchymal elements) within the mass [**Fig. 5.17**]. At sonography, cystic portions of the tumor may contain low-level echoes related to their gelatinous composition. Although vessels may be visible within septae on color Doppler,

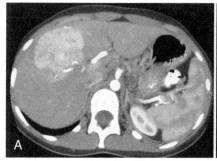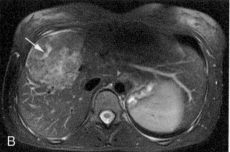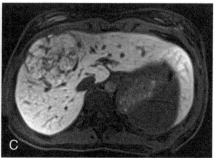

Figure 5.18 Focal nodular hyperplasia incidentally found in a 15-year-old girl. A, An axial contrast-enhanced computed tomography image shows a lobulated, heterogeneously enhancing mass. **B,** An axial T2-weighted magnetic resonance (MR) image with fat saturation shows a heterogeneously hyperintense mass with a hyperintense central scar (*arrow*). **C,** An axial T1-weighted MR image with fat saturation obtained 20 minutes after the intravenous injection of gadoxetic acid disodium shows accumulation of contrast in hepatocytes within the lesion.

overall relatively little tumor vascularity is present. Contrast-enhanced CT shows a complex cystic mass with enhancement of septae and stromal elements. On MRI, cystic portions of the mass demonstrate T2 hyperintensity because of high water content and variable T1 signal based on the presence of proteinaceous material within the cysts. As with CT, there will be mild contrast-enhancement of septae and solid stromal components.

Focal Nodular Hyperplasia. Focal nodular hyperplasia (FNH) is uncommon in young children, most frequently occurring in adolescents and adults. It represents approximately 2% of all primary hepatic tumors in children younger than 20 years. The female/male ratio is as high as 4:1 in the pediatric age group. The tumor commonly presents as an incidental finding at imaging or surgical exploration for other reasons.

FNH typically manifests as a solitary, well-circumscribed, lobulated, solid lesion that is commonly subcapsular in location. A stellate focus of fibrosis is seen centrally [**Fig. 5.18**]. Histologic examination demonstrates ectatic vessels in the central scar and benign lobules of hyperplastic hepatocytes containing bile ducts surrounding the scar.

At sonography, FNH appears as a homogeneous, well-circumscribed mass with variable echogenicity relative to normal liver parenchyma. When present, the central scar is hyperechoic relative to the remainder of the mass. On unenhanced CT, FNH is typically well circumscribed and isodense to slightly hypodense relative to normal surrounding liver. The scar is hypodense. After intravenous contrast administration, FNH typically shows early, uniform enhancement, becoming isodense to the liver during the late venous phase. Although the MRI appearance of FNH is variable, delayed scanning after the intravenous injection of a hepatocyte-selective, gadolinium-based contrast agent such as gadoxetic acid disodium (Eovist) may be useful in identifying the presence of normal hepatocytes within a lesion. These agents are taken up by normal hepatocytes and eliminated through bile. On delayed scanning (20 minutes after injection), there is accumulation of contrast in normal liver parenchyma and in focal liver lesions containing hepatocytes such as FNH. This results in relatively high signal on T1-weighted images. Lesions that do not contain hepatocytes appear hypointense after the administration of these contrast agents.

Malignant Lesions

Hepatoblastoma. Hepatoblastoma is the most common primary hepatic neoplasm of childhood, accounting for approximately 75% of all liver tumors. Patients typically present between the ages of 18 months and 3 years with an asymptomatic abdominal mass. Markedly elevated α-fetoprotein levels are seen in almost all patients. An increased incidence is seen in patients with Beckwith-Wiedemann syndrome, other hemihypertrophy syndromes, and familial adenomatous polyposis coli.

Hepatoblastoma is a tumor of epithelial and mesenchymal cell origin. It is usually a solitary, large (>10 cm), well-circumscribed lesion with a nodular surface and is most commonly seen in the right hepatic lobe [**Fig. 5.19**]. Multifocal liver lesions have been reported in up to 15% of patients. Calcifications can be seen in up to 50% of cases, and areas of hemorrhage or necrosis may be present. Tumor vascularity may be identified on ultrasound. The portal and hepatic vasculature should be carefully examined for intravascular tumor thrombus. Hepatoblastoma is usually hypodense on noncontrast CT imaging. With the administration of contrast material, there is slight enhancement relative to normal liver early on, with the tumor becoming isodense to hypodense relative to normal liver on delayed imaging. On MRI, most lesions are hypointense to adjacent liver parenchyma on T1-weighted images and heterogeneously hyperintense on T2-weighted images. Areas of intralesional fibrosis appear as bands of hypointense signal on both T1-and T2-weighted sequences. Hepatoblastoma typically shows heterogeneous enhancement.

Approximately 10% of patients will have metastatic disease at the time of diagnosis. This usually involves local lymph nodes and the lung, with rare involvement of the skeleton and brain.

Cure generally depends on complete resection of the primary tumor. Up to 85% of the liver can be safely resected with hepatic regeneration noted within 3 to 4 months after surgery. Chemotherapy increases the chance of long-term survival. In low-stage tumors, survival rates exceeding 90% can be achieved with multimodal treatment. When hepatoblastoma is multifocal, nonresectable, or metastatic at diagnosis, survival rates decline considerably. α-Fetoprotein levels can be used to measure disease response to therapy. Importantly, α-fetoprotein levels are normally elevated at birth, reaching adult levels by about 6 months of age.

Liver transplant is a viable option for unresectable primary hepatic malignancies. However, it is much more effective as primary treatment as opposed to salvage therapy.

Hepatocellular Carcinoma. HCC is the second most common malignant liver tumor encountered in children. Unlike hepatoblastoma, HCC is more common in older children and adolescents, with a peak incidence between 12 and 14 years of age. Patients present with abdominal distention and a palpable mass in the right upper quadrant. The serum α-fetoprotein level is elevated in up to 80% of patients. Most patients

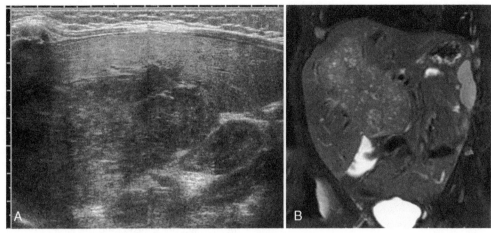

Figure 5.19 Hepatoblastoma in a 5-month-old infant with an abdominal mass. A, A composite sagittal ultrasound image of the right hepatic lobe shows a complex, heterogeneously hypoechoic solid mass compressing surrounding liver parenchyma. **B,** A coronal T2-weighted magnetic resonance image with fat saturation shows a heterogeneous, hyperintense mass extending into the porta hepatis and causing intrahepatic biliary ductal dilatation.

have underlying cirrhosis of the liver. Conditions predisposing to cirrhosis in pediatric patients include biliary atresia, infantile cholestasis, viral hepatitis, glycogen storage disease, hemochromatosis, α1-antitrypsin deficiency, Wilson disease, and single-ventricle disorders treated with Fontan shunts.

On ultrasound, smaller lesions (<3 cm) typically appear as circumscribed hypoechoic foci, whereas larger lesions appear more heterogeneous or hyperechoic. Up to 40% of lesions demonstrate internal calcification. Tumor invasion of the portal vein and/or inferior vena cava may result in tumor thrombus.

On multiphase CT, HCC demonstrates intense enhancement in the arterial phase, with rapid washout on delayed imaging save persistent capsular enhancement. On MRI, HCC usually appears hypointense to isointense with respect to the liver on T1-weighted images and isointense to hyperintense on T2-weighted images. The postgadolinium enhancement pattern is similar to that seen on CT, with early arterial phase enhancement of the mass followed by rapid washout with persistent capsular enhancement on delayed imaging.

Surgical management of HCC depends on whether disease is localized or multifocal, and also on the presence or absence of underlying liver disease. Complete surgical resection is accomplished in only 30% to 40% of cases. Tumors are typically poorly responsive to chemotherapy. Even with complete surgical resection, long-term survival is seen in only 30% of cases.

Rhabdomyosarcoma. Biliary rhabdomyosarcoma occurs almost exclusively in children. It represents only 1% of all pediatric liver tumors. Increasing abdominal distension and jaundice are the most common presenting symptoms. Laboratory evaluation typically reveals elevated direct bilirubin and alkaline phosphatase, with a normal α-fetoprotein level. This tumor is generally very large at the time of diagnosis and most often involves the major extrahepatic bile ducts with secondary invasion into the intrahepatic bile ducts. Polypoid or grapelike projections of tumor can sometimes be seen projecting into the lumen of the bile ducts, analogous to the appearance of botryoid rhabdomyosarcoma involving the bladder.

The imaging appearance can be variable based on tumor size and location. There are no pathognomonic imaging features described. The bile ducts are usually dilated. There may be mass effect on the portal vein, without vascular invasion by tumor or the presence of tumor thrombus. On CT and MRI, the tumor may be homogeneous or heterogeneous, with a

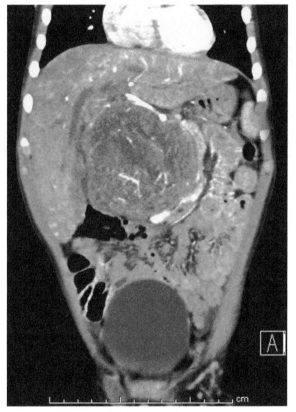

Figure 5.20 Biliary rhabdomyosarcoma in a 2-year-old with abdominal pain and jaundice. A coronal contrast-enhanced computed tomography image shows a large, heterogeneously enhancing mass arising from the porta hepatis.

variable pattern of enhancement demonstrated [**Fig. 5.20**]. MRCP can be particularly helpful to demonstrate involvement of the bile ducts.

Complete surgical resection is desirable but is achieved in only 20% to 40% of patients. Advances in multimodal therapy with surgery, radiation, and chemotherapy have led to markedly improved outcomes, with a 78% survival rate among patients with localized disease at diagnosis.

Metastatic Lesions. The liver is a common site for malignant spread of neoplasm due to its rich vascular supply. In children, the most common tumors that metastasize to the liver are neuroblastoma (particularly stage IV-S in children younger than 1 year) and Wilms tumor. Hepatic involvement by lymphoma and leukemia is less common.

The ultrasound appearance of metastatic disease can be variable, ranging from focal hypoechoic lesions to diffuse parenchymal infiltration. Notably, ultrasound has up to a 20% false-negative rate for the detection of metastatic lesions. CT is a more sensitive modality to delineate the extent of disease. Most liver metastases are hypointense on T1-weighted images. Even very tiny metastases may be clearly depicted as hyperintense lesions on T2-weighted, fat-saturated images [**Fig. 5.21**]. Diffusion-weighted imaging may be helpful in the detection of small metastatic foci.

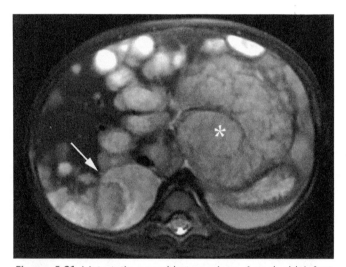

Figure 5.21 Metastatic neuroblastoma in a 6-week-old infant with hepatomegaly. An axial T2-weighted image with fat saturation through the upper abdomen shows multiple T2 bright metastatic hepatic nodules, with a large metastatic lesion in the left hepatic lobe (*asterisk*). A right adrenal primary tumor is shown (*arrow*).

PANCREAS

Anatomy and Embryology

The pancreas develops from ventral and dorsal anlagen that arise from the endodermal lining of the duodenum [**Fig. 5.22**]. The dorsal anlage develops at approximately 4 weeks' gestation as a bud from the dorsal side of the duodenum. The ventral anlage develops at approximately 5 weeks' gestation as a bud from the ventral side of the duodenum at the same level as the bile duct.

As the GI tract rotates into its final position in the seventh week of gestation, the ventral pancreatic anlage rotates in a counterclockwise direction. It moves posteriorly and to the left within the abdominal cavity, reaching its final position in the midabdomen.

The two pancreatic anlagen join into a single gland, with the ventral anlage forming the uncinate process and posterior part of the pancreatic head, and the larger dorsal anlage forming the anterior pancreatic head, body, and tail. Each pancreatic bud develops its own ductal system. The dorsal pancreatic ductal component drains the tail, body, and anterior portion of the pancreatic head, whereas the ventral component drains the posterior aspect of the pancreatic head and uncinate process. When the two pancreatic anlagen join, their ductal systems fuse. The ventral duct usually persists as the major drainage pathway, combining with the distal portion of the dorsal duct to form the main pancreatic duct (of Wirsung). This drains into the duodenum through the major papilla. The proximal portion of the dorsal duct may disappear or may persist to form the accessory pancreatic duct (of Santorini), draining the anterior portion of the pancreatic head through the minor papilla.

Normal Pancreas

The pancreas grows exponentially during the first year of life, with slower growth later in childhood. The pancreatic head is relatively more prominent than the body in children. This should not be mistaken for pathology. The pancreatic duct is often slightly more prominent in children than in adults, measuring up to 1.5 to 2 mm in normal patients. Prominence of the pancreatic duct should always be correlated with clinical history, physical examination, and laboratory values because this finding may be associated with acute pancreatitis.

At sonography, the normal pediatric pancreas is well marginated with echogenicity equal to or slightly greater than that of

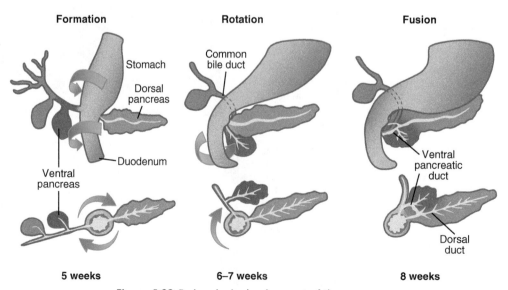

Figure 5.22 Embryologic development of the pancreas.

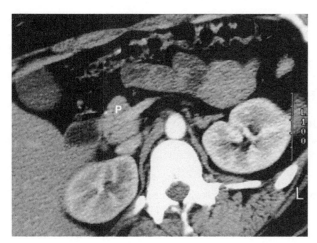

Figure 5.23 Congenital short pancreas (*P*). A small, globular pancreatic head is demonstrated, with absence of the body and tail.

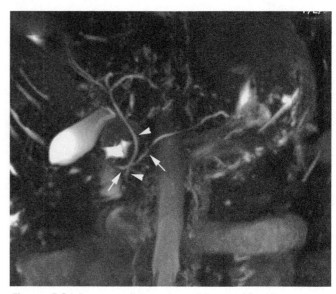

Figure 5.24 Pancreas divisum in a 16-year-old with recurrent pancreatitis. A coronal image from magnetic resonance cholangiopancreatography shows the common bile duct (*arrowheads*) crossing over the main duct (*arrows*) to join the duct of Wirsung.

the liver. In premature infants, the pancreas may be particularly echogenic, presumably related to the relative paucity of glandular tissue present at this age. The pancreas gradually diminishes in echogenicity to normal adult levels over the first 3 to 4 years of life.

At 1.5 Tesla, the MRI signal intensity of the normal pancreas is equal to that of the liver on both T1- and T2-weighted images. At 3.0 Tesla, the normal pancreas increases in signal intensity. Intensity also increases with advancing age of the child. CT imaging of the pancreas is often of limited value in young infants because of a paucity of surrounding mesenteric fat.

Developmental Anomalies

Congenital Short Pancreas

Congenital short pancreas occurs when there is failure of development of either the ventral or dorsal primordium. Associations of congenital short pancreas with polysplenia alone and of congenital short pancreas with polysplenia, bilobed lungs, malrotation, and congenital heart disease have been described. These associations are thought to be related to the development of both the pancreas and the spleen in the mesogastrium.

With failure of development of the dorsal pancreatic bud, only the smaller, ventral pancreas is present. The neck, body, and tail of the pancreas are absent, with only a portion of the head and the uncinate process remaining. Patients present with abdominal pain, pancreatitis, or diabetes, with the latter related to the relative lack of islet cells in the pancreatic head.

On cross-sectional imaging with ultrasound, CT, or MRI, only a small globular pancreatic head of variable size is identified [**Fig. 5.23**]. Treatment is focused on symptomatic relief of abdominal pain and support for diabetes and its complications.

Pancreas Divisum

Pancreas divisum is the most common anatomic variant of the pancreas, occurring in approximately 5% to 10% of the population. In this anomaly, there is absent or incomplete fusion between the ventral duct of Wirsung and the dorsal duct of Santorini. As a result, the majority of pancreatic secretions drain via the duct of Santorini into the minor papilla, with only the pancreatic head and uncinate process draining via the duct of Wirsung through the major papilla. Although pancreas divisum may be clinically silent, functional stenosis at the minor papilla can result in acute pancreatitis limited to the dorsal portions of the gland (the body and tail).

Notably, regardless of the presence of a congenital ductal anomaly, the duct of Wirsung always drains the pancreatic tail, the duct of Santorini always drains to the minor papilla, and the common bile duct always drains to the major papilla where it meets the duct of Wirsung.

A definitive diagnosis can be made on MRCP, which allows visualization of the two separate pancreatic ducts. The "crossing sign" describes the common bile duct crossing over the main duct to join the duct of Wirsung [**Fig. 5.24**]. Treatment options in symptomatic patients include sphincterotomy of the minor papilla and stenting of the duct to improve pancreatic drainage.

Annular Pancreas

Annular pancreas occurs when a ring of pancreatic tissue encircles the second portion of the duodenum. Pancreatic tissue may either partially (75%) or completely (25%) surround the duodenum. This abnormality is thought to be due to either incomplete rotation of the ventral pancreatic anlage or abnormal fixation of the tip of the ventral pancreatic anlage to the duodenum before normal rotation begins. Importantly, annular pancreas is associated with other congenital anomalies in up to 70% of infants. Associated anomalies include tracheoesophageal fistula and congenital heart disease.

Roughly half of patients with annular pancreas will present in the neonatal period with high-grade duodenal obstruction. On upper GI evaluation, a circumferential impression on the second portion of the duodenum is seen.

Ultrasound can demonstrate an abnormal, concentric course of the pancreatic duct around a dilated, fluid-filled duodenum. In patients with an incomplete ring of pancreatic tissue, the diagnosis can be suggested by the presence of excess pancreatic tissue anterior to the duodenum containing an anomalous branch of the pancreatic duct.

MRI with MRCP is the imaging modality of choice, demonstrating a complete or partial ring of pancreatic tissue around the duodenum as well as the encircling pancreatic ducts. Treatment involves surgical bypass of the obstruction by duodenoduodenostomy or laparoscopic gastrojejunostomy.

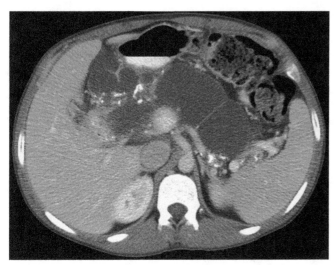

Figure 5.25 Pancreatic cystosis in a 23-year-old with cystic fibrosis. An axial contrast-enhanced computed tomography image demonstrates complete cystic replacement of the pancreas.

Systemic Disease With Pancreatic Involvement

Cystic Fibrosis

CF is the most common life-threatening recessive genetic disease in Caucasians. It is caused by defective function of the cystic fibrosis transmembrane conductance regulator (CFTR) protein, leading to impaired transport of chloride and sodium across the cell membrane, altered water diffusion out of the cell and into the mucous layer, and highly viscous epithelial secretions. The condition primarily affects the lungs and the pancreas, with exocrine pancreatic insufficiency affecting approximately 85% of patients with the disease. Protein-rich exocrine fluid in the pancreatic duct becomes viscous and inspissated, leading to duct obstruction. Retained pancreatic enzymes damage the pancreatic parenchyma, eventually leading to fatty replacement and fibrosis of the gland or diffuse glandular cystosis. The severity of pancreatic involvement in CF is variable. Patients present with signs and symptoms of malabsorption, with bulky stools and steatorrhea. CF-related diabetes is also quite common as patients with CF age. It is seen in approximately 35% of patients, with a peak onset between 18 and 24 years of age.

As the pancreatic parenchyma is replaced by fat, it becomes diffusely increased in echogenicity on ultrasound. Areas of glandular fibrosis appear hypoechoic. The pancreas may also be atrophic, with or without fatty replacement. The fatty pancreas is well demonstrated on CT and MRI.

With pancreatic cystosis, there is complete replacement of the gland by multiple macroscopic cysts [**Fig. 5.25**]. This is less commonly seen. Pathogenesis involves duct obstruction, with resultant duct ectasia and cyst formation. Macrocysts appear simple on all imaging modalities. Other less common pancreatic manifestations of CF include diffuse glandular calcification and single or multiple macroscopic parenchymal cysts.

Shwachman-Diamond Syndrome

Shwachman-Diamond syndrome (SDS) is a rare autosomal recessive disease, but the second most common cause of exocrine pancreatic insufficiency in children. SDS is associated with varying degrees of bone marrow dysfunction and skeletal anomalies. Intermittent neutropenia and pancytopenia may be seen, in addition to metaphyseal dysplasia.

In this disease, true lipomatosis of the pancreas occurs. This results in complete fatty replacement of the pancreas and glandular enlargement. Although there is near-complete pancreatic exocrine insufficiency, ductal architecture is preserved and can be well demonstrated on ultrasound and MRI.

Fatty replacement of the pancreas may also be seen in the setting of obesity and prolonged use of steroids.

Beckwith-Wiedemann Syndrome

Beckwith-Wiedemann syndrome is characterized by the classic triad of omphalocele, macroglossia, and hemihypertrophy. In this syndrome, variable degrees of organomegaly can be seen, and the pancreas may be involved. About half of the infants have hypoglycemia caused by hyperinsulinemia in the setting of islet cell hyperplasia. Although hypoglycemia is typically transient, the islet cell hyperplasia may persist. Because of abnormal cellular growth patterns, patients with Beckwith-Wiedemann syndrome are at increased risk for the development of abdominal visceral malignancies including pancreatoblastoma. Thus they are followed with routine surveillance abdominal ultrasounds from a young age.

Pancreatic Cysts

True congenital cysts of the pancreas are rare. They are most often seen in females. An isolated congenital cyst may present as an asymptomatic, palpable epigastric mass or may be associated with symptoms related to compression of the adjacent structures in the upper abdomen. Vomiting may be seen because of gastric outlet obstruction, jaundice and hyperbilirubinemia may result from biliary obstruction, and epigastric pain can develop in the setting of local mesenteric ischemia. Congenital cysts are typically simple and unilocular, and can range in size from microscopic to multiple centimeters.

Multiple congenital cysts of the pancreas may be seen as part of von Hippel-Lindau (VHL) disease, occurring in up to 30% of patients. Pancreatic cysts may be the first manifestation of disease. Involvement can range from a single cyst to innumerable cysts virtually replacing the normal pancreatic parenchyma. Cysts in VHL are typically simple but may have peripheral calcification. Other abdominal manifestations of VHL include cysts of the liver, spleen, kidneys, and mesentery. Importantly, patients with VHL are at risk for development of renal adenomas and renal cell carcinoma.

Pancreatic cysts are present in approximately 10% of patients with autosomal dominant polycystic kidney disease, a hereditary disorder with 100% penetrance but variable expressivity. Even though renal cysts are the major feature of the disease, cysts may also be seen in the liver, spleen, pancreas, and adrenal glands.

Other cystic pancreatic lesions reported in children include dermoid cysts, teratomas, and intestinal duplications.

Acquired Conditions

Acute Pancreatitis

Acute pancreatitis occurs in all age groups including infants. The incidence of acute pancreatitis in the pediatric population has increased in recent years to approach that seen in adults. This condition may be due to a wide variety of causes that lead to premature activation of pancreatic enzymes and resultant autodigestion and destruction of the pancreatic parenchyma. The subsequent inflammatory response may involve both adjacent and distant tissues and organs. The most common causes of acute pancreatitis are listed in **Table 5.1**.

Patients typically present with upper abdominal pain that is often associated with nausea and vomiting. Fever is uncommon. The most widely accepted laboratory criterion for acute pancreatitis is a greater than or equal to 3-fold elevation in the serum amylase and lipase levels. Although a clear underlying cause is

TABLE 5.1 Causes of Acute Pancreatitis in Children

COMMON
- Trauma (10%–40%)
- Biliary disorders/obstruction (10%–30%)
- Idiopathic (13%–34%)
- Medications: L-asparaginase, 6-mercaptopurine, valproic acid (<25%)

LESS COMMON
- Systemic conditions: sepsis, hemolytic-uremic syndrome, systemic lupus erythematosus (<30%)
- Infection (<10%)
- Genetic/hereditary disorders (5%–8%)
- Metabolic disease (2%–7%)

RARE
- Autoimmune pancreatitis
- Anatomic pancreaticobiliary abnormalities: pancreas divisum, annular pancreas

present in almost 25% of patients with acute pancreatitis, blunt abdominal trauma should be considered in patients with an unclear or confusing history. Gallstone pancreatitis should be suspected in the setting of elevated transaminase levels or hyperbilirubinemia.

Ultrasound is the primary imaging modality for the detection of pancreatic abnormalities in children. Important sonographic findings of pancreatitis include a focally or diffusely enlarged gland [**Fig. 5.26**] with abnormal echogenicity. Peripancreatic fluid is also a common finding in acute pancreatitis and is easily assessed with ultrasound. The most useful diagnostic feature of pancreatitis on ultrasound is dilation of the pancreatic duct [**Fig. 5.26**]. The normal pancreatic duct is less than 1.5 mm in diameter in children younger than 7 years and up to 2 mm in patients up to 15 years of age.

CT findings in acute pancreatitis include focal or diffuse enlargement of the pancreas, heterogeneous enhancement of the gland, an irregular or shaggy contour of the pancreatic margins, blurring of the peripancreatic fat planes with streaky soft tissue stranding, thickening of fascial planes, and the presence of intraperitoneal or retroperitoneal fluid collections. MRI and MRCP are excellent tools for the evaluation of pancreatitis and its complications. Peripancreatic edema and inflammation associated with acute pancreatitis are best visualized on T2-weighted sequences.

Outcomes in acute pancreatitis in pediatric patients are slightly better than in adults and notably are not correlated with initial amylase and lipase levels.

Complications of Acute Pancreatitis

Acute pancreatitis may be complicated by pseudocyst formation, abscess formation, or pancreatic necrosis [**Fig. 5.26**]. Pancreatic pseudocysts occur in up to 10% of cases of acute pancreatitis. Pseudocysts are associated with disruption of the pancreatic parenchyma and pancreatic duct, with extravasation of pancreatic enzymes. These enzymes destroy adjacent tissues and result in the formation of a fluid collection encapsulated by a thick fibrous wall. Pancreatic pseudocysts are a common complication of traumatic pancreatic injury in children.

Acute pancreatitis with necrosis is a severe form of disease that is usually associated with increased morbidity and mortality. On ultrasound, necrotic pancreatic tissue demonstrates diffusely decreased echogenicity. However, the full extent of pancreatic necrosis is often best appreciated on contrast-enhanced CT or MRI, which typically demonstrates geographic areas of nonenhancing, necrotic tissue [**Fig. 5.26**].

Complications of acute pancreatitis may involve adjacent structures and can include inflammation of the transverse colon, a reactive left pleural effusion, thrombosis of the splenic vein or left renal vein, or the development of an inflammatory pseudoaneurysm of the splenic artery.

Treatment for acute pancreatitis is generally supportive and is aimed at pain control and the reduction of pancreatic secretions through fasting and parenteral nutrition. Pseudocysts and pancreatic abscesses are typically treated with endoscopic or percutaneous drainage.

Chronic Pancreatitis

Chronic pancreatitis is unusual in children. It may be seen in patients with anatomic anomalies associated with ductal obstruction, inflammatory bowel disease, CF, and SDS.

The imaging appearance of chronic pancreatitis in children is similar to that seen in adults. Cross-sectional imaging may demonstrate heterogeneous or atrophied pancreatic parenchyma, irregular dilation of the pancreatic or common bile duct, and coarse pancreatic calcifications [**Fig. 5.27**]. MRCP can be used to better evaluate irregularity of the main and branch pancreatic ducts, sometimes replacing the need for ERCP.

Hereditary chronic pancreatitis is a rare form of chronic pancreatitis characterized by a young age at diagnosis and slow disease progression. This disease is indistinguishable from other forms of chronic pancreatitis by imaging and must be clinically suspected.

Autoimmune pancreatitis is a form of chronic disease caused by an inflammatory lymphoplasmacytic infiltrate. The typical appearance of autoimmune pancreatitis is a sausage-shaped enlargement of the entire gland; however, focal or segmental involvement can be seen.

Pancreatic Tumors

Primary pancreatic tumors are rare in childhood. Tumors can be classified into three major categories: exocrine, endocrine, or cystic tumors. Like primary tumors, metastases to the pancreas are uncommon. They can occasionally be seen with neuroblastoma, lymphoma (particularly Burkitt), and other aggressive primary tumors. Marked enlargement of the pancreas may be seen in the setting of leukemic infiltration.

Exocrine Tumors. The most common pediatric exocrine tumor is pancreatoblastoma, although it represents less than 1% of all epithelial tumors of the pancreas. There is a relatively high incidence in East Asia, and boys are affected twice as often as girls. There is a well-known association with Beckwith-Wiedemann syndrome. Even though the mean age at presentation is 4 years, the tumor may occur from the newborn period well into adulthood. Symptoms are nonspecific and typically include epigastric pain, anorexia, vomiting, diarrhea, weight loss, and obstructive jaundice in the setting of a palpable abdominal mass. α-Fetoprotein levels are elevated in up to 55% of patients. The tumor may also secrete adrenocorticotropic hormone.

Cross-sectional imaging typically reveals a solitary, large, well-defined, often multilobulated mass in any segment of the pancreas. It may entirely replace the gland or may be exophytic. Secondary pancreatic or biliary ductal obstruction may be seen. The lesion is typically heterogeneous at sonography, with focal hypoechoic areas noted. CT shows a heterogeneous mass with patchy areas of hypoattenuation and mild contrast enhancement. Calcifications are common. MRI characteristics include high signal intensity on T2-weighted images and low-to-intermediate signal on T1-weighted images. The tumor can be locally invasive, but metastatic disease is rare at presentation. When metastatic disease is present, the prognosis is poor.

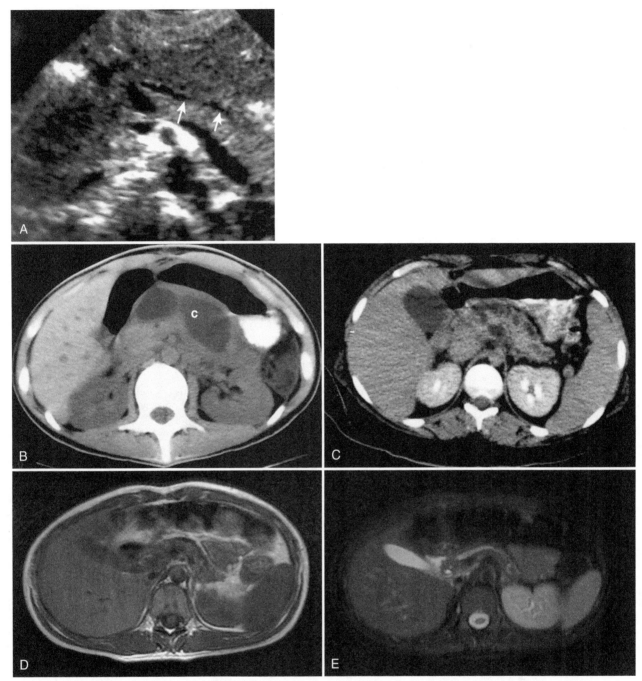

Figure 5.26 Pancreatitis. A, A transverse ultrasound image shows diffuse enlargement of the pancreas with a dilated pancreatic duct (*arrows*). **B,** An axial computed tomography (CT) image demonstrates a multiloculated pseudocyst (**C**) within the pancreas. **C,** An axial contrast-enhanced CT image shows multiple areas of necrosis in the setting of chronic pancreatitis. **D** and **E,** Axial magnetic resonance images demonstrate a shrunken, nodular pancreas with pancreatic ductal dilatation.

Endocrine Tumors. Adenomas or islet cell tumors of the pancreas are classified as functioning or nonfunctioning. Functioning tumors are further classified based on the type of hormone secreted by the predominant cell type within the tumor, and include insulinoma, gastrinoma, vasoactive intestinal peptide–producing tumor, and glucagonoma. This group of tumors accounts for approximately 20% of malignant pancreatic tumors in children, compared with only 5% in adults.

Insulin-secreting tumors (insulinomas) tend to manifest early, with symptoms secondary to hyperinsulinemia. Seizures or unexplained hypoglycemia may be seen shortly after birth. Insu-

linomas are benign in more than 90% of cases, whereas gastrinomas are benign in only 50% of cases.

Insulinoma and gastrinoma are typically small at presentation and very difficult to detect on imaging studies. They tend to be hypoechoic on ultrasound. On MR, they are hypointense on T1-weighted images and hyperintense on T2-weighted images. Hypervascularity is demonstrated with contrast administration.

Pancreatic endocrine tumors may be associated with specific syndrome complexes such as multiple endocrine neoplasia type I. This is an autosomal dominant disorder with a high degree of penetrance. Tumors are typically present in at least two of the following organs: pituitary gland, parathyroid gland, adrenal gland (cortex), thyroid gland, and pancreas. Pancreatic involvement is usually multifocal. Pancreatic endocrine tumors may also be seen in VHL disease.

Cystic Tumors. Solid-cystic papillary tumor accounts for less than 3% of all nonendocrine tumors of the pancreas in patients of all ages. This tumor has a strong predilection for women in their third decade of life, as well as individuals of Asian and African descent. Approximately 20% of cases occur in children in the second decade of life. Solid-cystic papillary tumor typically presents as a painful, palpable abdominal mass.

Common ultrasound and CT features include a large, well-defined lesion with variable solid, cystic, and necrotic components. Calcifications are occasionally noted. On MRI, central T1 hyperintense regions may be seen because of hemorrhagic necrosis or debris. A low signal rim is often demonstrated, corresponding to a fibrous capsule or residual compressed pancreatic tissue. On T2-weighted images, signal intensity varies considerably [**Fig. 5.28**].

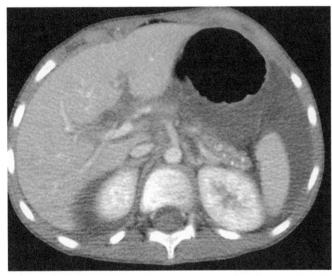

Figure 5.27 Chronic hereditary pancreatitis in a 7-year-old with recurrent abdominal pain. An axial contrast-enhanced computed tomography image shows an atrophic pancreatic tail, dilatation of the pancreatic duct, and several coarse calcifications.

A specific diagnosis is often difficult due to overlapping features between this and other pancreatic tumors with respect to laboratory values and imaging appearance. The prognosis in the pediatric population is better than that seen in adults. Children have a lower frequency of metastatic disease at presentation and a lower incidence of local recurrence after surgical resection. Surgical treatment is therefore typically less aggressive in pediatric patients.

SPLEEN

Anatomy and Embryology

The spleen develops around the fifth week of gestation from mesenchyme arising from the dorsal mesentery. As the dorsal mesentery rotates within in the abdominal cavity, the spleen is carried into the left upper quadrant.

During fetal development, the spleen functions as a primary source of hematopoiesis. After birth, the spleen primarily functions as an important secondary organ of the immune system and as a filter of blood as part of the reticuloendothelial system. Notably, the spleen retains the capacity to produce blood cells well into adult life, and it can be stimulated as a source of extramedullary hematopoiesis in the setting of extreme anemia.

Histologically, the spleen is composed of a combination of vascular and lymphatic tissue, termed the "red pulp" and the "white pulp." The red pulp consists of blood-filled sinusoids that act as a filter for the blood and a storage site for iron, erythrocytes, and platelets. The white pulp is lymphatic tissue arranged in and around the red pulp as perivascular lymphatic sheaths containing T cells and embedded germinal centers with B cells and macrophages.

The spleen is tethered in place in the abdomen by peritoneal ligaments that connect the spleen to the left kidney, stomach, diaphragm, and transverse colon.

Developmental Anomalies

Splenules, also known as supernumerary or accessory spleens, are small nodules of splenic tissue that fail to fuse with the larger splenic mass during embryologic development. They are seen in up to 16% of abdominal CT scans and up to 30% of autopsies, and are considered a normal anatomic variant. Splenules may vary in size and number. They are typically located within the splenic hilum along the course of the gastrosplenic ligament, but may be located anywhere in the abdomen. They have an imaging appearance that is similar to normal splenic parenchyma on ultrasound, CT, and MRI.

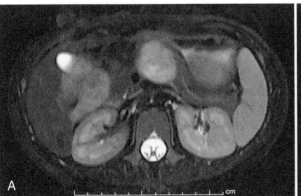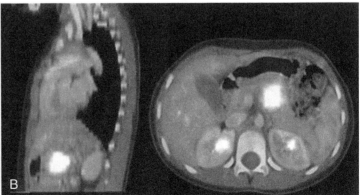

Figure 5.28 Solid-cystic papillary tumor in a 7-year-old girl with abdominal pain. A, An axial T2-weighted magnetic resonance image with fat saturation shows a hyperintense mass in the body of the pancreas. **B,** Sagittal and axial fused positron emission tomography computed tomographic images show a metabolically active pancreatic mass.

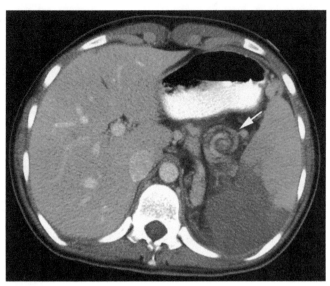

Figure 5.29 Splenic volvulus in a 15-year-old with acute left upper quadrant pain. An axial contrast-enhanced computed tomography image shows a partially ischemic spleen with volvulus of the splenic hilar vessels (*arrow*).

Asplenia and polysplenia are often part of the heterotaxy syndrome [see Figures 3.7 and 3.8]. In heterotaxy with asplenia, there is "duplication" of the right-sided viscera. Patients may have bilateral trilobed (right-sided) lungs, a large central liver, and a stomach in indeterminate position. A small, rudimentary spleen may be seen, or there may be complete asplenia. Heterotaxy with asplenia is more commonly associated with complex congenital heart disease.

Asplenia can also occur after infarct, most commonly in patients with sickle cell anemia. Patients can easily live without a functional spleen. However, given the role of the spleen in innate immunity, asplenic patients are considered "immunocompromised."

A wandering spleen exists when the spleen is absent from its normal position in the left upper quadrant and instead is demonstrated elsewhere in the abdomen. Importantly, the wandering spleen retains its relationship with the splenic vessels. The malpositioned spleen has a long vascular pedicle, which predisposes to vascular torsion and infarct. In splenic torsion, a classic "swirling" appearance of the twisting vascular structures can be seen, with abnormal splenic enhancement demonstrated [**Fig. 5.29**]. The treatment of choice is splenopexy, with splenectomy required in cases of infarction.

Splenogonadal fusion is a rare congenital anomaly in which a nodule of ectopic splenic tissue is fused to the left gonad—in males, the left testis, epididymis, or spermatic cord, and in females, the left ovary. Ultrasound is the imaging modality of choice for evaluation of the scrotum and adnexa. Ectopic splenic tissue is seen as an oval or rounded soft tissue mass with a similar appearance to normal splenic parenchyma and abundant vascularity.

Acquired Conditions
Splenomegaly

Enlargement of the spleen may signify an underlying pathologic process and requires further investigation. Ultrasound is the imaging modality of choice for the initial evaluation of splenomegaly. The spleen should be measured in maximal craniocaudal dimension, and this measurement should be compared with established normal values for age. As a rule of thumb for

children, average splenic length (in centimeters) = 6 + 1/3 patient age in years.

Viral infection is by far the most common cause of splenomegaly in children. Epstein-Barr virus and cytomegalovirus are most widely known to be associated with splenomegaly, but many other common viral infections may be responsible. In the setting of a viral infection, splenic enlargement will be mild to moderate in degree and transient in nature. The enlarged spleen typically retains a normal, homogeneous appearance on ultrasound.

Other causes of splenomegaly in children include autoimmune disease such as juvenile rheumatoid arthritis and inflammatory bowel disease, portal hypertension, splenic sequestration crisis in patients with sickle cell disease, storage disorders such as Gaucher disease or Niemann-Pick disease, and leukemia and lymphoma.

Small Spleen

A small spleen is much less common and is seen primarily in the setting of chronic splenic infarction in patients with sickle cell disease. The spleen may shrink to a very small size (<1 cm) or may completely autoinfarct. The chronically infarcted spleen may be densely calcified, and thus easily detected on radiographs or CT. On MRI, a small, chronically infarcted spleen will have decreased signal intensity on T1- and T2-weighted images related to iron deposition or calcification.

Infection or Abscess

Pyogenic splenic abscesses are almost always seen in immunocompromised patients because of the high concentration of phagocytic immune cells in the white pulp of normal individuals. Candidiasis is the opportunistic infection that most frequently affects the spleen. Multiple tiny microabscesses are seen disseminated throughout the spleen, with the liver typically also involved. The appearance is similar to that seen with hepatosplenic fungal infections [**Fig. 5.12**].

Granulomatous infections caused by *Histoplasma*, *Bartonella henselae* (cat-scratch fever), *Pneumocystis jiroveci*, *Francisella tularensis* (tularemia), and neonatal TORCH (toxoplasmosis, other agents, rubella, cytomegalovirus, herpes simplex virus) infections may also involve the spleen. In the acute and subacute phases of infection, splenic granulomas can have a variable appearance on imaging. Healed granulomata typically calcify and are frequently seen as an incidental finding on imaging in older children and adults.

Neoplasms

A hemangioma is the most common primary benign neoplasm of the spleen. It may be isolated or may be seen as part of generalized angiomatosis in syndromes such as Klippel-Trenaunay-Weber. This tumor is usually asymptomatic and discovered incidentally. Rarely, a splenic hemangioma can be quite large and may result in Kasabach-Merritt syndrome, with sequestration of blood and resulting anemia, thrombocytopenia, and coagulopathy. Splenic hemangiomas have a similar appearance to hepatic hemangiomas on cross-sectional imaging.

A splenic hamartoma is a nonneoplastic, solid lesion consisting of a mixture of normal red and white pulp. It is typically an isolated lesion, although it may be associated with hamartomas elsewhere in the body. It can be seen in patients with tuberous sclerosis. The majority of splenic hamartomas are detected incidentally on imaging. On ultrasound and CT, a solid mass is seen appearing nearly identical to surrounding normal splenic tissue [**Fig. 5.30**]. On MRI, hamartomas are isointense to normal splenic tissue on T1-weighted images and heterogeneously hyperintense on T2-weighted images.

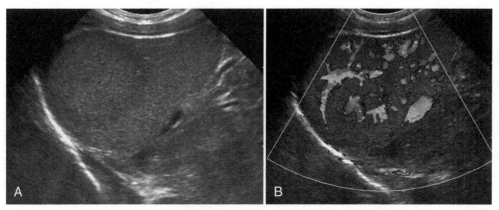

Figure 5.30 Splenic hamartoma in a 2-week-old infant with splenomegaly. A, A sagittal ultrasound image of the spleen shows a soft tissue mass which is isoechoic to the remainder of the splenic parenchyma with a hypoechoic halo. **B,** A sagittal color Doppler ultrasound image shows distinct tumor vascularity within the hamartoma.

Splenic Cysts

A true splenic cyst is typically an epidermoid cyst with an endothelial lining that produces a central fluid component. True cysts account for 10% to 25% of all solitary splenic cysts. Acquired pseudocysts are much more common, accounting for approximately 80% of solitary splenic cysts. Pseudocysts typically develop after trauma at the site of a focal splenic hematoma. These lesions lack an inner cellular lining and instead have a thin fibrous capsule.

The imaging appearance of congenital and acquired cysts is nearly identical. Both appear as solitary, simple, well-defined cystic lesions on cross-sectional imaging. Epidermoid cysts may have thin, avascular septations and may contain cholesterol crystals, inflammatory debris, or hemorrhage. Posttraumatic pseudocysts may demonstrate dense rim calcification.

TRAUMA

General Considerations

Traumatic injury in children results in more than 500,000 hospital admissions and 20,000 deaths each year. The abdomen is the second most common site of injury after head injury, and approximately 80% of abdominal injuries are due to blunt force trauma as opposed to penetrating injury. Children are most commonly injured as passengers in motor vehicle accidents, followed by automobile versus pedestrian injuries, injuries from falls, and bicycle injuries. In young children and particularly in infants, nonaccidental trauma is an important cause of blunt injury. In this population, the ribs are flexible and easily deformed by external forces. Thus the immature chest wall offers relatively less protection to the upper abdominal organs, and liver, spleen, and kidney injuries may be present in the absence of overlying rib fractures.

Certain physical examination findings may be associated with underlying abdominal injury, and thus have been used as clinical indicators for imaging after blunt trauma. These include the presence of abdominal tenderness, seat-belt ecchymoses, gross hematuria, and hemodynamic instability. Seat-belt ecchymoses across the lower abdomen or flank represent a specific high-risk marker for injury to bowel, bladder, and lumbar spine.

CT is the imaging method of choice in North America for the evaluation of abdominal and pelvic injury after blunt trauma in hemodynamically stable children. CT allows for the accurate detection and characterization of injury to both solid and hollow viscera. This modality also well demonstrates the presence of intraperitoneal and extraperitoneal free fluid and, importantly, any sites of active bleeding.

Established roles of CT in the assessment of injured children include the evaluation of visceral and bony injury, identification of injuries that require close monitoring and operative or endovascular intervention, and the estimation of associated blood loss. CT findings change initial management after clinical assessment in almost 50% of children imaged in the setting of blunt abdominal trauma.

Children should be hemodynamically stable before CT. Images should be obtained from the lung bases to the pubic symphysis after the intravenous administration of contrast material by rapid bolus injection. Additional noncontrast and multiphase postcontrast sequences contribute additional radiation exposure with little added diagnostic value. Oral contrast is not routinely used after blunt abdominal injury.

Sonography has been shown to have high sensitivity and specificity for the detection of peritoneal fluid and remains widely used in the screening of injured children. However, it has limited value in the detection and characterization of solid-organ injuries and in the identification of the cause of fluid accumulation (blood, urine, or intestinal contents). Sonography does have a potential role in the hemodynamically unstable patient. A rapid bedside ultrasound examination may serve as a quick, noninvasive substitute for diagnostic peritoneal lavage. The use of intravenous ultrasound contrast agents has been shown to improve the accuracy of sonography for the assessment of parenchymal injury; however, it is not yet recommended as an initial tool for the assessment of blunt trauma in children.

Spleen Injury

The spleen is one of the most frequently injured intraperitoneal organs in both children and adults, accounting for up to 45% of all traumatic visceral injuries. Splenic injury results in an intraparenchymal contusion or complex laceration, with or without an associated subcapsular hematoma. Associated injuries to adjacent structures such as the left kidney and left lung may be seen. Hemoperitoneum is observed with approximately 75% of splenic injuries.

Splenic lobulations or clefts may mimic a laceration. These normal variants typically have smooth, continuous contours, unlike the irregular contours seen with splenic lacerations.

A commonly used grading scale for quantification of injury to the spleen has been developed by the American Association for the Surgery of Trauma (**Table 5.2**). This scale is based on the anatomic extent of the injury, including the extent of parenchymal disruption, involvement of the vascular pedicle, capsular integrity, and the extent of subcapsular collection [**Fig. 5.31**]. In children, the severity of splenic injury is not predictive of the

TABLE 5.2 American Association for the Surgery of Trauma Splenic Injury Scale

Grade	Injury	Injury Description
I	Hematoma Laceration	Subcapsular hematoma <10% of surface area Capsular tear <1 cm parenchymal depth
II	Hematoma Laceration	Subcapsular hematoma 10%–15% of surface area Intraparenchymal hematoma <5 cm in diameter Capsular tear, 1-3 cm parenchymal depth, does not involve trabecular vessels
III	Hematoma Laceration	Subcapsular hematoma >50% surface area or expanding Ruptured subcapsular or intraparenchymal hematoma Intraparenchymal hematoma >5 cm or expanding Capsular tear, >3 cm parenchymal depth or involving trabecular vessels
IV	Laceration	Laceration involving segmental or hilar vessels producing major devascularization (>25% of spleen)
V	Laceration Vascular injury	Complete splenic parenchymal-capsular rupture Hilar vascular injury devascularizes spleen

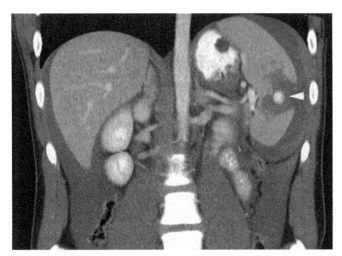

Figure 5.31 Grade IV splenic laceration with active bleeding in a 16-year-old injured playing football. A coronal contrast-enhanced computed tomography image shows a pancreatic laceration with active extravasation of contrast-containing blood (*arrowhead*).

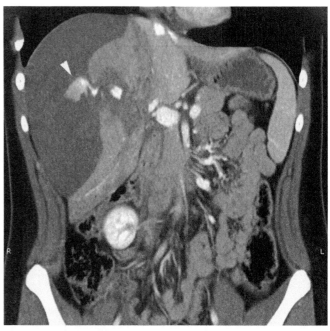

Figure 5.32 Hepatic laceration in a 16-year-old injured as a passenger in a motor vehicle crash. A coronal contrast-enhanced computed tomography image shows a large subcapsular hematoma deforming the liver, with active extravasation of contrast containing blood (*arrowhead*).

need for operative management. Most splenic injuries can be successfully managed nonoperatively regardless of severity because bleeding typically stops spontaneously. However, injury grading scales are frequently used as a guide in patient management decisions regarding intensity and duration of hospitalization and activity restriction that may be necessary.

Follow-up imaging has generally not been shown to significantly change management or affect patient outcomes, and is usually not necessary. Notably, posttraumatic splenic artery pseudoaneurysm is a rare but dangerous complication that may develop after splenic injury of any grade. Pseudoaneurysm formation is far less common in pediatric patients than in the adult population, and most lesions in children will spontaneously resolve or self-tamponade. Other sequelae of splenic trauma include splenosis and pseudocyst formation.

Liver Injury

The liver is the second most frequently injured organ in children in the setting of blunt trauma. A hepatic laceration appears as a nonenhancing, linear or branching area of abnormal parenchyma. An associated parenchymal or subcapsular hematoma may be present [**Fig. 5.32**]. Left lobe injury is typically more severe and harder to detect, and is often associated with trauma to the pancreas and duodenum. Because of its posterior location, the caudate lobe is only rarely involved in trauma.

Hepatic injury is associated with hemoperitoneum in approximately two-thirds of cases. Hemoperitoneum may extend throughout the entire peritoneal cavity including the pelvis. Hepatic artery pseudoaneurysm is a rare complication that may develop over time.

Regions of periportal low attenuation do not necessarily indicate hepatic injury. Most often, this finding represents distended periportal lymphatics related to intravascular third-space losses that occur after fluid resuscitation.

As with splenic injury, CT grading scales have been proposed to quantify the severity of hepatic injury and are most useful for nonoperative medical decision making. The majority of hepatic injuries can be safely treated without operative intervention, and grading scales are not predictive of the need for operative management.

Rarely, blunt abdominal trauma is associated with biliary injury. When present, findings may include hematobilia, biloma

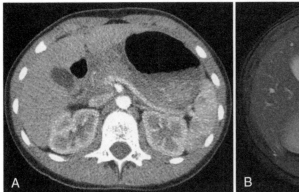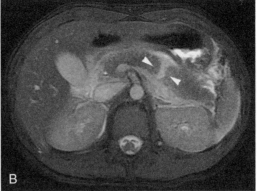

Figure 5.33 Pancreatic laceration in a 12-year-old injured by a bicycle handlebar. A, An axial contrast-enhanced computed tomography image shows diffuse edema of the pancreas. **B,** An axial steady-state gradient echo magnetic resonance image shows complete transection of the pancreas (*arrowheads*).

formation, or bile duct disruption. Gallbladder injury from blunt abdominal trauma is rare in children.

Pancreas Injury

Injury to the body of the pancreas is relatively uncommon in children and typically results from direct compression of the gland against the vertebral column. This may occur in the setting of bicycle handlebar injuries and falls. Direct signs of injury may be poorly shown on CT because of the small size of the gland, the lack of surrounding mesenteric fat, and close apposition of fracture fragments. Indirect imaging signs of pancreatic injury and subsequent pancreatitis include edema of the pancreas [**Fig. 5.33**], focal or diffuse gland enlargement, stranding of the peripancreatic and/or mesenteric fat, thickening of the anterior renal fascia, and free intraperitoneal fluid.

On CT, unexplained peripancreatic fluid in the anterior pararenal space or lesser sac is the most sensitive indicator of pancreatic injury. Notably, this finding may also be seen in the setting of third-space fluid loss, duodenal injury, and high-grade renal injury.

Peripancreatic fluid collections may develop soon after pancreatic injury. Although spontaneous resolution is fairly common, pancreatic pseudocysts develop in approximately 50% of cases. Pseudocysts are most commonly located within the substance of the pancreas or in the peripancreatic anterior pararenal space. Approximately 50% of these lesions resolve spontaneously, and the remaining 50% require percutaneous or surgical drainage.

Sonography is the modality of choice for monitoring the size and extent of peripancreatic fluid collections. MR and retrograde endoscopic cholangiopancreatography can both be very useful in the initial and subsequent imaging evaluation of pancreatic injury, especially in patients with transection of the pancreatic duct [**Fig. 5.33**].

In the setting of pancreatic duct injury, nonoperative management includes fasting, parenteral nutrition, and gastric intubation. Distal pancreatectomy may be performed for injuries to the left of the spine.

Bowel and Mesentery

Bowel and mesenteric injuries occur in 6% to 16% of children injured in the setting of blunt trauma. Bowel rupture most commonly occurs in the mid to distal small intestine and may be the result of a direct force to the abdomen, shear injury between fixed and mobile portions of bowel, or acutely increased intraluminal pressure leading to intestinal rupture. Significant bowel

and mesenteric injury is most often related to motor vehicle crashes, handlebar injuries, nonaccidental trauma, and falls. The combination of a seat belt ecchymosis in association with an acute hyperflexion (Chance) fracture of the lumbar spine has a strong and significant association with bowel and mesenteric injury. Nonaccidental injury should always be included in the differential diagnosis for a child with a history of minor blunt trauma and a bowel perforation.

CT plays an important role in early and accurate diagnosis because clinical signs may be absent or minimal at presentation. Delayed diagnosis can result in bowel ischemia, peritonitis, and rarely, death caused by sepsis.

The most frequent CT finding associated with bowel rupture and mesenteric injury is unexplained peritoneal fluid, defined as a moderate to large amount of free fluid in the absence of solid viscous injury or bony pelvic fracture [**Fig. 5.34**]. Although nonspecific, approximately 50% of children with significant peritoneal fluid as the only finding on CT after blunt trauma have serious intestinal injury. The presence of unexplained peritoneal fluid should be considered an important marker of potentially serious bowel or mesenteric injury.

CT findings that are specific to bowel or mesenteric injury include the extravasation of oral contrast material, abrupt termination of the mesenteric vessels, and mesenteric vascular extravasation. These findings are uncommon in children. Pneumoperitoneum is a highly specific finding that is relatively more common, seen in 20% to 30% of children with bowel injury [**Fig. 5.34**]. Notably, the absence of pneumoperitoneum does not exclude the possibility of serious bowel injury. Several other CT findings such as focal bowel wall thickening and mesenteric fluid or stranding are common in injured patients, but less specific for significant bowel injury.

Using current generation CT scanners, the sensitivity of CT for the diagnosis of bowel and mesenteric injury is reported to be between 80% and 95%. However, reported specificity values of 48% to 84% remain a challenge in clinical practice. Repeat CT imaging in patients with persistent abdominal symptoms and high-risk mechanisms of trauma may improve the detection of intestinal injury.

Hypoperfusion Complex

Severely injured children with partially compensated hypovolemic shock may have a characteristic constellation of findings on CT referred to as the hypoperfusion complex. CT findings in children with the hypoperfusion complex include diffuse intestinal dilation with fluid; abnormally intense contrast enhancement of

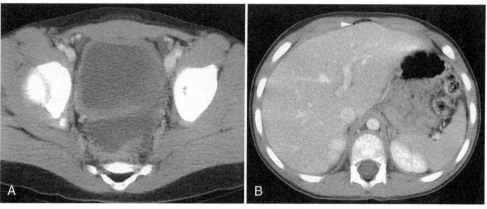

Figure 5.34 Jejunal perforation in a 5-year-old injured as a passenger in a motor vehicle crash. A, An axial computed tomography (CT) image through the pelvis shows "unexplained" peritoneal fluid in the cul-de-sac. **B,** An axial contrast-enhanced CT image through the liver shows a tiny collection of free air anterior to liver (*arrowhead*).

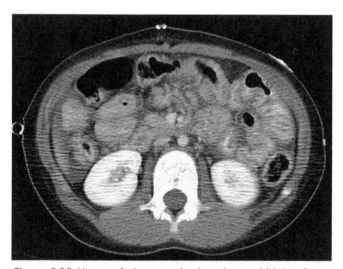

Figure 5.35 Hypoperfusion complex in a 6-year-old injured as a passenger in a motor vehicle crash. An axial contrast-enhanced computed tomography image shows a narrow-caliber aorta and inferior vena cava; fluid-filled, thickened bowel; and peritoneal fluid.

the bowel wall, mesentery, kidneys, aorta, and inferior vena cava; and diminished caliber of the aorta and inferior vena cava [**Fig. 5.35**]. Less common findings include areas of periportal low attenuation; intense adrenal, pancreatic, and mesenteric enhancement; decreased pancreatic and splenic enhancement; peritoneal and retroperitoneal fluid; and bowel wall thickening.

The hypoperfusion complex is a marker for a hemodynamic instability and a predictor of a poor outcome. The mortality rate in children with this constellation of CT findings approaches 80%.

SUGGESTED READINGS

Bai HX, Lowe ME, Husain SZ. What have we learned about acute pancreatitis in children? *J Pediatr Gastroenterol Nutr.* 2011;52:262-270.

Bixby SD, Callahan MJ, Taylor GA. Imaging in pediatric blunt abdominal trauma. *Semin Roentgenol.* 2008;43:72-82.

Brofman N, Atri M, Epid D, et al. Evaluation of bowel and mesenteric trauma with multi-detector CT. *Radiographics.* 2006;26:1119-1131.

Cagini L, Gravante S, Malaspina GM, et al. Contrast enhanced ultrasound (CEUS) in blunt abdominal trauma. *Crit Ultrasound J.* 2013;5(suppl 1):S9.

Chung EM, Cube R, Lewis RB, et al. Pediatric liver masses: radiologic-pathologic correlation part 1. Benign tumors. *Radiographics.* 2010;30:801-826.

Chung EM, Lattin GE, Cube R, et al. Pediatric liver masses: radiologic-pathologic correlation part 2. Malignant tumors. *Radiographics.* 2011;31:483-507.

Coley BD, ed. *Caffey's Pediatric Diagnostic Imaging.* 12th ed. Philadelphia, PA: Elsevier-Saunders; 2013.

Debray D, Priente D, Urvoas E, et al. Sclerosing cholangitis in children. *J Pediatr.* 1994;124:49-56.

Feldstein AE, Perrault J, El-Yussif M, et al. Primary sclerosing cholangitis in children: a long-term follow-up study. *Hepatology.* 2003;38:210-217.

Hansen K, Horslen S. Metabolic liver disease in children. *Liver Transpl.* 2008;14:391-411.

Karabulut N, Elmas N. Contrast agents used in MR imaging of the liver. *Diagn Interv Radiol.* 2006;12:22-30.

Lynn KN, Werder GM, Callaghan RM, et al. Pediatric blunt splenic trauma: a comprehensive review. *Pediatr Radiol.* 2009;39:904-916.

Mortelé KJ, Segatto E, Ros PR. The infected liver: radiologic-pathologic correlation. *Radiographics.* 2004;24:937-955.

Nijs E, Callahan MJ, Taylor GA. Disorders of the pediatric pancreas: imaging features. *Pediatr Radiol.* 2005;35:358-373.

Paterson A, Frush DP, Donnelly LF, et al. A pattern-oriented approach to splenic imaging in infants and children. *Radiographics.* 1999;19:1465-1485.

Rozel C, Garel L, Rypens F, et al. Imaging of biliary disorders in children. *Pediatr Radiol.* 2011;41:208-220.

Rumack CM, Wilson SR, Charboneau WJ, et al., eds. *Diagnostic Ultrasound.* 4th ed. Philadelphia, PA: Elsevier-Mosby; 2011.

Sharma OP, Oswanski MF, Kaminski BP, et al. Clinical implications of the seat belt sign in blunt trauma. *Am Surg.* 2009;75:822-827.

Siegel MJ, ed. *Pediatric Sonography.* 3rd ed. Philadelphia, PA: Lippincott Williams & Wilkins; 2002.

Skandalakis JE, Gray SW, eds. *Embryology for Surgeons.* 2nd ed. Baltimore, MD: Williams & Wilkins; 1994.

Turkbey B, Ocak I, Daryanani K, et al. Autosomal recessive polycystic kidney disease and congenital hepatic fibrosis. *Pediatr Radiol.* 2009;39:100-111.

Chapter 6
Genitourinary Imaging

Rama S. Ayyala, Cassandra Sams, George A. Taylor, and Jeanne S. "Mei-Mei" Chow

This chapter provides an introduction to pediatric genitourinary imaging for the radiology resident. It will focus on diseases commonly encountered in or specific to children and congenital anomalies. Diseases more commonly seen in adults will not be covered extensively in this chapter.

The goal of this chapter is not only to describe genitourinary diseases, but also to convey a systematic approach for imaging evaluation of these entities. Most imaging of the genitourinary system starts with ultrasound, and imaging algorithms should always respect the "as low as reasonably achievable" (ALARA) principle.

IMAGING TECHNIQUES

Ultrasound

In children, ultrasound is the first-line imaging modality for evaluation of the genitourinary system. It is readily available, making it easily accessible for fast and effective evaluation of the kidneys and urinary bladder. The lack of ionizing radiation makes this an optimal imaging tool in children. However, one of the disadvantages of ultrasound is the inability to acquire functional information. In addition, image quality is operator dependent, creating variability among examinations.

The parameters of imaging are optimized based on the age and size of the child. The kidneys and urinary bladder are imaged with the patient in the supine position [**Fig. 6.1**]. Additional imaging in the prone position is routine in children because the kidneys are not obscured by bowel gas, and some children are more comfortable when prone and thus more compliant. Transducer choice in children is optimized to patient size, with high-frequency linear transducers commonly used for neonates and lower-frequency curved transducers used for older children [**Fig. 6.2**].

Color Doppler imaging is used as an adjunct to grayscale imaging to provide information regarding movement and vascularity. This can be effective in delineating specific pathologies, such as the absence of a ureteral jet in a ureter obstructed by a stone or the absence of blood flow in a torsed testicle. Arterial and venous Doppler waveform analysis is helpful in evaluating entities such as renal artery stenosis (RAS) and renal vein thrombosis (RVT).

Prenatal ultrasound imaging can give valuable information about the kidneys and urinary bladder. This screening test provides the first indication that congenital genitourinary abnormalities may exist and allows for early diagnosis of diseases such as ureteropelvic junction obstruction (UPJO), bladder exstrophy, and multicystic dysplastic kidney (MCDK). Correlating postnatal imaging studies with prenatal imaging is very helpful in the diagnosis and workup of patients, and it should be done whenever possible. Most congenital anomalies are evaluated nonurgently in the first month of life. One exception is the case of suspected posterior urethral valves. In this setting, imaging evaluation and workup should be done in the hospital soon after birth [**Fig. 6.3**].

Ultrasound contrast agents, commonly used in adults and internationally, are now available for use in children in the United States. Voiding urosonography is one potential use for contrast material.

Fluoroscopy

Voiding Cystourethrography

Voiding cystourethrography (VCUG) is a common imaging study to evaluate the genitourinary system in children. Unlike ultrasound, VCUG can assess anatomy as well as function. It is the best test to evaluate both reflux and lower urinary tract anatomy and function.

After sterile catheterization of the urinary bladder, contrast is instilled via gravity. An 8 French feeding tube is commonly used for catheterization because it is generally the appropriate diameter for a newborn urethra and has a radiopaque strip for easy visualization. While instilling contrast into the bladder, early filling images are obtained to assess for ureteroceles or other potential filling defects [**Fig. 6.4**]. The expected bladder capacity is estimated based on the child's age and is used as a guide for volume of contrast instillation. After the urinary bladder is adequately filled, bilateral oblique views of the urinary bladder are obtained to assess the vesicoureteral junctions. This is particularly useful in cases of vesicoureteral reflux (VUR), where it is important to document the insertion site of the ureter. In cases of VUR, an AP image of the abdomen centered at the kidneys showing the highest grade of reflux observed is standard. The international reflux grading system classifies reflux from mild (grade 1) to severe (grade 5) [**Fig. 6.5**].

As implied by the name of the examination, all patients should void during the course of this study. This is vital not only in evaluation of the urethra, but also increase detection of reflux which may occur only during voiding. Because males are much more likely to have urethral abnormalities than girls, it is important to obtain dedicated lateral views of the entire male urethra, specifically to evaluate for the presence of posterior urethral valves. In children younger than 1 year, a cyclic examination is performed. This entails imaging the patient during three separate filling and voiding cycles. Studies have shown that this increases the sensitivity of the test for the detection of VUR. Postvoid images of the kidneys and ureters should also be obtained to assess for adequate drainage of refluxed contrast material, and thus evaluate for the possibility of concomitant obstruction. Another study that can be used to evaluate for VUR is a radionuclide cystogram (RNC), which is described later in the Nuclear Medicine section.

Retrograde Urethrogram

The retrograde urethrogram (RUG) is a contrast study that evaluates the appearance of the anterior urethra in males. The most urgent indication for an RUG is assessment for acute urethral injury after trauma. The urethra may be damaged from a straddle injury or in the setting of pelvic fracture(s). Patients present with blood per meatus and/or inability to void. An RUG is also used to assess for urethral stricture when patients present with a decreased urinary stream, difficulty with urination, or hesitancy. Strictures are commonly associated with prior trauma and, rarely, infections in children. An RUG is also commonly used to evaluate the postoperative urethra, such as after hypospadias or epispadias repair [**Fig. 6.6**].

With the patient in a steep oblique position, a small catheter is inserted into the anterior urethra, and contrast is injected while the distal urethra is occluded. A Foley catheter balloon inflated within the fossa navicularis or external pressure from fingers or a Zipser clamp can prevent contrast from leaking during injection under pressure. This allows for optimal distension of the urethra to the level of the external sphincter, which is identified by its smooth, conical contour.

Genitogram

In patients with ambiguous genitalia, a careful physical examination of the perineum is performed. Depending on the appearance of the perineum, water-soluble contrast is subsequently instilled through the appropriate orifice(s) to determine the patient's internal anatomy. This test is useful in studying specific clinical entities such as ambiguous genitalia (ie, distinguishing females with congenital adrenal hyperplasia [CAH] from males with severe hypospadias) or the cloacal malformation.

Nuclear Medicine

Nuclear medicine examinations are used in conjunction with ultrasound and VCUG in the workup of genitourinary anomalies, as these examinations have the advantage of providing functional information about the urinary tract. The RNC is a sensitive test for VUR. Cortical scintigraphy can evaluate for functional renal parenchyma. Diuretic scintigraphy is used in evaluation of urinary tract dilatation, specifically to distinguish obstructive versus nonobstructive causes.

Radionuclide Cystogram

Similar to VCUG, this study entails instilling contrast material into the urinary bladder (in this case, Technetium 99m pertechnetate) and performing dynamic imaging of the kidneys and

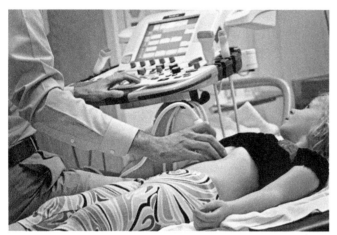

Figure 6.1 Ultrasound is the first-line imaging modality for evaluation of the genitourinary system in children given its ease of use, accessibility, noninvasive nature, and lack of ionizing radiation exposure.

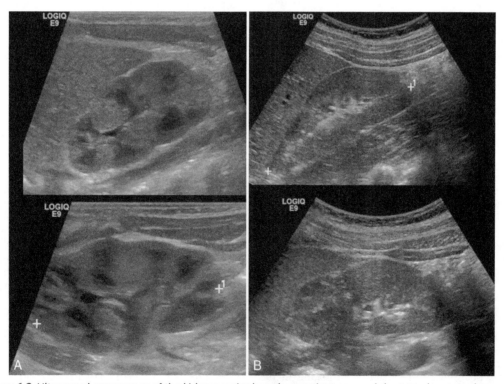

Figure 6.2 Ultrasound appearance of the kidneys varies based on patient age and the transducer used to evaluate the kidneys. **A,** Renal ultrasound in a 2-month-old performed using a linear transducer demonstrates fetal lobation (undulating outer contour of the kidneys) and hypoechoic medullary pyramids. These are normal characteristics of kidneys in infants and young children. Given the young age and small size of this child, a high-frequency linear transducer is ideal for evaluation. **B,** Renal ultrasound in an 8-year-old using a curved transducer. There are no longer hypoechoic medullary pyramids, and the outer contour of the kidneys is smooth. The lower-frequency curved transducer provides a larger footprint and better penetration for imaging of the kidneys in older children.

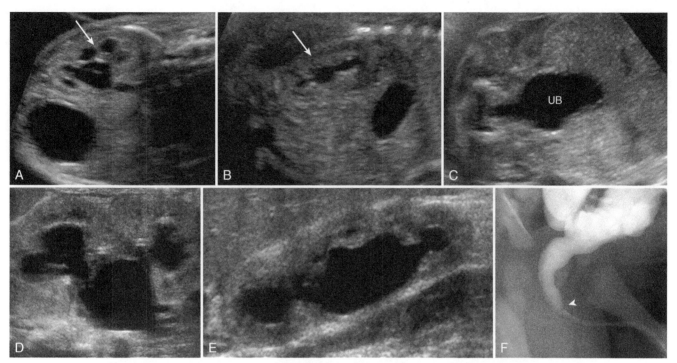

Figure 6.3 Posterior urethral valves. A and B, Fetal ultrasound images in the coronal plane demonstrate bilateral hydronephrosis (*white arrows*). **C,** The fetal urinary bladder (*UB*) is dilated with the typical keyhole configuration. **D and E,** Immediate postnatal renal ultrasound shows bilateral hydronephrosis, with thinning of the renal cortices. **F,** Voiding image from a voiding cystourethrogram demonstrates a dilated posterior urethra above the level of the posterior urethral valves (*arrowhead*), with an irregular, trabeculated appearance of the urinary bladder.

urinary bladder during filling and voiding to evaluate for VUR [**Fig. 6.7**]. With an RNC, reflux is graded 1 to 3 as opposed to the five-point international reflux study grading scale used for VCUGs. Although VCUGs provide better anatomic clarity, RNCs generally have a lower radiation dose, and perhaps, higher sensitivity. The indication for VCUG versus RNC varies by institution. It is common to first study patients for reflux with a VCUG, then perform follow-up studies with the lower-dose RNC study. Males should always first be studied by VCUG because only a VCUG provides imaging of the urethra during voiding.

Cortical Scintigraphy

Cortical scintigraphy determines the amount of functioning renal tissue. A cortical localizing agent, technetium-99m-dimer-captosuccinic acid (DMSA), is used for optimal visualization of the renal cortex. Uptake is seen in the renal cortex, with relative areas of photopenia in the renal medulla and sinus.

Indications for this examination include assessment for renal scar as a result of prior infections or chronic reflux [**Fig. 6.8**]. It is also used in the setting of acute pyelonephritis for cortical localization of the infection. Acute pyelonephritis may appear as a focus of photopenia with no associated volume loss. Follow-up imaging 6 months after resolution of the infection can help evaluate for scarring, characterized by a focus of photopenia with associated volume loss.

Congenital anomalies, such as ectopic kidney, horseshoe kidney, or ectopic fused kidney, can be seen with cortical scintigraphy because the renal parenchyma and anatomic location can be identified [**Fig. 6.9**]. Scintigraphy is useful in distinguishing MCDK from severe hydronephrosis because an MCDK has no functioning renal tissue.

Diuretic Renography

In contrast with cortical scintigraphy, renography evaluates urine formation and excretion by the kidney. Technetium-99m-mercaptoacetyltriglycine (MAG3) or technetium-99m-diethylene triamine pentaacetic acid (DTPA) may be used for this examination. MAG3 is the preferred agent, particularly in patients with impaired renal function, because it has a higher first-pass extraction.

This study is indicated to differentiate obstructive versus non-obstructive urinary tract dilatation. After administration of the tracer intravenously, imaging of the kidneys is performed to visualize cortical uptake, urine formation, and urine excretion. If urinary tract dilatation is identified in a renal collection system, a diuretic challenge is performed with the administration of furosemide (1 mg/kg, max 40 mg). The rate of urinary excretion from the renal pelvis and ureter after a diuretic challenge is calculated and compared with a normal standard, often the contralateral kidney. The time required for half of the tracer to pass the ureteropelvic junction (UPJ) is calculated ($t_{1/2}$). A $t_{1/2}$ of less than 10 minutes is considered normal, and a $t_{1/2}$ of greater than 20 minutes is considered abnormal. A $t_{1/2}$ between 10 and 20 minutes is deemed equivocal.

In infants and young children, the diagnosis of obstructive versus nonobstructive urinary tract dilatation is difficult due to the high capacity of the renal pelvis and relatively low urine output. Therefore, evaluation of dynamic images is important. This allows assessment of the function of the kidney, evaluation

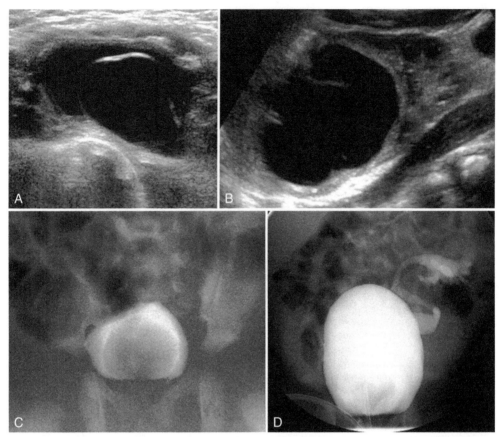

Figure 6.4 Ultrasound and voiding cystourethrography (VCUG) of a completely duplicated collecting system in a 3-week-old male with a prenatal diagnosis of unilateral hydronephrosis. **A,** Transverse ultrasound image of the urinary bladder shows a ureterocele, a thin-walled cystic structure noted along the left lateral bladder wall. Although ureteroceles can be seen in a single collecting system, they are more frequently associated with the upper pole of a duplex kidney, especially in girls. **B,** Sagittal image of the left kidney in the same patient. The upper pole is markedly hydronephrotic and dysplastic, with an echogenic renal cortex. The lower pole has a normal sonographic appearance, with no hydronephrosis and preservation of normal corticomedullary differentiation. **C,** Coned down view of the bladder obtained during a VCUG during the early filling phase demonstrates a large ovoid filling defect located centrally within the bladder, compatible with the ureterocele noted on ultrasound. As in this case, it may be difficult to determine the laterality of a large ectopic ureterocele on a VCUG. **D,** A spot radiograph taken later during the course of the same VCUG demonstrates contrast refluxing from the urinary bladder into a dilated and tortuous left ureter and into the dilated lower pole renal collecting system. The dilated collecting system has a "drooping" appearance because of visualization of only the lower pole calyces and mass effect from the obstructed, dilated upper pole.

of changes in hydronephrosis before and after diuretic administration, and visualization of the overall washout curve of the kidney [**Fig. 6.10**].

Computed Tomography

Computed tomography (CT) is readily accessible and images can be acquired quickly, reducing the need for sedation that may be required for MRI. However, CT should be used judiciously in children because it has the disadvantage of exposing patients to ionizing radiation. When performing CT scans in children, the ALARA principle should always apply. One should scan only when necessary, and pediatric protocols should be used. Low-dose pediatric protocols are now routine in pediatric hospitals, thereby decreasing the amount of ionizing radiation exposure per examination and the potential overall risk to children. Ultrasound, rather than CT, is the primary imaging modality for the urinary tract in children. However, CT is useful in certain clinical situations. Although ultrasound is the initial study of choice to evaluate for renal stones, noncontrast CT is useful when further

clarification is needed [**Fig. 6.11**]. Computed tomography angiography (CTA) and CT venography can provide exquisite detail regarding renal perfusion and drainage. Contrast-enhanced CT is useful in assessing the renal parenchyma, as well as in detecting underlying renal masses. Delayed postcontrast imaging demonstrates excretion of contrast material through the urinary system, highlighting the ureters and the urinary bladder. This may be particularly useful in the setting of trauma. Unlike the multiphase protocols frequently used in adults, a single imaging phase tailored to the specific clinical question typically suffices in children.

Magnetic Resonance Imaging

Aside from the specific indications for CT stated earlier, after ultrasound as the initial screening modality, magnetic resonance imaging (MRI) is typically the most commonly used cross-sectional examination for assessment of the genitourinary system. Similar to CT, MRI can show anatomic detail of the genitourinary system with the added ability to perform multiplanar

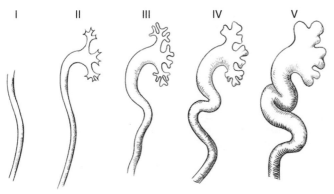

Grades of Reflux

Figure 6.5 The international reflux grading system. The standard grading of reflux is from 1 to 5, with 1 representing the mildest grade of reflux into the ureters and 5 the most severe grade with reflux into a tortuous ureter and dilated renal pelvis and calyces. The radionuclide cystogram grading system for reflux is from 1 to 3. (Courtesy of Robert L. Lebowitz, MD.)

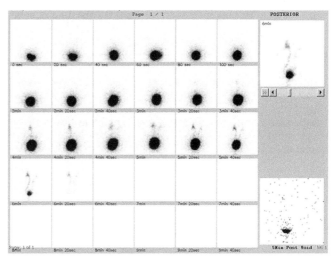

Figure 6.7 This radionuclide cystogram (RNC) was performed in a 2-year-old for follow-up of vesicoureteral reflux seen on prior voiding cystourethrography. RNC images in the posterior projection demonstrate radiotracer extending into the bilateral ureters and renal collecting systems, consistent with bilateral RNC grade 2 reflux (RNC grading: grade 1—activity limited to the ureter and not involving the collecting system; grade 2—activity reaching the collecting system; grade 3—activity in a dilated collecting system and a dilated, tortuous ureter).

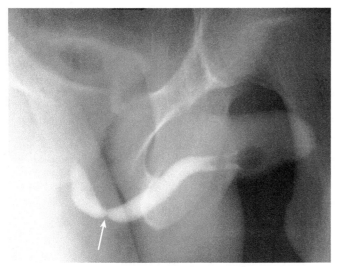

Figure 6.6 Seventeen-year-old male with a remote history of a straddle injury as a child and recurrent stricture of the bulbar urethra. Fluoroscopic image from a retrograde urethrogram demonstrates a focal area of significant narrowing of the bulbar urethra (*arrow*), with mild dilatation proximal to the stricture. In this example, a 10 French Foley catheter was inserted into the urethra. Three cubic centimeters of air were instilled into the Foley balloon. The balloon rests in the fossa navicularis, holding the catheter in place.

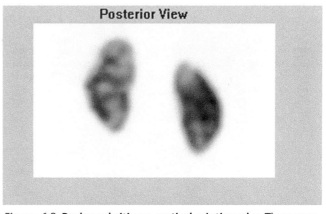

Figure 6.8 Pyelonephritis on cortical scintigraphy. Three-year-old girl diagnosed with bilateral pyelonephritis 2 months prior. Technetium-99m-dimercaptosuccinic acid scan demonstrates multiple cortically based areas of relatively decreased uptake in the left kidney and upper pole right of the kidney, suggesting areas of persistent pyelonephritis or resultant scarring.

acquisition. Additional advantages of MRI include lack of ionizing radiation exposure and superb soft tissue contrast resolution. One of the primary disadvantages of MRI is the long scan time, which necessitates sedation or anesthesia in some children. Pediatric patients with poor renal function should not receive intravenous gadolinium-based contrast agents because of the risk for nephrogenic systemic fibrosis, a rare disease that can affect the skin and various organs. In these patients, MR evaluation of the kidneys must be limited to noncontrast examinations.

Magnetic resonance urography (MRU) is a useful tool in evaluating the genitourinary system, both for anatomic detail and for functional information. Traditional T1- and T2-weighted imaging is performed, in addition to postcontrast sequences after the administration of intravenous gadolinium-based contrast material. This imaging technique not only helps in the assessment of the kidneys, urinary bladder, and vasculature, but also allows for the measurement of functional parameters of the kidney such as glomerular filtration rate and differential renal function.

Radiography

Radiographs are not typically performed as part of the initial imaging assessment of the kidneys and urinary bladder. However, pediatric patients may present with generalized, vague abdominal symptoms that may prompt clinicians to begin with radiographs. The KUB (kidneys, ureters, and bladder) provides a global view of the abdomen and is easily accessible and rapidly acquired.

Depending on the age and size of the patient, the outline of the normal renal shadows can be seen in the paraspinal region bilaterally at the L1-L2 level. Sometimes the renal shadows may be difficult to see secondary to overlying densities. Displacement of the normal bowel gas pattern by abnormal soft tissue may suggest the presence of an intraabdominal mass, including masses arising from the kidney. Radiopaque densities such as calcifications or renal stones may be best evaluated on radiographs. Although not always first obtained to evaluate the

genitourinary system, radiographs often serve as a useful adjunct to other imaging modalities.

NORMAL GENITOURINARY SYSTEM IN CHILDREN

Kidneys

The imaging appearance of the kidneys is variable in children of different ages, with a typical pattern observed from the newborn period to adulthood. On ultrasound, the kidneys of infants typically have markedly hypoechoic medullary pyramids, and it is important not to mistake this finding for the dilated calyces of hydronephrosis. Over time, the echogenicity of the pyramids becomes more isoechoic to that of the surrounding cortex. Fetal lobation is seen in infancy, with the renal margins becoming smoother over time. It is notably possible to see remnant hypoechoic pyramids and fetal lobation even in teenagers [**Fig. 6.12**].

Although the cortex of the adult kidney is normally hypoechoic compared with the liver and spleen, renal echogenicity is more variable in children and changes with age. In premature and term infants up to a few months of age, normal kidneys may be echogenic in comparison with the adjacent liver or spleen. Later in life, normal kidneys may be isoechoic or relatively hypoechoic to the adjacent viscera [**Fig. 6.13**]. Loss of normal echogenicity and/or diminished corticomedullary differentiation are signs of medical renal disease.

As the child grows, so should the kidney. Charts are readily available to ensure that renal size is appropriate for the age the child. Renal growth should be relatively symmetric from side to side, with the left kidney typically slightly longer than the right. If the kidneys are larger or smaller than expected or if they are abnormally asymmetric in size, suspicion for underlying renal pathology should increase.

The normal CT and MRI appearance of pediatric kidneys, both with and without contrast, is very similar to that seen in adults. On T1-weighted images, the renal cortex is similar in signal intensity to the spleen, with the medullary pyramids relatively

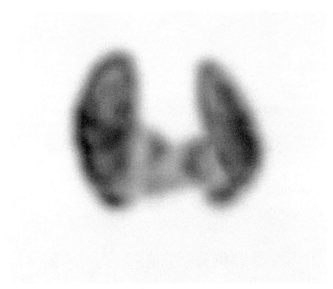

Figure 6.9 Horseshoe kidney. Five-month-old with recurrent urinary tract infections. Technetium-99m-dimercaptosuccinic acid scan demonstrates fusion of the kidneys inferiorly by an isthmus, forming a horseshoe kidney.

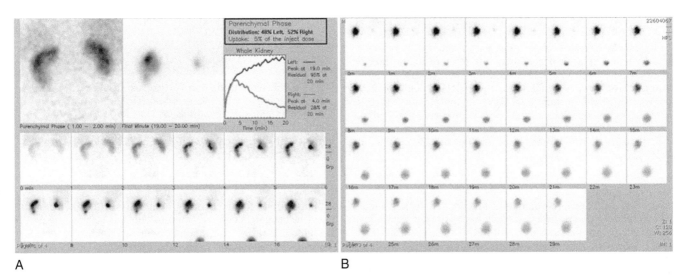

A   B

Figure 6.10 Left ureteropelvic junction obstruction (UPJO). Diuretic renography using technetium-99m-mercaptoacetyltriglycine in a seventeen-year-old boy with intermittent flank pain. **A,** Initial imaging demonstrates normal cortical uptake of radiotracer in the bilateral kidneys. The right kidney demonstrates normal time to peak activity with urine formation and excretion. The left kidney demonstrates delayed urine formation and excretion, with dilatation of the renal pelvis. **B,** After the administration of furosemide, there is delayed spontaneous drainage of the left renal collecting system, with intermittent to obstructive parameters with diuresis (renal washout half-time 18 minutes). Surgery revealed a crossing vessel as the cause of intermittent UPJO.

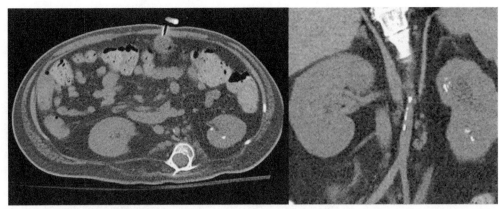

Figure 6.11 Computed tomography (CT) of renal stones. Twenty-four-year-old with a history of nephrolithiasis, status post lithotripsy, with continued flank pain. Axial and coronal noncontrast CT images show multiple high-density foci in the left kidney consistent with urinary calculi. There is associated mild fullness of the collecting system. The patient has a gastrostomy tube.

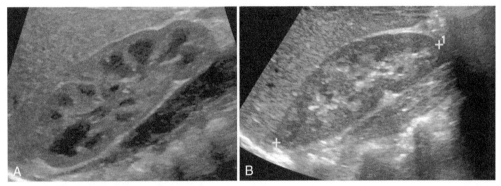

Figure 6.12 Normal ultrasound of the kidneys at different ages: sagittal ultrasound images in two different patients shows the changes in the appearance of the kidney from infancy to later in childhood. **A,** In neonates, the kidneys are lobulated in contour because of normal fetal lobation, with hypoechoic renal pyramids. **B,** Later in childhood, the contour of the kidney becomes smooth. The renal pyramids are less hypoechoic, and the echogenicity of the renal parenchyma is more homogeneous.

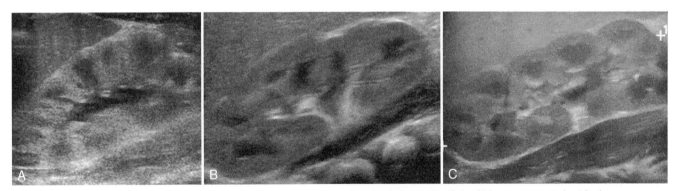

Figure 6.13 Normal renal echogenicity in infants: the normal echogenicity of the kidneys compared with the adjacent liver or spleen is variable in infants. The kidneys can be (**A**) hyperechoic, (**B**) isoechoic, or (**C**) hypoechoic relative to the adjacent viscera. All of these infants had normal renal function.

hypointense. On T2-weighted images, the renal parenchyma is overall hyperintense [**Fig. 6.14**]. Fluid signal may be seen in the collecting systems and the ureters because of the presence of urine. Fetal lobations may be visible on these imaging modalities and should not be mistaken for renal scarring.

The renal collecting system is well profiled by a variety of imaging studies. In the past, intravenous pyelograms (IVPs) were frequently used. Today, CT and MRU have largely supplanted IVPs. In a normal, single-system kidney, 9 to 12 calyces should be present.

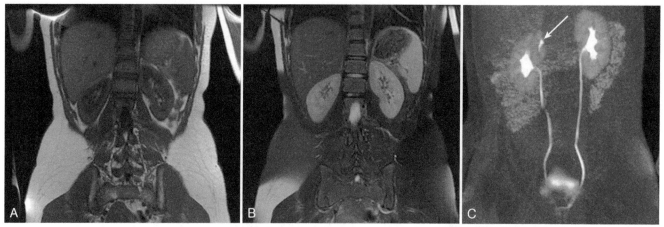

Figure 6.14 Magnetic resonance imaging (MRI) of the genitourinary system. A, Coronal T1 and (**B**) coronal T2 images demonstrate the normal MRI appearance of the kidneys. On T1 imaging, the renal parenchyma is similar in signal to the spleen. On T2, imaging the renal parenchyma is high in signal. **C,** Coronal MRU image in a different patient shows the urographic phase, with contrast in the collecting systems and the ureters. This female presented with constant urinary dribbling. She has a right upper pole ectopic ureter (*arrow*), which inserts ectopically into the vagina and causes her constant wetness.

Ureters

The normal ureter is made up of musculature that allows peristalsis to promote antegrade flow of urine. On dynamic imaging, the normal, peristalsing ureter may be seen intermittently. It is more commonly seen when it is abnormally dilated. On ultrasound, a dilated ureter appears as a thin-walled, anechoic, tubular structure. Dilated ureters can typically be seen proximally at the level of the renal pelvis and distally in the deep pelvis. The ureteral insertion should be visualized to assess whether it is normal or ectopic. The middle portion of a dilated ureter may be difficult to see on ultrasound secondary to overlying bowel gas. A posterior approach may be helpful to bypass the bowel. Alternatively, a coronal approach using the kidney as an acoustic window may allow better visualization of the midureter. If there is concern for a possible ureteral abnormality that cannot be resolved by ultrasound the entire course of the ureters can be well seen on cross-sectional imaging. On MRI, for example, a dilated ureter appears as a T2 bright tubular structure that enhances on delayed postcontrast imaging.

Bladder

The normal urinary bladder is situated in the midline of the pelvis, just above the pubic symphysis and posterior to the rectus abdominous muscles. It is directly anterior to the uterus in females and anterior to the rectum in males. The bladder normally appears as a fluid-filled structure on all imaging modalities. The expected bladder capacity can be calculated based on the patient's age, with older patients having larger bladder capacities.

The bladder wall should be thin but may become thickened in the setting of inflammation or hypertrophy from bladder outlet obstruction. On postvoid images or studies performed with a partially distended bladder, the wall may appear thickened because of redundant, collapsed tissue.

Urethra

The female urethra is shorter than the male urethra. The longer male urethra is anatomically divided into the anterior and posterior urethra. The anterior urethra is made up of penile and bulbar segments, whereas the posterior urethra is made up of membranous and prostatic portions. The prostatic urethra passes through

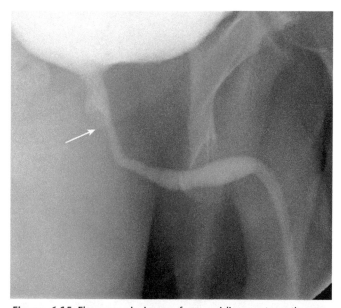

Figure 6.15 Fluoroscopic image from voiding cystourethrography in a male child demonstrates the normal anatomy of the male urethra. The verumontanum (*arrow*) is a mound of tissue along the posterior wall of the prostatic urethra through which the ducts of the prostate gland, paired ejaculatory ducts, and single midline prostatic utricle drain. When present, posterior urethral valves are encountered just inferior to the verumontanum.

the prostate, and the membranous urethra passes through the urogenital diaphragm.

The verumontanum is a mound of tissue along the posterior wall of the prostatic urethra [**Fig. 6.15**]. This mound contains the orifices of three different structures: (1) the midline prostatic utricle, a Müllerian duct remnant; (2) paired ejaculatory ducts; and 3) the many ducts of the prostate gland. Posterior urethral valves are located at the base of the verumontanum.

The male urethra may be evaluated by both the RUG and the VCUG. The RUG evaluates only the anterior urethra and is useful for revealing strictures or disruption. Both the anterior and the posterior urethra are opacified during a VCUG, and this is the only test to reveal the presence of posterior urethral valves.

CONGENITAL ANOMALIES OF THE KIDNEYS AND URETERS

Embryology

Although an in-depth discussion of the embryology of the genitourinary system is beyond the scope of this text, certain points of embryogenesis are important to understand in appreciating the development of congenital anomalies. The kidney progenitor, the pronephros, is a transitory structure which develops in the fourth week of gestation and involutes during the fifth week. From this structure, the mesonephros arises and forms the primitive kidney and the mesonephric duct. While the primitive kidney involutes, the mesonephric or Wolffian duct persists. Its final form differs based on the sex of the developing fetus. In both sexes, the mesonephric duct forms a portion of the bladder and ureter (discussed later). In females, the mesonephric duct otherwise involutes, whereas in males, it is responsible for the development of the seminal vesicles, epididymis, and vas deferens.

The final form of the kidney arises as a bud from the mesonephric duct. This ureteric bud or diverticulum interacts with the metanephric blastema to form the kidney. The ureteric bud develops into the renal collecting system. The metanephric blastema forms the renal parenchyma.

The transformation from the pronephros into the final form of the kidney occurs in the pelvis. By the ninth week of gestation, the kidneys ascend to their typical position in the retroperitoneum [**Fig. 6.16**].

Renal Anomalies

Abnormalities of Development, Ascent, and Fusion

During any of the earlier developmental steps, a mishap may occur resulting in a specific congenital anomaly. If the ureteric bud fails to develop off the mesonephric duct, renal agenesis may occur. Although unilateral renal agenesis may occur in a number of syndromes as well as sporadically, it is generally a benign entity. In females, there is a frequent association with Müllerian duct abnormalities, which will be discussed in a subsequent section of this chapter called *Anomalies of the Female Genital Tract*. Bilateral renal agenesis is incompatible with life due to the severe oligohydramnios and pulmonary hypoplasia that will ensue. In utero, development of the lungs is inextricably linked with development of the kidneys. Normal lung development depends on the presence of adequate amniotic fluid, which is mainly composed of fetal urine produced by the kidneys. Therefore, if fetal renal function is significantly impaired, there will be insufficient amniotic fluid production for normal lung development.

If the kidney fails to ascend appropriately, it remains in the pelvis as an ectopic pelvic kidney. Rarely, the kidney may ascend higher than normal, producing a thoracic kidney. This is a benign entity, but may be a source of confusion and concern on a chest radiograph.

If there is abnormal coalition of the metanephric blastema, fusion of the kidneys will occur. When the lower poles of the kidneys are fused in the midline, they are unable to ascend properly and a horseshoe kidney results [see **Fig. 6.9**]. The band of parenchymal tissue joining the lower poles is referred to as the isthmus. This anomaly is frequently an incidental finding on imaging studies. However, horseshoe kidneys are predisposed to urinary stasis, stone formation, and injury in the setting of relatively minor trauma [**Fig. 6.17**]. Whether horseshoe kidneys are predisposed to the development of malignancy remains a point of debate.

If the metanephric blastemas fuse off midline, cross-fused renal ectopia will result. There are a variety of manifestations of cross-fused renal ectopia, depending on both where the kidneys fuse and how far superiorly the fused renal mass is able to ascend [**Fig. 6.18**]. This condition is frequently an incidental finding, and there are no deleterious effects on renal function. If surgery is planned in the setting of a fusion anomaly, close attention should be paid to the arterial supply and venous drainage because these are frequently aberrant.

Multicystic Dysplastic Kidney

An MCDK is a dysplastic, nonfunctioning kidney that is composed of multiple cysts. These cysts involute over time leaving a tiny soft tissue remnant. MCDK may present prenatally as a complex cystic structure in the expected location of the kidney, and may present postnatally as an abdominal mass. Although this condition typically involves the entirety of the kidney, segmental forms of MCDK can be seen.

Two different mechanisms have been proposed for the development of this condition. The first is related to abnormal induction of the metanephric blastema by the ureteric bud, with abnormal development of the renal parenchyma. The second involves atresia of the renal pelvis or proximal ureter early in the course of gestation, resulting in severe obstruction of the developing kidney.

On imaging studies, it is important to differentiate a severely hydronephrotic kidney from an MCDK. Whereas a hydronephrotic kidney may regain some function, an MCDK will not. This differentiation is made by determining whether the fluid-filled structures observed within the kidney communicate with one another. With hydronephrosis, the "cysts" (representing the severely dilated calyces) communicate, whereas with MCDK, they do not. Ultrasound cine clips are vital to assess this relationship as a single, static image may be misleading.

If the MCDK appears atypical or does not involute, a DMSA scan may be performed. There should be no cortical uptake of radiotracer by an MCDK, whereas faint radiotracer uptake will be seen in even a severely hydronephrotic kidney [**Fig. 6.19**].

Abnormalities of the Ureters

Ureteropelvic Junction and Ureterovesical Junction Obstruction

Congenital obstruction of the ureter occurs most frequently at the UPJ and ureterovesical junction (UVJ). Congenital UPJO is postulated to most commonly result from abnormal development of the upper segment of the ureter, resulting in intrinsic narrowing. External compression from a crossing vessel is also a cause, although rare. Patients with intrinsic obstruction tend to present earlier. The fixed obstruction that causes hydronephrosis is often first detected on prenatal ultrasound. Patients with a crossing vessel have intermittent obstruction, and tend to present later in childhood or adolescence with recurrent abdominal pain. The kidneys are hydronephrotic only during episodes of obstruction, and frequently appear normal otherwise. Imaging should be done during the painful obstructive crisis to visualize hydronephrosis.

Prenatally, UPJO may present with hydronephrosis. Postnatally, if the obstruction is severe enough, it can present as a palpable abdominal mass because of the markedly dilated renal pelvis. Older children and even adults may present with intermittent abdominal or flank pain, recurrent infections, or hypertension. The diagnosis is most frequently made with ultrasound. A dilated renal pelvis and hydronephrosis are seen with a normal-caliber distal ureter [**Fig. 6.20**]. Diuretic renal scintigraphy with MAG3 can determine whether there is a true obstruction. Depending on clinician preference, cross-sectional imaging with CT or MR may be performed to assess for a crossing vessel as

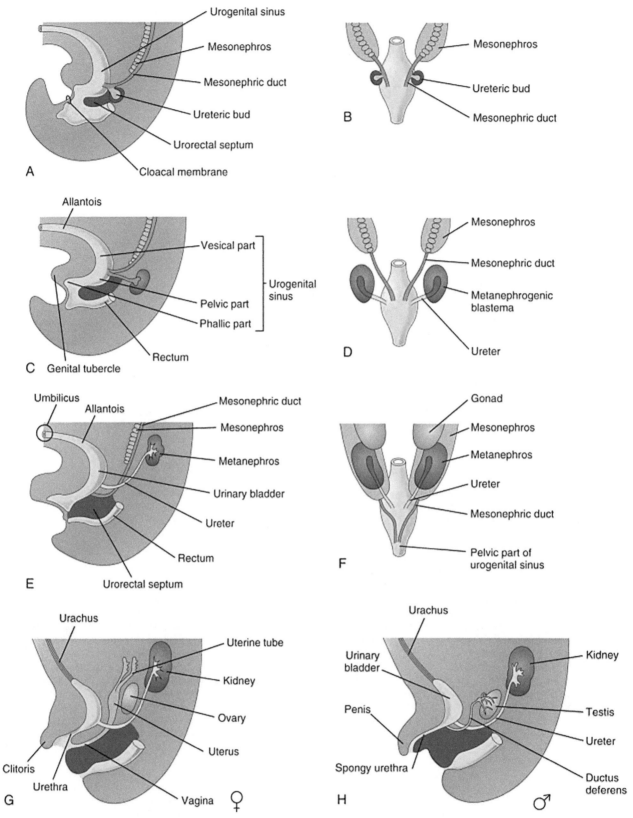

Figure 6.16 Development of the urinary system in the male and female between 5 and 12 weeks' gestation (top to bottom). Diagram showing division of the cloaca into urogenital sinus and rectum, absorption of the mesonephric ducts, development of the urinary bladder, urethra, and urachus, and changes in the location of the ureters. **A, C, E, G, and H,** Lateral views of the caudal half of the embryo. **B, D, and F,** Dorsal views. The stages shown in (**G**) and (**H**) are reached at about 12 weeks' gestation. (From Moore KL. *The Developing Human: Clinically Oriented Embryology,* 9th ed. Philadelphia, PA: Elsevier; 2011.)

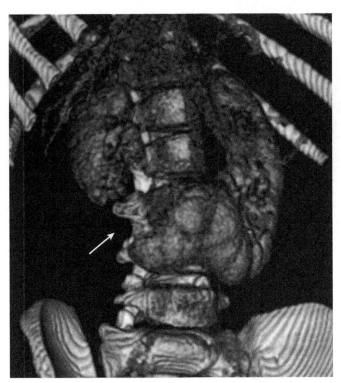

Figure 6.17 Horseshoe transection. This 10-year-old boy had a handlebar injury to his midabdomen. Three-dimensionally reformatted images from a computed tomography scan demonstrate complete transection through the right side of a horseshoe kidney. The cleft is marked by an *arrow*.

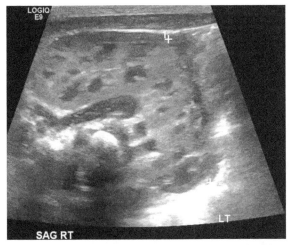

Figure 6.18 Cross-fused renal ectopia. Three-month-old with a prenatal diagnosis of "renal abnormalities." On this sagittal ultrasound image of the abdomen, two renal moieties are seen fused together. The calipers demarcate the "left kidney" that is fused to the lower pole of the right kidney. Note that even though the contour of the fused kidney is abnormal, there is normal corticomedullary differentiation. Renal function in cross-fused ectopia is typically normal.

the cause of obstruction. Recently, increased attention has been paid to dynamic MRU as a tool to help determine need for surgery. Treatment for this condition is typically with pyeloplasty, with resection of the intrinsically narrowed segment of ureter and creation of an anastomosis between the pelvis and ureter.

More rarely, congenital UVJ obstruction (UVJO) may occur. In a single-system kidney, this is most commonly due to primary megaureter. In this condition, a functional obstruction of the distal ureter prevents the normal egress of urine from the ureter into the bladder. This results in hydroureteronephrosis. Greater than 70% of cases of primary megaureter improve with time. Thus patients rarely require surgery. Although the ureter in UVJO typically inserts normally into the bladder at the trigone, UVJO may also be associated with ectopic sites of ureteral insertion. This is the case both for a single system and for the upper pole ureter of a duplex system.

Other forms of obstruction may occur anywhere along the length of the ureter. These are even rarer than UVJO. A midureteral valve may be seen, or a retrocaval ureter can be present with the right ureter coursing posterior to the inferior vena cava (IVC) (preureteral vena cava). This latter anomaly causes medial displacement of the ureter on urographic studies such as an IVP or MRU.

Vesicoureteral Reflux

Another congenital anomaly of the UVJ is VUR, thought to occur because of an abnormal width and length of the distal ureter as it inserts into the bladder wall. With this abnormality, the normally competent UVJ fails, allowing retrograde movement of urine from the urinary bladder up the ureter. This is thought to damage the kidney over time, predominantly because of recurrent infections. The extent of damage to the kidneys is directly related to the degree of reflux. VUR is often found during the evaluation of infections or prenatal hydronephrosis, but it may also be clinically silent.

VUR is most commonly detected and graded by two different imaging modalities: the VCUG and the RNC. In the United States the VCUG is the most commonly used modality. This technique is described in the *Imaging Techniques* section earlier in this chapter. Occasionally, there is concomitant reflux and obstruction, either at the level of the UPJ or the UVJ. If there is coexisting reflux and obstruction, reflux cannot be graded using the standard system. Refluxed contrast material will appear diluted when it enters a dilated, obstructed collecting system because it mixes with trapped urine. On delayed images, there will be prolonged retention of contrast material proximal to the obstruction, most commonly at the level of a UPJO. Thus delayed images are important for making the diagnosis of reflux coexisting with obstruction [**Fig. 6.21**].

The treatment for reflux varies widely depending on the age of the patient, the severity of the reflux, and the preference of the individual practitioner. Therapeutic options include watchful waiting with antibiotic prophylaxis and surgery. Low-grade reflux in the infant and young child typically can be observed. As the patient matures and grows, the UVJ most often becomes competent and reflux resolves. For refractory cases, surgical reimplantation of the ureters or submucosal injection of a synthetic material (such as Deflux by Salix Pharmaceuticals) below the ureteral orifice is offered. The surgically created Deflux mounds may seem similar to soft tissue masses within the bladder and should not be confused for malignancy. Deflux may occasionally calcify. At the UVJ, this may mimic distal ureteral calculi. Knowledge of a history of Deflux injection is helpful to avoid diagnostic confusion [**Fig. 6.22**].

Duplicated Collecting Systems

A duplicated collecting system results from either a bifid ureteric bud that arises from the mesonephric duct or two separate buds that meet the metanephros. Duplex collecting systems exist along a spectrum. At one end of the spectrum, just the renal pelvis may be bifid, with a single ureter exiting the kidney. This is frequently an incidental finding with no clinical significance.

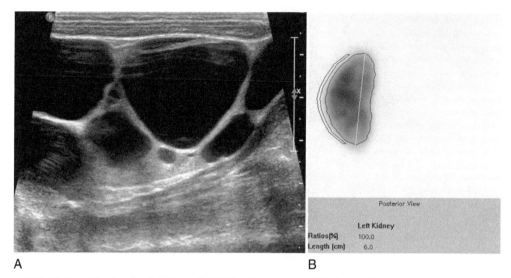

A   B

Figure 6.19 Multicystic dysplastic kidney (MCDK). One-month-old infant with a prenatal diagnosis of MCDK. **A,** Sagittal ultrasound image of the patient's right kidney demonstrates cysts of varying size replacing the renal parenchyma. No normal renal parenchyma is seen. Notably, a severely hydronephrotic kidney could have a similar appearance on a static image. Cine ultrasound clips are essential in differentiating severe hydronephrosis from MCDK. **B,** Posterior planar image from a technetium-99m-dimercaptosuccinic acid renal scan. Uptake is seen only in the left kidney, compatible with the diagnosis of a nonfunctioning right MCDK. Some uptake of radiotracer is expected even in a severely hydronephrotic kidney.

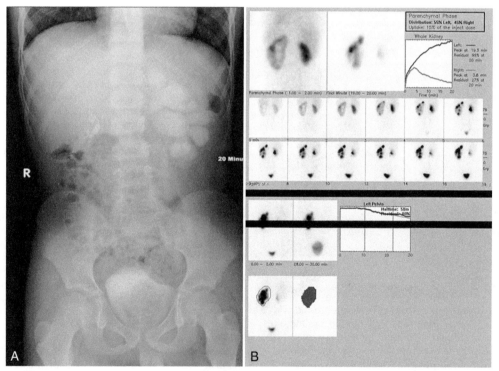

Figure 6.20 Congenital ureteropelvic junction (UPJO) obstruction. Twelve-year-old male with intermittent flank pain. **A,** Radiograph obtained during an intravenous pyelogram (IVP) 20 minutes after the injection of intravenous contrast. The normal right kidney excretes contrast into a normal-sized collecting system, whereas the left collecting system is markedly dilated with distention of the calyces. Although the left ureter is visible, there is an abrupt change in caliber at the level of the UPJ, compatible with UPJO. The bladder is partially filled with contrast material. The concavity along the left side of the bladder dome is due to adjacent stool-filled bowel. **B,** Posterior planar images obtained during a technetium-99m-mercaptoacetyltriglycine (MAG3) Lasix study. The initial images demonstrate relatively symmetric uptake of radiotracer, with asymmetric renal size. Radiotracer is subsequently seen to accumulate in the dilated left collecting system. The associated graphs show minimal excretion from the left kidney before the administration of Lasix. Delayed images after Lasix administration show minimal excretion of radiotracer, compatible with a true obstructive process.

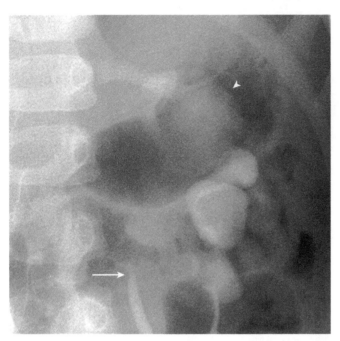

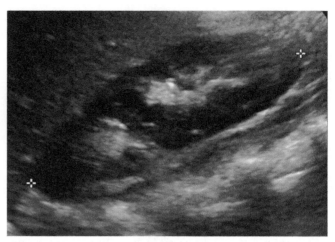

Figure 6.23 Seven-year-old female with abdominal pain. Sagittal ultrasound image of the left kidney shows a band of renal parenchyma bifurcating the echogenic renal sinus. The upper and lower moieties demonstrate similar behavior; that is, neither moiety is hydronephrotic nor scarred. This appearance is most compatible with an incomplete ureteral duplication. This is most frequently an incidental finding with no clinical significance.

Figure 6.21 This ten-year-old had intermittent flank pain and a urinary tract infection. Voiding cystourethrography demonstrates reflux into the left ureter with hesitation at the ureteropelvic junction (UPJ) (*arrow*). Contrast is dilute within the dilated collecting system, with prolonged retention on delayed images (*arrowhead*). This patient has reflux and concomitant UPJ obstruction. Reflux cannot be graded using the 1 to 5 scale because collecting system distention reflects the obstruction, not just the reflux.

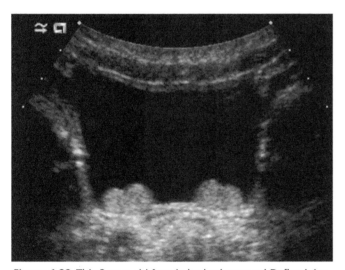

Figure 6.22 This 8-year-old female had submucosal Deflux injections for bilateral reflux. Transverse image of the bladder shows two lobulated, echogenic mounds along the posterior wall of the bladder, representing the Deflux injections. These should not be confused for other soft tissue masses in the setting of this surgical history. Occasionally these mounds may calcify, mimicking distal ureteral calculi.

At the other end of the spectrum, a complete duplication may be seen, with two distinct renal moieties and separate ureters that insert at different locations in the urinary bladder.

When there is complete ureteral duplication, the upper pole ureter is abnormal and inserts medial and inferior to the orthotopic orifice. The lower pole ureter is the analog of the single-system ureter and inserts normally. This relationship was

originally described by pathologists Weigert and Meyer, giving us the *Weigert-Meyer rule.*

While the insertion site of the upper pole ureter is always medial and inferior to that of the normal lower pole ureter, the exact location of the insertion varies. It may insert into the bladder proper, potentially extending inferiorly to the level of the bladder sphincter. In females, the insertion site may be below the urinary sphincter, into the distal urethra, vagina, or perineum. In males, the insertion site may include the urethra, but it is always proximal to the external sphincter and the Wolffian duct derivatives. The morphology of the upper pole ureteral insertion may also be abnormal, which can predispose to obstruction and reflux. The upper pole ectopic ureter may end in a ureterocele, a common cause of obstruction. A ureterocele is a dilation of the intravesical portion of the distal ureter, and it is seen as a thin-walled, ovoid structure protruding into the bladder lumen [see **Fig. 6.4**]. Ureteroceles seen in association with the upper pole of a duplex kidney are more common in females. They may also be seen in single-system kidneys, more commonly in males.

A duplicated system is most frequently initially detected with ultrasonography. The presence of a duplicated collecting system is suggested when a band of normal renal parenchyma is seen bifurcating the renal sinus fat [**Fig. 6.23**]. If the duplex kidney appears otherwise normal, no further evaluation is needed. An incomplete ureteral duplication is likely present.

When imaging findings suggest that the upper and lower poles of a duplex kidney are functioning independently, a complete duplication is likely. An example of this is lower pole hydronephrosis with a normal-appearing upper pole. The presence of a ureterocele, particularly in a female, is also suggestive of a duplicated collecting system.

Patients with suspicion of complete ureteral duplication should undergo further evaluation with a VCUG. RNC has no role in the initial workup of these patients because it provides insufficient anatomic detail. A ureterocele is best detected with a minimum amount of contrast material in the bladder and appears as an ovoid filling defect [see **Fig. 6.4**]. Because of its thin wall, a ureterocele can collapse or efface once the bladder is full. It may also evert or intussuscept, mimicking a bladder diverticulum. Thus early filling views are essential for accurate detection.

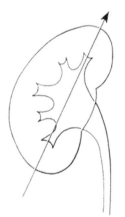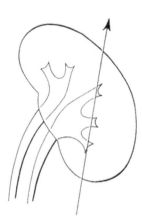

Figure 6.24 Axis of calyces on voiding cystourethrography: the axis, a line drawn from the lowest to the highest calyx of the collecting system, normally points to the contralateral shoulder in a single-system kidney. When there is isolated lower pole reflux, only lower pole calyces are opacified, and the axis of these calyces points to the ipsilateral shoulder. (Courtesy of Robert L. Lebowitz, MD.)

A careful evaluation for reflux should be performed. Lower pole reflux is a frequent finding in complete ureteral duplication. This may be mistaken for reflux into a single system, particularly if there is no prior imaging such as ultrasound for comparison. Certain characteristics of the opacified collecting system can be helpful in differentiating reflux into the lower pole of a duplex system from reflux into a single-system kidney. In a single-system kidney, when the refluxed contrast extends to the level of the collecting system, 9 to 12 calyces should fill, and the longitudinal orientation of the calyces should point toward the contralateral shoulder. If contrast fills a smaller number of calyces and the longitudinal axis of the kidney points toward the ipsilateral shoulder [**Fig. 6.24**], the presence of a duplicated collecting system with lower pole reflux should be considered. The appearance of lower pole reflux has been compared with that of a "drooping lily" [**Fig. 6.25**]. This appearance is related to mass effect from a hydronephrotic upper pole system and the orientation of the calyces (petals) toward the ipsilateral shoulder. Reflux can also rarely occur into the upper pole of a duplex system.

Functional imaging, either by nuclear medicine or MRU, is useful in assessing the degree of function of the upper and lower poles, and also in the evaluation for obstruction. Typically, the more ectopic the ureter, the more dysplastic and dysfunctional the associated upper pole. The lower pole may have decreased function or scarring from dysplasia or reflux.

The clinical presentation of a duplicated collecting system can vary widely. Most frequently, particularly in the case of an incompletely duplicated system, there are no clinical ramifications. With a completely duplicated system, patients may present with recurrent infections because of reflux or obstruction. Hydronephrosis may also be discovered, also related to reflux or obstruction. Obstruction will typically involve the upper pole.

A duplicated collecting system with an ectopic upper pole ureteral insertion can be a cause of incontinence in a female. Males do not experience this type of incontinence, because the ectopic ureter always inserts above the external urinary sphincter. As discussed earlier, in females the ectopic ureter may insert below the level of the sphincter, either into the urethra or the vagina. With these forms of ectopic insertion, there is constant leakage of urine. Thus an ectopic ureter causing incontinence may be diagnosed with the clinical history of a girl who has never been dry, day or night. Physical examination will show dribbling of urine at the perineum. In this setting, the goal of the radiologist is to find the offending upper pole ureter [see **Fig. 6.14**].

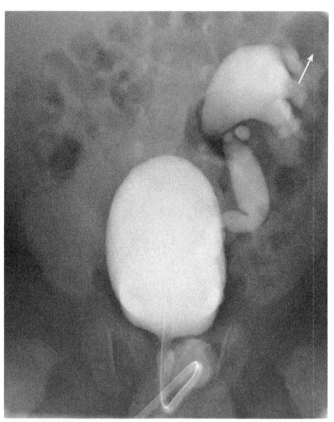

Figure 6.25 Lower pole reflux. This voiding cystourethrography image demonstrates reflux into the lower pole of a duplex system, with the axis of the calyces pointing to the ipsilateral shoulder (*arrow*). The appearance of the calyces mimics that of a drooping lily.

CONGENITAL ANOMALIES OF THE BLADDER AND URETHRA

Embryology

While the kidneys and ureters arise from the ureteric bud, the bladder and urethra arise predominantly from the cloaca. Early in fetal life there is a single orifice for the bladder, rectum, and in females, the vagina. This is the cloaca. By the sixth week of gestation, a urorectal septum develops, dividing the cloaca into the urogenital sinus ventrally and the rectum dorsally. The cephalic portion of the urogenital sinus unites with the caudal end of the mesonephric duct, and together these structures form the bladder and ureteral orifices. The caudal portion of the urogenital sinus forms the urethra in males, and both the urethra and the vagina in females [see **Fig. 6.16**].

Congenital Anomalies of the Bladder
Urachal Anomalies

The allantois is a structure that drains the fetal bladder during the first trimester. It extends from the bladder dome to the umbilicus. In most cases it eventually involutes, leaving the urachus or median umbilical ligament. Portions of the duct may remain patent postnatally. When the entirety of the duct remains open, a patent urachus results. This presents with drainage of urine through the umbilicus. A blind ending pouch extending inferiorly from the umbilicus is a urachal sinus, which can present with infection. A portion of the urachus that remains fluid filled with both ends closed is a urachal cyst. This entity may present with infection or, if large enough, a palpable

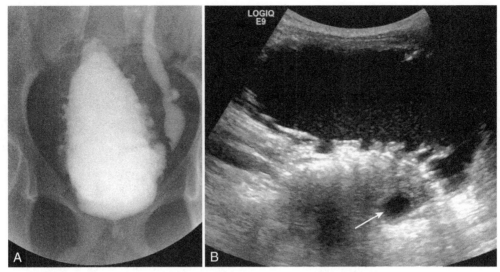

Figure 6.26 Neurogenic bladder. Teenage female with myelomeningocele. **A,** Coned down spot image of the urinary bladder obtained during a voiding cystourethrography. The urinary bladder has a very irregular appearance and an elongated, conical shape. This is described as a pinecone or Christmas tree appearance. Irregularity is due to marked bladder wall hypertrophy in the setting of bladder sphincter dyssynergia. Contrast is seen refluxing into the left ureter, a frequent coexisting finding. **B,** Transverse ultrasound image of the bladder in the same patient shows the markedly irregular bladder wall. The dilated distal left ureter is also shown (*arrow*).

abdominal mass. Finally, the urachus may remain open at the level of the bladder dome, resulting in a urachal diverticulum. Urachal anomalies may be visualized with ultrasound and sometimes with cystography (both CT and fluoroscopic) as fluid-filled tubular structures following the expected trajectory of the median umbilical ligament.

Neurogenic Bladder

Neurogenic bladder, although not a congenital anomaly resulting from maldevelopment of the bladder or urethra, is an anomaly that can be present at birth secondary to an abnormality of the spinal cord such as myelomeningocele or tethered cord. In the setting of such an abnormality, the bladder does not receive appropriate innervation, and two different problems may result. The bladder sphincter may be weak, leading to incontinence and a low capacitance bladder. The bladder wall will be of normal thickness. Alternatively, bladder sphincter dyssynergia may result, where the bladder contracts but the sphincter does not relax. This results in marked hypertrophy and trabeculation of the bladder wall. The thickened, trabeculated, elongated appearance of the bladder on VCUG in this setting has been likened to that of a pinecone or Christmas tree [**Fig. 6.26**].

Management for these patients includes intermittent catheterization to empty the bladder completely and regularly, as well as anticholinergics to relax the bladder wall. Not infrequently, however, the bladder may need to be surgically augmented. Augmentation is most commonly performed using ileum, followed by other segments of bowel including colon or stomach. The classic configuration of an augmented bladder is a hollow viscous with the appearance of the bladder inferiorly and bowel segment superiorly. Often the original valvulae conniventes or haustra can be appreciated in the augmented section.

Bladder Diverticula

Bladder diverticula can be seen in patients of all ages. The younger the patient, the more likely the diverticulum is to be congenital in etiology. Congenital diverticula are due to abnormalities of the detrusor muscle of the bladder wall, allowing for outpouching of the urothelium through a muscular defect. Congenital diverticula frequently occur near the ureteral orifice, creating a periureteral or Hutch diverticulum. Acquired diverticula may be multiple and occur most frequently in the setting of bladder outlet obstruction because of increased intraluminal pressure. They may occur in patients with a neurogenic bladder (discussed earlier). Rarely, multiple bladder diverticula may be seen in Menkes kinky hair syndrome, Williams syndrome, or Ehlers-Danlos syndrome.

Abnormalities of the Urethra

Posterior Urethral Valves

Continuing the march down the urinary tract, we will end our discussion of congenital anomalies with the urethra. Congenital bladder outlet obstruction is seen predominantly in males due to posterior urethral valves. Although the exact embryologic mechanism responsible for the development of valves remains a point of debate, they result from abnormality in the formation of the urethra. Posterior urethral valves are overwhelmingly the most common form, although anterior urethral valves may also exist and cause obstruction. With advances in fetal imaging, posterior urethral valves are frequently suspected before birth. Postnatally, patients may present with recurrent infections and hydronephrosis in more mild forms of PUV, or urosepsis in more severe forms. If not diagnosed early in life, patients are at risk for development of renal failure caused by chronic obstructive uropathy.

Prenatal ultrasonography may demonstrate a dilated, thick-walled urinary bladder with a keyhole appearance, representing the dilated urinary bladder and posterior urethra [see **Fig. 6.3**]. Hydronephrosis or hydroureteronephrosis is a frequent coexisting finding due to obstruction and/or reflux. The degree of dilation is typically asymmetric between the right and left sides. If the obstruction causes forniceal rupture, urinomas may form or urinary ascites may be seen. In severe cases, PUV causes decreased urine production, oligohydramnios, and pulmonary hypoplasia. On postnatal ultrasound, one may see a dilated, thick-walled urinary bladder with a variable presence and degree of hydroureteronephrosis.

Although findings on ultrasound may be suggestive of PUV, the diagnosis ultimately depends on lateral voiding images of the urethra obtained during a VCUG. Valves are seen as thin slips of tissue and are located at the base of the verumontanum (discussed in the earlier section of this chapter called *Normal Genitourinary System in Children*.) Because the valves are anteriorly positioned within the urethral lumen, the stream of contrast will be eccentrically positioned along the posterior aspect of the urethra. The urethra will be dilated proximal to the valves. The degree of proximal urethral dilation, bladder wall thickening, and reflux depend on the severity of the valves [see **Fig. 6.3**]. Treatment for this condition is surgical endoscopic fulguration of the valves.

OTHER CONGENITAL ANOMALIES OF THE GENITOURINARY SYSTEM

Anomalies with a short urethra and abnormal location of the urethral meatus include hypospadias and epispadias. The meatus is located on the ventral surface of the urethra in hypospadias, and along the dorsal surface in epispadias. Hypospadias occurs only in boys, whereas epispadias occurs in both boys and girls.

Hypospadias

Hypospadias occurs because of abnormal development of the urethral groove. The degree of hypospadias may vary widely, with the site of urethral exit seen anywhere from immediately inferior to the expected position to a more proximal position along the penile shaft to the anal verge. The prostatic utricle, a midline diverticular structure arising from the verumontanum, is a normal Müllerian duct remnant that becomes enlarged in patients with hypospadias. The more severe the hypospadias, the larger the associated prostatic utricle. Hypospadias most frequently occurs as a sporadic, isolated malformation, but it may occur in constellation with other abnormalities such as cryptorchidism or imperforate anus. Hypospadias is diagnosed on physical examination. Preoperative VCUG is useful to evaluate for the presence of a refluxing prostatic utricle that may require excision. RUG is helpful postoperatively to assess for complications. In severe hypospadias, the dysmorphic physical appearance is on the spectrum of ambiguous genitalia. The distinction between severe hypospadias and other forms of ambiguous genitalia, such as CAH, is made based on a combination of radiologic findings

(ultrasound and genitogram), physical examination, and laboratory data.

Exstrophy-Epispadias Complex

Epispadias is secondary to failure of midline fusion of the urethra, a problem occurring much earlier in embryogenesis than hypospadias. It is a part of the continuum of the exstrophy-epispadias complex. In patients with complete bladder exstrophy, the normally spherical bladder forms instead as a flat plate, a process termed *detubularization*. The bladder mucosa is exposed on the anterior surface of the abdominal wall. The urethra is similarly detubularized and forms a urethral plate. When only the urethra is detubularized, the result is epispadias. There are many associated anomalies. One is diastasis of the pubic symphysis, which occurs because of outward rotation of the pelvis and bony deficiency, as well as a change in the pelvic floor muscular configuration [**Fig. 6.27**]. The genitalia also have an abnormal appearance, with a bifid clitoris in females and separation of the corporal tissue in boys, which is mild in epispadias and more severe in exstrophy. In patients with bladder exstrophy, the ureteral insertions are abnormal. Once the bladder is closed, VUR is nearly universal.

Epispadias is suspected on prenatal imaging by ambiguous genitalia, with the phallus typically much shorter than normal in males. It may be occult in females. Bladder exstrophy is a more obvious diagnosis on prenatal imaging and is considered when one does not visualize the normal fluid-filled bladder consistently during the course of the examination. Other findings suggestive of the diagnosis include widening of the pubic symphysis and visualization of an abnormal mass reflecting the bladder plate along the anterior wall of the pelvis.

Postnatally, the diagnosis of epispadias in boys and bladder exstrophy in boys and girls is clinically obvious. The role of imaging, if any, is primarily for surgical planning. Epispadias is often missed in females because the only visible sign on physical examination may be a bifid clitoris. MRI is useful in evaluating the pelvic musculature, bladder plate, and pubic diastasis in patients with bladder exstrophy. After the bladder has been reconstructed and the epispadias repaired, cystography is frequently performed to assess the size and integrity of the bladder and urethra. Ultrasound is used to monitor the appearance of the entire genitourinary system, particularly the kidneys, which are prone to scarring from reflux.

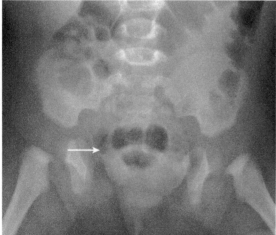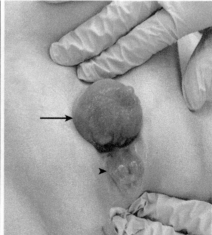

Figure 6.27 This baby boy was born with bladder exstrophy. A, The radiograph demonstrates wide diastasis of the pubic symphysis. The opacity in the pelvis represents the exstrophied bladder (*arrow*) seen on physical examination. **B,** The epispadiac urethra (*arrowhead*) is exposed, with retraction below the bulbous bladder plate (*arrow*).

Prune Belly Syndrome

Prune belly, or Eagle Barrett syndrome, is a rare disorder characterized by the presence of three major findings: marked dilatation of the ureters, cryptorchidism, and significant deficiency of the abdominal musculature. Abdominal wall muscular deficiency is responsible for the characteristic physical examination finding of a wrinkled or prunelike belly. The etiology of this condition is unknown, but it is thought to be due to abnormalities of the mesenchyme early in gestation. The developing fetus is unable to expel urine appropriately, resulting in obstructive uropathy, maldeveloped kidneys, oligohydramnios, and pulmonary hypoplasia.

Early postnatal radiographs of affected infants will have an unusual appearance. The abdominal contents will be splayed laterally because of the lack of normal musculature. Ultrasound will show markedly dilated ureters, associated hydronephrosis, and a dilated urinary bladder. The kidneys are typically dysplastic and appear echogenic. Ultrasound can also aid in the diagnosis of cryptorchidism. With VCUG, one will see an enlarged urinary bladder with reflux up massively enlarged, tortuous ureters into dilated renal collecting systems. A urachal diverticulum is a frequent coexisting finding. The posterior urethra is typically dilated due to deficiency of the prostate gland. Occasionally, the anterior urethra is dilated ("megalourethra").

The prognosis for these patients greatly depends on the degree of urinary tract abnormalities and pulmonary hypoplasia. In terms of genitourinary care, patients frequently undergo clean intermittent catheterization or vesicostomy to improve the egress of urine, decompress the urinary system, and avoid further injury to the kidneys. Patients are prescribed antibiotic prophylaxis because of the severity of VUR.

ACQUIRED ABNORMALITIES OF THE GENITOURINARY SYSTEM

Infections of the Genitourinary System

Urinary tract infections (UTIs) are very common in children, surpassed only in frequency by upper respiratory tract infections. The term *UTI* generally refers to an infection anywhere along the urinary tract. Pyelonephritis is distinguished from cystitis by high fever (>101.3°F), systemic symptoms, and flank pain.

The clinical presentation of an infant with a UTI is nonspecific but typically includes fever and irritability. As part of the workup for a fever without a clear source, a urine sample is often obtained. Ideally, a catheterized specimen is collected in non-toilet-trained children, and a clean catch specimen is obtained in toilet-trained children. This minimizes the risk for contamination. The diagnosis is made when a single organism grows more than 50,000 colony-forming units. The clinician must then decide whether to pursue further imaging to determine the cause of the UTI. One approach is to routinely perform both renal ultrasound and VCUG after the initial infection. The purpose of these studies is to assess for the presence of VUR (discussed earlier in this chapter). Recommendations from the American Academy of Pediatrics in 2011 state that a renal ultrasound should be performed after the initial infection in children aged 2 to 24 months, but that a VCUG need not be performed unless there are abnormalities on ultrasound or the patient experiences recurrent febrile UTIs. That said, many studies have shown that a normal ultrasound does not exclude the presence of VUR, even high grade, and is a poor screening test for reflux.

Pyelonephritis

When infected, the kidney may appear enlarged with loss of corticomedullary differentiation. With power Doppler, regions of relative hypoperfusion may be demonstrated [**Fig. 6.28**]. On CT or MRI, the kidney is noted to be enlarged, with variable amounts of perinephric fluid. On postcontrast images, a "striated nephrogram" pattern may be observed. Poorly defined regions of hypoenhancement may also be seen. On a DMSA study, regions of diminished uptake are noted. These can remain for weeks to months after the infection, and may reflect areas of scarring if they persist.

Imaging is most beneficial when signs and symptoms of pyelonephritis have not resolved as expected after appropriate antibiotic therapy. Persistent signs and symptoms may be related to complications of infection such as a renal or perirenal abscess. An underlying congenital anomaly such as a UPJO may also be contributory. An ultrasound is the most frequent imaging study obtained to assess for complications of infection and underlying congenital anomalies.

A renal abscess appears as a rounded hypoechoic region within the renal parenchyma, frequently with surrounding

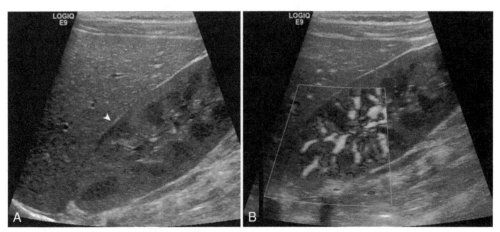

Figure 6.28 Pyelonephritis. Three-year-old girl with fever. **A and B,** Grayscale and power Doppler images of the right kidney obtained with a linear transducer. On the grayscale image, there is a subtle, wedge-shaped area of hypoechogenicity in the renal cortex (*arrowhead*), which does not demonstrate flow with power Doppler. These findings are suggestive of a focal region of pyelonephritis.

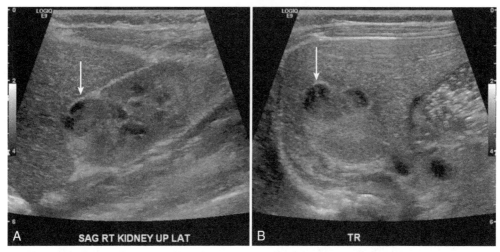

Figure 6.29 Renal abscess. Two-year-old with a urinary tract infection not responsive to antibiotics. **A and B,** Sagittal and transverse images of the superior pole of the right kidney show a round, heterogeneous lesion centered in the cortex (*arrow*). In this clinical setting, this appearance is most suggestive of a renal abscess. However, in the absence of signs of infection, this may be confused with a neoplasm.

hyperemia [**Fig. 6.29**]. A perirenal abscess occurs when the infection has breached the renal capsule but remains contained within Gerota's fascia. Sonographically, a perirenal abscess is seen as a complex fluid collection abutting the kidney. The perirenal fat is frequently echogenic. On contrast-enhanced cross-sectional imaging, renal and perirenal abscesses demonstrate rim enhancement, and extensive inflammatory change is seen involving the kidney and retroperitoneum. An area of infection may appear very masslike on all imaging studies and can be mistaken for a neoplastic process. It is important to keep in mind that infection is overwhelmingly more common than tumor in the pediatric population.

In individuals who have suffered multiple episodes of pyelonephritis, the kidneys may develop focal regions of scarring with loss of normal corticomedullary differentiation. If this appearance is seen during routine ultrasonography of the kidneys in a pediatric patient, the ordering clinician should be notified. If not worked up previously, further imaging with a VCUG or DMSA study should be considered. The DMSA study is notably much more sensitive for detecting scarring than renal ultrasound.

Pyonephrosis

A specific type of infection occurs in the setting of obstruction. In pyonephrosis, pus fills an obstructed collecting system. This is a rare entity in the pediatric population. When it occurs, it is a medical emergency. Clinically, patients with pyonephrosis are very ill and present with flank pain. On imaging, hydronephrosis or hydroureteronephrosis will be present. Fluid within the dilated collecting system may appear complex, with debris demonstrated on ultrasound or CT.

Urethral Strictures

In the pediatric population, urethral strictures are most frequently congenital or related to prior trauma. In adolescents, they can also be seen in the setting of a sexually transmitted disease. Regardless of the causative factor, patients present clinically with urinary retention and hesitancy. The diagnosis is typically made with an RUG because strictures are most commonly seen along the anterior urethra [see **Fig. 6.6**]. If the diagnosis of a urethral stricture is made by VCUG, a subsequent RUG may be needed to better assess the length of the stricture.

Abnormalities of Calcium Deposition

Nephrocalcinosis

Nephrocalcinosis refers to the deposition of calcium in the kidneys. This deposition occurs most frequently in the medullary pyramids (>90%), termed *medullary nephrocalcinosis*, but can also occur in the cortex, termed *cortical nephrocalcinosis*. Typically, cortical calcification is related to a prior renal insult such as cortical necrosis or chronic glomerulonephritis. Broadly speaking, medullary nephrocalcinosis is due to abnormalities in the excretion of calcium, phosphate, and oxalate. The exact cause of this abnormal excretion varies widely. Rarely cortical and medullary nephrocalcinosis may coexist, as seen in oxalosis or Alport syndrome.

Preterm infants are particularly susceptible to the development of medullary nephrocalcinosis. Predisposing factors include underdeveloped renal function, parenteral nutrition, and prolonged administration of loop diuretics such as Lasix. The long-term impact of this condition is unknown, but the imaging findings typically resolve after the cessation of diuretics. Occasionally, affected infants may experience the development of true renal stones. Medullary sponge kidney, or ectasia of the renal tubules, is also a cause of medullary nephrocalcinosis occasionally encountered in the pediatric population. Rarer causes include hypophosphatemic rickets, primary hyperparathyroidism, and distal renal tubular acidosis. Transient medullary echogenicity is a mimicker of medullary nephrocalcinosis in neonates. This is of unknown cause and was previously thought to be due to the presence of Tamm-Horsfall proteins [**Fig. 6.30**]. Regardless of etiology, this finding is of no clinical significance and typically resolves within the first week of life.

In most cases, patients with nephrocalcinosis are asymptomatic, and findings are seen incidentally on imaging studies. On all imaging modalities, the diagnosis is made by the presence of abnormal calcific density within the kidney. In medullary nephrocalcinosis, a portion or the entirety of the medulla may demonstrate increased echogenicity [**Fig. 6.31**]. This appearance may sometimes be mistaken for echogenic renal sinus fat.

Nephrolithiasis

As with medullary nephrocalcinosis, metabolic abnormalities may contribute to the development of nephrolithiasis. Additional risk factors for the development of renal stones include a family history, infection, and urinary stasis caused by congenital anomalies such as UPJO or UVJO. Renal stones are a common finding in patients with chronic medical conditions such as inflammatory bowel disease. Although once considered relatively rare, renal stones in otherwise healthy children are being seen with increased frequency.

The clinical presentation of nephrolithiasis is similar to that seen in adults. Patients present with intermittent flank pain and/or hematuria. In younger children presenting symptoms may be more nonspecific, with abdominal pain or fussiness. Ultrasound is the initial imaging modality used in the assessment for nephrolithiasis. As in adults, renal calculi are seen as echogenic, shadowing foci, although smaller stones may not shadow. With color Doppler, calculi may demonstrate a "twinkle" artifact. If a stone obstructs a ureter, the urinary tract will be dilated proximal to the level of the stone. Given the smaller body habitus of many pediatric patients, an obstructing ureteral stone is frequently visualized with ultrasound.

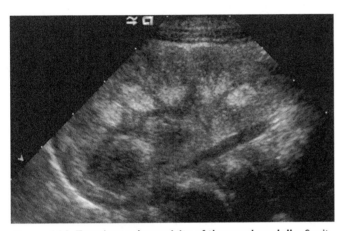

Figure 6.30 Transient echogenicity of the renal medulla. Sagittal grayscale image of a kidney in a neonate. The medullary pyramids are echogenic, mimicking the appearance of medullary nephrocalcinosis. This is a benign, transient finding that typically resolves within the first week of life.

If ultrasound results are equivocal, a CT scan can be used in the evaluation for potential nephrolithiasis. Currently, very-low-dose CT protocols are used, taking advantage of the inherent contrast differences between a calcified stone and the surrounding soft tissues. As in adults, a stone is seen as a hyperdense structure within the renal collecting system, along the course of the ureters, within the bladder, or rarely, within the urethra [see **Fig. 6.11**]. Radiographs may be used to follow up previously documented stones, although visibility may be suboptimal for certain stone compositions.

Bladder Stones

In the United States primary bladder stones are infrequently encountered in the pediatric population. Most bladder stones originate from the kidneys. Primary bladder stones are typically associated with an underlying anatomic anomaly of the urinary tract, such as a bladder diverticulum. They may also occur as a result of recurrent catheterization, which introduces a nidus for stone formation.

The diagnosis of a bladder stone may be suggested on abdominal radiographs when a calcific density is seen within the pelvis [**Fig. 6.32**]. Phleboliths in pelvic veins are unusual in children, so when a calcification is seen in the lower pelvis, the possibility of a bladder calculus should be considered. Ultrasound demonstrates an echogenic, shadowing, mobile mass within the bladder lumen. On CT, bladder stones are typically fairly obvious.

MASSES OF THE GENITOURINARY SYSTEM

In comparison with the renal masses typically seen in adults, a distinct group of pathologies is encountered in the pediatric population. To evaluate a renal mass in a child, the age of the child at presentation should be considered in conjunction with the imaging characteristics of the mass. Unilateral versus bilateral involvement is important to discern [**Table 6.1** and **Box 6.1**]. Using this approach, a targeted differential diagnosis for a renal mass can be provided.

Masses may also arise from the urinary bladder. It is important to differentiate primary bladder lesions from other pelvic masses that may arise from various primary organs and pelvic soft tissues. There are also potential mimickers of pelvis masses, as will be discussed later in this section.

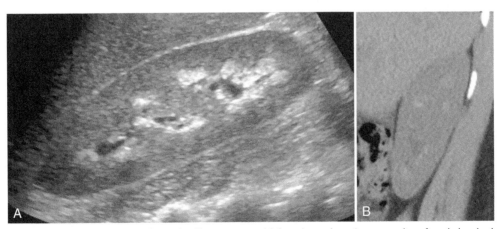

Figure 6.31 Medullary nephrocalcinosis. Sixteen-year-old female undergoing a workup for abdominal pain. **A,** Sagittal image of the right kidney demonstrates marked echogenicity of the renal medulla, compatible with medullary nephrocalcinosis. **B,** Sagittal reconstruction from a noncontrast computed tomography of the same patient shows subtle, amorphous calcific densities along the renal medulla, corresponding to the findings better depicted on ultrasound. Medullary nephrocalcinosis can be caused by a wide variety of etiologies, including medullary sponge kidney and abnormalities in the excretion of phosphate and calcium.

Ultrasound is usually the first-line imaging modality for evaluation of masses of the genitourinary system, followed by contrast-enhanced cross-sectional imaging, either CT or MRI. Although CT has been favored in the past for the initial diagnosis of renal masses, MRI is now often used in both the initial diagnosis and in follow-up because of lack of ionizing radiation. This is an especially important consideration in patients who will require frequent imaging.

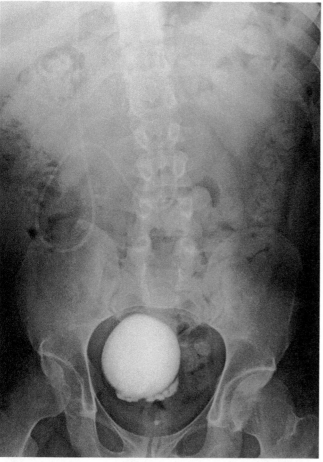

Figure 6.32 KUB (kidneys, ureters, and bladder) in a patient born with a myelomeningocele demonstrates multiple small and large stones within the pelvis, known to be in the urinary bladder. A small stone is seen in the region of the right ureter. The patient has lumbosacral spinal dysraphism and a ventriculoperitoneal shunt.

Unilateral Renal Masses
Mesoblastic Nephroma

Mesoblastic nephroma is the most common solid renal tumor in neonates. Most cases are diagnosed within the first few months of life in the setting of a palpable abdominal mass, although some tumors are detected on prenatal ultrasound. Pathologically, this is a benign lesion containing nephrogenic mesenchyme. For this reason, it has also been referred to as fetal renal hamartoma and leiomyomatous hamartoma.

On ultrasound, this lesion appears as a heterogenous mass arising from the kidney. Contrast-enhanced CT shows a large, infiltrative, heterogenously enhancing mass with ill-defined borders and no capsule. Necrotic and hemorrhagic regions can be seen within this tumor. The renal sinus is commonly involved [**Fig. 6.33**]. This is typically a solitary lesion. Wide surgical resection is the treatment of choice and is usually curative. Metastases are rare; however, they have been reported in the lungs, brain, and bones. Aggressive behavior and paraneoplastic syndromes may occur with the cellular subtype of this tumor. Recurrence is rare, but can occur in instances of incomplete resection. Prognosis is good overall, with the best prognosis in patients diagnosed and treated before 6 months of age.

Wilms Tumor

Wilms tumor is the most common renal malignancy seen in children and represents 87% of all pediatric renal tumors. The mean age of diagnosis is 3 to 4 years. Between 4 and 13% of patients present with bilateral disease.

Wilms tumor arises from nephrogenic rests in the renal parenchyma. The tumor can arise sporadically or in patients with a genetic predisposition. Wilms tumor has been associated with WAGR (Wilms, aniridia, genitourinary abnormalities, and mental retardation), Denys-Drash syndrome (male pseudohermaphroditism and progressive glomerulonephritis), and Beckwith-Wiedemann syndrome. For patients with these entities, screening imaging is recommended. An initial CT is performed at 6 months of age, followed by interval ultrasound

---

BOX 6.1 Bilateral Renal Masses in Children

Infection
Lymphoma
Leukemia
Metastases
Bilateral Wilms tumor
Nephroblastomatosis

TABLE 6.1 Unilateral Renal Masses by Age

	Solid	Cystic	Rare Tumors in the Pediatric Population
Neonate	Mesoblastic nephroma	Multicystic dysplastic kidney	• Renal medullary carcinoma (hemoglobin SC disease) • Rhabdoid tumor • Clear cell sarcoma • Angiomyolipoma
Toddler	Wilms tumor	• Wilms tumor • Multilocular cystic nephroma	
Schoolage	Wilms tumor		
Teenager	Renal cell carcinoma (rare)		

Always consider infection when seeing a mass.

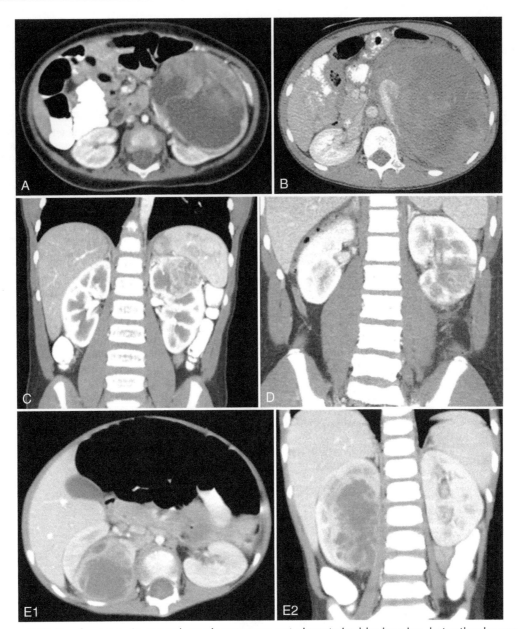

Figure 6.33 Renal masses. In general, renal masses are not characterized by imaging, but rather by age at presentation and clinical history. **A,** This heterogeneous mass presenting in a newborn is a mesoblastic nephroma. **B,** The large mass in the left kidney of this toddler is a Wilms tumor, the most common tumor seen in toddlers and young children. **C,** This 12-year-old with a left renal mass has renal cell carcinoma. Although it is unusual for children of this age to have a primary renal mass, after the age of 11 years, renal cell carcinoma is more commonly seen than Wilms tumor. **D,** This patient with hemoglobin SC disease has a renal medullary carcinoma, a rare tumor specific to this patient population. **E1 and E2,** This 5-year-old with a fever has a right renal abscess. When evaluating a renal mass, clinical context is important. Infection should be considered in the appropriate setting.

performed every 3 months until the age of 7 years. After age 7, no additional imaging is needed because the risk for development of Wilms tumor is significantly decreased.

Patients usually present with a painless, palpable abdominal mass. Symptoms are rare. Wilms tumor is usually found incidentally on physical examination or imaging. A small percentage of patients present with hypertension secondary to renin-producing cells within the tumor.

Ultrasound demonstrates a large, heterogenous mass centered within the kidney, with distortion and displacement of adjacent structures [see **Fig. 6.33**]. Tumor thrombus may occur and

extend into the renal vein, IVC, and right atrium. Mass effect on local structures should be assessed, and evaluation for synchronous contralateral renal lesions and metastatic disease should be performed. Although staging can be predicted by cross-sectional imaging, it is based on findings at surgery [**Table 6.2**].

In patients with unilateral Wilms tumor, treatment includes radical nephrectomy with adjuvant chemotherapy. When there is bilateral renal involvement [**Fig. 6.34**], each side is staged independently. Patients with bilateral involvement are initially treated with chemotherapy with the goal of decreasing tumor burden in preparation for surgical resection. Unlike patients with unilateral Wilms tumor, patients with bilateral Wilms may be considered for partial nephrectomy. A risk associated with surgical resection is tumor spillage, which can lead to peritoneal spread of disease and potential upstaging of the tumor. Prognosis is better in patients with more favorable histology rather than anaplastic histology. Most tumor recurrences occur within the first 3 years after completion of chemotherapy; therefore, interval follow-up imaging during this period is crucial. The highest recurrence is seen in patients with incomplete surgical resection, vascular invasion, or lymph node metastases.

TABLE 6.2 **Staging of Wilms Tumor**

Stage	Description
I	Limited to the kidney and completely resectable with renal capsule intact: renal sinus may be infiltrated but not beyond hilum
II	Tumor infiltrates beyond kidney, completely resected: includes tumor with local spillage confined to flank
III	Residual tumor confined to abdomen, nonhematogenous: includes (a) positive abdominal nodes; (b) diffuse peritoneal contamination by direct growth, implants, or spillage; (c) positive margins; or (d) residual nonresected tumor
IV	Hematogenous disease (added: lungs, lymph nodes, liver)
V	Bilateral disease: each side should be staged separately, because prognosis is dependent on the higher individual stage

From Paulino, AC. Current issues in the diagnosis and management of Wilms' tumor. *Oncology.* 1996;10:1553-1565.

Multilocular Cystic Renal Tumor

The predominantly cystic and septated appearance of the multilocular cystic renal tumor distinguishes it from other renal lesions. The tumor is typically well circumscribed and insinuates into the renal hilum. There is no excretion of contrast material into the cystic portion of the lesion on delayed imaging, distinguishing it from the collecting system. When the cystic components are small, the mass can appear solid because of the enhancing intervening soft tissue.

Histologically this tumor represents two separate lesions: a cystic nephroma and a cystic partially differentiated nephroblastoma. Radiologically, these are indistinguishable from each other. Both can occur in children, although traditionally a cystic nephroma is seen in middle-aged women, whereas a cystic partially differentiated nephroblastoma is seen in young boys [**Fig. 6.35**].

The first line of treatment is complete surgical resection. Recurrence is rare and occurs in the setting of incomplete surgical resection. If recurrence occurs, further treatment with local radiation or chemotherapy is recommended.

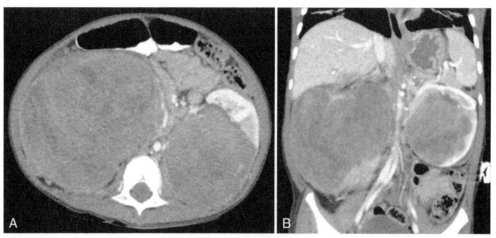

Figure 6.34 Bilateral Wilms tumor: 3-year-old girl with bilateral renal masses. A, Axial and (**B**) coronal contrast-enhanced computed tomography images demonstrate large bilateral heterogeneously enhancing renal masses. The differential diagnosis includes nephroblastomatosis, leukemia, and lymphoma.

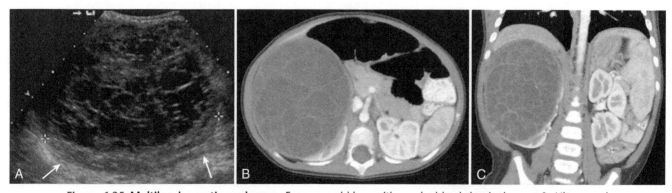

Figure 6.35 Multilocular cystic nephroma. Four-year-old boy with a palpable abdominal mass. **A,** Ultrasound demonstrates a large complex cystic mass in the right renal fossa. The normal renal parenchyma (*arrows*) is noted to be distorted by the mass. **B,** Axial and (**C**) coronal contrast-enhanced computed tomography images demonstrate a large, complex cystic mass in the right kidney, with multiple enhancing intervening septations.

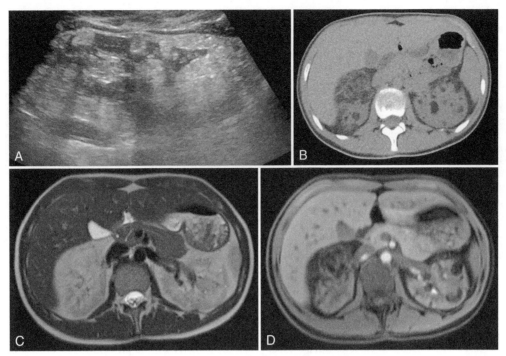

Figure 6.36 Angiomyolipoma (AML). Seventeen-year-old girl with tuberous sclerosis and multiple angiolipo-mata. **A,** Renal ultrasound shows multiple rounded, cortically based echogenic masses. **B,** Non-contrast-enhanced computed tomography shows multiple bilateral low-density renal lesions, the same attenuation as the subcutaneous fat. **C,** Axial T1 image shows multiple high signal renal lesions bilaterally, consistent with fat-containing tumors. **D,** T1 fat-saturated postcontrast image shows low-signal, nonenhancing renal lesions.

Renal Cell Carcinoma

Although this is the most common primary renal tumor in adults, renal cell carcinoma (RCC) is uncommon in young children. After the age of 11 years, the incidence of RCC surpasses that of Wilms tumor. At this stage, patient age is more important than the appearance of the mass in considering the diagnosis [see **Fig. 6.33**]. A diagnosis of RCC in a young child can suggest the presence of von Hippel-Lindau syndrome. Imaging is important to assess the extent of the primary mass and evaluate for local lymph node involvement and metastatic lesions to the lungs, bones, and liver. Disease confined to the renal fossa and regional lymph nodes can be treated with radical nephrectomy and lymph node dissection. RCC is more aggressive than Wilms tumor, and metastatic disease is more resistant to chemotherapy.

Angiomyolipoma

An angiomyolipoma (AML) is a benign renal mass composed of smooth muscle, vascular elements, and fat. The presence of fat on imaging studies helps distinguish this from other renal masses. This lesion may be seen sporadically or in children with tuberous sclerosis. AMLs are not typically the presenting feature of tuberous sclerosis and are commonly found later in childhood. On ultrasound, an AML is typically echogenic with internal vascularity. Intralesional fat on CT or MRI is pathognomonic [**Fig. 6.36**]. Complications associated with this lesion include intratumoral bleeding and aneurysm formation. Renal artery angiography demonstrates a tangle of vessels throughout the lesion. Multiple small aneurysms may be seen. Larger lesions (>4 cm) are at highest risk for intratumoral hemorrhage and are therefore treated with catheter embolization or partial nephrectomy. AMLs rarely become aggressive. When they do, they invade local structures such as the vasculature or lymph nodes.

Renal Medullary Carcinoma

Although exceedingly rare in the general population, renal medullary carcinoma may be seen in children with sickle cell trait or hemoglobin SC disease. This lesion is not seen in patients with homozygous hemoglobin SS disease. This is an aggressive renal neoplasm. Patients present with gross hematuria, flank pain, weight loss, fever, or a palpable abdominal mass. At presentation, this lesion is often large with invasion of the adjacent vasculature. The tumor typically arises centrally within the kidney near the renal sinus. There may be mass effect on and obstruction of the collecting system [see **Fig. 6.33**]. Peripheral satellite nodules may be present. On postcontrast CT, heterogeneous enhancement is demonstrated. Prognosis is poor overall because response to chemotherapy and radiation is limited.

Infection

As discussed previously, infection can appear very masslike on imaging and should be considered in the differential diagnosis for a solitary renal mass. Distinguishing focal pyelonephritis or renal abscess from a true neoplasm is critical to implement appropriate treatment. Correlation of imaging findings with clinical presentation is key to making the correct diagnosis. In patients with suspected focal pyelonephritis or a renal abscess, imaging should be performed after treatment to exclude the presence of an underlying renal mass [see **Fig. 6.33**].

Other Renal Neoplasms

Less common renal masses that may be seen in the pediatric population include rhabdoid tumor and clear cell sarcoma. Rhabdoid tumor is a rare but highly aggressive neoplasm. It typically presents early in life, with a mean age at diagnosis of 18 months. About 10% to 15% of patients have synchronous or metachronous primary brain tumors, which are usually of primary neuroectodermal origin. Imaging characteristics are similar to other renal neoplasms. Often, subcapsular fluid collections can be seen in association with this mass; however, this finding is not pathognomonic. The subcapsular fluid is thought to represent necrotic material. Rhabdoid tumor metastasizes early and quickly, and has one of the poorest prognoses of all childhood renal masses.

Like rhabdoid tumor, clear cell sarcoma is highly aggressive and has nonspecific imaging characteristics. It is indistinguishable from other renal masses on imaging alone. This tumor is heterogenous and may contain cystic components thought to represent necrosis or hemorrhage. Like rhabdoid tumor, clear cell sarcoma commonly metastasizes. Bone metastases are most common, with other areas of involvement including the lymph nodes, lungs, liver, and brain.

Bilateral Renal Masses

Many of the entities discussed earlier can present as bilateral renal masses. For example, bilateral AMLs can be seen in patients with tuberous sclerosis, and multifocal fungal pyelonephritis may appear as bilateral renal masses. However, there are distinct entities that present almost exclusively with bilateral disease rather than unilateral involvement, such as nephroblastomatosis, lymphoma, and leukemia [see **Box 6.1**]. These entities can present with multifocal renal masses or bilateral diffuse renal enlargement.

Nephroblastomatosis

Renal parenchyma is formed from the mesoblastic cells, with development usually complete by the 36th gestational week. The persistence of nephrogenic cells beyond the 36th week of gestation is termed *nephroblastomatosis*. Nephrogenic rests can occur anywhere in the kidney and are usually bilateral. They are categorized as intralobar (within the renal lobe) or perilobar (cortically based). Depending on location, syndromic associations, and histologic features, the incidence of malignant degeneration to Wilms tumor varies. Intralobar rests are less common and have a higher incidence of malignant degeneration. Intralobar rests are associated with Denys-Drash syndrome, WAGR syndrome, and sporadic aniridia. Perilobar nephrogenic rests are more common and less likely to undergo malignant degeneration. They are associated with hemihypertrophy, Beckwith-Wiedemann syndrome, and trisomy 18.

Nephrogenic rests are homogenous in appearance on imaging [**Fig. 6.37**]. In the presence of these lesions, the kidneys appear markedly enlarged. Nephrogenic rests can appear isoechoic or hypoechoic to adjacent renal parenchyma on ultrasound. Diffuse, multifocal nephrogenic rests may be challenging to discern on ultrasound because they may essentially replace the entire kidney. On contrast-enhanced CT, nephrogenic rests enhance relatively less than the normal renal parenchyma. Normal parenchyma may be distorted due to mass effect. On MRI, nephrogenic rests present as T1 isointense, T2 isointense to hyperintense lesions, with little enhancement on postcontrast images.

In patients with nephrogenic rests or syndromes associated with nephroblastomatosis, close imaging surveillance is recommended given the high risk for development of Wilms tumor. Although no consensus exists on the guidelines for surveillance, baseline cross-sectional imaging with CT or MRI is recommended at the time of diagnosis, followed by serial ultrasounds every 3 to 4 months until the age of 7 years. After the age of 7, the risk

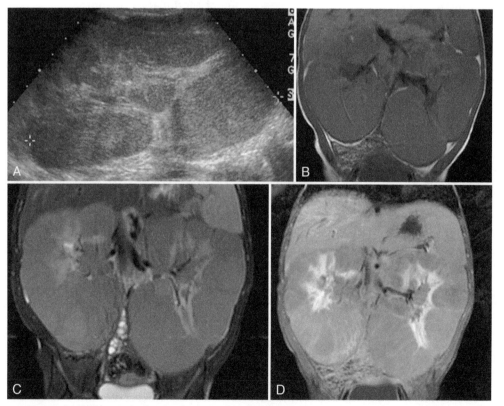

Figure 6.37 Nephroblastomatosis. A, Ultrasound of the right kidney in this 5-year-old demonstrates lack of normal corticomedullary differentiation, with an overall lobulated contour and renal enlargement. **B,** T1-and (**C**) T2-weighted magnetic resonance imaging (MRI) demonstrate multiple cortically based lobular masses which are T1 isointense and T2 hyperintense. **D,** Postcontrast MRI shows little enhancement relative to normal renal parenchyma.

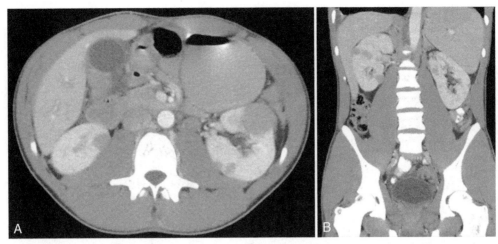

Figure 6.38 Lymphoma. Eighteen-year-old male with T cell lymphoma. **A,** Axial and (**B**) coronal contrast-enhanced computed tomography images demonstrate multiple round, cortical, nonenhancing masses within the kidneys.

for development of Wilms tumor is significantly decreased. On surveillance imaging, rapid growth of a nephroblastoma and/or development of heterogeneous imaging characteristics are suspicious for degeneration to Wilms tumor.

Lymphoma

Primary renal lymphoma is rare given the lack of lymphoid tissue in the kidneys. Renal lymphomatous involvement is usually secondary to hematogenous spread of disease or local extension from the retroperitoneum. Non-Hodgkin lymphoma is the most common type in children and usually presents beyond age 5 years. Renal involvement is typically clinically silent and is identified on surveillance imaging studies. Occasionally, patients may present with hematuria or flank pain.

On imaging, multiple bilateral renal masses are typically present. Sonographic characteristics can be variable, with isoechoic, hypoechoic, or hyperechoic masses identified. Lymphoma may be very uniform and hypoechoic on ultrasound, mimicking the appearance of renal cysts. On contrast-enhanced CT, multiple homogenous, nonenhancing masses are seen in the renal parenchyma [**Fig. 6.38**]. Associated perinephric findings include thickening of Gerota's fascia and plaquelike soft tissue nodules. On MRI, lymphomatous masses are T1 and T2 hypointense, with homogenous enhancement that is less avid than the remainder of the renal parenchyma.

Leukemia

The most common malignancy in children is acute lymphoblastic leukemia. Leukemic involvement of the kidneys can manifest as diffuse infiltration of the parenchyma. On imaging, this presents with marked bilateral renal enlargement and loss of corticomedullary differentiation. In some instances, leukemic infiltrates can present as solitary or multiple bilateral renal masses, with imaging characteristics similar to lymphoma.

Pelvic Masses

When evaluating a pelvic mass in a child, the age and sex of the patient should be considered to formulate a useful list of diagnostic considerations. Masses can arise from any of the organs and soft tissues in the pelvis. In females, ovarian and uterine masses should be considered. In males, masses may be related to prostate or testicular pathology. These entities are discussed

in detail later in this chapter in the sections called *Male Genital Tract* and *Female Genital Tract*.

Pelvic masses can be cystic or solid. One of the most common solid neoplasms in the pelvis in children is rhabdomyosarcoma, which can arise from the bladder, uterus, vagina, or prostate gland [**Fig. 6.39**]. A pelvic mass unique to newborns is a sacrococcygeal teratoma, which may be cystic or solid. This typically large tumor is often first diagnosed in utero. It arises from the coccyx and may be predominantly intrapelvic, extrapelvic, or both. This tumor is best evaluated in the postnatal period with MRI.

Various other lesions may be encountered on imaging studies that may mimic a primary neoplasm of the pelvis. An abscess appears as a complex cystic mass. In this setting, correlation with clinical history and patient presentation is important [**Fig. 6.40**]. Other cystic structures that may be seen in the pelvis include mesenteric cysts, enteric duplication cysts, and lymphatic malformations. In females, a Müllerian anomaly can present as fluid-filled structure in the pelvis and may be mistaken for a cystic mass.

Bladder Masses

Bladder tumors, both benign and malignant, are rare in children. Benign pathologies include hemangioma, neurofibroma, fibromatous polyp, inflammatory processes, and abscesses. The most common and worrisome malignant mass encountered is rhabdomyosarcoma. Other less commonly seen malignancies include lymphoma, adenocarcinoma, and leiomyosarcoma. Deflux injections at the UVJs [see **Fig. 6.22**] and hematomas can be confused for tumors.

A patient with a bladder mass may present with gross hematuria or obstructive voiding symptoms. Diagnostic workup includes urinalysis and culture, urine cytology, and imaging studies. Ultrasound is the initial imaging study to evaluate the bladder; however, contrast-enhanced CT or MRI can help define a bladder lesion further. Cystoscopy is the ultimate diagnostic study, allowing not only direct visualization, but also potential biopsy of the lesion.

RENAL CYSTS

Solitary Cysts

Compared with adults, it is relatively rare for a child to have a single renal cyst. When a single cyst is identified, an important

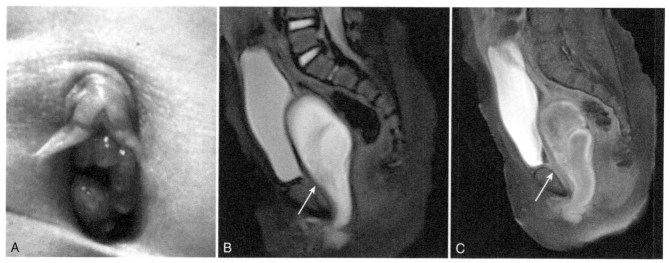

Figure 6.39 Vaginal rhabdomyosarcoma. Two-year-old girl with a mass growing out of the vagina. **A,** On physical examination, a grapelike mass is seen arising from the vaginal orifice. **B,** Sagittal T2 image of the pelvis demonstrates a heterogenous, high-signal mass posterior to the urinary bladder, extending into the vagina (*arrow*). **C,** Sagittal postcontrast image demonstrates heterogenous enhancement (*arrow*). Surgical pathology confirmed vaginal rhabdomyosarcoma, sarcoma botryoides type.

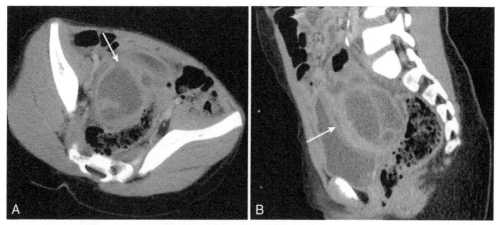

Figure 6.40 Perforated appendicitis mimicking a pelvic mass. Six-year-old girl with fever and abdominal pain. **A,** Axial and **(B)** sagittal contrast-enhanced computed tomography images demonstrate a heterogeneously enhancing, cystic and solid mass in the pelvis posterior to the urinary bladder (*arrows*). Image-guided drainage of this lesion confirmed perforated appendicitis with abscess formation.

differential consideration is a calyceal diverticulum. These two lesions may be difficult to differentiate, particularly on ultrasound. Communication between the "cyst" and the underlying collecting system suggests a calyceal diverticulum. On delayed postcontrast CT and MR images, contrast material excreted into the collecting system will fill a calyceal diverticulum, but not a simple cyst.

Because both cysts and renal tumors are relatively uncommon in children, the Bosniak criteria used in adults are not used for classification of cystic renal masses in children.

Polycystic Kidney Disease

The presence of multiple renal cysts in a child should raise suspicion for polycystic kidney disease. Polycystic kidney disease is a heterogeneous group of hereditary disorders caused by primary defects in ciliary motility. Multiple disorders are associated with ciliary abnormalities, and the kidneys are the organ most commonly affected. We will present the two most common forms of polycystic kidney disease seen in children.

Autosomal Recessive Polycystic Kidney Disease

Autosomal recessive polycystic kidney disease (ARPKD) is the most common ciliopathy affecting infants and young children. This disease commonly manifests as massively enlarged kidneys because of the presence of dilated tubules and innumerable tiny cysts. This is associated with congenital hepatic fibrosis. ARPKD is typically diagnosed in the prenatal period during routine ultrasound imaging. When hepatic involvement predominates, disease may present later in childhood. Renal and liver involvement are thought to be inversely related, with severe renal disease but little hepatic involvement in some individuals, and hepatic fibrosis and portal hypertension with relatively mild renal disease in others.

On prenatal ultrasound imaging, enlarged, echogenic kidneys are seen, sometimes with small subcortical cysts. Poor renal function leads to oligohydramnios, and possibly pulmonary hypoplasia and limb deformities. After birth, ultrasound performed with a high-frequency linear transducer will better resolve the multiple dilated tubules and cysts. Radiographs typically show a small, bell-shaped thorax, with an enlarged abdomen

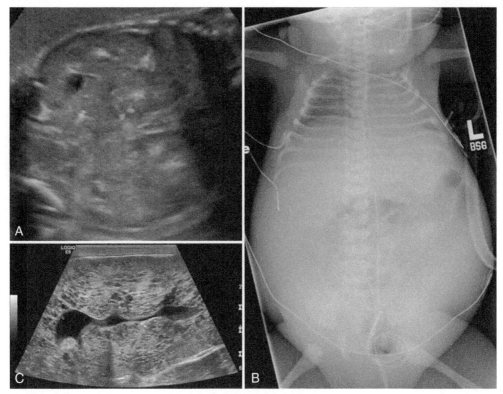

Figure 6.41 Autosomal recessive polycystic kidney disease (ARPKD). This infant was born with respiratory distress. **A,** In utero, both kidneys were enlarged and echogenic, with reversal of the normal corticomedullary differentiation pattern. There was oligohydramnios (not shown) due to poor renal function and low urine output. **B,** The babygram shows intubation, with hypoplastic lungs and a markedly distended abdomen. The lungs are hypoplastic due to oligohydramnios and mass effect from the distended abdomen. The abdomen is filled with markedly enlarged kidneys. **C,** On postnatal ultrasound, each kidney measured 12 cm in length (normally 4.5 cm at birth).

and bulging flanks secondary to marked renal enlargement [**Fig. 6.41**]. Patients presenting later in childhood may have less severe cystic change or only segmental involvement.

Although ultrasound is typically sufficient, MRI may be performed for further characterization of renal and liver disease. The use of contrast may be limited because of renal insufficiency. On MRI, enlarged, T2 hyperintense kidneys are noted, with multiple tiny T2 bright lesions within the parenchyma corresponding to dilated tubular and cystic structures. Macrocysts measuring 1-2 cm may be present; however, these are uncommon. Liver findings may include hepatomegaly, fibrosis, dilated ducts, and cysts. Hepatic cysts may show communication with the biliary ducts. Sequelae of portal hypertension can be seen, including splenomegaly, varices, and a recanalized umbilical vein.

Autosomal Dominant Polycystic Kidney Disease

Autosomal dominant polycystic kidney disease (ADPKD) is the most common inherited cause of end-stage renal disease. This autosomal dominant disease has been linked to mutations in the *PKD1* gene on chromosome 16 and the *PKD2* gene on chromosome 4. Most patients present in adulthood, with findings seen incidentally on imaging studies performed for other indications. Disease may also first be detected in the setting of screening in patients with a strong family history of ADPKD. Correlation with family history is important to distinguish ADPKD from ARPKD, and specific genetic testing should be performed. Some imaging characteristics can help differentiate ADPKD and ARPKD. In ADPKD, renal cysts are typically larger and round, as opposed

to the tubular cystic changes seen with ARPKD. In addition, ADPKD is associated with cysts in other organs, including the liver, pancreas, and spleen. However, the two diseases do overlap in their appearances.

Initial imaging is performed using ultrasound. Children with a family history of ADPKD may have normal-appearing kidneys, a single renal cyst, or multiple renal cysts, which may be unilateral or bilateral [**Fig. 6.42**]. Cysts become more numerous over time. Both ultrasound and MRI are used to follow these patients because the cysts are well seen with these imaging modalities that avoid the use of ionizing radiation. MRI shows T2 bright, round, well-circumscribed lesions in the kidneys. As children get older, renal cysts typically increase in size and number, with associated progressive enlargement of the kidneys. As cysts proliferate and grow, they replace the normal renal parenchyma, ultimately leading to renal failure.

VASCULAR ABNORMALITIES OF THE KIDNEYS

Renal Artery Stenosis

Hypertension is an uncommon diagnosis in the pediatric population. When present, a workup is warranted. Although rare in adults, renovascular hypertension is one of the more common forms of hypertension seen in the pediatric population. Renovascular hypertension may be related to a vascular cause such as renal artery stenosis (RAS), which may be seen in the setting of fibromuscular dysplasia, neurofibromatosis, Kawasaki disease, middle aortic syndrome, and Takayasu arteritis. Renovascular

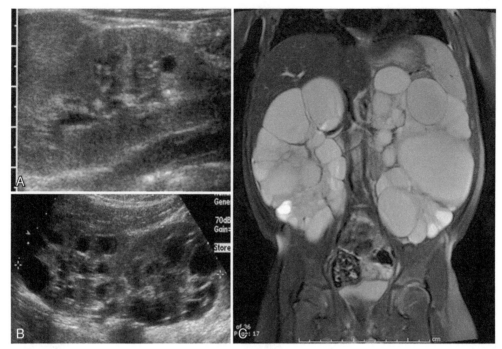

Figure 6.42 Autosomal dominant polycystic kidney disease (ADPKD). Renal imaging in three different patients with ADPKD demonstrates the variability of renal involvement. **A,** The first patient has a single renal cyst at the lower pole of the kidney. **B,** The second patient has multiple noncommunicating cysts throughout the kidney. **C,** Coronal T2 magnetic resonance image in a 6-year-old demonstrates replacement of the normal renal parenchyma with multiple cysts of varying size.

hypertension may also be related to causes such as obstructive uropathy or polycystic kidney disease.

Ultrasound is typically the initial imaging modality used for the assessment of renovascular hypertension and specifically RAS. Grayscale signs of underlying renal dysfunction or "medical renal disease" that may predispose to renovascular hypertension include small renal size for age, increased renal echogenicity, or an underlying congenital anomaly. These findings may be asymmetric in the setting of unilateral RAS. Color Doppler imaging may show a focal area of narrowing of the renal artery with aliasing present. The waveform at the site of the stenosis may show turbulent flow, whereas the waveform within the peripheral renal parenchyma may demonstrate the classic "parvus tardus" waveform with a dampened systolic upstroke. Direct Doppler interrogation of the aorta should be performed. A renal artery-to-aorta peak systolic velocity of greater than 3.5 is highly suggestive of RAS.

Transcatheter angiography remains the gold standard for evaluation of RAS. Pressure gradients can be assessed, and blood from the renal arteries, renal veins, and aorta can be sampled to determine differential renin secretion. For specific causative factors of RAS such as fibromuscular dysplasia, treatment with balloon angioplasty can be performed in the interventional radiology suite. CTA, and increasingly magnetic resonance angiography, are used for surgical planning to better visualize the site and extent of narrowing in RAS, and also to evaluate for the presence of accessory renal vessels.

Renal Vein Thrombosis

Renal vein thrombosis (RVT) is uncommonly seen in the pediatric population. When it occurs, it is typically encountered in the neonatal population. This is likely due to the relative dehydration and polycythemia present in these patients. Thrombus is typically confined to the intrarenal veins but may propagate from

the IVC to the renal veins as in the case of thrombosis caused by central venous line placement.

Ultrasound is the primary imaging modality used in both the diagnosis and follow-up of this condition. On grayscale ultrasound images, the affected kidney is frequently enlarged and echogenic. With Doppler imaging, the presence of an echogenic intraluminal thrombus may variably be seen. However, nonvisualization of a clot does not exclude thrombosis because the small intrarenal veins are most often primarily involved. Indirect signs of RVT include elevated resistive indices caused by obstruction of normal venous outflow, as well as loss of or reversal of diastolic flow [**Fig. 6.43**].

GENITOURINARY TRAUMA

Renal Trauma

Blunt force trauma to the abdomen accounts for the majority of renal injuries. After the liver and spleen, the kidneys are the most frequently injured solid viscera in the abdomen. Children are particularly susceptible to renal injury due to the relatively large size of the kidneys compared with the size of the abdomen and pelvis. Children also have less perinephric fat than adults, providing less of a cushion. Clinically, patients who have sustained renal trauma present with hematuria and flank pain. Renal injuries rarely occur in isolation and may be associated with injuries to other abdominal viscera or injuries to the lower thorax.

Although ultrasound performed in the trauma bay may be used for detection of free fluid in the abdomen, CT is the mainstay for evaluation of the solid abdominal viscera after trauma. CT should be performed after the administration of intravenous contrast material, with images obtained during the mixed venous phase. If injury to the renal collecting system is suspected, delayed imaging should be performed to assess for the presence of contrast extravasation.

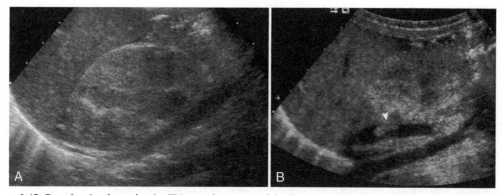

Figure 6.43 Renal vein thrombosis. This newborn was dehydrated and developed hematuria. **A,** Ultrasound demonstrates an enlarged, echogenic right kidney with poor corticomedullary differentiation. **B,** A thrombus was present in the inferior vena cava (*arrowhead*).

TABLE 6.3   Kidney Injury Scale

Stage*	Type of Injury	Description of Injury
I	Contusion	Microscopic or gross hematuria, urologic studies normal
	Hematoma	Subcapsular, nonexpanding without parenchymal laceration
II	Hematoma	Nonexpanding perirenal hematoma confined to retroperitoneum
	Laceration	<1.0 cm parenchymal depth of renal cortex without urinary extravasation
III	Laceration	<1.0 cm parenchymal depth of renal cortex without collecting system rupture or urinary extravasation
IV	Laceration	Parenchymal laceration extending through renal cortex, medulla, and collecting system
	Vascular	Main renal artery or vein injury with contained hemorrhage
V	Laceration	Completely shattered kidney
	Vascular	Avulsion of renal hilum which devascularizes kidney

*Advance one grade for bilateral injuries up to grade III.
Data from Moore EE, Shackford SR, Pachter HL, et al. Organ injury scaling - spleen, liver and kidney. *J Trauma.* 1989;29:1664.

The American Association for the Surgery of Trauma (AAST) grading system for renal trauma used in adults is also used in the pediatric population [**Table 6.3**]. The most mild form of renal injury is a contusion, seen as a patchy hypodensity in the renal parenchyma. A laceration is the next highest grade of injury, the severity of which depends on depth of extension into the collecting system. The most severe injuries involve trauma to the renal hilum, affecting the renal artery, renal vein, renal pelvis, and/or proximal ureter. A perinephric fluid collection seen on CT may represent a hematoma or a urinoma. On mixed venous phase imaging, a hematoma will appear hyperdense because of the presence of acute blood. The attenuation of a urinoma will depend on the phase of CT scanning. It may appear relatively hypodense on a scan obtained during the mixed venous phase because of the presence of extravasated urine, but will become extremely dense during delayed phase imaging because of the presence of excreted contrast material [**Fig. 6.44**].

In recent years, there has been more emphasis on conservative management of renal trauma even when it is high grade. As long as a patient is hemodynamically stable, supportive care is becoming the mainstay treatment. A more extensive renal laceration with ongoing bleeding may be treated with transcatheter embolization as an alternative to an open surgical approach.

Bladder Trauma

Bladder rupture is not an uncommon finding in the setting of blunt force trauma. This diagnosis can be suspected on the initial trauma CT scan when pelvic fractures are present and there is free fluid in the pelvis. However, lack of free fluid does not exclude the diagnosis. The diagnosis is most frequently made with a CT cystogram, but can also be made using fluoroscopy. With either technique, it is essential to exclude a urethral injury before inserting a catheter. The volume of contrast instilled into the bladder depends on the patient's age, size, and expected bladder capacity. Notably, a delayed CT scan performed after contrast from an initial trauma scan has been excreted into the bladder is not adequate for excluding bladder rupture.

If extravesical contrast has been identified on cystogram indicating a bladder rupture, the determination must be made whether the rupture is intraperitoneal or extraperitoneal. Intraperitoneal rupture occurs most frequently because of acute compression of the pelvis in the setting of a distended urinary bladder, with the tear occurring at the bladder dome. Extraperitoneal bladder rupture frequently coexists with pelvic fractures, and the tear is located below the level of the peritoneal reflections. Differentiating these two entities on imaging studies is important because extraperitoneal rupture can be managed conservatively, whereas intraperitoneal rupture requires urgent surgical repair. With intraperitoneal rupture, contrast is seen surrounding loops of bowel and extending into the posterior cul-de-sac. Extraperitoneal rupture is less frequently seen in children. Contrast is seen around the perivesical spaces, extending anteriorly into the space of Retzius, and possibly extending inferiorly into the scrotal sac in males.

Bladder rupture in patients who have undergone bladder augmentation is worthy of special mention. These patients can present with bladder rupture with no history of antecedent trauma. A very high level of suspicion is needed because the patient's symptoms may be nonspecific and abdominal pain may be relatively mild. As in a typical patient with suspected bladder rupture, either a CT or fluoroscopic cystogram can be used for evaluation. The bladder will have an atypical contour related to augmentation with some form of hollow viscous (most frequently ileum, rarely rectosigmoid colon or stomach). The most common site of bladder rupture in this setting is the posterior margin of the anastomosis. This type of rupture is intraperitoneal and requires prompt surgical intervention because it may be a life-threatening emergency [**Fig. 6.45**].

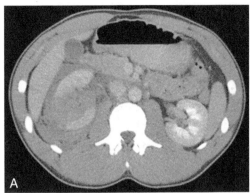
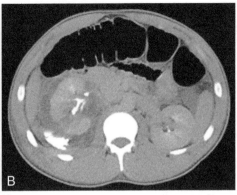
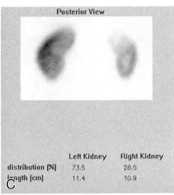

Figure 6.44 Renal trauma. Teenager involved in an motor vehicle collision. **A,** Axial computed tomography (CT) image obtained through the kidneys during the arterial phase demonstrates relative hypoenhancement of the right kidney, with a large laceration through the renal cortex extending to the renal hilum. There is high attenuation fluid surrounding the kidney, likely reflecting a combination of urine and blood. **B,** Axial CT image at the same level during the excretory phase demonstrates high attenuation material in the disrupted renal collecting system with extension posterior to the kidney, where a urinoma is seen. This is compatible with a grade IV injury. Despite this high grade, this patient was managed with supportive measures and surgery was not needed. **C,** Renal DMSA scan performed 3 years later demonstrates that, although there is asymmetrically decreased function of the superior pole of the right kidney, some degree of renal function is maintained.

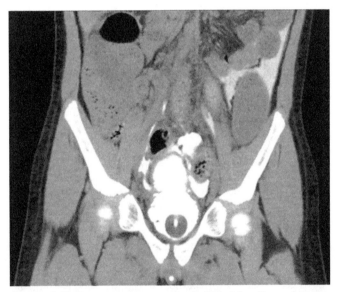

Figure 6.45 Rupture of an augmented bladder. Coronal image from a computed tomography cystogram demonstrates extravasation of contrast from an augmented bladder. This type of rupture is typically intraperitoneal and must be repaired immediately because it is a life-threatening emergency. The base of the bladder is native and the superior portion is augmented, giving the appearance of a peanut. The Foley catheter balloon is inflated at the base of the bladder. (Courtesy of Micheál Breen, MD.)

Urethral Trauma

Urethral injuries are seen almost exclusively in males and may occur in the setting of blunt force trauma to the pelvis or with straddle injury. Urethral injury is suspected in the presence of hematuria, particularly when a patient presents with blood at the meatus or inability to void. In a patient with this history, an RUG must be performed before bladder catheterization.

Urethral injury may be classified as anterior or posterior based on the portion of the urethra affected. Posterior urethral injury is more commonly seen with a direct blow to the pelvis, whereas anterior injury is more frequently seen with straddle injury. Urethral injury is staged according to the same classification system used for adults. Urethral strictures may develop as a result of trauma. Evaluation for strictures is typically performed with an RUG.

Scrotal Trauma

The clinical presentation of scrotal injury is usually straightforward. Patients present with acute-onset scrotal pain after some form of trauma. Ultrasound is the primary imaging modality used to assess for injury. Testicular hemorrhage/contusion may appear as poorly defined regions of hypoechogenicity, often with a masslike appearance. A discrete fracture line with disruption of the testicular parenchyma is rarely seen. Complex fluid may surround the testicle, representing a hematocele. A hematocele may be secondary to injury to the testicle itself, or it may be related to intraabdominal trauma with blood extending through a patent processus vaginalis. Testicular rupture refers to violation of the integrity of the tunica albuginea, with extrusion of the seminiferous tubules through the defect. The tunica is normally seen as a thin, echogenic structure closely apposed to the testis, and should be visualized circumferentially [**Fig. 6.46**]. Testicular rupture requires prompt surgical repair. Efficient, accurate diagnosis is the key to testicular salvage.

THE ADRENAL GLAND

The adrenal gland is an endocrine organ with a triangular configuration reminiscent of a Napoleonic hat, perched atop the kidney [**Fig. 6.47**]. Histologically, the gland is composed of a cortex and medulla and is responsible for the secretion of specific steroids, hormones, and catecholamines.

In the fetus and neonate, the adrenal gland is relatively larger because of the size of the cortex. The normal adrenal gland can routinely be seen with ultrasound in neonates. The cortex is typically hypoechoic, with an echogenic medulla located centrally. As the fetal cortex is replaced with the adult cortex, the adrenal gland rapidly shrinks, decreasing by up to 50% its original size in the first 3 weeks of life. As the patient ages, the adrenal gland assumes the size and configuration seen in adults.

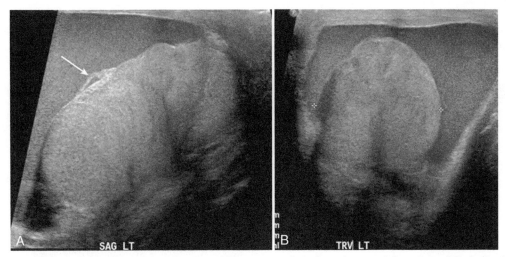

Figure 6.46 Testicular trauma. Fourteen-year-old boy presenting after a lacrosse injury. **A and B,** Sagittal and transverse images of the left testis. Complex fluid surrounds the left testis, compatible with a hematocele. The normally smooth, echogenic tunica albuginea surrounding the testicle is disrupted. There is a flap in the tunica, indicated by the *arrow* in (**A**). A bulge is seen in the normally rounded contour of the testis, best appreciated on the transverse view. The echogenicity of the testis is heterogeneous, compatible with contusion. At surgery, there was a near-circumferential tear in the tunica with extrusion of the seminiferous tubules through the defect.

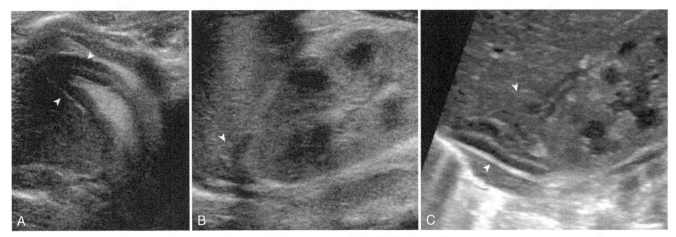

Figure 6.47 Normal adrenal gland. A, Transverse and (**B, C**) Sagittal ultrasound images demonstrate the adrenal gland (*arrowheads*). It is a triangular structure that is shaped like a Napoleonic hat and located immediately superior to the upper pole of the kidney. It can normally be seen in infants.

Morphologic Abnormalities

The triangular configuration of the adrenal gland as an inverted Y is thought to be related to the presence of the kidney splaying apart the limbs of the gland. In ipsilateral renal agenesis or renal ptosis, the adrenal gland assumes a linear or "lying-down" configuration and tends to be somewhat longer and thicker than the normal gland [**Fig. 6.48**]. This morphologic appearance has no impact on function.

Congenital Adrenal Hyperplasia

CAH refers to a group of disorders in which there is an enzymatic defect in the pathway for the synthesis of cortisol, most frequently a deficiency in 21-hydroxylase. Clinically, patients present with abnormalities in sexual development (in its most severe form, ambiguous genitalia), as well as life-threatening salt-wasting crises. In females with CAH, the urethra and vagina join to form a common distal channel called a *urogenital sinus*. These patients have one external orifice through which both

structures empty. The configuration of the urogenital sinus can be evaluated with a genitogram.

In the setting of CAH, the adrenal gland may be uniformly enlarged. Although the diagnosis of CAH is based on laboratory data, the presence of an enlarged adrenal gland on antenatal or postnatal imaging can suggest this diagnosis. Postnatally, a gland is considered enlarged with a length of greater than 20 mm or a limb width of greater than 4 mm. In contrast with the smooth configuration of the normal adrenal gland, a gland affected by CAH has a more crenellated contour and may be described as "cerebriform" [**Fig. 6.49**].

Masses and Pseudomasses

In the neonate, the most commonly encountered adrenal mass is adrenal hemorrhage, with the second most common being neuroblastoma. Beyond the neonatal period, neuroblastoma and tumors of neural crest origin are most frequently encountered.

Adrenal Hemorrhage

Adrenal hemorrhage typically occurs in the setting of perinatal stress or a traumatic delivery. The sonographic appearance varies based on the age of the hemorrhage. As seen elsewhere in the body, the hematoma is initially echogenic. As it involutes, it becomes progressively more hypoechoic with a variable presence of echogenic septations. An adrenal hematoma will frequently calcify. It should be avascular, with no flow detected on color Doppler evaluation. If it is at all difficult to differentiate an adrenal hematoma from a tumor on initial imaging, follow-up ultrasonography is recommended for further evaluation. An adrenal hemorrhage will demonstrate progressive involution [**Fig. 6.50**].

Neuroblastoma

Neuroblastoma is the most common extracranial solid neoplasm in children. This tumor may originate anywhere along the sympathetic chain, although the majority arise from the adrenal medulla. Tumors of neural crest origin exist along a spectrum and include neuroblastoma (malignant), ganglioneuroblastoma (variable behavior), and ganglioneuroma (benign).

Neuroblastoma most frequently presents as a palpable mass, particularly when arising from the adrenal gland or elsewhere in

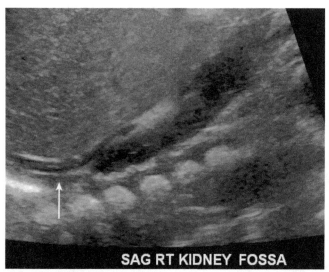

Figure 6.48 Lying-down adrenal gland. Neonate with a prenatal diagnosis of a dysplastic right kidney. Sagittal ultrasound image of the right renal fossa demonstrates a linear configuration to the adrenal gland (*arrow*), as opposed to the normal triangular configuration. This is seen when the ipsilateral kidney does not develop normally to splay the limbs of the adrenal gland.

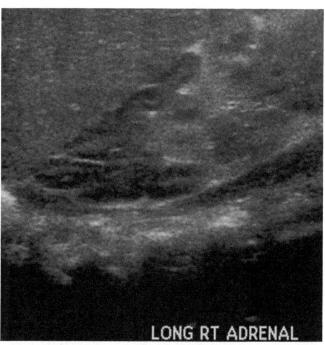

Figure 6.49 Congenital adrenal hyperplasia (CAH). Female neonate with ambiguous genitalia. Sagittal ultrasound image of the right adrenal gland demonstrates an enlarged gland with a cerebriform appearance compatible with CAH. A limb length of more than 20 mm or limb thickness of more than 4 mm suggests adrenal gland enlargement. The left adrenal gland had an identical appearance.

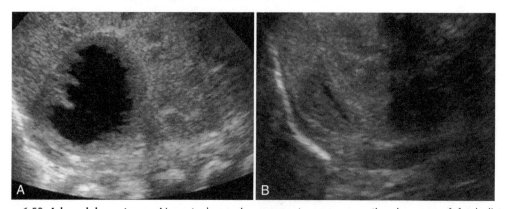

Figure 6.50 Adrenal hematoma. Neonate born via emergent cesarean section because of fetal distress. **A,** Sagittal image obtained through the left suprarenal area shows a circumscribed, thick-walled anechoic structure felt to most likely represent an adrenal hematoma given the clinical context. **B,** Sagittal image of the same area 1 month later demonstrates decreased size of this structure and more uniform echogenicity with only a thin hypoechoic area remaining. This follows the expected involution of an adrenal hematoma. Although a neuroblastoma could potentially have a similar appearance on initial imaging, involution would not be expected on a follow-up examination.

TABLE 6.4A Image-Defined Risk Factors in Neuroblastic Tumors

Ipsilateral tumor extension within two body compartments
 Neck-chest, chest-abdomen, abdomen-pelvis

Neck
 Tumor encasing carotid and/or vertebral artery and/or internal jugular vein
 Tumor extending to base of skull
 Tumor compressing the trachea

Cervico-thoracic junction
 Tumor encasing brachial plexus roots
 Tumor encasing subclavian vessels and/or vertebral and/or carotid artery
 Tumor compressing the trachea

Thorax
 Tumor encasing the aorta and/or major branches
 Tumor compressing the trachea and/or principal bronchi
 Lower mediastinal tumor, infiltrating the costo-vertebral junction between T9 and T12

Thoraco-abdominal
 Tumor encasing the aorta and/or vena cava

Abdomen/pelvis
 Tumor infiltrating the porta hepatis and/or the hepatoduodenal ligament
 Tumor encasing branches of the superior mesenteric artery at the mesenteric root
 Tumor encasing the origin of the coeliac axis, and/or of the superior mesenteric artery
 Tumor invading one or both renal pedicles
 Tumor encasing the aorta and/or vena cava
 Tumor encasing the iliac vessels
 Pelvic tumor crossing the sciatic notch

Intraspinal tumor extension whatever the location provided that:
 More than one third of the spinal canal in the axial plane is invaded and/or the perimedullary leptomeningeal spaces are not visible and/or the spinal cord signal is abnormal

Infiltration of adjacent organs/structures
 Pericardium, diaphragm, kidney, liver, duodeno-pancreatic block, and mesentery

Conditions to be recorded, but *not* considered IDRFs
 Multifocal primary tumors
 Pleural effusion, with or without malignant cells
 Ascites, with or without malignant cells

IDRS, image-defined risk factors.
From Monclair T, Brodeur GM, Ambros PF, et al; INRG Task Force. The International Neuroblastoma Risk Group (INRG) staging system: an INRG Task Force report. *J Clin Oncol.* 2009;27(2):298-303.

TABLE 6.4B International Neuroblastoma Risk Group Staging System

Stage	Description
L1	Localized tumor not involving vital structures as defined by the list of image-defined risk factors and confined to one body compartment
L2	Locoregional tumor with presence of one or more image-defined risk factors
M	Distant metastatic disease (except stage MS)
MS	Metastatic disease in children younger than 18 months with metastases confined to skin, liver, and/or bone marrow

NOTE. Patients with multifocal primary tumors should be staged according to the greatest extent of disease as defined in the table.
From Monclair T, Brodeur GM, Ambros PF, et al; INRG Task Force. The International Neuroblastoma Risk Group (INRG) staging system: an INRG Task Force report. *J Clin Oncol.* 2009;27(2):298-303.

metastatic disease is found exclusively in patients younger than 18 months. This is referred to as stage 4S neuroblastoma (*S* for "special"). Metastatic disease is confined to the skin, liver, and/or bone marrow. This form is "special" because in most cases, the disease resolves without therapy.

Radiographs are frequently the initial imaging study obtained in the workup of an abdominal mass. Findings on radiographs are nonspecific, but mass effect may be seen with displacement of bowel gas or visceral contours. Calcifications are variably noted.

Ultrasound is also a first-line imaging modality used in the workup of an abdominal mass. Neuroblastoma will appear as a heterogeneous mass that is usually suprarenal in location, with possible inferior displacement of the kidney [**Fig. 6.51**]. Not uncommonly, it may be difficult to differentiate a suprarenal mass from a renal mass with ultrasound. An adrenal mass will typically form an acute angle with the kidney, whereas a renal tumor will be surrounded by a claw of normal renal parenchymal tissue. Neuroblastoma often contains calcifications. This tumor typically encases and narrows vessels, as opposed to invading them. This is an important distinction from Wilms tumor.

Cross-sectional imaging with intravenous contrast is necessary for staging. Both CT and MRI may be used, although MRI is being performed more frequently because of lack of ionizing radiation exposure. On CT, a heterogenous, enhancing mass will be seen, with a variable presence of necrosis and hemorrhage. Calcification is often noted. MRI will show a heterogeneously T2 hyperintense, T1 hypointense mass with heterogeneous enhancement. The presence of calcification may be missed on MRI. Displacement of adjacent organs and displacement or encasement of blood vessels may be seen. Close inspection for the presence of enlarged lymph nodes and hepatic metastases is warranted.

A nuclear medicine metaiodobenzylguanidine (MIBG) scan is obtained as part of the staging workup. This is particularly important for detection of osseous metastases. MIBG is a norepinephrine analog taken up by adrenergic cells. Uptake of this tracer can be seen with both neuroblastoma and pheochromocytoma. MIBG may be paired with iodine 123 for diagnostic imaging, or with iodine 131 when a therapeutic dose is administered. Approximately 90% of neuroblastomas take up MIBG. When the tumor is not MIBG avid, evaluation for osseous metastases can be performed with a technetium bone scan or fluorodeoxyglucose (FDG) positron emission tomography scan.

A number of other adrenal masses are rarely seen in the pediatric population and include adrenal adenoma, pheochromocytoma, and adrenocortical carcinoma. The presentation of these

the abdomen. However, a wide range of clinical manifestations may be seen at initial presentation. A paraneoplastic syndrome known as opsoclonus-myoclonus may be seen, where a patient presents with ataxia and nystagmus or "dancing eyes." If a tumor arises in the mediastinum near the lung apex, a patient may present with Horner syndrome. Laboratory data obtained at the time of presentation frequently but not universally demonstrates elevated urinary catecholamines.

The prognosis of neuroblastoma depends on stage of disease at presentation. In recent years there has been a shift away from the International Neuroblastoma Staging System (INSS) created in the 1990s. The International Neuroblastoma Risk Group Staging System (INRGSS) is now more commonly used (**Table 6.4a**). This shift is of particular importance to radiologists, as it is based on a set of image defined risk factors (IDRF) (**Table 6.4b**) for tumor staging prior to surgery. The previously used INSS, in contradistinction, was based on surgical findings for staging of disease.

When metastases are present, they are most frequently found in the lymph nodes, liver, and bone. An interesting form of

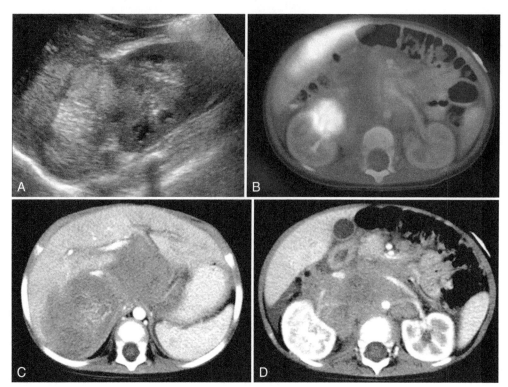

Figure 6.51 Neuroblastoma. Toddler with an abdominal mass. **A,** Sagittal ultrasound image of the right kidney shows a heterogeneous suprarenal mass. The kidney is displaced inferiorly. Echogenic foci noted centrally within the mass are compatible with calcifications, a frequent finding in neuroblastoma. **B,** Axial fused computed tomography (CT) and metaiodobenzylguanidine (MIBG) single-photon emission CT image shows intense MIBG avidity, another typical characteristic of neuroblastoma. Although most neuroblastomas are MIBG avid, they do not invariably take up this radiotracer. **C and D,** Two axial contrast-enhanced CT images show a right suprarenal mass that is heterogeneously enhancing with central calcifications, as seen on the corresponding ultrasound image. The mass surrounds and encases the vasculature but does not invade the vessels. This is a feature that helps to distinguish neuroblastoma from a Wilms tumor.

masses in the pediatric population is essentially identical to their presentation in the adult population.

MALE AND FEMALE GENITAL TRACTS

Embryology

Because the embryology of the male and female genital tracts is similar, they will be discussed together. Both the testis and the ovary develop from a portion of the intermediate mesoderm known as the gonadal ridge. At approximately the seventh week of gestation, this gonadal ridge begins to differentiate [**Fig. 6.52**].

In the presence of the SRY gene found on the Y chromosome, the male genital tract develops. Together with the gonadal ridge, the mesonephros or Wolffian duct forms the epididymis, vas deferens, and seminal vesicles. These structures form in the posterior portion of the abdominal cavity. A fascial band known as the gubernaculum extends from the caudal end of the developing gonad to the peritoneal floor. At approximately the 13th week of gestation, the processus vaginalis forms from an outpouching from the peritoneum of the abdominal cavity. The testis then begins to descend along the course of the gubernaculum through the processus vaginalis [**Fig. 6.53**].

During the second trimester, the maturing testis remains near the orifice of the processus vaginalis at the level of the inguinal ring. During the third trimester, both the testis and the epididymis descend into the scrotum. The patent processus vaginalis does not normally close until anywhere from the 37th to 40th week of gestation. This accounts for the frequency of indirect

hernias in preterm neonates. When descent fails to occur, cryptorchidism results.

In females, lack of suppression by the SRY gene allows for continued development of the paramesonephric or Müllerian ducts. In concert with the gonadal ridge, these structures form the female genital tract. Typically the paramesonephric ducts are located lateral to the mesonephric ducts. Fusion of the caudal aspect of the paramesonephric ducts with regression of the medial part leads to the development of a single uterus, cervix, and vagina. The caudal aspect fuses with the urogenital sinus, forming the vagina. The cranial aspect canalizes and moves laterally, ultimately forming the bilateral fallopian tubes. This sequence of formation can be interrupted at various stages, leading to various developmental anomalies (discussed later in this chapter).

External genitalia arise from the urogenital tubercle, urogenital swelling, and urogenital folds. In males, the presence of the SRY gene allows for the production of testosterone, ultimately leading to the formation of the testes, scrotum, and penis. In females, the lack of these hormones allows for the development of clitoris, labia majora, and labia minora. Anomalies in the sequence of formation of these structures can lead to ambiguous genitalia (discussed later in this chapter).

Male Genital Tract

Normal Anatomy of the Testis

Regardless of the clinical question, ultrasound is typically the imaging modality used for evaluation of the scrotum and its contents. On ultrasound, the testicle appears as an ovoid

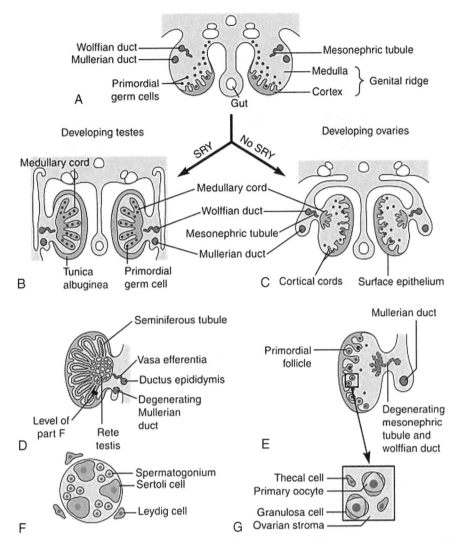

Figure 6.52 Diagram illustrating differentiation of indifferent gonads into testes or ovaries. A, Bipotential gonads from a 6-week-old embryo. **B,** At 7 weeks, showing testes developing under the influence of SRY. **C,** At 12 weeks, showing ovaries developing in the absence of SRY. **D,** Testis at 20 weeks, showing the rete testis and seminiferous tubules derived from medullary cords. **E,** Ovary at 20 weeks, showing primordial follicles. **F,** Section of a seminiferous tubule from a 20-week fetus. **G,** Section from the ovarian cortex of a 20-week fetus, showing two primordial follicles. (Reproduced from Jones RE, Lopez KH. Sexual differentiation. In: Jones RE, Lopez KH, eds. *Human Reproductive Biology,* 4th ed. San Diego, CA: Academic Press; 2014:87-102.)

structure with homogenous echotexture. A linear, hyperechoic band reflecting the mediastinum testis partially bisects the testicle. In prepubertal males, the testes can be quite small and mobile. Partial retraction into the inguinal canal is often noted during the course of sonographic evaluation. During puberty, the testicles grow to reach adult size. This growth may be asymmetric [**Fig. 6.54**].

The tunica albuginea is closely apposed to the testicular surface. Sonographically, this is seen as a thin, continuous, echogenic structure surrounding the testis. Trace free fluid can normally be seen surrounding the testis external to the tunica albuginea. The tunica vaginalis is the embryologic remnant of the processus vaginalis. This is a very thin structure exterior to the tunica albuginea and is not normally visualized as a distinct structure on ultrasound. The scrotal skin overlying the testis should be thin.

There should be uniform blood flow throughout the testicular parenchyma. Blood flow should be symmetric in both testicles and can be seen at all ages with modern ultrasound equipment.

Capsular vessels are present along the periphery of the testis. When evaluating for torsion, the central vessels should be interrogated. Evaluation of the capsular vessels alone may result in a false-negative study.

The epididymis is composed of a head, body, and tail. The head sits atop the cranial aspect of the testis, with the body extending along the posterior surface and the tail at the caudal end where it connects with the vas deferens. The epididymis has homogenous echotexture, with uniform blood flow. It should be smaller than the adjacent testis.

Cryptorchidism

When the testis fails to descend appropriately into the scrotal sac, cryptorchidism results. This may be unilateral or bilateral, and the undescended testis may be located anywhere along the path of descent described earlier. Although not routinely performed, ultrasound or MRI may be used to locate the undescended testis. Infants with cryptorchidism are typically observed

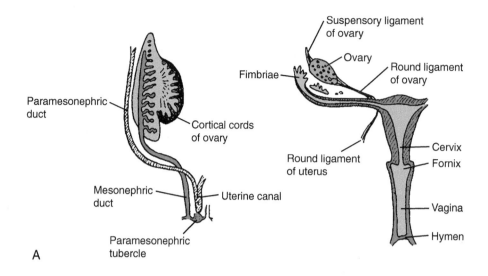

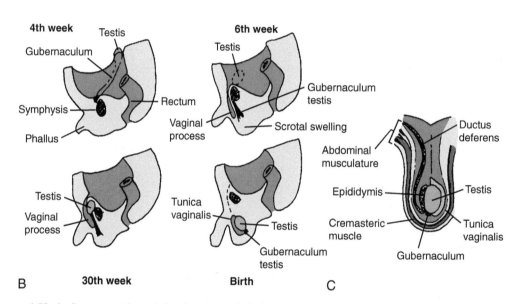

Figure 6.53 A, Representation of the female genital ducts at 8 weeks and their contribution to the female genital system. **B,** Descent of the testes. **C,** Adult relationship of the testes and their coverings. (Reproduced from Palastanga N, Field D, Soames R. Embryology. In: Palastanga N, Field D, Soames R, eds. *Anatomy and Human Movement,* 2nd ed. London, UK: Butterworth-Heinemann; 1994:23-44.)

for the first year of life, as the testis may descend without intervention. If the testis has failed to descend by 1 year of age, a surgical orchiopexy is performed. An undescended testis, even when surgically corrected, is at higher risk for development of a neoplasm in the future. If an undescended testis is not discovered early on, it may be a source of confusion on cross-sectional imaging in an older child because an abnormally located testis may be mistaken for an enlarged lymph node or other mass.

Acute Scrotal Pain

Scrotal pain is a frequent chief complaint in the pediatric emergency department. Ultrasound is the imaging study of choice and should be performed as expeditiously as possible because of the risk for possible testicular torsion.

Testicular Torsion. Although not the most common cause of scrotal pain, testicular torsion is the most worrisome. The most common form of torsion is known as intravaginal torsion, so named because the torsion occurs within the tunica vaginalis. A bell clapper deformity predisposes to this form of torsion. This occurs when the testis and epididymis are inadequately fixed to the tunica vaginalis. Because of this inadequate fixation, the testis is able to rotate freely and twist along the pedicle of the spermatic cord. When this twisting occurs, the vascular supply to the testis is cut off. Time is of the essence for diagnosis because the chance of salvage of the testis diminishes significantly after approximately 6 hours. Patients present with the acute onset of unilateral, intense scrotal pain and swelling. Frequently, the cremasteric reflex is absent on the affected side.

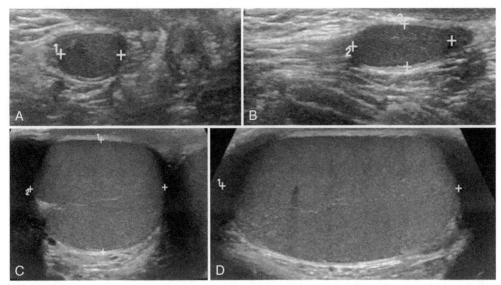

Figure 6.54 Normal testes. A and B, Transverse and sagittal ultrasound images of a normal prepubertal testis. The testicle has a homogenous echotexture. The mediastinum testis is noted, although subtle. The normal volume of a prepubertal testicle is typically less than 1.5 cc. **C and D,** Transverse and sagittal ultrasound images of a normal postpubertal testis. The postpubertal testicle also has a homogenous echotexture, with the exception of the mediastinum testis. Here, the mediastinum testis is best appreciated on the transverse (**C**) image. The normal volume of a postpubertal testis may range from 15 to 30 cc.

Extravaginal torsion is much less common, and it occurs when the tunica vaginalis does not have the appropriate attachments to the scrotal wall. In this setting, the entirety of the tunica and all of its contents may torse. This form of torsion occurs almost exclusively in the neonate. Patients present with pain and swelling. Extravaginal torsion may occur in utero and present as a firm mass during the initial newborn examination. Pain is typically absent because the torsion event is usually somewhat remote.

In the acute setting, these two forms of torsion may be impossible to distinguish before surgery. The difference is of little clinical significance because both forms are treated the same.

Ultrasound is currently the only imaging modality used to make the diagnosis of torsion. In the acute setting, the torsed testicle will be enlarged and hypoechoic on grayscale images. Changes may be subtle, and careful comparison with the contralateral asymptomatic testicle is important. Occasionally, twisting of the spermatic cord may be visualized. If presentation is delayed, grayscale changes will become more obvious. The testicle will become progressively more heterogeneous, and regions of necrosis will develop [**Fig. 6.55**]. With color Doppler evaluation, flow is frequently absent. However, if torsion is early and/or intermittent, flow may be preserved or even increased. Thus a high index of suspicion should be used when making this diagnosis, and if the grayscale findings are convincing, the presence of minimal flow should not necessarily be reassuring. Although historically radionuclide studies were used to make the diagnosis of torsion, this is not standard today.

Torsion of the Appendix Testis/Epididymis. Another frequent cause of acute scrotal pain is torsion of the appendix testis or appendix epididymis. These two entities are virtually impossible to distinguish from one another, so the terms are used interchangeably. Both the testicle and the epididymis can have an associated small soft tissue excrescence that is susceptible to torsion. The clinical presentation of a torsed appendix testis or epididymis is difficult to differentiate from testicular torsion. In all of these entities, the affected male will present with an acute onset of unilateral scrotal pain. In the setting of torsion of the

appendix testis, there will be a normal orientation of the testicle within the scrotal sac, and a "blue dot sign" may be seen, representing the necrotic and hemorrhagic torsed appendix visualized through the skin. These physical examination findings may help differentiate torsion of the appendix testis from testicular torsion.

On ultrasound, a normal appendix testis may occasionally be visualized, particularly in the presence of a hydrocele. It will have the same echotexture as the adjacent testis. In the setting of a torsed appendage, the appearance of the scrotum may be similar to that seen with epididymitis. There will be inflammation of the epididymis and scrotal soft tissues, and an associated hydrocele may be seen. The possibility of a torsed appendix should be considered in all cases of epididymitis. When torsed, the appendix will initially be enlarged with surrounding hyperemia and will later become atrophic and avascular. As the appendix involutes, it shrinks, becomes calcified, and detaches from its stalk, eventually forming a scrotal pearl [**Fig. 6.56**]. A torsed appendix may present as a paratesticular mass. The sonographic appearance and history of pain distinguish this entity from paratesticular neoplasms, which are painless. Torsed appendages are a nonsurgical diagnosis, and pain control is the mainstay of treatment.

Epididymitis/Orchitis. Infectious epididymitis, both with and without orchitis, is relatively rare in the pediatric population in comparison with the adult population. Clinically, an affected patient will present with pain, and the hemiscrotum may be enlarged and erythematous. Typically, the onset of pain is more gradual than with testicular torsion, although these entities may be difficult to distinguish clinically.

On ultrasound, the epididymis will be enlarged, sometimes markedly so. It can have a homogenous or heterogeneous echotexture. When the testicle is also involved, it will be enlarged with a variable echotexture. With color Doppler, marked hyperemia will be seen [**Fig. 6.57**]. A reactive hydrocele is frequently present, and the overlying scrotal skin may be thickened. As noted earlier, when these sonographic findings are present, one should carefully inspect for a torsed appendix testis.

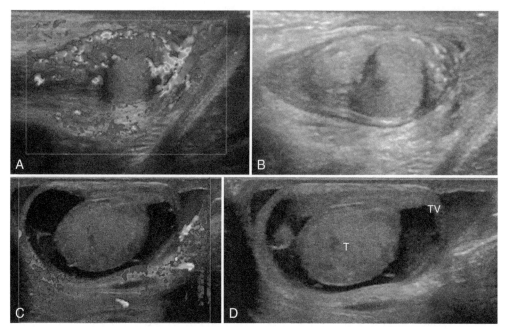

Figure 6.55 Testicular torsion. Seven-year-old boy with a 2-day history of testicular pain. **A and B,** Sagittal color Doppler and grayscale images of the left testicle. No flow is identified in the testis on the color Doppler image, although there is surrounding reactive hyperemia. On the grayscale image, the testicle is heterogeneous with an area of hypoechogenicity worrisome for necrosis. At surgery, the testicle was necrotic and nonviable. **C and D,** Neonate with a swollen left testicle. Sagittal color Doppler and grayscale images of the left testicle. The testis (*T*) is enlarged and heterogeneous, with little internal flow. A reactive hydrocele is noted. In addition, there is circumferential thickening of the tunica vaginalis (*TV*), with complex fluid noted between the tunica vaginalis and the scrotal skin. These findings are compatible with extravaginal testicular torsion because both the testicle and the tunica vaginalis are torsed and edematous.

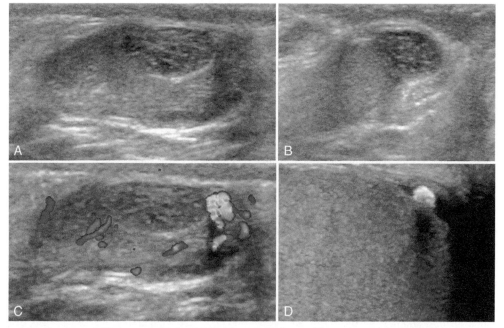

Figure 6.56 Torsion of the appendix testis. Eight-year-old boy with acute onset of scrotal pain. **A and B,** Sagittal (**A**) and transverse (**B**) grayscale ultrasound images of the left testis demonstrate an ovoid, heterogeneous structure superior to the testis. **C,** On the color Doppler image, the surrounding epididymis and testis demonstrate flow, but the ovoid, heterogeneous structure is avascular. This appearance is classic for torsion of the appendix testis. **D,** Ultrasound image in a different patient showing a small, echogenic, shadowing focus adjacent to the testis. This is a "scrotal pearl" and may represent the end stage of torsed appendix testis.

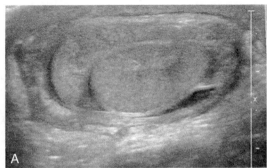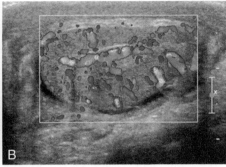

Figure 6.57 Epididymitis and orchitis. Ten-year-old boy with acute onset of scrotal pain. **A and B,** Sagittal grayscale and color Doppler images of the right testicle. The epididymis, seen superior to the testicle, is enlarged, heterogeneous, and hyperemic. On the color Doppler image, both the epididymis and the testis demonstrate increased blood flow. These findings are compatible with epididymitis and orchitis. There is a small hydrocele present.

Enlargement of the Scrotum/Testis

Most often, enlargement of the scrotal sac in a neonate or young child is due to an extratesticular cause such as a hernia or hydrocele. Primary testicular masses, both benign and malignant, are relatively rare in the prepubertal population.

Hernia. As described earlier in the *Embryology* section, the testicle normally descends through a patent processus vaginalis which typically closes before or immediately after birth. For unknown reasons, it may sometimes remain patent, and abdominal contents can protrude through this opening. This is referred to as an indirect hernia. Most frequently, fat alone protrudes through this defect. However, any abdominal contents may also extend through, including small bowel, colon, appendix, and even the bladder. Although the presence of a hernia may cause pain, if the hernia is reducible into the abdominal cavity, there is little cause for alarm in the acute setting. However, once the hernia becomes nonreducible or incarcerated, the contents are at risk for ischemia and necrosis.

Given its unparalleled real-time imaging capabilities, ultrasound is the most useful modality to assess for the presence of a hernia and reducibility. One may see fat and bowel protruding through the inguinal ring. During the course of the ultrasound examination, a patient should be asked to perform a Valsalva maneuver. The size of the hernia should increase with an increase in intraabdominal pressure. If there is clinical concern for incarceration, involved abdominal contents should be carefully interrogated. Bowel should be assessed for wall thickening and the presence of blood flow. Increased echogenicity of the surrounding soft tissue structures is suggestive of edema and inflammatory change.

Because patients may often present with abdominal pain in addition to scrotal swelling, abdominal radiographs may initially be obtained. An inguinal hernia may be seen as a soft tissue bulge over the groin or asymmetry in the size of the scrotum. A hernia is much more apparent when it contains gas-filled loops of bowel [**Fig. 6.58**]. When a hernia is present, one should always assess for signs of small-bowel obstruction. These may include the presence of dilated loops of bowel and air–fluid levels. Cross-sectional imaging, including both CT and MRI, can also be used to assess for the presence of a hernia. The presence of bowel wall thickening and surrounding inflammatory change are suggestive of possible incarceration. These modalities are particularly helpful when there is concern for possible small-bowel obstruction.

Hydrocele. Although generally an incidental finding, a large hydrocele may present as a scrotal "mass." A hydrocele

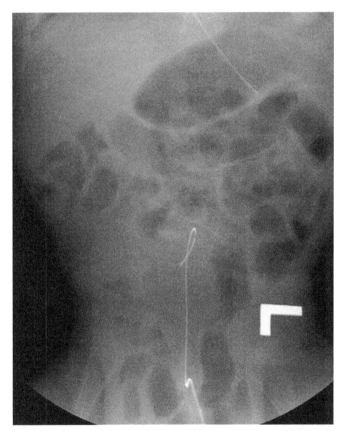

Figure 6.58 Inguinal hernia. KUB (kidneys, ureters, and bladder) of a preterm infant obtained during a voiding cystourethrography shows bilateral inguinal hernias containing large bowel. Loops of gas-filled bowel are seen inferior and lateral to the pubic symphysis. Inguinal hernias are a frequent finding in neonates, particularly preterm infants. This patient did not have clinical symptoms of obstruction, and the bowel gas pattern is otherwise normal.

frequently occurs in isolation but may also occur secondary to other intrascrotal pathology such as epididymitis or a tumor. There are various subtypes of hydroceles, classified according to location and communication with the abdominal cavity. As with urachal abnormalities, classification depends on which portion of the embryologic structure (the processus vaginalis) remains

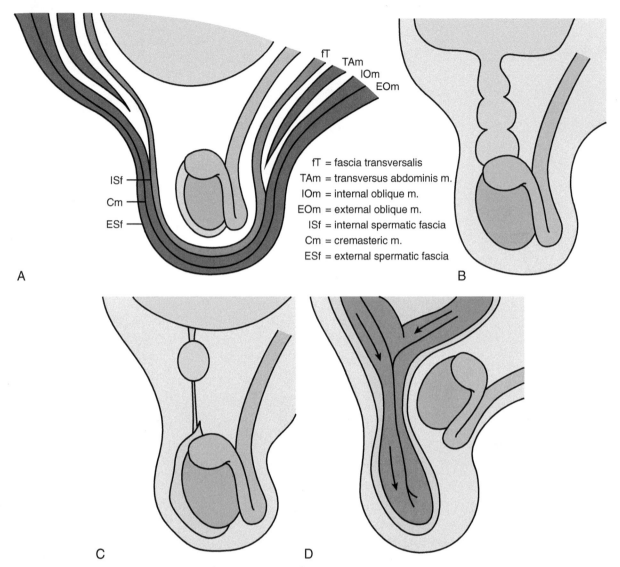

fT
TAm
IOm
EOm

ISf
Cm
ESf

fT = fascia transversalis
TAm = transversus abdominis m.
IOm = internal oblique m.
EOm = external oblique m.
ISf = internal spermatic fascia
Cm = cremasteric m.
ESf = external spermatic fascia

A

B

C

D

Figure 6.59 Illustration demonstrating the different types of anomalies associated with incomplete closure of the processus vaginalis. **A,** The normal layers of the wall of the scrotum. **B,** Funicular hydrocele. **C,** Encysted hydrocele, or hydrocele of the spermatic cord. **D,** Inguinal scrotal hernia. (Reproduced from Garriga V, Serrano A, Marin A, et al. US of the tunica vaginalis testis: anatomic relationships and pathologic conditions. *Radiographics.* 2009;29:2017-2032.)

patent. If the entirety of the processus vaginalis remains open, a communicating hydrocele results. One can sometimes demonstrate movement of fluid from the scrotal sac into the abdominal cavity with the application of pressure on ultrasound, although this is not always a reliable finding. If the processus vaginalis remains open at the level of the inguinal ring but is closed at the level of the testis, a funicular hydrocele develops. This is seen as an oblong structure centered in the groin that does not surround the testis but may communicate with the abdominal cavity. An encysted hydrocele occurs when the fluid collection does not communicate with the abdominal cavity or surround the testis. This is also referred to as a hydrocele of the spermatic cord. Finally, the most frequently seen hydrocele is a form that surrounds the testis but does not extend superiorly [**Fig. 6.59**].

Ultrasound is the primary imaging modality used in the detection of hydroceles. A simple hydrocele is seen as anechoic fluid surrounding the testis. In the setting of infection or

trauma, there may be debris noted dependently within the hydrocele. If the hydrocele is long standing, thin internal septations may develop. A rare type of hydrocele sometimes seen in the neonate is a meconium hydrocele. This develops in the setting of an intrauterine bowel perforation. This contains complex fluid and multiple echogenic foci reflecting partially calcified debris. The treatment for hydroceles varies widely based on the size, duration, and presence of related symptoms.

Varicocele. Varicoceles are infrequently seen in infants and young children, but they are not infrequent in teenagers. They occur because of dilatation of the pampiniform plexus of veins surrounding the spermatic cord. As in adults, they are most frequently seen on the left but may be bilateral. On sonographic evaluation, multiple anechoic, tubular structures are seen at the superior margin of the testis, which fill in with color Doppler. These vascular structures will change in size with variation in

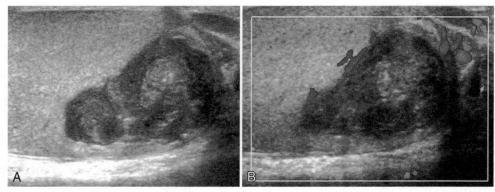

Figure 6.60 Epidermoid. Fourteen-year-old male with a painless, palpable testicular mass. **A and B,** Sagittal grayscale and color Doppler images of the testis show a lobulated, heterogeneous, avascular mass within the testicle with a lamellated internal architecture. This appearance is typical for an epidermoid. When an epidermoid is suspected before surgery, enucleation of the mass may be performed as opposed to an orchiectomy.

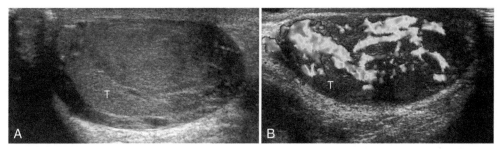

Figure 6.61 Paratesticular rhabdomyosarcoma. Seven-year-old boy with unilateral scrotal swelling. **A and B,** Sagittal grayscale and color Doppler images show a large, heterogeneous, highly vascular mass that is displacing the normal testicle (*T*) inferiorly. This is an extratesticular mass, but the normal testis may be difficult to distinguish from the mass because it is frequently compressed and distorted. A large, rapidly growing, painless extratesticular mass is concerning for rhabdomyosarcoma.

intraabdominal pressure. Because of the concern for potential associated infertility, patients undergo routine ultrasound surveillance to monitor testicular growth.

Benign Testicular Masses

Epidermoid. An epidermoid [**Fig. 6.60**] is one of the more common benign pediatric testicular masses. This lesion presents as a palpable, painless mass. It is a cystic lesion filled with layers of keratinous debris surrounded by squamous epithelium. The layers of keratin create a lamellated appearance on ultrasound, often likened to an "onion skin." Epidermoids are well-circumscribed and avascular. They may be multiple and even bilateral. Although ultrasound remains the mainstay for diagnosis, MRI is more frequently being used for evaluation. On MRI, an epidermoid is seen as a T2 hyperintense, T1 hypointense lesion with a surrounding rim of low signal intensity. On postcontrast imaging, there is no enhancement. If imaging findings are suggestive of an epidermoid, the patient may undergo testicular-sparing surgery with enucleation of the mass.

Adrenal Rests. An adrenal rest is a rare cause of a testicular mass in patients with CAH. In this clinical setting, it is important to consider this entity to avoid unnecessary surgery. On ultrasound, adrenal rests are seen as poorly defined regions of hypoechogenicity. They are frequently bilateral.

Microlithiasis. Testicular microlithiasis is seen on ultrasound as multiple punctate echogenic foci within the testicular parenchyma. The cause of this entity is uncertain. Microliths may be sparse or very numerous. Currently, long-term follow-up imaging is not routinely recommended because an increased risk for malignancy has not been definitely proven.

Malignant Testicular and Paratesticular Masses

Rhabdomyosarcoma. In children, the most common intrascrotal but extratesticular malignancy is rhabdomyosarcoma. Rhabdomyosarcoma is a soft tissue tumor that may arise anywhere in the body, with the genitourinary tract commonly involved. In the male, the tumor may arise from the bladder, prostate gland, or scrotum. In the scrotum, it arises from paratesticular soft tissues such as the epididymis or spermatic cord. Children present with painless scrotal swelling.

As with virtually all forms of scrotal pathology, ultrasound is the initial imaging modality used. Rhabdomyosarcoma may be quite large at presentation, and normal testicular parenchyma may be difficult to appreciate because of mass effect. The tumor is heterogeneous, with variable regions of necrosis present. There is often prominent internal vascularity. Hydroceles are a frequent coexisting finding [**Fig. 6.61**].

Cross-sectional imaging with CT or MRI is needed for staging. Disease often initially spreads to the retroperitoneal lymph nodes. Surgery is the primary mode of therapy, in conjunction with variable radiation and chemotherapy regimens. When localized to the scrotum, the prognosis for this malignancy is favorable.

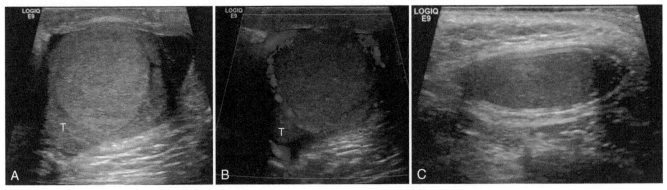

Figure 6.62 Yolk sac tumor. Five-year-old boy with unilateral scrotal swelling. **A and B,** Sagittal grayscale and color Doppler images show a large mass with a rim of normal testicular tissue (*T*) inferiorly. A yolk sac tumor is an intratesticular mass. It is more homogenous and circumscribed than rhabdomyosarcoma. Yolk sac tumors may be very large at presentation, and the testis may be difficult to identify. **C,** The normal contralateral testis provides a sense of scale for the size of the mass.

Primary Testicular Neoplasms. Intratesticular masses are more likely to be benign in prepubertal boys and malignant in postpubertal boys. Tumors may be divided into germ cell and non–germ cell tumors. Non–germ cell tumors, such as Sertoli and Leydig cell tumors, are rare in the pediatric population. Germ cell tumors may be further subdivided into seminomatous and nonseminomatous tumors. Seminomas are the most common testicular tumor in postpubertal males, and their clinical presentation and imaging appearance are essentially identical to that seen in the adult population. Nonseminomatous tumors, the most common of which are teratomas and yolk cell tumors, are more common in prepubertal males, with an average age of 2 years at diagnosis.

Like elsewhere in the body, teratomas have a heterogeneous appearance, with regions of fat and calcification often present. These are typically treated with testicular-sparing surgery in the prepubertal population. Yolk sac tumors may be very large at presentation, sometimes replacing the entirety of the testis [**Fig. 6.62**]. They may be heterogeneous, with regions of necrosis present. Serum α-fetoprotein levels are typically elevated. Treatment is with radical orchiectomy.

Some malignancies may metastasize to the testes. Because of the scrotal–blood barrier, the testis can be a haven for malignancy. It is one of the most common sites of recurrent disease, particularly for leukemia and lymphoma. The testes may be diffusely infiltrated with tumor, appearing enlarged and diffusely hypoechoic on ultrasound. Patchy, multifocal regions of hypoechogenicity may also be seen.

Female Genital Tract
Normal Anatomy of Uterus and Ovaries

The size and appearance of the uterus and ovaries are variable and depend on patient age. This is due to differences in hormonal influences at different stages of life. Neonates have a relatively large uterus and prominent ovaries because of the influence of maternal hormones in the postnatal period [**Figs. 6.63** and **6.64**]. From infancy until just before puberty, the uterus and ovaries are small. Although the ovaries remain small in prepubertal females, tiny ovarian follicles can be seen throughout childhood because of the presence of follicle-stimulating hormone. A small uterine growth spurt is seen in late childhood. During this period, the cervix can be equal to or greater than the size of the uterine fundus. At puberty, the uterine fundus elongates and thickens, ultimately becoming larger than the cervix [see **Fig. 6.63**]. The ovaries become more visible and are

capable of developing the dominant follicles and corpus luteum cysts that are seen in adult ovaries.

Anomalies of the Female Genital Tract

As described previously, anomalies of the female genital tract arise from abnormalities of fusion during the formation of the paramesonephric ducts. These are otherwise known as Müllerian duct anomalies. There is strong association of female genital tract anomalies with renal anomalies. These include unilateral renal agenesis, renal ectopia, and renal dysplasia. There is also an association with anorectal malformations. When a patient is diagnosed with an anomaly involving one of these systems, screening for associated anomalies should be performed.

Müllerian duct anomalies can range from complete agenesis to hypoplasia to abnormal formation of normal structures. Different classification systems exist to categorize the various anomalies. The American Society of Reproductive Medicine categorization is most widely used [**Fig. 6.65**].

Failure of resorption of the intervening tissue between the two Müllerian precursors leads to a septate uterus. This may be partial or complete, with extension to the internal cervical os. With this condition, the fundal contour is normal, and there is one cervix. An arcuate uterus is a mild variation of this and is presumably related to near-complete involution of the uterine septum. Thus a discrete septum is not seen. There is slight concavity to the endometrial contour subjacent to the uterine fundus, and the external uterine fundal contour is normal.

A bicornuate uterus is a result of partial nonfusion of the Müllerian precursors [**Fig. 6.66**]. Unlike a septate uterus, the external fundal contour is deeply indented. The dividing myometrium can extend to the internal cervical os (bicornuate unicollis) or to the external cervical os (bicornuate bicollis). Uterine didelphys results from complete nonfusion of the Müllerian precursors. There are two separate functional uterine cavities and two separate cervices. The presence of a vaginal septum predisposes to obstruction of one of the hemivaginas. In many of these patients, a solitary kidney is also seen. This constellation of findings is known as OHVIRA (obstructed hemivagina and ipsilateral renal agenesis) [**Fig. 6.67**]. A unicornuate uterus results from complete formation of only one Müllerian duct, with incomplete or failed development of the contralateral side.

Distal vaginal obstruction is seen in the setting of imperforate hymen and transverse vaginal septum. These entities present at birth with a bulging perineal mass, or in teenage years as amenorrhea with cyclic pelvic pain. An imperforate hymen is more

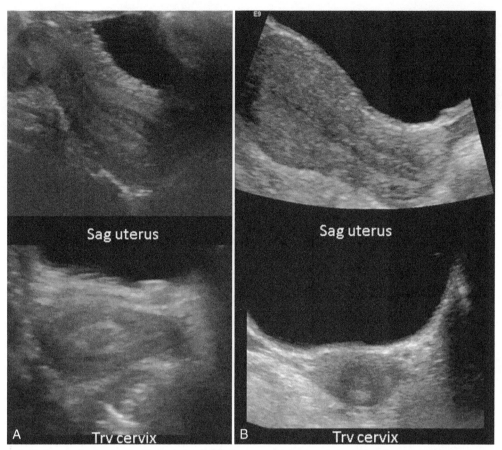

Figure 6.63 Normal uterus. A, Transabdominal ultrasound images of the pelvis in a neonate demonstrate a relatively large configuration of the uterus because of the influence of maternal hormones. Notably, the cervix is equal to or larger than the transverse dimension of the uterus. **B,** Transabdominal ultrasound images of the pelvis in a 14-year-old girl demonstrate elongation and thickening of the uterine fundus. Note that the cervix is smaller than the remainder of the uterus. Between the newborn period and puberty the uterus is long and thin, and more challenging to visualize.

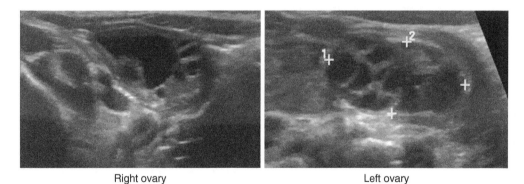

Right ovary   Left ovary

Figure 6.64 Normal ovaries in a neonate. Transabdominal ultrasound images of the pelvis in a neonate show easily visualized, relatively high-volume ovaries (right ovarian volume: 2.6 cc; left ovarian volume: 1.5 cc). This is due to the influence of residual maternal hormones in the early postnatal period. Later in childhood but before puberty, the ovaries are smaller and more difficult to visualize.

superficial, located between the caudal end of the Müllerian duct and the cranial end of the urogenital sinus where the two structures normally fuse. A transverse vaginal septum can be seen in a variety of locations within the vagina. Precise location is best determined with MRI. The septum represents a transverse band of fibrous tissue. It may be associated with atresia of a segment of the vagina. Ultrasound imaging demonstrates a dilated vagina (*colpo*) and possibly a dilated uterus (*metra*). These structures often contain heterogeneous echogenic material, representing a combination of fluid (*hydro*), secretions (*muco*), and blood (*hemato*).

Aplasia of the uterus and upper vagina is known as Mayer-Rokitansky-Küster-Hauser syndrome. The distal vagina and hymen may be normally formed, as these structures arise from the urogenital sinus. This syndrome can be associated with various Müllerian anomalies. Uterine rudiments may be present.

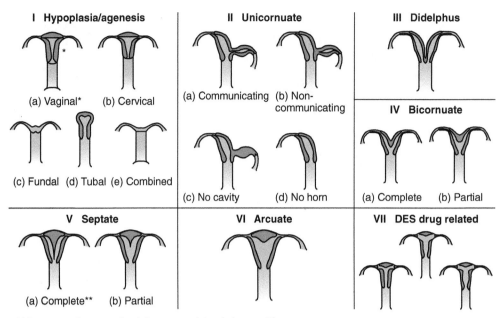

* Uterus may be normal or take on a variety of abnormal forms.
** May have two distinct cervices

Figure 6.65 Classification system of Müllerian duct anomalies. *DES,* diethylstillbestrol. (From American Fertility Society. The American Fertility Society classifications of adnexal adhesions, distal tubal occlusion, tubal occlusion secondary to tubal ligation, tubal pregnancies, Müllerian anomalies and intrauterine adhesions. *Fertil Steril.* 1988;49:952.)

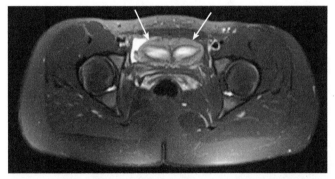

Figure 6.66 Bicornuate uterus. Fourteen-year-old girl with an incidentally noted bicornuate uterus on magnetic resonance imaging of the pelvis performed for trauma. On this axial T2 image, there are two distinct uterine horns (*arrows*). This was confirmed with subsequent pelvic ultrasound (not shown).

In some instances, it can also be associated with urologic, skeletal, auditory, and cardiac anomalies. Patients usually present in adolescence with primary amenorrhea. They may also present with difficulty during sexual intercourse because of underdevelopment of the vagina. If patients have uterine rudiments, endometrial proliferation can lead to hematometra.

Adolescents with primary amenorrhea and cyclic pelvic pain may also have distal vaginal atresia. This results from failure in formation of the distal third of the vagina from the urogenital sinus. On imaging, fluid and blood are seen filling the upper vagina, and to a lesser extent the uterine cavity. A transperineal ultrasound can be helpful with presurgical planning to estimate the distance between the proximal vagina and the introitus [**Fig. 6.68**].

Ambiguous Genitalia

Immediately after birth, a careful examination of the external genitalia should be performed as part of a complete physical examination. If there is concern for ambiguous genitalia, prompt further workup is imperative. This should include karyotyping, hormonal analysis, and imaging evaluation. First-line imaging is performed with ultrasound to determine the location and appearance of the gonads, evaluate for the presence of a uterus, and assess the adrenal glands for possible enlargement which may be seen in the setting of CAH. Patients with CAH must be diagnosed promptly because life-threatening salt-wasting crises may ensue.

Cloacal malformation occurs exclusively in girls. This results from incomplete separation of the urinary, genital, and gastrointestinal tracts. The cloaca is a common orifice that typically separates early in development into the urogenital sinus anteriorly and the hindgut posteriorly. Abnormalities in this process can lead to a persistent confluence for these tracts at the cloaca. This appears as a single perineal orifice on physical examination. As with other entities, there can be associated Müllerian anomalies. Ultrasound can be used to evaluate internal anatomy, although a genitogram will provide the most detailed anatomic information about the cloaca itself. Patients are studied fluoroscopically with the instillation of contrast material through a colostomy or through the common distal orifice to demonstrate the relationship of the urethra, vagina, and rectum to the cloaca [**Fig. 6.69**]. This information can provide helpful guidance for reconstructive surgery. It is important to note that the cloacal malformation and cloacal exstrophy are distinct entities.

Ovarian Masses

In children, various neoplastic and nonneoplastic processes can involve the ovaries. These are similar to entities seen in adults; however, the incidence may be different in the pediatric population. The most commonly encountered ovarian mass in a child

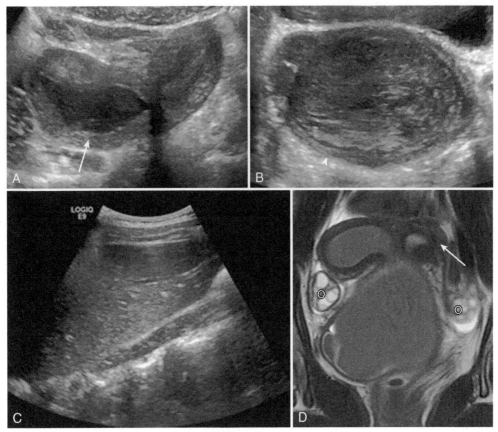

Figure 6.67 Uterine didelphys. Thirteen-year-old girl with pelvic pain. **A,** Sagittal and (**B**) transverse transabdominal pelvic ultrasound images demonstrate a dilated, fluid-filled endometrial cavity (*arrow*) and vagina (*arrowhead*), consistent with hematometrocolpos. **C,** There is an empty right renal fossa caused by renal agenesis. **D,** On subsequent magnetic resonance imaging of the pelvis, a dilated, fluid-filled right hemiuterus and vagina is noted, with a normal-appearing left hemiuterus (*arrow*). Findings are consistent with uterine didelphys. Here, a transverse septum caused right hemiuterus obstruction. Renal agenesis on the side of uterine obstruction is a common association. *O,* ovaries.

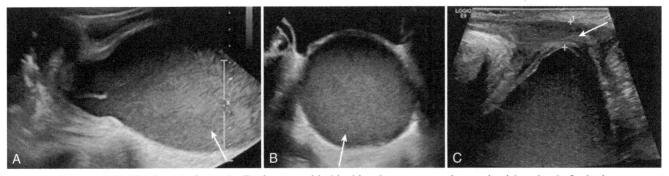

Figure 6.68 Distal vaginal atresia. Twelve-year-old girl with primary amenorrhea and pelvic pain. **A,** Sagittal and (**B**) transverse transabdominal ultrasound images demonstrate a dilated vagina containing echogenic material representing blood products (*arrows*). **C,** Transperineal ultrasound shows an introitus to skin distance of less than 1 cm (*arrow*). Findings are consistent with distal vaginal atresia.

is an ovarian cyst. Various primary ovarian neoplasms can also arise in children, with metastatic lesions much less frequently seen.

Ovarian Cysts. An ovarian cyst by definition measures greater than 3 cm in diameter. Ovarian cysts can arise at any age, including in fetal life when they may be seen with routine prenatal imaging. The early development of an ovarian cyst is related to stimulation by maternal and fetal gonadotropins. On ultrasound, these lesions appear as well-circumscribed, anechoic structures within the pelvis, with normal surrounding ovarian tissue variably seen. Some cysts may demonstrate complexity, containing internal echoes and/or septations. Hyperechoic material within a cyst suggests possible hemorrhage into the lesion. Simple cysts are typically asymptomatic. As with adults, hemorrhagic cysts may present with pelvic pain [**Fig. 6.70**].

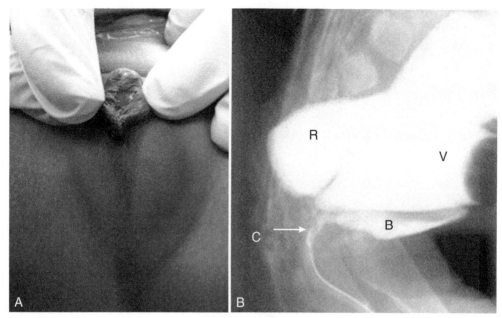

Figure 6.69 Cloacal malformation. A, On physical examination, there is a single perineal orifice. **B,** Genitogram performed via the single orifice demonstrates opacification of the rectum (*R*), vagina (*V*), and bladder (*B*), consistent with a single channel for these structures, the cloaca (*C, arrow*).

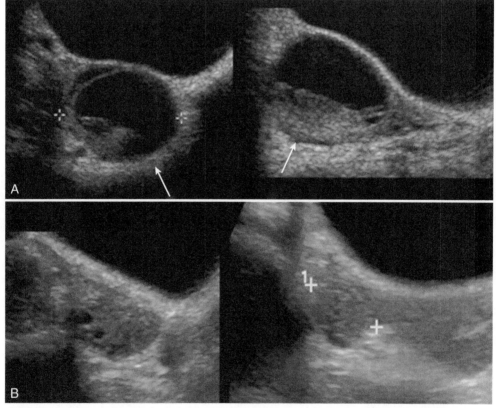

Figure 6.70 Ovarian cyst. Fourteen-year-old girl with pelvic pain. **A,** Transverse and sagittal images from a transabdominal pelvic ultrasound demonstrate a well-circumscribed cystic lesion in the right adnexa with a fluid–debris level (*arrows*). **B,** Follow-up imaging 6 weeks later demonstrates complete resolution of the cyst.

Primary Ovarian Neoplasms. Ovarian tumors are categorized based on the cell of origin: germ cell, epithelial cell, and stromal cell tumors. These tumors are commonly characterized as solid, cystic, or mixed lesions. Generally speaking, tumors with more solid elements are more apt to be malignant.

Germ cell tumors are the most common type of ovarian tumor encountered in children. Included in this category are teratoma, dysgerminoma, yolk sac tumor (endodermal sinus tumor), and choriocarcinoma. These tumors can have similar imaging characteristics. Specific laboratory values such as an α-fetoprotein level may be helpful in determining the nature of a lesion.

The majority of germ cell tumors in children are teratomas. The terms *mature cystic teratoma* and *dermoid cyst* are often used interchangeably. Sonographically, a teratoma appears heterogeneous, with areas of fat and calcification. Dense calcification can produce significant posterior shadowing, with the characteristic "tip of the iceberg" appearance. Additional findings on ultrasound may include linear echogenic foci representing hair, as well as a solid dermoid plug or Rokitansky nodule. The latter appears as an echogenic focus with associated posterior acoustic shadowing. The majority of teratomas are mature. Immature teratomas are more concerning given a higher incidence of recurrence and metastatic spread [**Fig. 6.71**].

Epithelial cell tumors include cystadenoma and cystadenocarcinoma, which are further classified into serous and mucinous subtypes. These tumors are typically seen in postpubertal girls and present with increasing abdominal girth because of their large size. Imaging characteristics are similar for tumors within this group. It can therefore be difficult to fully categorize a lesion based on imaging alone [**Fig. 6.72**]. Ultrasound demonstrates a large pelvic mass with mixed solid and cystic components,

including internal septations and papillary projections. Low-level echoes may be seen within cystic portions of mucinous lesions. Visualization of the ovaries and uterus is usually difficult because of large tumor size. Intraabdominal extension is typically seen. Definitive diagnosis is made by pathology after surgical resection. Before surgery, contrast-enhanced MRI can help with characterization of the lesion as well as delineation from surrounding structures.

Among primary ovarian neoplasms, stromal cell tumors are least commonly seen. Unlike epithelial cell tumors which present in postpubertal girls, these tumors are associated with hormone production, and therefore present earlier with premature development of secondary sex characteristics and precocious puberty. Included in this group are granulosa thecal cell tumor, Sertoli-Leydig cell tumor, and undifferentiated sex cord stromal tumors. In contrast with many other ovarian neoplasms, these are predominantly solid lesions [**Fig. 6.73**].

Secondary neoplasms of the ovary are rare in children. Metastases to the ovary can be caused by hematogenous spread, lymphatic spread, or direct extension of tumor. The most common primary tumors that metastasize to the ovary include Burkitt lymphoma, alveolar rhabdomyosarcoma, Wilms tumor, neuroblastoma, and retinoblastoma.

Ovarian Torsion

Like its counterpart in males, ovarian torsion is a surgical emergency. Prompt and accurate diagnosis is critical. The diagnosis is made with a combination of clinical and radiologic findings. Patients typically present with severe pain and nausea. Torsion can be idiopathic secondary to excess mobility of the ovary, or it can be related to the presence of a lead point such as a paraovarian cyst. Ovarian torsion can occur at any age, including in utero. Ultrasound imaging in infants with torsion will typically show a complex cystic and solid pelvic mass. There may be no internal vascularity, particularly if the torsion occurred in utero. If the torsed ovary is enlarged, it may appear to be an abdominal mass rather than a pelvic mass because of the relatively small size of the infant pelvis. In older patients, torsed ovaries appear enlarged, round, and displaced toward the midline [**Fig. 6.74**]. The absence or presence of flow on Doppler evaluation is not a reliable indicator of torsion or lack of torsion. Doppler flow may be present in early or intermittent torsion, and lack of vascularity does not necessarily indicate torsion when the ovary is otherwise normal in appearance. Ultrasound can be used to assess for a lead point, which is present in 50% of cases. Ultrasound findings must be correlated with clinical presentation for a diagnosis of ovarian torsion to be made. When there is diagnostic confusion, further evaluation with MRI may be helpful. A torsed ovary will appear as an enlarged, round, T2 hyperintense structure, and a twisted vascular pedicle may be seen.

Pelvic Inflammatory Disease

Pelvic inflammatory disease (PID) is commonly caused by sexually transmitted diseases. There is a spectrum of clinical manifestations, ranging from involvement of the endometrium (endometritis) to the fallopian tubes (salpingitis) to the ovaries (oophoritis). Although ultrasound may be normal in the setting of PID, it is a useful tool to evaluate for complications of PID. These include pyosalpinx and tuboovarian abscess. A dilated tubular structure filled with simple or complex fluid may be seen with hydrosalpinx or pyosalpinx. Notably, the echogenicity of the fluid is not a reliable indicator of the presence of infection. A thick-walled fallopian tube with increased echogenicity may be seen in salpingitis. A tuboovarian abscess is seen as a complex fluid collection in the adnexa [**Fig. 6.75**]. Normal ovarian tissue may be difficult to discern because it may be entirely replaced by infection. Free fluid in the pelvis is a nonspecific finding but

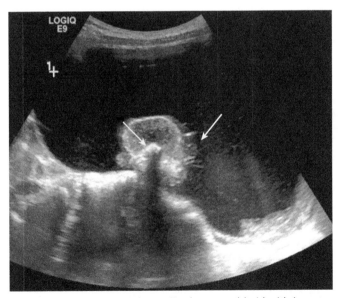

Figure 6.71 Mature teratoma. Twelve-year-old girl with increasing abdominal girth. Transabdominal pelvic ultrasound image demonstrates a large pelvic mass with cystic and solid components. There is a rounded echogenic area in the center of the large, hypoechoic cystic portion. A central dense echogenic focus (*yellow arrow*) demonstrates posterior acoustic shadowing, consistent with calcification. Tiny linear echogenic foci (*white arrow*) are also associated with the central echogenic mass, representing hair. This constellation of findings is seen with a mature teratoma or dermoid cyst.

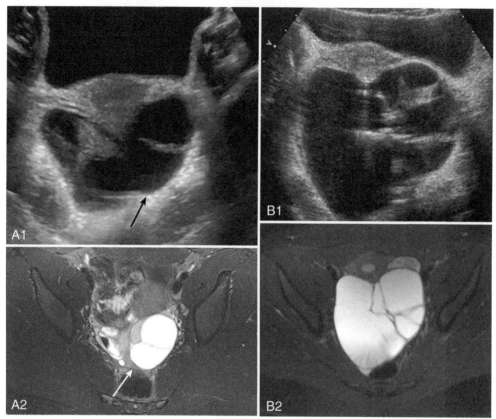

Figure 6.72 Serous cystadenoma and mucinous cystadenoma. A1 and A2, Twenty-year-old female with pelvic pain. **A1,** Transverse ultrasound and **(A2)** axial T2 fat-saturated magnetic resonance images (MRIs) demonstrate a complex cystic mass with septations in the left adnexa (*arrows*). This was removed and found to be a serous cystadenoma. **B1 and B2,** Fifteen-year-old girl with pelvic pain. **B1,** Transverse ultrasound and **(B2)** axial T2 fat-saturated MRIs demonstrate a cystic, septated mass posterior to the uterus. After surgical resection, pathology confirmed a mucinous cystadenoma. Note that the imaging appearances of serous and mucinous cystadenoma are similar. A specific diagnosis is difficult to discern based on imaging alone.

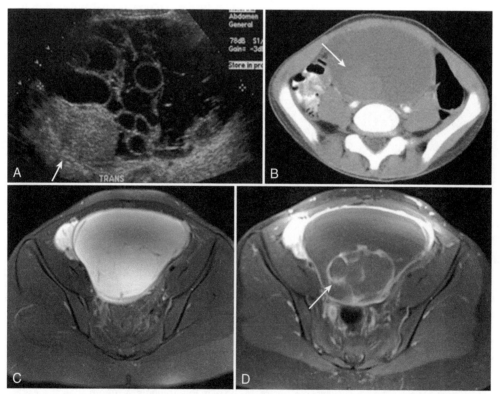

Figure 6.73 Sertoli-Leydig cell tumor. Two-year-old girl with a palpable pelvic mass and secondary sex characteristics. **A,** Transabdominal pelvic ultrasound demonstrates a complex cystic, septated mass, with a solid component posteriorly (*arrow*). **B,** Contrast-enhanced computed tomography shows a predominantly cystic mass, with an enhancing mural nodule along the posterior margin (*arrow*). **C,** T2-weighted and **(D)** contrast-enhanced magnetic resonance images in a different patient demonstrate a T2 hyperintense lesion in the pelvis, with enhancing internal solid components noted after contrast administration (*arrow*).

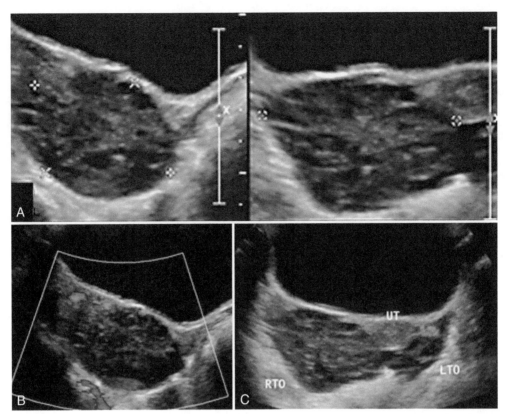

Figure 6.74 Ovarian torsion. Fifteen-year-old girl with acute-onset pelvic pain. **A,** Sagittal and transverse transabdominal pelvic ultrasound images demonstrate a rounded appearance of the right ovary, which is displaced medially and positioned posterior to the uterus. There is peripheralization of the ovarian follicles. **B,** Power Doppler imaging shows no demonstrable flow within the ovarian parenchyma. **C,** Transverse image of the pelvis shows marked asymmetric enlargement of the right ovary (*RTO*) in comparison with the normal left ovary (*LTO*). This patient went to surgery, and right ovarian torsion was confirmed. *UT,* uterus.

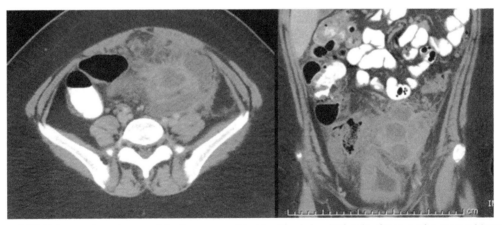

Figure 6.75 Tuboovarian abscess. Nineteen-year-old girl with abdominal pain, fever, and a recent history of sexually transmitted disease. Axial and coronal contrast-enhanced computed tomography images demonstrate a peripherally enhancing, multiloculated collection in the left lower quadrant, extending into the pelvis. This collection was in close proximity to the uterus, with the normal ovary difficult to visualize.

may be related to inflammation in the pelvis. Patients are treated aggressively with intravenous antibiotics. Surgical intervention is reserved for recalcitrant cases.

Polycystic Ovarian Syndrome

Polycystic ovarian syndrome (PCOS) is an endocrinopathy that affects adolescents. Patients present with primary amenorrhea.

Various criteria have been outlined for the accurate diagnosis of this entity. This diagnosis may have significant clinical implications, including the need for hormonal treatment and potential psychological distress. PCOS is thought to result from hyperandrogenism, which may be confirmed with hormonal testing. The hormonal imbalance leads to hirsutism, ovarian dysfunction, and ultimately amenorrhea. Sonographic findings are variable. A polycystic ovary has been described as having a volume greater than 10 cc with at least 12 follicles, each measuring 2 to 9 mm in diameter. Follicles may have a peripheral orientation, with a "string-of-pearls" configuration. Notably, the ovaries may also be normal in appearance in the setting of PCOS.

Rhabdomyosarcoma

As mentioned previously, rhabdomyosarcoma is an aggressive malignancy that arises from both the male and the female pelvic organs. In females, it may arise from the urethra, bladder, and vagina. When arising from the urethra or vagina, the mass may extrude into the perineum and present with bleeding [see **Fig. 6.39**]. Sarcoma botryoides is a subset of this malignancy that has a grapelike appearance. These tumors are treated with surgery and chemotherapy.

Acknowledgments

We give special thanks to Rhonda Johnson for her expertise and diligence, and for elevating our work.

SUGGESTED READINGS

Anthony EY, Caserta MP, Singh J, et al. Adnexal masses in female pediatric patients. *AJR Am J Roentgenol*. 2012;198:W426-W431.

Avni FE, Garel C, Cassart M, et al. Imaging and classification of congenital cystic renal diseases. *AJR Am J Roentgenol*. 2012;198:1004-1013.

Avni FE, Hall M. Renal cystic diseases in children: new concepts. *Pediatr Radiol*. 2010;40:939-946.

Balassy C, Navarro OM, Daneman A. Adrenal masses in children. *Radiol Clin North Am*. 2011;49:711-727, vi.

Baldisserotto M. Scrotal emergencies. *Pediatr Radiol*. 2009;39:516-521.

Chapman T. Fetal genitourinary imaging. *Pediatr Radiol*. 2012;42(suppl 1):S115-S123.

Chauvin NA, Epelman M, Victoria T, et al. Complex genitourinary abnormalities on fetal MRI: imaging findings and approach to diagnosis. *AJR Am J Roentgenol*. 2012;199:W222-W231.

Chung EM, Conran RM, Schroeder JW, et al. From the radiologic pathology archives: pediatric polycystic kidney disease and other ciliopathies: radiologic-pathologic correlation. *Radiographics*. 2014;34:155-178.

Dinan D, Epelman M, Guimaraes CV, et al. The current state of imaging pediatric hemoglobinopathies. *Semin Ultrasound CT MR*. 2013;34:493-515.

Epelman M, Chikwava KR, Chauvin N, et al. Imaging of pediatric ovarian neoplasms. *Pediatr Radiol*. 2011;41:1085-1099.

Fernbach SK, Feinstein KA, Spencer K, et al. Ureteral duplication and its complications. *Radiographics*. 1997;17:109-127.

Frush DP, Sheldon CA. Diagnostic imaging for pediatric scrotal disorders. *Radiographics*. 1998;18:969-985.

Kraus SJ, Lebowitz RL, Royal SA. Renal calculi in children: imaging features that lead to diagnoses: a pictorial essay. *Pediatr Radiol*. 1999;29:624-630.

Levin TL, Han B, Little BP. Congenital anomalies of the male urethra. *Pediatr Radiol*. 2007;37:851-862, quiz 945.

Lowe LH, Isuani BH, Heller RM, et al. Pediatric renal masses: Wilms tumor and beyond. *Radiographics*. 2000;20:1585-1603.

Milla SS, Chow JS, Lebowitz RL. Imaging of hypospadias: pre- and postoperative appearances. *Pediatr Radiol*. 2008;38:202-208.

Paltiel HJ, Phelps A. US of the pediatric female pelvis. *Radiology*. 2014;270:644-657.

Pierre K, Borer J, Phelps A, et al. Bladder exstrophy: current management and postoperative imaging. *Pediatr Radiol*. 2014;44:768-786, quiz 765-767.

Renjen P, Bellah R, Hellinger JC, et al. Advances in uroradiologic imaging in children. *Radiol Clin North Am*. 2012;50:207-218, v.

Shah RU, Lawrence C, Fickenscher KA, et al. Imaging of pediatric pelvic neoplasms. *Radiol Clin North Am*. 2011;49:729-748, vi.

Siegel MJ, Chung EM. Wilms' tumor and other pediatric renal masses. *Magn Reson Imaging Clin N Am*. 2008;16:479-497, vi.

Sivit CJ. Imaging children with abdominal trauma. *AJR Am J Roentgenol*. 2009;192:1179-1189.

Snow A, Estrada C, Chow JS. *Ultrasonography of the Pediatric Bladder*. New York, NY: Elsevier; 2013.

Chapter 7
Musculoskeletal Imaging

David W. Swenson and Michele M. Walters

IMAGING TECHNIQUES

Radiography

Conventional radiographs depict the bony detail of the skeletal system quite well and remain the mainstay in the evaluation of musculoskeletal disease. In the setting of acute trauma, radiographic views of the long bones are obtained in at least two projections, whereas joints are typically imaged in at least three projections. When bony injury to a digit is suspected, dedicated views of the digit alone should be obtained rather than views of the entire hand or foot. On occasion, comparison views with the contralateral asymptomatic side are useful, particularly when it is difficult to discern a suspected injury from a normal finding or normal variant. This may be helpful in the evaluation of the developing elbow in the setting of trauma, when patterns of apophyseal ossification and fusion may be confusing [**Fig. 7.1**]. Complete radiographic skeletal surveys are indicated in the workup of suspected child abuse in infants and small toddlers. In this setting, imaging is performed on a high detail system to demonstrate subtle injuries characteristic of abuse to best advantage.

Radiographs should first be obtained in the setting of suspected infection, although they may be negative early on. It is important to exclude the presence of other pathology that may be responsible for a patient's presenting symptoms, such as an underlying fracture or a primary osseous lesion.

Radiographs are essential in the evaluation of benign and malignant bone lesions. Although cross-sectional imaging is important in the diagnostic workup for many lesions, radiographic features are often more specific and helpful in narrowing differential diagnostic considerations. Radiographs are also helpful in planning advanced imaging once a lesion is identified.

Skeletal surveys are performed in the evaluation for dysplasia and in the assessment for multifocal bone disease seen with entities such as Langerhans cell histiocytosis (LCH). For these indications, a standard imaging system is typically used.

Ultrasound

Ultrasound has several applications in pediatric musculoskeletal imaging. It is the primary modality used in the evaluation for developmental dysplasia of the hip (DDH) from the newborn period until approximately 4 to 6 months of age, prior to ossification of the cartilaginous capital femoral epiphyses. It is used as a screening tool in infants with risk factors for DDH and also to monitor response to treatment once a diagnosis of DDH has been made.

In some centers, ultrasound is used to evaluate glenohumeral dysplasia in patients with a history of brachial plexus birth injury. The relationship of the humeral head to the glenoid can be assessed, and the angle of glenoid version can be calculated from ultrasound images.

Sonography is an effective tool in the evaluation of superficial soft tissue masses. Many common superficial lesions with characteristic sonographic features may be diagnosed by ultrasound alone. These include infantile hemangiomas, ganglion cysts, normal and abnormal lymph nodes, and popliteal cysts, among others [**Fig. 7.2**]. When a specific diagnosis cannot confidently be made, ultrasound is helpful in stratifying lesions into those that can be clinically followed, those that require short-term ultrasound follow-up, those that might be further characterized by computed tomography (CT) or magnetic resonance imaging (MRI), and those that warrant surgical excision or biopsy.

Ultrasound is frequently used to evaluate for a joint effusion in the setting of suspected infectious or inflammatory disease. If an effusion is identified and the cause is unclear, joint fluid may be sampled under sonographic guidance.

Computed Tomography

CT remains an important modality in the evaluation of the musculoskeletal system. Scan times are very short, allowing most examinations to be completed without the need for sedation or anesthesia. Low-dose protocols are now standard for many musculoskeletal applications. The capacity for reformatting and three-dimensional reconstruction is a major advantage and is often important in guiding surgical management.

CT is particularly useful in the setting of trauma when radiographic evaluation is believed to be inconclusive or incomplete. Subtle injuries such as nondisplaced fractures of the scaphoid bone may be challenging to detect on radiographs, but well demonstrated on CT. Intraarticular extension of injuries may be shown to best advantage, and intraarticular fragments not seen on radiographs may be well demonstrated on CT. Complex injuries that may require surgical management are well profiled, including the distal tibial triplane and Tillaux fractures. CT is often useful in assessing fracture complications, including nonunion and premature physeal fusion after injury to the growth plate. Potential sternoclavicular joint injury is well assessed with CT. The sternoclavicular joints can be evaluated for symmetry, and injury to subjacent mediastinal structures can be detected in the setting of subluxation/dislocation.

Although MRI is often the advanced imaging modality of choice for assessment of a bone lesion after identification on radiographs, certain lesions have a very characteristic CT appearance, which is helpful when there is diagnostic confusion. An example is the cortically based osteoid osteoma. The MRI appearance of this lesion may be misleading. The lesion itself is typically small and may be difficult to discern, and there is often significant surrounding marrow edema and possibly synovitis involving a neighboring joint. Although these MRI features may be

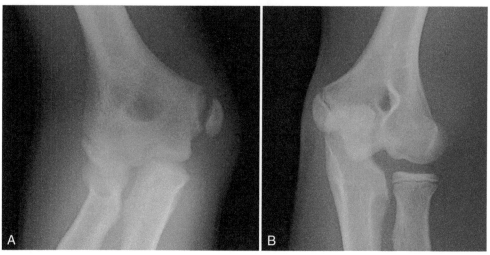

Figure 7.1 Medial epicondyle avulsion injury in a 14-year-old male baseball pitcher. **A,** Radiograph of the right elbow demonstrates a medial epicondyle avulsion fracture, with distraction of the medial epicondyle apophysis from the parent bone. **B,** Radiograph of the asymptomatic contralateral left elbow shows the medial epicondyle apophysis in normal position, more closely apposed to the parent bone.

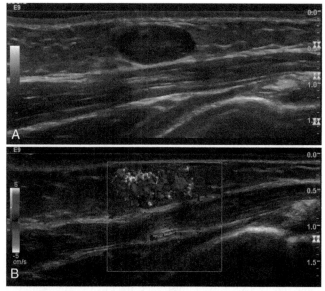

Figure 7.2 Infantile hemangioma in a 12-month-old girl with a palpable bluish soft tissue mass of the anterior chest wall. **A,** Grayscale and (**B**) color Doppler images of the chest wall in the transverse plane demonstrate a well-circumscribed, ovoid-shaped, heterogeneously hypoechoic mass confined to the subcutaneous tissues. Significant vascularity is seen throughout the lesion. Clinical presentation and sonographic features are diagnostic of an infantile hemangioma.

puzzling, a CT scan will demonstrate the classic appearance of this lesion and is most often diagnostic [**Fig. 7.3**].

CT is helpful in the assessment for congenital anomalies such as tarsal coalition. Coalition is sometimes radiographically evident, although the diagnosis is not always clear without cross-sectional imaging. Osseous coalition is well demonstrated on CT, and fibrous and cartilaginous coalitions are typically also evident.

CT is routinely used in the evaluation of alignment disorders, including abnormalities of femoral version and tibial torsion. Glenohumeral dysplasia related to brachial plexus birth injury

and patellofemoral tracking disorders also may be evaluated with CT. Multiplanar reformatting capabilities are particularly helpful for these indications, allowing quantitative measurements to be made that are useful in surgical planning.

Magnetic Resonance Imaging

There has been tremendous growth in the use of MRI in the pediatric population. Major applications include the imaging of infectious, inflammatory, neoplastic, metabolic, and sports-related pathology. Generally speaking, most children younger than 8 years require sedation or anesthesia to complete an MRI, which is managed by a dedicated team of sedation nurses and anesthesiologists (see Chapter 1).

Sequences used are tailored for the specific examination indication. A T1-weighted sequence is optimal for evaluation of the marrow and is particularly important in oncologic and metabolic imaging. Both T1-weighted and proton density sequences are useful for assessing trabecular architecture and demonstrating fractures to best advantage. Ligamentous anatomy, articular cartilage, and labra are well seen on proton density images.

Fluid-sensitive sequences include proton density with fat saturation, T2 with fat saturation, and short tau inversion recovery (STIR). These sequences are important in all musculoskeletal imaging, with marrow and soft tissue edema, myotendinous and ligamentous abnormality, and cartilage pathology all well demonstrated.

A gradient echo sequence is added to some protocols. This is useful to evaluate for anything that might cause susceptibility artifact, including blood products and intraarticular loose bodies. An example is the assessment for pigmented villonodular synovitis (PVNS). With this entity, there is often hemosiderin deposition in the synovium and joint space, with related blooming artifact demonstrated [**Fig. 7.4**].

Postcontrast imaging is important in several settings. It is routine in the initial evaluation of bone and soft tissue tumors, and also is important in follow-up to assess for residual or recurrent disease. Postcontrast imaging is standard in the workup of suspected musculoskeletal infection. Joint involvement and intraosseous, subperiosteal, and soft tissue abscesses are well demonstrated on postcontrast images, and MRI findings are used to guide medical and/or surgical management in this setting. Inflammatory joint disease is also well profiled on

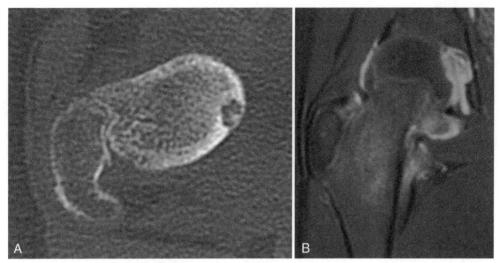

Figure 7.3 Osteoid osteoma of the femoral neck in a 9-year-old girl with hip pain and abnormal gait. **A,** Axial computed tomography image through the right proximal femur demonstrates a small, cortically based lucent lesion with a central sclerotic nidus and surrounding sclerosis, the classic appearance of an osteoid osteoma. **B,** Coronal T1 fat-saturated postcontrast magnetic resonance (MR) image demonstrates regional signal abnormality in the femoral neck, although the lesion itself is not clearly seen. There is a joint effusion, along with significant synovitis. In this case, MR imaging was obtained first, and the diagnosis was initially not clear.

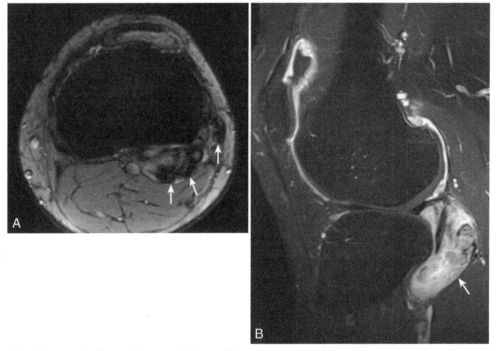

Figure 7.4 Pigmented villonodular synovitis in an 18-year-old male with knee pain and swelling. **A,** Axial gradient echo image of the left knee demonstrates prominent soft tissue masses in the posterior joint space (*arrows*). There is blooming artifact related to hemosiderin deposition. **B,** Sagittal T1 fat-saturated postcontrast image shows significant synovial thickening and hyperemia, with heterogeneous enhancement of the larger mass shown in (**A**) (*arrow*).

contrast-enhanced imaging, with abnormal synovial thickening and hyperemia noted at the affected joint(s).

Nuclear Imaging

With improvements in the diagnostic accuracy of CT and MRI for many musculoskeletal imaging applications, utilization of nuclear imaging has decreased. It remains a useful modality in certain clinical settings, including the evaluation for very early osteomyelitis and radiographically occult bony injury. Skeletal scintigraphy is primarily performed with technetium-99m methylene diphosphonate, a pharmaceutical agent that concentrates in regions of increased blood flow and bone turnover. Sensitivity of scintigraphy with this agent is higher than that for

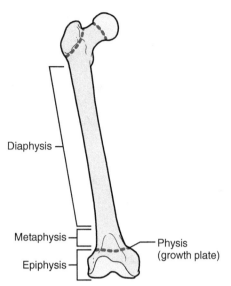

Figure 7.5 Illustration depicting the anatomy of a tubular bone in the developing skeleton.

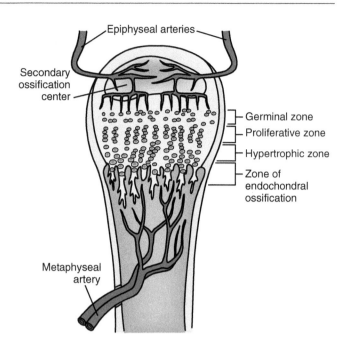

Figure 7.6 Illustration of the physis, the site of long bone growth by endochondral ossification.

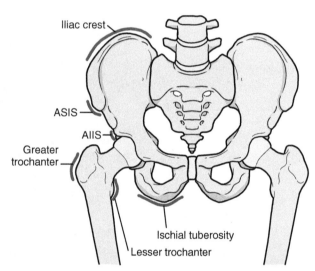

Figure 7.7 Illustration of the apophyses of the pelvis in the developing skeleton. *ASIS*, anterior superior iliac spine; *AIIS*, anterior inferior iliac spine.

radiography in the evaluation of pathology with osteoblastic activity, including infection, trauma, and neoplasia. Importantly, images obtained are nonspecific and do not provide anatomic detail.

Positron emission tomography (PET) imaging with fluorine-18-deoxyglucose offers high sensitivity for the detection of aggressive bone tumors, and also is useful in monitoring response to therapy. Fusion with CT or MRI improves spatial localization and allows for better characterization of lesions.

ANATOMY

The tubular bones of the extremities are composed of four parts: the diaphysis; metaphysis; epiphysis; and physis, or growth plate [**Fig. 7.5**]. Long, tubular bones have a physis at each end, whereas short tubular bones like the metacarpals and metatarsals have a physis at one end only. Generally, this is at the end of greater joint motion. The physis is composed of four layers of cartilage arranged in an organized fashion, and it is the site of long bone growth by endochondral ossification [**Fig. 7.6**]. The physis is the weakest part of a long bone in a skeletally immature child, and thus is prone to mechanical failure and fracture.

An apophysis is an ossification center at a site where a tendon inserts. It does not contribute to the longitudinal growth of bone and does not form an articular surface [**Fig. 7.7**]. Similar to physes, apophyses are points of relative weakness in the developing musculoskeletal system. Apophyseal injuries are relatively common in older children and adolescents, and are commonly seen involving the pelvis.

NORMAL VARIANTS

Physiologic Subperiosteal New Bone Formation

Subperiosteal new bone formation may be seen as a normal finding in about 50% of infants younger than 6 months of age. In this setting, new bone is thin (≤2 mm) and smooth, and parallels the diaphysis of long bones such as the humerus, radius, femur, and tibia [**Fig. 7.8**]. It is typically bilateral and symmetric. This finding disappears over the first weeks to months of life. There is a broad differential diagnosis for the finding of periosteal new bone formation in an infant [**Box 7.1**].

BOX 7.1 Differential Diagnosis: Subperiosteal New Bone Formation in an Infant

Physiologic new bone formation
Caffey disease (infantile cortical hyperostosis)
Hypervitaminosis A
Prostaglandin therapy
TORCH (toxoplasmosis, other [congenital syphilis and viruses], rubella, cytomegalovirus, and herpes simplex virus) infections
Metastatic neuroblastoma
Child abuse

Physiologic Sclerosis

In children younger than 6 years, physiologic sclerosis may be seen along the zone of provisional calcification (ZPC) at the metaphyses of rapidly growing bones such as the femur and tibia

[**Fig. 7.9A**]. These sclerotic metaphyseal bands may be difficult to distinguish from the "lead lines" seen in the setting of heavy metal intoxication. Lead lines are typically relatively broader, and are also seen in the metaphyses of more slowly growing bones such as the fibula [**Fig. 7.9B**].

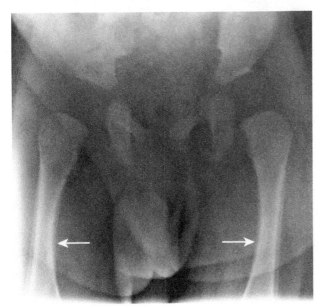

Figure 7.8 Physiologic subperiosteal new bone formation in an infant. Anteroposterior supine radiograph of the pelvis demonstrates thin, smooth, symmetric subperiosteal new bone formation along the proximal femurs (*arrows*).

Growth Recovery Lines

In the setting of stress, blood flow at the metaphysis of a long bone may be temporarily slowed and diverted. This can occur in a variety of settings, including prematurity, congenital heart disease, and trauma. Mineralization is disrupted, and a lucent band develops along the metaphysis [**Fig. 7.10A**]. When stress is relieved and bone growth resumes, a growth recovery line of Park will be seen as a curvilinear band of sclerosis at the metaphysis [**Fig. 7.10B**]. Over time this will migrate into the metadiaphysis and diaphysis, and fade into normal mineralization over months to years.

Epiphyseal Variants

Ivory epiphyses are sclerotic-appearing epiphyses most commonly seen in the distal phalanges and occasionally in the middle phalanges. This is often noted at the fifth digit [**Fig. 7.11A**]. This finding is seen in 1 in 300 children. *Cone-shaped epiphyses* are most commonly seen in the distal phalanges [**Fig. 7.11B**]. They may be a normal finding in 5% to 10% of children. When multiple, they may be associated with osteochondrodysplasias such as achondroplasia, Ellis–van Creveld syndrome, and cleidocranial dysostosis. They may also be associated with metabolic bone disease. *Pseudoepiphyses* may be seen in the proximal aspect of the second through fifth metacarpals and metatarsals or distal aspect of the first metacarpals and metatarsals [**Fig. 7.11C**]. These form by 4 to 5 years of age and fuse with the underlying bony shaft at the time of skeletal maturation. Histologically, a true physis is not identified, and pseudoepiphyses contribute little or nothing to linear growth. They are more commonly seen in children with hypothyroidism and cleidocranial dysostosis. *Epiphyseal clefts or fissures* may be seen, most commonly in the great toe, and should not be mistaken for fracture [**Fig. 7.11D**].

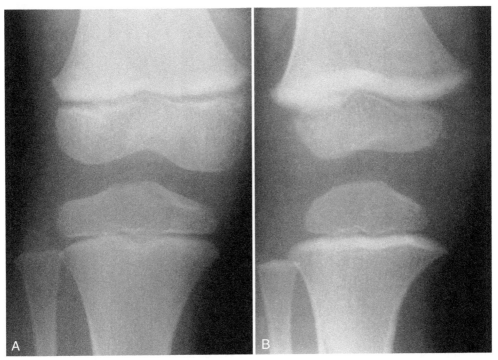

Figure 7.9 Physiologic *versus* pathologic metaphyseal sclerosis. A, Anteroposterior (AP) radiograph of the right knee demonstrates physiologic sclerosis along the metaphyses of the distal femur and proximal tibia. **B,** AP radiograph of the right knee in a different patient with lead poisoning shows thicker "lead lines" along the metaphyses of all bones of the knee, including the more slowly growing fibula.

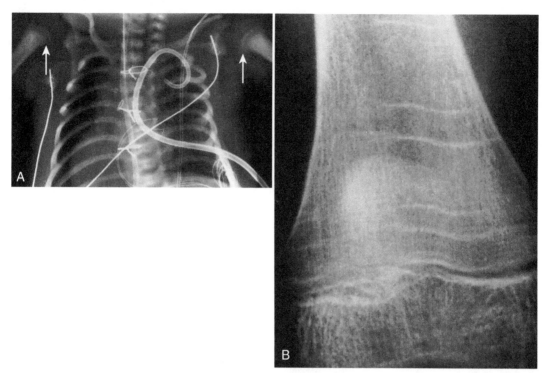

Figure 7.10 Growth arrest and recovery lines. A, Portable chest radiograph of an infant in the intensive care unit with complex congenital heart disease. Prominent lucent bands are seen along the proximal humeral metaphyses (*arrows*) reflecting disordered endochondral ossification in the setting of illness. **B,** Anteroposterior radiograph of the distal femur in a patient with cystic fibrosis and recurrent bouts of pulmonary infection demonstrates multiple thin, curvilinear, sclerotic growth recovery lines along the metaphysis and metadiaphysis.

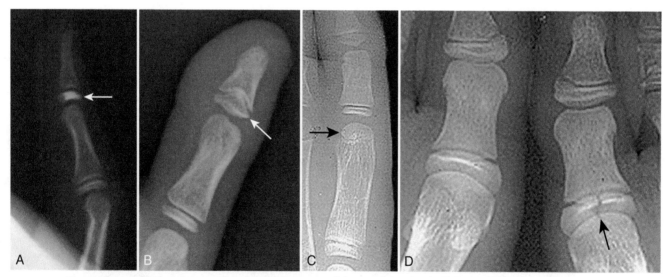

Figure 7.11 Epiphyseal normal variants. A, Ivory epiphysis at the distal phalanx of the fifth digit (*arrow*). **B,** Cone-shaped epiphysis at the distal phalanx of the fifth digit (*arrow*). **C,** Pseudoepiphysis at the distal aspect of the thumb metacarpal (*arrow*). **D,** Cleft epiphysis at the base of the proximal phalanx of the thumb (*arrow*).

Metaphyseal Variants

Metaphyseal irregularity is commonly seen in the bones of the knee and wrist. A metaphyseal step-off, spur, or "beak" may be noted [**Fig. 7.12**]. It is important to recognize these variants and be able to distinguish them from the classic metaphyseal lesions or bucket handle fractures seen in infants in the setting of child abuse.

Apophyseal Variants

The apophyses of the developing skeleton can have a widely varied appearance, and apophyseal irregularity is common. The apophysis at the fifth metatarsal base is a common source of confusion. This apophysis first appears during puberty. It may be in close approximation to the parent bone, or it may be somewhat distracted in the normal setting. A normal apophysis

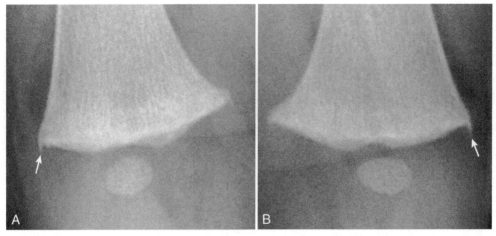

Figure 7.12 **Prominent periosteal collars in a 5-month-old infant born at 23 weeks' gestational age.** This infant presented with respiratory distress, and a skeletal survey was performed because of concern for possible child abuse. Radiographs of the bilateral knees demonstrate normal variant metaphyseal "beaking" at the distal femoral metaphyses (*arrows*).

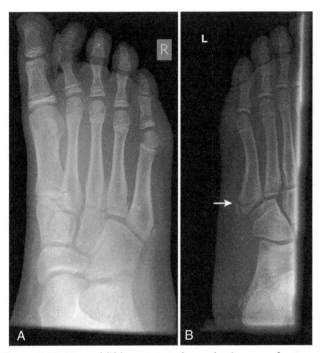

Figure 7.13 **Normal fifth metatarsal apophysis versus fracture. A,** Oblique radiograph of the right foot shows a normal apophysis at the fifth metatarsal base. **B,** Oblique radiograph of the left foot in a different patient demonstrates an unfused apophysis at the fifth metatarsal base and an additional transverse lucency reflecting a nondisplaced fracture (*arrow*).

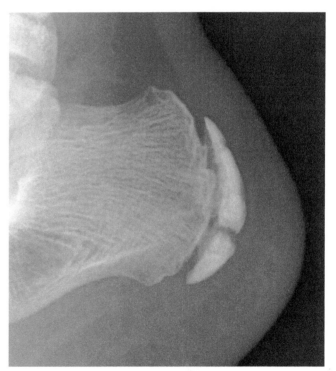

Figure 7.14 **Normal calcaneal apophysis.** Lateral radiograph of the ankle demonstrates a sclerotic and somewhat fragmented calcaneal apophysis in a patient with no symptoms referable to the hindfoot.

may be bifid or even somewhat fragmented. Attention to the surrounding soft tissues and correlation with focal symptoms and physical examination findings are important for diagnostic accuracy [**Fig. 7.13**].

The calcaneal apophysis first appears around 7 years of age. It forms from the coalescence of multiple ossifications centers which fuse in the teenage years. Before fusion with the body of the calcaneus, the normal apophysis may be quite fragmented and sclerotic [**Fig. 7.14**]. This appearance sometimes raises concern for calcaneal apophysitis, or Sever disease. This diagnosis is best made on clinical grounds rather than radiographic findings. MRI may be supportive, demonstrating apophyseal edema.

Irregular Ossification

Ossification of cartilage is not a smooth, uninterrupted process; thus irregular ossification patterns are common. This is classically seen in the epiphysis of the distal femur in younger children. Rapid growth and ossification of this epiphysis typically occurs in children between 2 and 6 years of age. During this time, the medial and lateral ends of the epiphysis may appear shaggy and irregular [**Fig. 7.9B**]. This is a normal appearance that should not be mistaken for pathology.

In older children, focal areas of irregular ossification can be seen along the posterior femoral condyles and may mimic

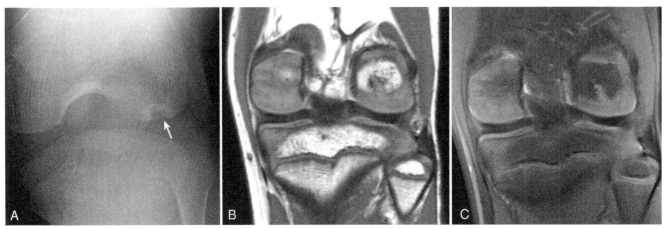

Figure 7.15 **Normal variant focus of irregular ossification. A,** Notch view of the left knee demonstrates a crescentic-shaped focus of lucency with surrounding sclerosis along the posterior aspect of the lateral femoral condyle (*arrow*). **B,** Coronal proton density (PD) and (**C**) coronal PD fat-saturated magnetic resonance images show a corresponding focus of unossified cartilage, without evidence of undercutting fluid or surrounding marrow signal abnormality. The overlying bony cortex and cartilage are normal.

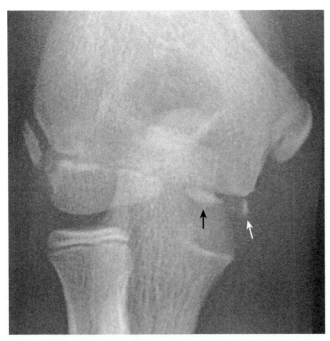

Figure 7.16 **Normal trochlear ossification.** Anteroposterior view of the right elbow shows an irregular, fragmented trochlear ossification center (*arrows*), a normal finding.

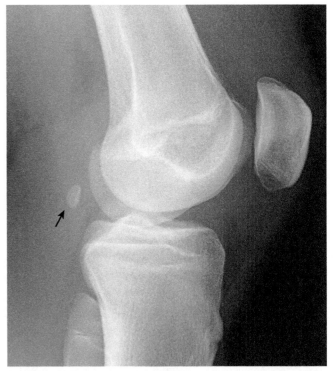

Figure 7.17 **Normal variant fabella.** Lateral radiograph of the left knee demonstrates a prominent sesamoid bone within the lateral head of the gastrocnemius muscle along the posterior aspect of the lateral femoral condyle (*arrow*).

osteochondritis dissecans (OCD) [**Fig. 7.15**]. This normal variant is seen in up to 30% of children, most commonly between 8 and 10 years of age. It is most frequent along the posterior aspect of the lateral femoral condyle. OCD typically affects somewhat older children, and it is most common along the lateral aspect of the medial femoral condyle. With a normal variant, MRI will show a focal area of residual normal-appearing, unossified cartilage overlying the focal area of irregular ossification [**Fig. 7.15**]. The characteristic MRI findings of OCD, including undercutting fluid, cystic change, overlying cartilage abnormality, and surrounding marrow edema, will not be present.

Irregular ossification patterns are also often seen at the proximal humeral epiphysis, proximal femoral epiphysis, and navicular bone. The ossification centers at the elbow may

also be irregular as they come in, most notably the trochlea [**Fig. 7.16**].

Sesamoid Bones

Sesamoid bones lie within tendinous insertion sites. The largest sesamoid bone in the body is the patella, which lies within the tendon of the quadriceps muscle. Two other sesamoid bones of the knee are the more common fabella within the lateral head of the gastrocnemius muscle [**Fig. 7.17**] and the

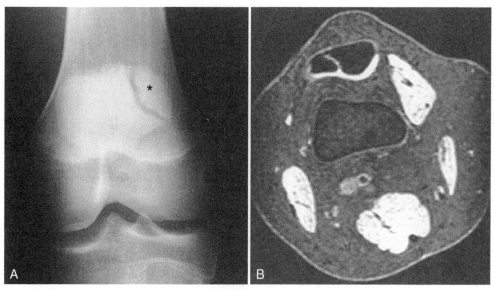

Figure 7.18 Bipartite patella. A, Anteroposterior radiograph of the left knee demonstrates a large unfused accessory ossicle along the superolateral aspect of the patella (*asterisk*). **B,** Axial gradient echo magnetic resonance image shows normal signal in the synchondrosis between this ossicle and the parent bone, and no marrow edema in the patella.

less common cyamella within the tendon of the popliteus muscle.

Sesamoid bones are very common in the hands and feet. At the first ray of the foot, sesamoids are seen within the medial and lateral slips of the hallux brevis tendon at the level of the first metatarsal head. The medial sesamoid is frequently bipartite, which may be challenging to distinguish from fracture in the setting of trauma. Chronic stress-related change, or sesamoiditis, is often seen in this location. MRI is helpful in the evaluation of acute trauma and also chronic inflammatory change.

Accessory Ossicles

Accessory ossicles are common and may be unilateral or bilateral. They may be asymptomatic and discovered incidentally, or may be associated with pain and/or susceptible to trauma. A *bipartite patella* is one example. This typically develops between 10 and 12 years of age and may persist into adulthood. The accessory ossicle is superolateral in position and appears after the ossification centers of the main body of the patella have fused [**Fig. 7.18**]. This variant is seen in 1% to 6% of the population. It is much more common in males (90%) and is bilateral in 40% of cases. Stress injury or acute fracture may occur at the synchondrosis between the accessory ossicle and the parent bone, producing symptoms.

The *accessory navicular ossicle* is also common. This is seen in more than 20% of individuals, and is frequently bilateral. The ossicle is seen along the medial aspect of the parent navicular bone where the tibialis posterior tendon inserts. Three types are described [**Fig. 7.19**]. A type I variant is a rounded ossicle measuring 2 to 6 mm. It is a true sesamoid bone, lying within the tibialis posterior tendon. It is usually asymptomatic, and typically does not fuse with the parent bone. The type II variant is larger, measuring 9 to 12 mm. It is connected to the parent navicular by a fibrous or cartilaginous synchondrosis. It is often symptomatic, and usually ultimately fuses with the parent navicular. A type III variant is also referred to as a cornuate navicular. There is no separate ossicle; rather, there is medial and plantar elongation of the navicular bone. This variant may be symptomatic.

An *os trigonum* is seen at the posterior aspect of the talus in approximately 15% of individuals [**Fig. 7.20**]. This ossicle may predispose to posterior ankle impingement, the so-called os trigonum syndrome. This is particularly common in athletes who participate in activities that require repetitive forced plantar flexion, such as ballet dancers who dance en pointe.

Upper Extremity

The *supracondylar process* of the humerus is a pedunculated bony excrescence emanating from the medial aspect of anterior humeral shaft 5 to 7 cm proximal to the medial epicondyle [**Fig. 7.21**]. This structure "points" to the joint. It is seen in 1% of individuals. It is most often asymptomatic but may be associated with a median nerve neuralgia.

An *os styloideum*, or *carpal boss*, is an accessory ossicle at the dorsal aspect of the wrist between the trapezium, capitate, and base of the second and third metacarpals [**Fig. 7.22**]. It is seen in 1% to 3% of individuals and presents as a palpable mass.

Lower Extremity

Irregularity of the posteromedial aspect of the distal femoral metaphysis is very common [**Fig. 7.23**]. It is sometimes referred to as a *cortical desmoid*. This is a "tug" lesion related to the origin of the medial head of the gastrocnemius muscle or adductor muscle insertion. It is important to be familiar with this entity, as it can sometimes appear quite irregular and may be mistaken for pathology.

A *dorsal defect of the patella* is a focal anomaly of ossification at the superolateral aspect of the dorsal patella. It is seen as a well-circumscribed lucency on radiographs [**Fig. 7.24A**]. On MRI, the cartilage overlying this defect is intact [**Fig. 7.24B**]. This lesion is typically asymptomatic. It must be differentiated from an OCD of the patella.

Accessory ossification centers may be seen inferior to the medial malleolus (*os subtibialis*) or lateral malleolus (*os subfibularis*) [**Fig. 7.25**]. These accessory ossicles typically have a smooth contour and corticated margins. The differential diagnostic consideration is an avulsion injury.

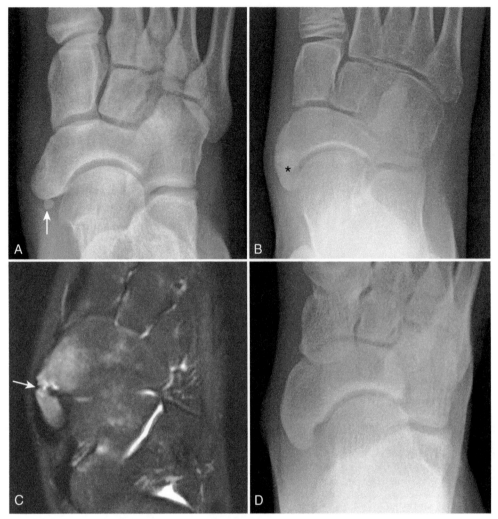

Figure 7.19 Accessory navicular ossicles. A, Anteroposterior (AP) radiograph of the foot demonstrates a small type I accessory navicular ossicle (*arrow*). This was an incidental finding in a patient without symptoms referable to this area. **B,** AP radiograph and (**C**) coronal footprint fast spin-echo inversion-recovery magnetic resonance (MR) image of the foot in a different patient demonstrate a larger type II accessory navicular ossicle (*asterisk*). On MR imaging, there is increased fluid signal in the synchondrosis between the ossicle and the parent bone (*arrow*), and surrounding marrow edema is seen. This patient was symptomatic with pain. **D,** AP radiograph demonstrates a type III accessory navicular with a cornuate configuration in an asymptomatic patient.

A *calcaneal pseudocyst* presents as a triangular-shaped area of radiolucency in the anterior calcaneus [**Fig. 7.26A**]. This appearance is due to a relative deficiency of spongy bone in this location, rather than the presence of a true bony lesion. A simple bone cyst or an intraosseous lipoma may have a similar appearance [**Fig. 7.26B and C**]. When the diagnosis is not clear, CT or MRI may be helpful to distinguish these entities.

Pelvis

An accessory ossification center may develop in the cartilage of the acetabular rim, referred to as an *os acetabuli.* This typically appears in the second decade of life and subsequently fuses with the parent bone. This entity must be distinguished from an acetabular rim fracture.

The *ischiopubic synchondrosis* forms from two metaphyseal equivalents at the ischial and pubic bones. Irregularity and asymmetry of the synchondrosis is very commonly seen before fusion [**Fig. 7.27**]. This is most often an incidental, asymptomatic finding. Fusion/ossification is highly variable, but usually occurs by the teenage years.

CONSTITUTIONAL DISORDERS OF BONE

Skeletal Dysplasias

Skeletal dysplasias are defined as congenital disturbances of bone growth, structure, and modeling. Shortening of the limbs or the spine below the third percentile for a normal newborn constitutes congenital dwarfism.

Short stature may be symmetric or asymmetric. Symmetric short stature includes short-limb dwarfism, short-trunk dwarfism, and proportionate short stature.

Short-limb dwarfism is classified according to the appendicular skeletal segment involved. *Rhizomelia* involves the proximal appendicular skeleton, with shortening of the humeri and femurs. *Mesomelia* involved the middle appendicular segments, with shortening of the bones of the forearms and lower legs. With *acromelia,* there is shortening of the distal portions of the appendicular skeleton, including the metacarpals, metatarsals, and phalanges of the hands and feet.

Short-trunk dwarfism may be seen in the neonatal period as fatal achondrogenesis. In surviving infants it manifests as the

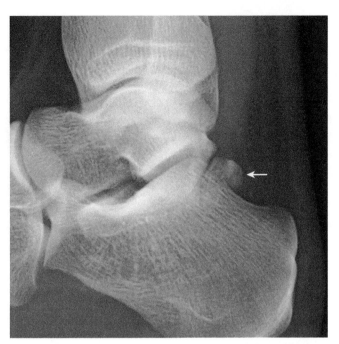

Figure 7.20 Os trigonum. Lateral radiograph of the ankle demonstrates a prominent ossicle along the posterior aspect of the talocalcaneal joint (*arrow*).

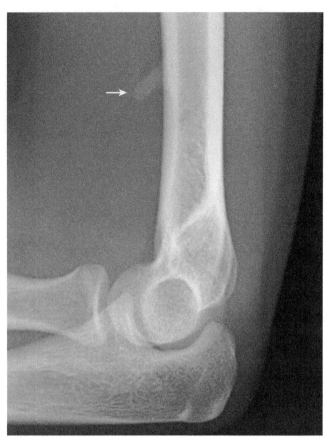

Figure 7.21 Supracondylar process. Lateral radiograph of the elbow shows a small bony excrescence arising from the anterior aspect of the distal humeral shaft and "pointing" toward the elbow joint (*arrow*).

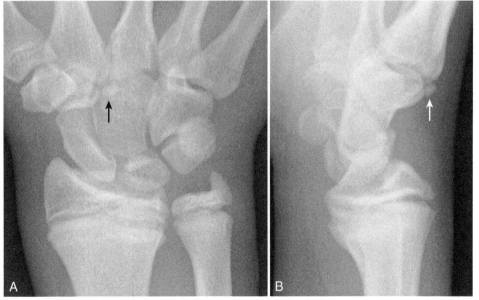

Figure 7.22 Os styloideum/carpal boss. A, Posteroanterior and (**B**) lateral radiographs of the right wrist demonstrate a small ossicle at the dorsal aspect of the wrist at the base of the second and third metacarpals (*arrows*). This patient presented with a palpable lump.

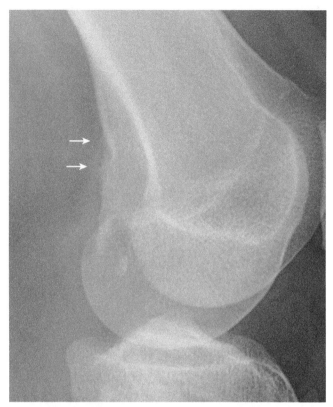

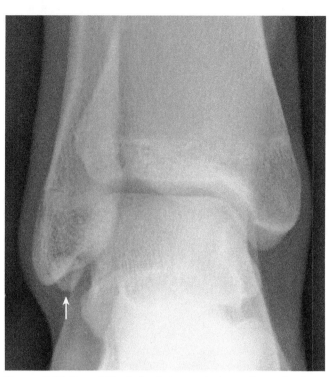

Figure 7.25 Os subfibularis. Anteroposterior radiograph of the right ankle demonstrates a prominent ossicle inferior to the lateral malleolus (*arrow*).

Figure 7.23 Distal femoral metaphyseal irregularity/cortical desmoid. Lateral radiograph of the knee demonstrates irregularity at the medial aspect of the distal femoral metaphysis (*arrows*), a normal variant appearance related to the insertion of the medial head of the gastrocnemius muscle or adductors.

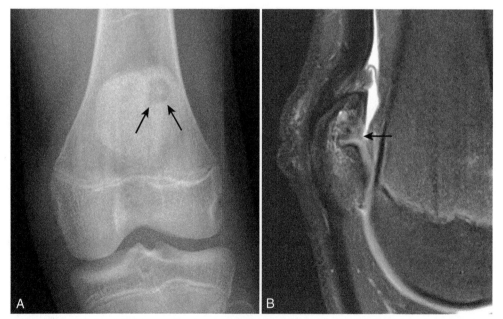

Figure 7.24 Dorsal defect of the patella. A, Anteroposterior radiograph of the left knee demonstrates a well-circumscribed lucency in the superolateral aspect of the patella (*arrows*). **B,** Sagittal T2 fat-saturated magnetic resonance image shows intact cartilage invaginating into and lining this defect (*arrow*).

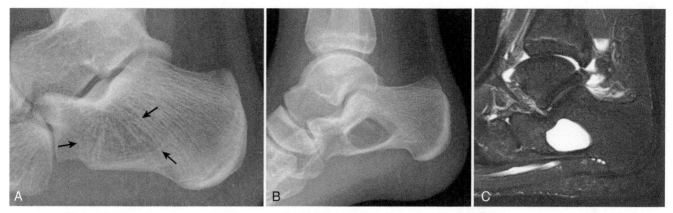

Figure 7.26 Calcaneal pseudocyst versus simple bone cyst. A, Lateral radiograph of the ankle demonstrates a normal area of rarefaction in the trabecular matrix of the calcaneus (*arrows*). **B,** Lateral view of the ankle in a different patient demonstrates a well-circumscribed, benign-appearing lucent lesion in the calcaneus. **C,** Sagittal T2 fat-saturated magnetic resonance image of the patient in **B** confirms a simple-appearing fluid-filled lesion compatible with a unicameral bone cyst.

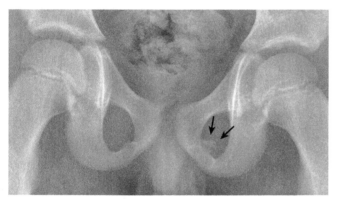

Figure 7.27 Ischiopubic synchondrosis. Anteroposterior radiograph of the pelvis shows marked irregularity of the left ischiopubic synchondrosis (*arrows*), with an asymmetric appearance to the right side. The patient did not have symptoms referable to this area, and a smooth, symmetric appearance developed over time.

metaphyseal chondrodysplasias, and in developing children as the mucopolysaccharidoses, the mucolipidoses, or spondyloepiphyseal dysplasia.

Proportionate short stature may be normal, may result from a variety of systemic conditions, or may be seen in the setting of entities such as cleidocranial dysostosis.

Asymmetric short stature is seen in entities such as osteogenesis imperfecta (OI) and multiple hereditary exostoses.

Symmetric Short Stature

Short-Limb Dwarfism

Rhizomelic Shortening. Thanatophoric dysplasia, achondroplasia, and hypochondroplasia are forms of rhizomelic dwarfism. These entities develop because of variable mutations in the *fibroblast growth factor receptor type 3 (FGFR3)* gene, which encodes a protein responsible for the velocity of endochondral growth.

Thanatophoric ("death-bearing") dwarfism is the most common lethal skeletal dysplasia. This condition is nearly uniformly fatal, although there are rare cases of survival. Classic features include a "cloverleaf skull" caused by in utero craniosynostosis, curved long bones, dysmorphic femurs with a

"French telephone receiver" appearance, and severe platyspondyly [**Fig. 7.28**].

Achondroplasia is the most common skeletal dysplasia overall. This form of dwarfism is characterized by autosomal dominant inheritance, although the majority of cases are sporadic. Affected individuals have a normal or near-normal life span and normal mentation. An enlarged skull is seen, with frontal bossing and midface hypoplasia. The skull base is small, with a tight foramen magnum predisposing to cervicomedullary compression and related symptoms. The thorax is small, and the ribs are shortened and splayed anteriorly. The pedicles of the spine are short, and there is narrowing of the interpediculate distances progressing inferiorly along the spine. These features are associated with an increased risk for spinal stenosis. There is posterior vertebral body scalloping, kyphoscoliosis with gibbus deformity, and a profound lumbar lordosis. The iliac bones have a square shape and the acetabular roofs are flattened, leading to a "tombstone" configuration. The sacroiliac notches are narrow, giving the pelvic inlet a "champagne glass" appearance. The humeri and femurs are short, and the fibulas appear overgrown. Metaphyseal cupping is seen, with a V-shaped physeal margin ("chevron deformity") [**Fig. 7.29**].

Hypochondroplasia is a relatively milder form of rhizomelic dwarfism. This entity typically manifests in late childhood with clinical and radiographic findings that are similar to but less severe than those seen in achondroplasia.

Mesomelic/Acromelic Shortening. The mesomelic dysplasias are rare. Acromelic dysplasias are relatively more common and include asphyxiating thoracic dystrophy (Jeune syndrome) and chondroectodermal dysplasia (Ellis–van Creveld syndrome). *Asphyxiating thoracic dystrophy* is a genetically heterogeneous disorder with a variable prognosis. Patients may present in infancy with respiratory distress caused by significantly shortened ribs with a small chest. Recurrent pulmonary infections, hypertension, and renal failure caused by progressive nephropathy may develop later in life. Characteristic radiographic findings include short, horizontal ribs with bulbous anterior ends and a long, tubular thorax. The iliac wings are small, short, and flared, and "trident acetabula" are seen [**Fig. 7.30**]. The tubular bones of the hands and feet are shortened, and polydactyly is seen in up to one third of affected individuals.

Similar findings are seen in *chondroectodermal dysplasia,* an autosomal recessive, nonlethal disorder that is relatively common in the Amish community. Additional clinical manifestations include hypoplastic, brittle nails; thin, sparse hair; and dental

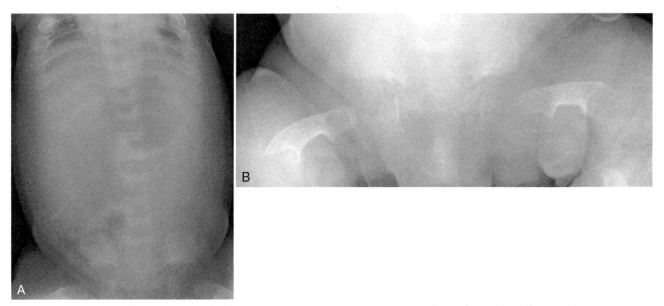

Figure 7.28 Thanatophoric dysplasia. A, Anteroposterior (AP) supine radiograph of the abdomen demonstrates diffuse platyspondyly. **B,** AP radiograph of the pelvis shows the characteristic "French telephone receiver" appearance of the femurs.

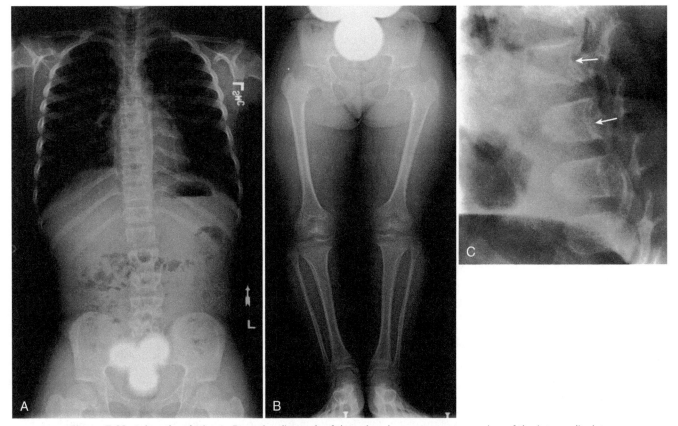

Figure 7.29 Achondroplasia. A, Frontal radiograph of the spine demonstrates narrowing of the interpediculate distances progressing inferiorly along the lumbar spine. The iliac bones have a "tombstone" configuration, and the acetabular roofs are flattened. **B,** Frontal radiograph of the lower extremities from the hips to the ankles shows relatively short femurs, overgrown fibulas, and a "chevron deformity" along the distal femoral physes. The pelvic inlet has a "champagne glass" appearance. **C,** Lateral radiograph of the lumbar spine demonstrates posterior vertebral body scalloping (*arrows*).

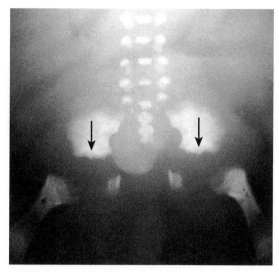

Figure 7.30 **Asphyxiating thoracic dystrophy/Jeune syndrome.** Anteroposterior radiograph of the pelvis demonstrates small, short iliac wings with characteristic "trident acetabula" (*arrows*).

abnormalities. Congenital heart disease is seen in two thirds of patients, with an atrial or ventricular septal defect being most common. Polydactyly is almost always present [**Fig. 7.31**].

Short-Trunk Dwarfism

Achondrogenesis/Hypochondrogenesis. Several forms of short-trunk dwarfism exist with varied levels of severity. The most severe form is *achondrogenesis*, which is fatal in the neonatal period. Affected infants have a large skull, a small thorax with short ribs, lack of mineralization of the spine and ischial and pubic bones of the pelvis, and significant micromelia (shortening of the proximal and distal segments of the appendicular skeleton). *Hypochondrogenesis* is a less severe variant, with infants typically surviving a few months.

Metaphyseal Chondrodysplasias. In surviving infants with short-trunk dwarfism, four types of metaphyseal chondrodysplasias are seen which vary in severity. Affected infants have a large head, severe micromelia, and bowed limbs. With the autosomal dominant *Jansen and Schmid types,* irregular metaphyses and widened physes are seen. With the autosomal recessive *McKusick type* and *Shwachman-Diamond dysplasia,* epiphyseal flattening and metaphyseal irregularity are noted.

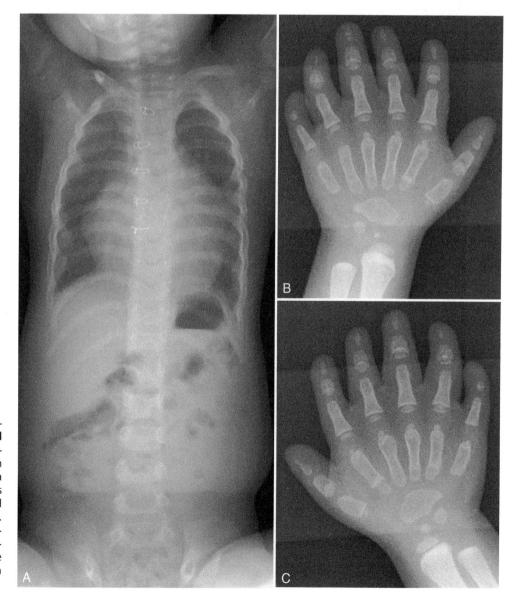

Figure 7.31. **Chondroectodermal dysplasia/Ellis–van Creveld syndrome. A,** Frontal radiograph of the chest and abdomen demonstrates short ribs and a long, tubular thorax. The heart is enlarged, with changes related to prior cardiac surgery noted. **B** and **C,** Posteroanterior radiographs of the hands show bilateral postaxial polydactyly. The carpus appears dysmorphic on both sides.

Rarer forms of short-trunk dwarfism which manifest early in life include *Kniest dysplasia* and *spondylometaphyseal dysplasia,* both with autosomal dominant inheritance. Radiographic findings include platyspondyly, anterior vertebral body wedging, and abnormal kyphosis, lordosis, or scoliosis. The metaphyses are irregular, and ossification of the epiphyses is often delayed.

Dysostosis Multiplex. Dysostosis multiplex refers to a group of storage diseases associated with skeletal dysplasia. This group includes the mucopolysaccharidoses *Hurler syndrome, Hunter syndrome,* and *Morquio syndrome.* The mucopolysaccharidoses typically present in late infancy or early childhood. Definitive diagnosis is made by a geneticist with documentation of a specific enzymatic deficiency; however, the radiologist may first suggest the presence of a mucopolysaccharidosis. Radiographic findings are similar for Hurler and Hunter syndromes. A J-shaped sella turcica is often noted. The ribs are oar or paddle shaped, thin posteriorly and thickened anteriorly. There is characteristic inferior beaking at the anterior aspect of the vertebral bodies with a gibbus deformity, or focal kyphosis at the level of the thoracolumbar junction [**Fig. 7.32**]. The acetabular roofs are often steep and irregular. At the hands, the proximal metacarpals are tapered. Some imaging features of Morquio syndrome overlap with those seen in Hurler and Hunter syndromes. A notable distinction is beaking of the central (rather than inferior) portion of the anterior vertebral bodies [**Fig. 7.33**].

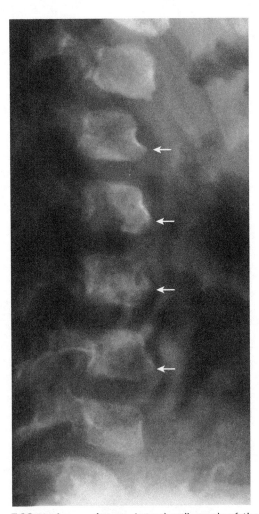

Figure 7.32 Hurler syndrome. Lateral radiograph of the spine demonstrates beaking at the anterior, inferior aspect of the vertebral bodies (*arrows*).

Proportionate Short Stature. Proportionate short stature may be normal, as approximately 2% of all children measure below the third percentile on growth charts. It may also be seen in the setting of various systemic conditions including renal and nutritional disorders. Proportionate short stature is also often seen in children with chromosomal abnormalities.

Cleidocranial dysostosis is a relatively common autosomal dominant disorder characterized by cranial, clavicular, rib, and pelvic abnormalities. There is delayed closure of the fontanelles, and the cranial sutures are wide with wormian bones often present. The cranium is enlarged and brachycephalic. There is hypoplasia or absence of the clavicles. Eleven pairs of ribs are often seen, which may be shortened and downsloping. Delayed ossification of the symphysis pubis is common, with apparent widening on radiographs [**Fig. 7.34**]. Affected patients develop normally and have a normal life span.

Asymmetric Short Stature

A relatively common entity associated with asymmetric short stature is osteogenesis imperfecta (OI). OI is an inherited disorder characterized by abnormal formation of type I collagen. Boys and girls are equally affected. Many different mutations have been identified, and there is a wide spectrum of clinical presentations. Historically, this condition has been divided into an autosomal recessive congenital form, which is often fatal (10%), and an autosomal dominant "tarda" form, which is clinically less severe (90%). Many types are now described. All forms of disease are characterized by osteopenia and a propensity for fractures. In the congenital form, thickened, tubular bones are seen as a result of multiple healing fractures. In the tarda from, the bones have a thin, gracile appearance. Other clinical manifestations of disease include blue sclera, poor dentition, and deafness related to otosclerosis. Radiographic findings may include diffuse osteopenia, multiple fractures of different ages, long bone bowing deformities, and wormian bones in the skull [**Fig. 7.35**].

Tarda forms of disease are often treated with bisphosphonate therapy to increase bone calcium deposition. Intramedullary rods are used to correct bowing deformities and help prevent new fractures.

Chromosomal Disorders

Skeletal abnormalities are often seen in association with chromosomal disorders. *Trisomy 21/Down syndrome* is the most common chromosomal syndrome overall. Skeletal manifestations include short stature, atlantoaxial instability, 11 pairs of ribs, hypersegmentation of the sternum, flared iliac wings, and hip dysplasia, which may be seen in up to 40% of affected individuals [**Fig. 7.36**]. *Turner syndrome* is seen in the setting of a 45, XO chromosomal pattern. Short stature, short fourth metacarpals, Madelung deformity, and osteopenia are characteristic.

Focal Congenital Anomalies of Bone

Proximal focal femoral deficiency is a congenital disorder consisting of a spectrum of abnormalities that may range from mild shortening and hypoplasia of the proximal femur to complete absence of the acetabulum, femoral head, and proximal femur [**Fig. 7.37**]. It is bilateral in 15% of cases. This abnormality is thought to result from abnormal development and proliferation of chondrocytes in the proximal femoral physis in prenatal life. The acetabulum is secondarily affected. Ipsilateral fibular hemimelia (see the following paragraph) is present in more than 50% of cases. Ipsilateral foot deformities such as equinovalgus deformity are also often associated. Goals for management include maximizing the length of the affected extremity, optimizing alignment, and promoting joint stability.

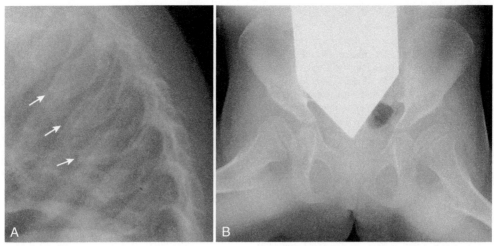

Figure 7.33 Morquio syndrome. A, Lateral radiograph of the thoracic spine demonstrates beaking of the central portion of the anterior vertebral bodies (*arrows*). **B,** Frog-leg lateral image of the pelvis shows steep acetabula and flattened, broad femoral heads.

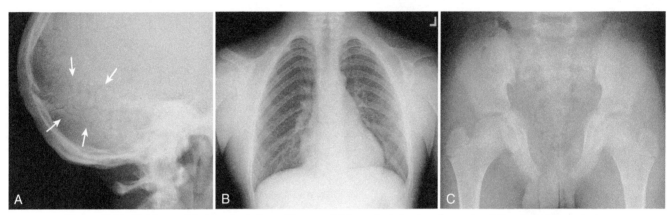

Figure 7.34 Cleidocranial dysostosis in a 13-year-old boy. A, Lateral radiograph of the skull demonstrates multiple wormian bones in the lambdoid sutures (*arrows*). **B,** Frontal radiograph of the chest shows absent clavicles. **C,** Anteroposterior image of the pelvis demonstrates apparent widening of the symphysis pubis related to delayed ossification.

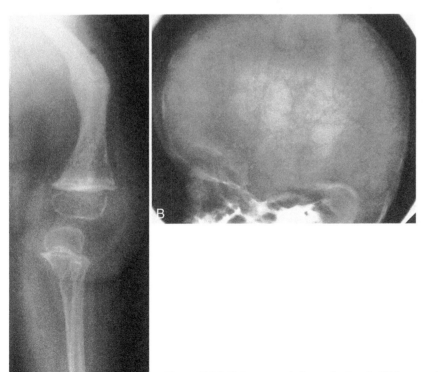

Figure 7.35 Osteogenesis imperfecta. A, Oblique radiograph of the lower extremity demonstrates a healing fracture of the distal femoral diaphysis with significant angulation/bowing deformity. The long bones have a gracile appearance, and there is diffuse osteopenia. **B,** Lateral radiograph of the skull demonstrates multiple prominent wormian bones.

Hemimelia is defined as the congenital absence of all or part of a limb. *Fibular hemimelia* is most common overall. Fibular abnormality may range from mild deficiency of the proximal fibula to complete absence of the bone [**Fig. 7.38**]. Associated abnormalities of the ipsilateral lower extremity are common and may include a short, bowed tibia, femoral shortening or

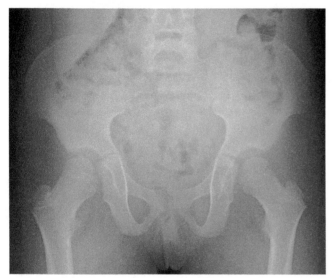

Figure 7.36 Trisomy 21/Down syndrome. Anteroposterior radiograph of the pelvis demonstrates flared iliac wings.

hypoplasia, tarsal coalition, clubfoot deformity, and absent lateral rays of the foot.

Radial dysplasia consists of a spectrum of abnormalities involving the upper extremity. Complete absence of the radius is most common, although hypoplasia may also be seen. The forearm is typically short and bowed, and there is radial deviation of the hand. The first metacarpal and/or thumb is often hypoplastic or absent [**Fig. 7.39**]. Bilateral abnormality is seen in up to 50% of cases. Radial dysplasia is seen in association with a number of syndromes, including Holt-Oram syndrome (associated with congenital heart disease), VACTERL association (*v*ertebral anomalies, *a*nal atresia, *c*ardiac anomalies, *t*racheo-esophageal fistula, *r*enal anomalies, and *l*imb anomalies), Fanconi anemia, and thrombocytopenia-absent radius syndrome. Management includes serial casting or splinting to improve radial deviation of the hand, surgical centralization of the hand over the ulna, and reconstruction of the thumb with pollicization of the index finger.

Amniotic band syndrome results when constricting amniotic bands form in utero and disrupt the amnion from the chorion. As the amnion separates, adhesions form which can entrap and constrict parts of the developing fetus. This may result in amputations, soft tissue syndactyly, and less commonly bony syndactyly [**Fig. 7.40**]. Surgical treatment is primarily cosmetic.

Tarsal coalition is an abnormal connection between two or more tarsal bones due to a congenital failure of segmentation. The connection may be osseous, cartilaginous, or fibrous in nature. Talocalcaneal and calcaneonavicular coalitions are most common. Coalition affects approximately 1% of the population and is bilateral in more than 50% of affected individuals. Patients most often present in the second decade of life with pain. There

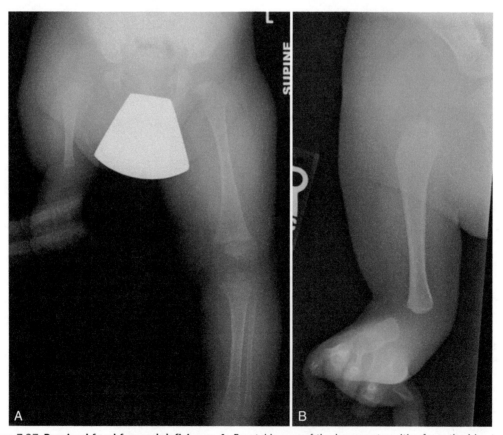

Figure 7.37 Proximal focal femoral deficiency. A, Frontal image of the lower extremities from the hips to the ankles and (**B**) coned down image of the right lower extremity demonstrate significant right-sided abnormality. The acetabulum is absent, the femoral head ossification center is small, the femur is hypoplastic, the bones of the lower leg are absent, and foot deformities are present.

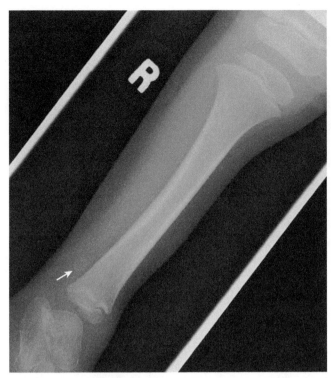

Figure 7.38 Fibular hemimelia. Anteroposterior radiograph of the right lower leg shows a very small, rudimentary distal fibula (*arrow*). The tibia is short and somewhat broad, with undertubulation distally.

may also be flatfoot deformity, limited range of motion, and a propensity for ankle and foot injury.

An osseous coalition may be evident on radiographs. A calcaneonavicular coalition is typically well demonstrated on an oblique radiograph of the foot. An "anteater sign" may be seen on the lateral view, with abnormal elongation of the anterior process of the calcaneus [**Fig. 7.41**]. A talocalcaneal coalition is often more subtle on radiographs, although sometimes a "C sign" can be seen on a lateral view [**Fig. 7.42**]. Secondary radiographic signs of tarsal coalition include pes planus deformity and a talar beak, or dorsal extension of the talar head. A cartilaginous or fibrous coalition is suggested on radiographs by a narrowed joint space between the involved bones, with irregularity of the articular margins.

Cross-sectional imaging is helpful to determine the nature and extent of a tarsal coalition. Osseous coalition is well demonstrated on CT scan [**Figs. 7.41** and **7.42**]. Osseous cartilaginous, and fibrous coalitions are all well seen on MRI, and associated findings such as marrow edema may be noted.

Conservative management includes immobilization with casting or orthotics, nonsteroidal antiinflammatory drugs, and physical therapy. Surgical resection is performed for symptomatic coalition refractory to conservative management. The coalition is excised, with interposition of fat graft or extensor digitorum brevis tendon to halt regrowth. Subtalar arthrodesis or triple arthrodesis (subtalar, calcaneocuboid, and talonavicular) may be performed for advanced cases with a suboptimal response to management with resection.

Sclerosing Bone Dysplasias/Disorders of Increased Bone Density

Osteopetrosis may be caused by several different genetic mutations, all ultimately leading to osteoclast dysfunction. There is a

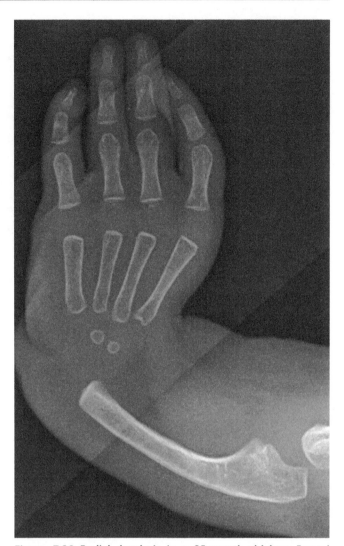

Figure 7.39 Radial dysplasia in a 25-month-old boy. Frontal radiograph of the left forearm and hand demonstrates an absent radius, a short, bowed ulna, radial deviation of the hand, and absence of the first metacarpal and thumb.

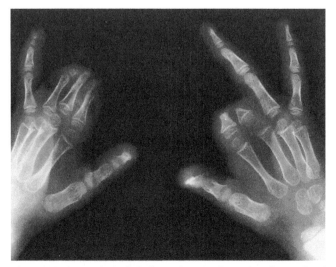

Figure 7.40 Amniotic band syndrome. Frontal radiograph of both hands shows amputation of multiple digits bilaterally.

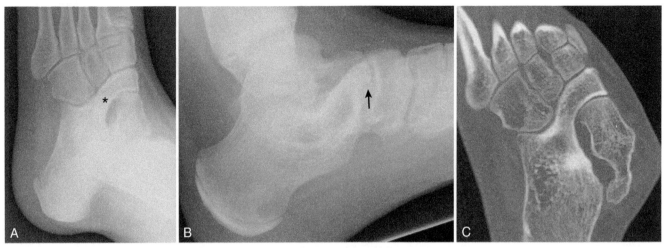

Figure 7.41 Calcaneonavicular coalition. A, Oblique radiograph of the left foot demonstrates an osseous coalition between the calcaneus and the navicular bone (*asterisk*). **B,** Lateral radiograph of the foot shows elongation of the anterior process of the calcaneus, the "anteater sign" (*arrow*). **C,** Oblique axial reformatted computed tomography image shows a calcaneonavicular coalition with patchy surrounding sclerosis.

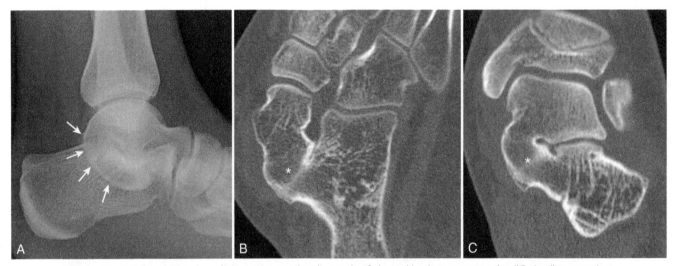

Figure 7.42 Talocalcaneal coalition. A, Lateral radiograph of the ankle demonstrates the "C-sign" suggestive of talocalcaneal coalition (*arrows*). **B,** Axial oblique and (**C**) coronal oblique reformatted computed tomography images confirm an osseous coalition (*asterisks*).

failure of resorption of cartilage and bone matrix, with resultant dense, brittle bones with marrow underdevelopment and a propensity for fractures. For clinical purposes, the different forms of osteopetrosis are distinguished by age at onset. Early-onset, infantile disease is characterized by autosomal recessive inheritance and is most severe. Patients present in infancy with hepatosplenomegaly, pancytopenia, multiple infections, and leukemia. Prognosis is poor, and early death is common. Later-onset ("tarda") forms of disease are characterized by autosomal dominant inheritance and may present in childhood or adolescence. Affected individuals sustain multiple fractures but have a normal life span.

Characteristic radiographic findings of osteopetrosis include diffusely increased bone density, "Erlenmeyer flask" deformity of the metaphyses caused by undertubulation, and a characteristic "bone-within-bone" or "picture frame" appearance [**Fig. 7.43**]. The skull base is thickened, with obliteration of the mastoid air cells and paranasal sinuses and encroachment on the cranial nerves. Although total body calcium levels are typically high, serum calcium levels are often paradoxically low because

nearly all calcium present is bound in highly mineralized, dense bone. Thus superimposed rachitic changes can be seen. Bone marrow transplantation may be curative, replenishing the marrow with normally functioning osteoclasts.

Pyknodysostosis is an autosomal recessive disorder that usually presents in infancy. It is a form of short-limbed, acromelic dwarfism. Patients have short stature, short, broad hands and feet, and micrognathia. Fractures are frequent. On radiographs, there is diffuse osteosclerosis. The cranium is enlarged due to significantly delayed closure of the fontanelles and sutures, and wormian bones may be seen. In the extremities, there is resorption of the phalangeal tufts with an appearance similar to acro-osteolysis. Bony resorption may also be seen at the distal clavicles.

Osteopoikilosis is an autosomal dominant condition characterized by multiple small foci of sclerosis predominantly involving the cancellous bone of the carpal and tarsal bones, pelvis, and scapulae in a periarticular distribution [**Fig. 7.44**]. It is asymptomatic, often picked up incidentally, and does not progress. Lesions may show increased uptake on bone scan.

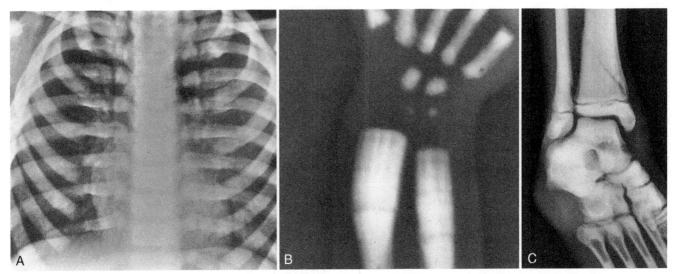

Figure 7.43 Osteopetrosis. A, Frontal radiograph of the chest and (**B**) Posteroanterior image of the right wrist demonstrate diffusely dense bones in a young child with osteopetrosis. **C,** Mortise view of the right ankle in an older child shows a pathologic fracture through the distal tibia in the setting of diffusely increased bone density. The "bone within bone" or "picture frame" appearance is noted, most pronounced in the metatarsals.

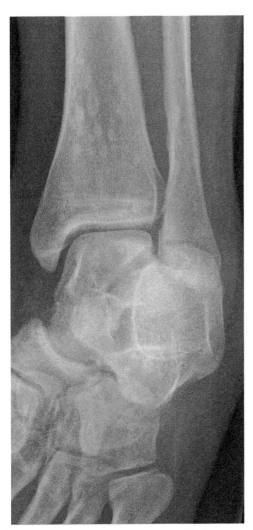

Figure 7.44 Osteopoikilosis in a 16-year-old boy. Mortise radiograph of the left ankle demonstrates numerous small, benign-appearing sclerotic foci in all bones of the ankle.

Osteopathia striata is an asymptomatic entity characterized by bilateral, symmetric, lucent, linear striations in the metadiaphysis of long bones. This may be an isolated finding in the sporadic form of this condition. Alternatively, there may be associated cranial sclerosis in the X-linked dominant form of this entity.

Melorheostosis is an uncommon condition that may be sporadic or may be associated with autosomal dominant inheritance. Disease is usually limited to a single extremity, with the lower extremities more frequently affected than the upper extremities. Children present with limb asymmetry which may be painless or associated with bone pain and joint stiffening. On radiographs, there is dense, linear cortical hyperostosis along the long axis of the bone, often likened to the appearance of dripping candle wax. This entity is associated with increased uptake on bone scan.

Caffey disease (infantile cortical hyperostosis) is an idiopathic condition that occurs in the first few months of life. The average age at onset is 9 weeks, and it is seldom seen beyond the age of 6 months. Boys and girls are equally affected. Clinically, infants present with irritability, low-grade fever, and soft tissue swelling surrounding involved areas. The erythrocyte sedimentation rate may be elevated. On radiographs, there is symmetric periosteal new bone formation with overlying soft tissue edema. The mandible, clavicles, ribs, humeri, ulnae, femurs, scapulae, and radii are most often involved [**Fig. 7.45**]. Disease is usually self-limited, resolving over several months.

SYSTEMIC SKELETAL DISORDERS

Metabolic Disorders

Rickets

Rickets develops because of a relative or absolute deficiency in vitamin D or its derivatives, resulting in failure of mineralization of the normal growing cartilage into bone. There are several causes of rickets. It may be related to nutritional deficiencies, malabsorption of vitamin D, or renal osteodystrophy. It is almost always diagnosed in children younger than 2 years. The clinical manifestations of rickets include failure to thrive, weakness, short stature, bowing deformities, and a predisposition to fractures.

In one third of patients, the radiographic manifestations of rickets may be seen before it is clinically evident. Classic radiographic findings are seen after 4 to 6 weeks of vitamin D deficiency. The rapidly growing physes of the knees and wrists are typically abnormal, with disruption of regulated chondrocyte apoptosis at the ZPC resulting in abnormal endochondral ossification. Mineralization does not occur, and the hypertrophic zone widens. Radiographically, there is physeal widening and cupping, fraying, and irregularity of the metaphysis [**Fig. 7.46**]. Generalized osteopenia is seen. Craniotabes, or a "ping-pong ball" deformity of the skull, may be noted. The classic "rachitic rosary" at the anterior rib ends is not commonly seen today. With treatment, there is mineralization of the ZPC and physeal thickness normalizes. This results in a dense metaphyseal band.

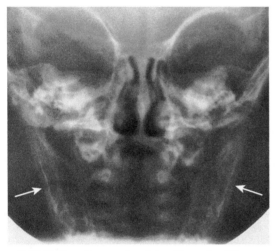

Figure 7.45 **Caffey disease.** Frontal radiograph of the mandible demonstrates symmetric, smooth periosteal new bone formation (*arrows*).

Hyperparathyroidism

Primary hyperparathyroidism is caused by increased parathyroid hormone (PTH) secretion in the setting of a parathyroid adenoma or diffuse parathyroid hyperplasia. These entities are relatively rare in children and are most often associated with the multiple endocrine neoplasia (MEN) syndromes. In secondary hyperparathyroidism, PTH secretion is increased due to chronic hypocalcemia. This is most often caused by chronic renal failure in children, but may also be related to other disorders of calcium metabolism. PTH stimulates the osteoclasts and leads to resorption of bone at multiple sites. The most specific radiographic manifestation of hyperparathyroidism is bony resorption along the radial aspect of the middle phalanges of the second, third, and fourth digits. With more advanced disease, resorption may be seen along the distal clavicles and medial aspects of the humeral and femoral necks and proximal tibial metaphyses [**Fig. 7.47**]. Characteristic brown tumors (osteoclastomas) may be seen, reflecting localized, intraosseous accumulation of fibrous tissue. Generalized osteopenia is characteristic.

Renal Osteodystrophy

Renal osteodystrophy comprises the variety of changes that occur in the skeleton in patients with chronic renal insufficiency. With decreased glomerular filtration, there is retention of phosphate and a slight decrease in calcium levels. This stimulates PTH and results in the mobilization of calcium and phosphate from bone. When there is severe growth failure in the setting of renal osteodystrophy, the radiographic changes of hyperparathyroidism predominate. With skeletal growth, the changes of rickets may be seen. Osteosclerosis is often demonstrated. This may be generalized or may be most pronounced along the vertebral body endplates with the characteristic "rugger jersey spine" appearance [**Fig. 7.48**].

Hypothyroidism

Hypothyroidism is the most common metabolic abnormality diagnosed with routine newborn screening. It most often results

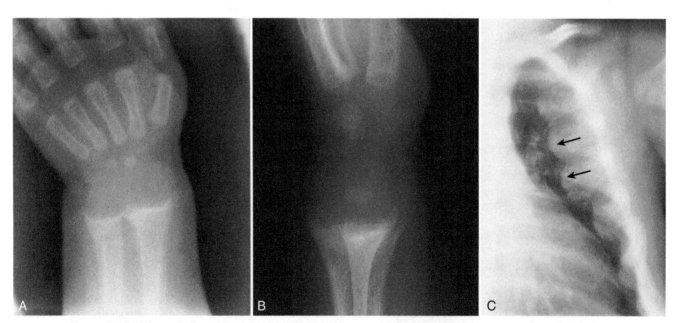

Figure 7.46 **Rickets. A,** Posteroanterior and (**B**) lateral images of the left wrist demonstrate physeal widening and abnormal cupped, frayed, and irregular metaphyses at the distal radius and ulna. **C,** Frontal radiograph of the chest shows the classic "rachitic rosary" appearance of the anterior rib ends (*arrows*). (**C,** From Merten DF. *Pediatric Learning File.* Reston, VA: American College of Radiology Institute; 1987.)

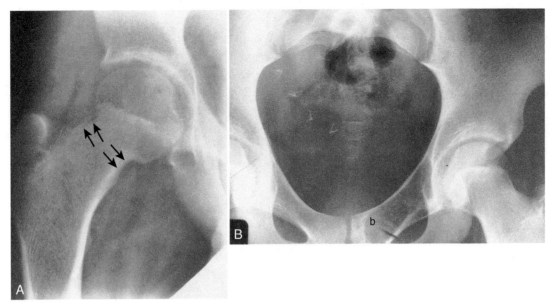

Figure 7.47 **Hyperparathyroidism. A,** Anteroposterior radiograph of the right hip shows subperiosteal resorption along the femoral neck (*arrows*). **B,** Anteroposterior radiograph of the pelvis shows a well-defined lucent lesion in the left superior pubic ramus reflecting a brown tumor (*b*). Surgical sutures are seen in the right lower quadrant related to renal transplantation for chronic glomerulonephritis.

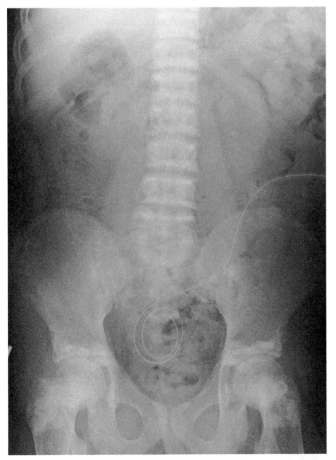

Figure 7.48 **Renal osteodystrophy in a 21-year-old male.** Anteroposterior view of the abdomen demonstrates sclerosis along the superior and inferior vertebral body endplates, with the characteristic "rugger jersey spine" appearance. Patchy sclerosis is also seen in the bones of both hips. A peritoneal dialysis catheter is coiled in the pelvis.

from congenital absence or hypoplasia of the thyroid gland. It occurs three times more frequently in girls than in boys. Thyroid hormone is essential for bone growth and maturation, and also for development of the central nervous system. With deficiency of thyroid hormone, skeletal maturation is delayed out of proportion to linear growth. The bone age is typically greater than two standard deviations below the mean. Epiphyseal dysgenesis is characteristic. Ossification of the epiphyses is delayed, and the pattern of ossification is often irregular. Multiple, fragmented ossification centers may be seen, which eventually coalesce. Epiphyseal margins are typically irregular. There is delay in closure of the cranial sutures, and wormian bones are common. The sella may be enlarged due to pituitary hyperplasia, and brachycephaly may result from decreased growth at the spheno-occipital synchondrosis.

Hypervitaminosis A

Hypervitaminosis A has become rare in the pediatric population. Historically, it has been attributed to the use of fish liver oil and other similar preparations used in the treatment and prevention of xerophthalmia. More recently, it has been linked to high-potency vitamin A analogs used to treat dermatologic disorders. Vitamin A toxicity typically develops at least 6 months after excess intake begins. Clinically, patients present with anorexia, irritability, dry, pruritic skin with desquamation, lip fissuring, focal areas of swelling and pain along the extremities, and hepatomegaly.

Radiographically, exuberant periosteal new bone formation is seen along the ulnae, metatarsals, and phalanges. Undulating cortical thickening may be noted. The main differential diagnostic consideration is infantile cortical hyperostosis, or Caffey disease. These two entities may be distinguished based on patient age and distribution of disease. Caffey disease is most often seen in the first few months of life, whereas hypervitaminosis A most commonly presents between 1 and 3 years of age. With Caffey disease, hyperostosis along the mandible and clavicles is classically seen. A unique radiographic feature of vitamin A toxicity is premature central growth plate closure, resulting in a cone-shaped epiphysis with invagination into the metaphysis.

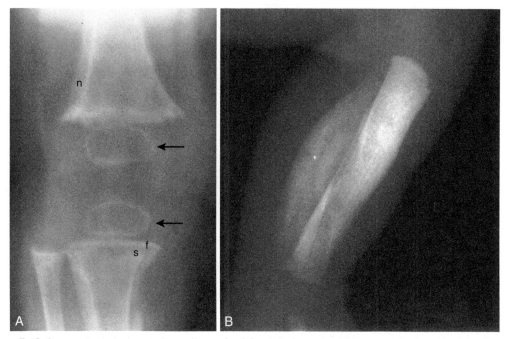

Figure 7.49 Scurvy. A, Anteroposterior radiograph of the right knee demonstrates a dense white line of scurvy/ white line of Frankel (*f*) along the metaphyses related to diminished resorption of calcified cartilage. Subjacent to this, the lucent scurvy zone (*s*) is seen. Corresponding to these metaphyseal findings, a "Wimberger ring" is seen at the distal femoral and proximal tibial epiphyses (*arrows*). A rim of calcified cartilage surrounds a central area of lucency. There is subperiosteal new bone formation (*n*) along the distal femur and proximal tibia, and the bones are diffusely osteopenic. **B,** Sequelae of remote fracture of the distal tibial metaphysis are demonstrated, with subperiosteal hemorrhage and subsequent mineralization.

Clinical symptoms and radiographic abnormalities resolve with cessation of vitamin A intake.

Scurvy

Scurvy is a metabolic bone disease that is rarely seen today. It is caused by a dietary deficiency of vitamin C. Historically, it was seen in babies fed pasteurized or boiled milk. Today, it is occasionally seen in children with highly selective diets. It almost always presents after 6 months of age. Lack of vitamin C results in poor bone matrix/collagen formation, with several characteristic radiographic findings. Resorption of calcified cartilage is diminished on the metaphyseal end of the physis. This results in a thick, opaque ZPC, referred to as the white line of scurvy or white line of Frankel. Subjacent to this, a lucent band designated the scurvy zone is seen. Corresponding findings are seen in the epiphysis, with a thick, peripheral shell of calcified cartilage surrounding a central region of lucency. This produces the "Wimberger ring" that is characteristic of scurvy [**Fig. 7.49A**].

Both the thickened ZPC and the lucent scurvy zone are prone to fracture. Metaphyseal fractures are common, with associated subperiosteal hemorrhage. Subperiosteal hemorrhage is initially seen as a soft tissue opacity along the shaft of a tubular bone, which eventually mineralizes and becomes the new cortex [**Fig. 7.49B**]. A prominent metaphyseal spur ("Pelkan spur") may be seen after a fracture, with lateral extension of the dense, thickened ZPC.

Lead Poisoning

Lead poisoning is the most common type of heavy metal poisoning seen in children. It is usually related to the ingestion of lead-based paint chips found in older homes. Clinically, patients may present with abdominal pain, encephalopathy, peripheral neuropathy, and anemia. On abdominal radiographs, lead-based

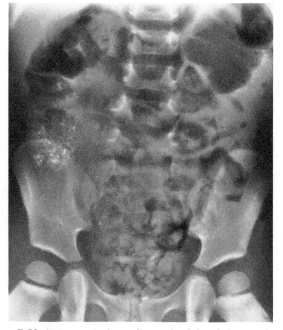

Figure 7.50 Anteroposterior radiograph of the abdomen demonstrates retention of radiopaque lead-based paint chips within bowel, predominantly clustered in the ascending colon. Dense "lead lines" are noted in the proximal femoral metaphyses.

paint chips may be visualized in the bowel [**Fig. 7.50**]. Bony manifestations are typically a late finding of chronic lead exposure. Lead toxicity interferes with the resorption of calcified cartilage in the primary spongiosa. This accumulates and leads to the formation of the dense, radiopaque metaphyseal bands ("lead lines") that are characteristic of this disease [**Figs. 7.9** and **7.50**]. The major differential diagnostic consideration is the normal, physiologic dense bands that are typically seen in the metaphyses of the more rapidly growing long bones in young children. Lead lines will be seen in all metaphyses, including those of the more slowly growing bones such as the fibula.

Anemias and Coagulopathies

Sickle Cell Disease

Sickle cell disease is an inherited hemoglobinopathy with autosomal recessive inheritance. The homozygous form of disease, HbSS, is seen in 1 in 650 African Americans. The mutation is a substitution of valine for glutamic acid on the beta chain of hemoglobin, resulting in deformed, "sickled" red blood cells, intravascular sludging of blood, and chronic hemolytic anemia. In the musculoskeletal system, the main manifestations of disease include hematopoietic marrow hyperplasia, vasoocclusive crises/osteonecrosis, and osteomyelitis. Osteomyelitis is most often caused by *Staphylococcus aureus,* although infection with salmonella is seen with greater frequency (20 times more often) in patients with sickle cell disease in comparison with the general pediatric population.

In the first 6 months of life, the presence of fetal hemoglobin is protective and symptoms are not typically seen. Approximately one-third of patients experience symptoms between 6 months and 2 years of age. Swollen fingers (dactylitis) and possibly also toes (hand-foot syndrome) may be seen. On radiographs, mild marrow expansion, periosteal new bone formation, and soft tissue swelling are noted involving the digits [**Fig. 7.51**]. Distinction from osteomyelitis can be difficult.

Presentation with bone and joint pain becomes more common through childhood. In the spine, infarction may occur along the central portion of the vertebral endplates, creating H-shaped vertebral bodies, or the characteristic "Lincoln log" deformity [**Fig. 7.52**]. This is thought to be related to the formation of rouleaux, or stacks of deformed red blood cells in the small vessels supplying the central endplates. Infarction of the long bones is common and appears similar to osteonecrosis related to other causes. The femur often is involved. On radiographs, patchy, geographic areas of sclerosis are demonstrated. Characteristic MRI findings of avascular necrosis include geographic areas of serpiginous low signal intensity on T1-weighted sequences, with abnormal high signal intensity on T2-weighted and STIR sequences. MRI is the modality of choice to detect avascular necrosis in its earliest stage when it may be radiographically occult. Changes related to marrow reconversion in the setting of chronic anemia are well demonstrated on MRI. Diffuse hypointensity of the marrow on T1-weighted sequences and hyperintensity on T2-weighted and STIR sequences are typically seen.

Vasoocclusive crises are treated with supportive care and pain management. Infections are managed with antimicrobial therapy which must be tailored for coverage of pathogens more commonly seen in sickle cell disease.

Thalassemia

Thalassemia is an inherited hemoglobinopathy most frequently seen in individuals of Eastern Mediterranean descent. There is a more severe homozygous form of disease referred to as *thalassemia major* and a less severe heterozygous form of disease called *thalassemia minor*. Disease is characterized by ineffective erythropoiesis, intramedullary hemolysis, and chronic anemia.

Radiographic changes are primarily related to marrow hyperplasia. In the skull, there is widening of the diploic space with a so-called "hair-on-end" appearance of the calvarium

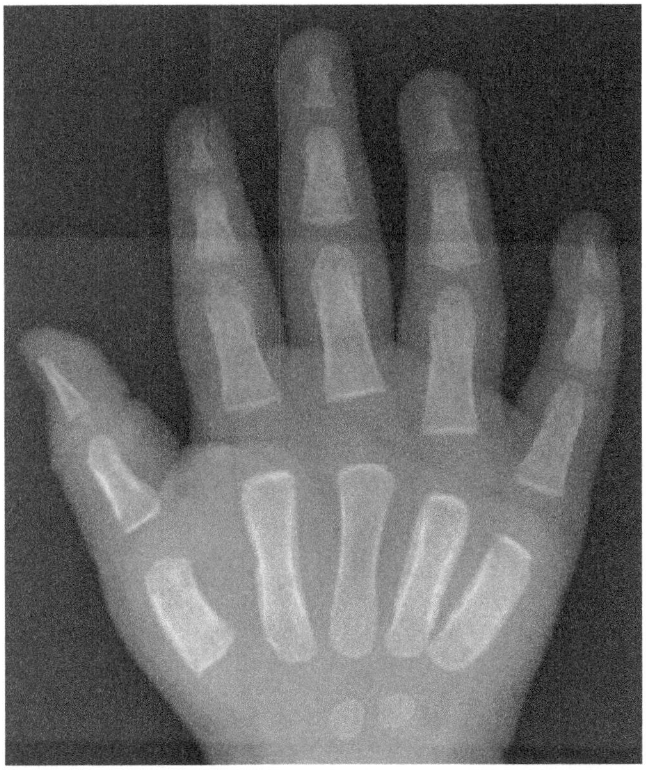

Figure 7.51 Dactylitis in an 11-month-old with sickle cell anemia. Posteroanterior radiograph of the right hand demonstrates subperiosteal new bone formation along the second, fourth, and fifth metacarpals, and also along the proximal phalanx of the thumb.

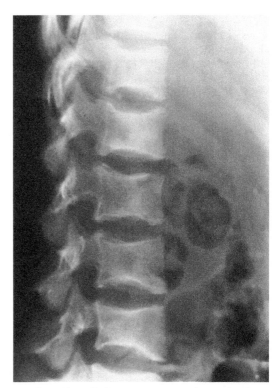

Figure 7.52 Sickle cell disease. Lateral radiograph of the spine demonstrates superior and inferior vertebral body endplate concavities, with the characteristic H-shaped vertebral bodies or "Lincoln log" deformity.

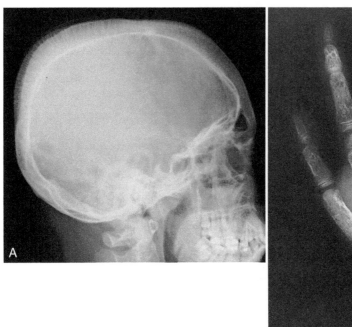
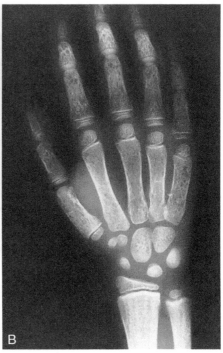

Figure 7.53 **Thalassemia. A,** Lateral radiograph of the skull in an 18-month-old boy demonstrates widening of the diploic space caused by marrow hyperplasia, with a "hair-on-end" appearance to the calvarium. **B,** Posteroanterior radiograph of the right hand in a different patient demonstrates widening of the medullary cavities and a coarsened trabecular pattern. The metacarpals and phalanges have a squared-off configuration.

[**Fig. 7.53A**]. The paranasal sinuses may fail to develop, or progressive obliteration of the sinuses may occur. In the hands and feet, the medullary cavities are widened, a coarsened trabecular pattern is seen, and the metacarpals and phalanges have a squared-off configuration [**Fig. 7.53B**]. Undertubulation of the long bones is typical, with an "Erlenmeyer flask" deformity. Generalized osteopenia is often seen in the axial skeleton. Extramedullary hematopoietic tissue along the spine may cause spinal cord compression.

Thalassemia is managed with transfusion therapy to suppress marrow hyperplasia and allow normal hematopoietic to fatty marrow conversion. This leads to iron overload, a complication which is reduced by chelation therapy. Bone marrow transplantation can be pursued as a potentially curative treatment for severe cases of thalassemia.

Hemophilia

Hemophilia is an X-linked recessive disorder of coagulation. Classic hemophilia (hemophilia A) is due to a deficiency of factor VIII, whereas Christmas disease (hemophilia B) is related to a deficiency of factor IX. Hemophilia primarily affects the large joints, with the knee, elbow, and ankle most frequently involved. Recurrent hemarthrosis leads to inflammation, with hemosiderin deposition and fibrosis. Synovial hypertrophy and overgrowth result, with subsequent cartilage and subchondral bone destruction, bony erosion, and subchondral cyst formation. Avascular necrosis may be seen due to occlusion of epiphyseal vessels in the setting of hemarthrosis. Pseudotumor formation occurs in about 1% of patients with severe hemophilia. Pseudotumors are often intramuscular and manifest as painless, slowly expanding masses.

On radiographs, findings related to joint hyperemia may be seen. These include premature ossification of the epiphyses, epiphyseal overgrowth, and premature fusion of the growth plates. At the knee, classic findings include a joint effusion,

squaring of the femoral condyles, a widened intercondylar notch, and squaring of the inferior aspect of the patella. Secondary degenerative change may be evident, with joint space narrowing, subchondral cyst formation, and bony erosions.

MRI shows hemarthrosis, with joint fluid of variable signal intensity based on the acuity of hemorrhage. Gradient echo sequences are most sensitive for the detection of hemosiderin deposition within the synovium; however, synovium-containing hemosiderin will appear abnormally low in signal intensity on all sequences. Although the extent of synovial abnormality is nicely demonstrated on postcontrast sequences, contrast administration is not usually necessary or routine in the evaluation of hemophilic arthropathy. Red marrow recruitment and hyperplasia occur in the setting of hemophilia; thus the expected normal conversion of red marrow to yellow marrow will be delayed.

Ultrasound has been increasingly used in the assessment of hemophilic arthropathy. A major advantage over MRI is the lack of susceptibility artifact related to hemosiderin deposition, potentially affording better visualization of the extent of synovial hypertrophy.

Neurofibromatosis

Neurofibromatosis (NF) is an autosomal disorder with variable penetrance and an almost 50% mutation rate. Chromosomal mutations have been mapped to 17q21 (NF-1) and 22q12 (NF-2). NF may involve any organ system in the body. Classic clinical manifestations include café-au-lait spots, axillary or inguinal freckles, Lisch nodules/hamartomas of the iris, neurofibromas of the peripheral nerves, and skeletal deformities. Musculoskeletal involvement is seen in about 80% of individuals with NF. Anterolateral bowing of the tibia is characteristic. A congenital pseudarthrosis of the tibia or fibula is also often seen, resulting from fracture with incomplete healing and subsequent nonunion [**Fig. 7.54A**]. Cortical erosions may be noted related to mass effect from adjacent enlarged nerves [**Fig. 7.54B**]. The ribs often have a twisted, ribbonlike appearance. Kyphoscoliosis is seen in about 20% of patients with NF-1. Posterior vertebral body scalloping may be present in the setting of dural ectasia or multiple spinal neurofibromas. "Dumb-bell neurofibromas" may extend through and widen the neural foramina of the spine.

HIP DISORDERS

Developmental Dysplasia of the Hip

Developmental dysplasia of the hip (DDH) reflects a spectrum of abnormalities that may range from ligamentous laxity to primary

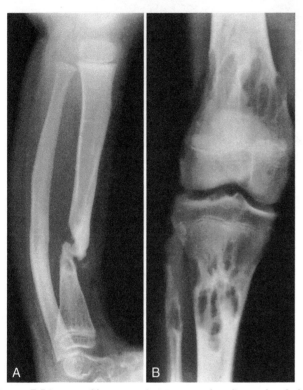

Figure 7.54 Neurofibromatosis. A, Lateral radiograph of the lower leg shows a pseudarthrosis of the distal tibia and significant bowing of the fibula. **B,** Anteroposterior radiograph of the right knee shows multiple bony erosions caused by mass effect from adjacent enlarged nerves.

acetabular dysplasia with femoral head subluxation or dislocation. It is relatively common, with an incidence as frequent as 1 in 200 live births. Girls are affected far more frequently than boys. There is often a family history of hip dysplasia. DDH is more common on the left side, and may be bilateral in up to 30% of cases. Several prenatal factors may contribute to the development of DDH due to in utero constriction. These include breech presentation, being large for gestational age, and oligohydramnios. DDH may be associated with torticollis or congenital knee dislocation. DDH is also associated with myelodysplasia, arthrogryposis, proximal focal femoral deficiency, neuromuscular disorders, mucopolysaccharidoses, and chromosomal abnormalities.

For proper development, the normal relationship of the femoral head and acetabulum must be maintained with congruity along the articular surface. DDH most often develops in the setting of primary structural abnormality involving the acetabulum and/or femoral head. Combined with ligamentous laxity, this leads to the development of an abnormal incongruent hip, possibly with subluxation or dislocation of the femoral head.

Ultrasound is the modality of choice for screening for hip dysplasia in young infants. In babies at risk for DDH who do not have concerning physical examination findings, ultrasound is generally performed at or after 6 weeks of age. In the first few weeks of life, there is some degree of physiologic laxity of the hips due to the influence of maternal hormones, and it is often difficult to exclude the presence of dysplasia. Ultrasound is performed early (before 6 weeks of age) for infants with concerning physical examination findings who may benefit from early treatment. Worrisome findings may include a hip "click" or "clunk," gluteal or thigh fold asymmetry, or a clinically obvious dislocated hip.

Coronal and transverse images of the hip are acquired using a high-resolution linear transducer. With the hip in flexion, it has the appearance of a "lollipop" in the coronal plane and a "seagull" in the transverse plane [**Fig. 7.55**]. Two important measurements are made on coronal images. The cartilaginous femoral head should be at least 50% covered by the bony acetabulum. This is assessed by a line drawn along the long axis of the iliac bone. More than half of the femoral head should lie deep to this line. The alpha angle is drawn to assess acetabular depth. This is the angle created by the iliac bone and the bony acetabulum and should measure at least 60 degrees. Stress maneuvers are performed in the transverse plane, similar to the Barlow maneuver performed on physical examination to assess whether a hip can be dislocated. Qualitative features of hip immaturity and

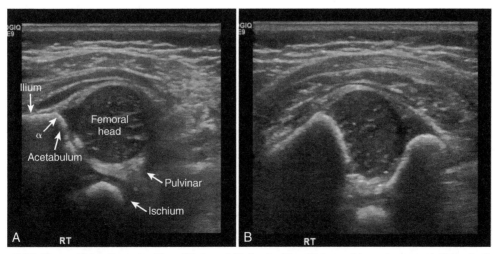

Figure 7.55 Normal hip ultrasound in a 72-day-old infant with a history of breech presentation. A, Coronal and (**B**) transverse images of the right hip demonstrate greater than 50% coverage of the cartilaginous femoral head by the bony acetabulum with a normal alpha angle measuring greater than 60 degrees.

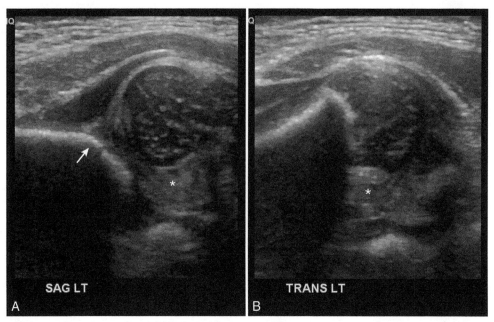

Figure 7.56 Developmental dysplasia of the hip in a 16-day-old girl with left hip instability on physical examination. A, Coronal and (**B**) transverse ultrasound images of the left hip demonstrate deficient coverage of the femoral head by the bony acetabulum and a shallow alpha angle. The acetabular roof is rounded (*arrow*), and the pulvinar is thickened (*asterisks*).

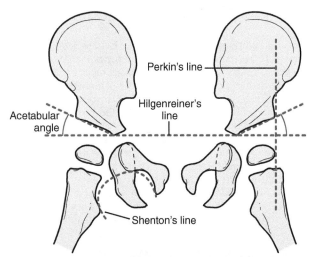

Figure 7.57 Illustration depicting the lines drawn in the radiographic assessment for hip dysplasia.

dysplasia that may be seen on ultrasound include a rounded acetabular roof and a prominent, thickened fibrofatty pulvinar [**Fig. 7.56**].

At about 6 months of age, femoral head ossification is often present. From this time forward, evaluation for DDH is performed with radiography rather than ultrasound. An anteroposterior (AP) supine radiograph of the pelvis is obtained, with several lines drawn to assess for dysplasia [**Fig. 7.57**]. The horizontal line of Hilgenreiner is drawn through the superior aspect of the triradiate cartilages. A perpendicular line of Perkins is drawn intersecting this, passing along the ossified rim of the acetabular roof. In a normal hip, the femoral head should lie in the inferior, medial quadrant created by these lines. The acetabular angle is created by the acetabular roof and the Hilgenreiner line. This angle is typically just under 30 degrees at birth and decreases to about 20 degrees or less by age 2 years. At any given age, the normal angle is slightly higher in girls than in boys.

Shenton's line is a curvilinear arc connecting the medial cortex of the proximal femoral metaphysis and the inferior edge of the superior pubic ramus. This arc is continuous and smooth in a normal hip, but discontinuous in subluxation and dislocation. Radiographic findings of DDH may include a shallow bony acetabulum, delayed ossification of the capital femoral epiphysis, and superolateral subluxation of the femoral head. In the setting of subluxation or dislocation, a frog-leg lateral view or von Rosen view (AP pelvis with hip abduction and internal rotation) is helpful to assess for femoral head reduction [**Fig. 7.58**].

Treatment of DDH is variable depending on severity of disease. Patients with immaturity or mild DDH may be watched with close clinical follow-up and serial ultrasounds. Conservative treatments may include bracing with a device such as a Pavlik harness. More severe DDH with subluxation or dislocation often requires surgical management with a closed or open reduction of the hip followed by spica cast placement. In the setting of a late diagnosis or persistent DDH despite treatment, a pelvic and/or femoral osteotomy may be required.

Cross-sectional imaging is useful in the postoperative setting. Both CT and MRI may be used to evaluate femoral head position after reduction. Contrast-enhanced MRI affords the added benefit of an assessment of femoral head perfusion. This may help identify patients at risk for avascular necrosis, the most common serious complication of surgical hip reduction.

Legg-Calve-Perthes Disease

Legg-Calve-Perthes disease (LCP), or idiopathic avascular necrosis of the femoral head, is the most common cause of hip pain in the young child. It most often develops between 4 and 8 years of age, is much more common in boys (4:1), and is most often seen in Caucasians. It may be bilateral in up to 20% of affected individuals. Patients typically present with hip pain, knee pain, or a limp. Skeletal maturity is often delayed.

Radiographs may show an asymmetric, small, ossified femoral epiphysis and a curvilinear subchondral lucency reflecting a fracture through necrotic bone ("crescent sign"). The subchondral fracture is often seen to best advantage on a frog-leg lateral

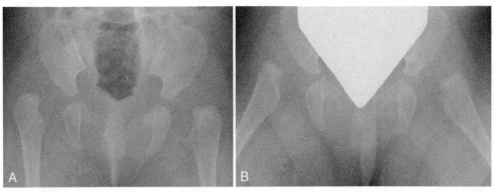

Figure 7.58 **Bilateral developmental dysplasia of the hip in a 6-month-old girl. A,** Anteroposterior and (**B**) von Rosen images of the pelvis show subtle, early femoral head ossification. The femoral heads are dislocated from shallow bony acetabula and do not reduce with von Rosen positioning.

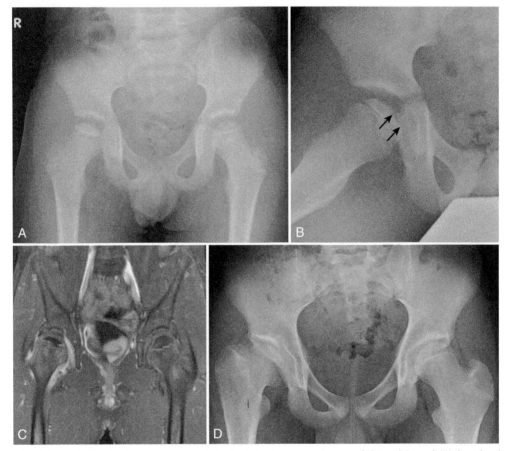

Figure 7.59 **Legg-Calve-Perthes disease (LCP). A,** Anteroposterior image of the pelvis and (**B**) frog-leg lateral image of the right hip show a flattened, sclerotic right femoral head, with a "crescent sign" reflecting a subchondral fracture (*arrows*). **C,** Coronal T1 postcontrast image with fat saturation through the pelvis shows asymmetrically decreased femoral head enhancement and striking synovitis on the right. **D,** Anteroposterior radiograph of the pelvis in a 16-year-old boy with a history of LCP with onset at 8 years of age. The right hip is significantly abnormal, with coxa magna, plana, and breva deformities and significant elevation of the greater trochanter. The acetabulum is shallow.

view [**Fig. 7.59A** and **B**]. The joint space may be widened due to the presence of a joint effusion and/or synovitis. With long-standing disease, patchy lucency and sclerosis may be seen within the femoral head, with fragmentation and flattening.

MRI is sensitive for the detection of early disease when radiographs may be nondiagnostic. Marrow edema is seen in the epiphysis, physis, and metaphysis on T2-weighted sequences, with loss of normal fatty marrow on T1-weighted sequences.

Curvilinear low signal will be demonstrated in the setting of subchondral fracture. With contrast administration, asymmetrically decreased femoral head enhancement will be seen. Synovitis is also well demonstrated on postcontrast images [**Fig. 7.59C**].

The treatment for LCP is rest until the patient is asymptomatic, with restriction of high-impact activities during the healing phase of the disease. Healing is present when fragmentation and

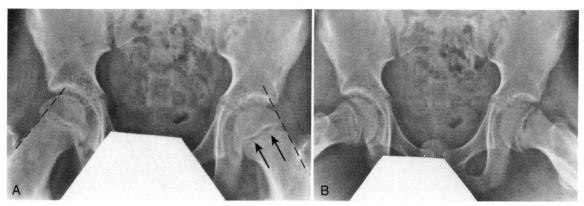

Figure 7.60 **Slipped capital femoral epiphysis. A,** Anteroposterior radiograph of the pelvis shows asymmetric physeal widening on the left (*double arrows*). Klein's line (*dotted lines*) does not cross the epiphysis on the affected side. **B,** Frog-leg lateral image confirms inferomedial slip of the femoral head relative to the proximal femoral metaphysis.

collapse of the femoral head have stabilized and reossification is evident.

Chronic LCP may lead to loss of normal femoroacetabular congruity. Coxa magna (epiphyseal enlargement), coxa plana (epiphyseal flattening), and coxa breva (shortened femoral neck) deformities can develop, and the greater trochanter may be elevated because of relative overgrowth. This may result in inadequate coverage of the dysmorphic femoral head and a predisposition to CAM-type femoral-acetabular impingement, with possible secondary degenerative change [**Fig. 7.59D**]. Ultimately, surgical reconstruction with pelvic and/or femoral osteotomies may be required.

Slipped Capital Femoral Epiphysis

Slipped capital femoral epiphysis (SCFE) is a Salter-Harris I injury of the proximal femoral physis. This occurs most commonly in adolescent boys who are overweight and is most frequently seen in the African American population. The left hip is more commonly affected, and SCFE may be bilateral in up to one-third of patients. Patients present clinically with groin and thigh pain. Knee pain is also fairly common. Importantly, symptoms are often present for weeks to months before a diagnosis is made.

Standard radiographic assessment for suspected SCFE includes AP and frog-leg lateral views of the pelvis with careful attention to both hips. If a patient cannot bear weight on presentation, instability is a concern. In this setting, a shoot-through lateral radiograph should be obtained in lieu of the frog-leg lateral view. In relatively more subtle or earlier cases of SCFE, there is asymmetric widening and/or lucency of the proximal femoral physis on the affected side. In later or more advanced stages, patients present with posterior and inferomedial displacement of the femoral head relative to the femoral neck [**Fig. 7.60**]. This appearance has been likened to a "scoop of ice cream falling off of a cone." On an AP radiograph, Klein's line may be drawn to assess femoral head positioning. This line is drawn along the lateral aspect of the femoral neck and should intersect the capital femoral epiphysis. When it does not, a slip is suggested and may be shown to better advantage on the frog-leg lateral view.

MRI is occasionally helpful in the diagnosis of very early, subtle SCFE. A few short sequences with both hips in the field of view will show asymmetric fluid in the physis and possibly also periphyseal edema on the affected side. Subtle asymmetric physeal widening may be seen, even if not well-profiled on radiographs. A joint effusion and synovitis are often present.

Treatment most often consists of in situ pinning of the affected hip. In some acute cases, a limited closed reduction may be performed before pinning. There is controversy surrounding

prophylactic pinning of the contralateral hip; this practice is practitioner and patient/family dependent. Late complications of SCFE include avascular necrosis of the femoral head and chondrolysis. The latter is more common when the fixation pin traverses the subchondral cortex of the femoral head.

INFECTION

Acute Osteomyelitis

Acute hematogenous osteomyelitis is primarily a disease of children. The incidence is approximately 1 in 5000 in children younger than 13 years of age. Half of all cases occur in the first 5 years of life, and boys are affected more often than girls (2:1). The highly vascularized metaphyses of the fastest growing bones are most frequently affected, including the distal femur, proximal tibia, proximal humerus, and distal radius. The most common organism involved is *Staphylococcus aureus* (85%). Infections with *Streptococcus pneumoniae* and *Haemophilus influenzae* are less commonly seen due to routine vaccination against these pathogens. In older children with sickle cell disease, infection with salmonella is relatively common.

Blood-borne organisms flourish in the metaphyses because of the large, slow-flowing terminal capillary sinusoids in the medullary cavity of this region of bone. Small abscesses first form, with destruction of adjacent bone. These abscesses eventually coalesce. In the setting of significant inflammatory change, intraosseous pressure increases, and infection may spread deeper into the medullary cavity, into the subperiosteal space, and into the adjacent soft tissues, with possible abscess formation. Infection can spread across the physis to involve the epiphysis and possibly the joint. Diaphyseal extension may also be seen.

Clinically, patients present with fever, pain, decreased range of motion, and reduced weightbearing. A history of trauma is provided in up to 30% of patients. The erythrocyte sedimentation rate is always elevated, but white blood cell count elevation and positive blood cultures are seen in only 50% of cases.

Radiographs should be obtained first, particularly to exclude an alternative diagnosis such as trauma or neoplasm. Although deep soft tissue swelling may be evident early in the course of acute osteomyelitis, bony changes are typically not seen on radiographs until the second week of disease. The earliest finding is typically one or more focal areas of subtle radiolucency in the metaphysis of a long bone, reflecting sites of bone destruction and necrosis. These areas may enlarge and become confluent and more well-defined over time [**Fig. 7.61A** and **B**]. Subperiosteal new bone next develops, usually 2 to 3 weeks after the onset of infection.

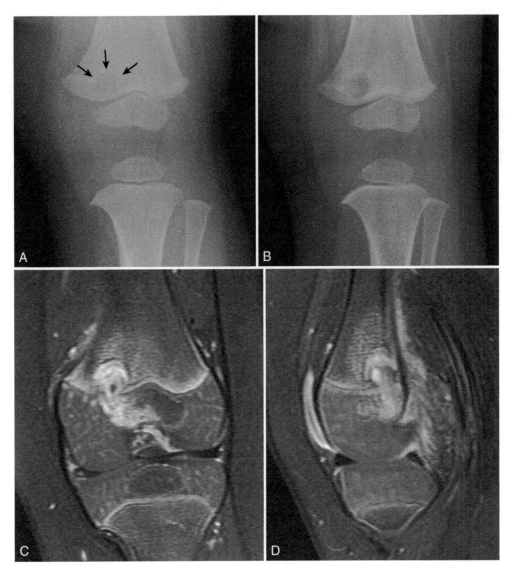

Figure 7.61 Osteomyelitis in a 16-month-old girl presenting with a limp. A, Anteroposterior radiograph of the left knee on initial presentation shows a subtle, ill-defined lucency in the medial aspect of the distal femoral metaphysis (*arrows*). **B,** This was not initially appreciated, and the patient returned nearly 3 weeks later with persistent symptoms. Anteroposterior image of the left knee shows a well-defined circular lucency with a sclerotic rim in the distal femoral metaphysis, consistent with a Brodie abscess in the setting of subacute/chronic osteomyelitis. **C,** Coronal and (**D**) sagittal T1 postcontrast images with fat saturation demonstrate abnormal edema and enhancement in the distal femoral metaphysis, crossing the physis to involve the epiphysis. There is surrounding marrow edema and deep soft tissue edema. Synovitis is demonstrated, with intraarticular spread of infection difficult to exclude.

Radionuclide bone scans are more sensitive than radiographs in the detection of early acute osteomyelitis. A multiphase bone scan will typically be positive 24 to 48 hours after the onset of symptoms. The affected area of bone demonstrates increased tracer activity reflecting hyperemia and bone turnover characteristic of infection. Pitfalls include cold defects related to focal ischemia in the setting of infection, potential difficulty in distinguishing osteomyelitis from septic arthritis, and simulation of infection by fracture or other pathology.

CT scan is of limited utility in the imaging of acute osteomyelitis but may be helpful in demonstrating several characteristic features of subacute and chronic disease (see subsequent section).

MRI is helpful to confirm a diagnosis of osteomyelitis, particularly early in the course of disease when radiographs may be normal. Inflammatory change will be seen in the involved marrow, with homogeneous high signal on T2-weighted sequences and corresponding areas of enhancement after contrast administration [**Fig. 7.62**]. Postcontrast sequences are helpful to evaluate for intraosseous, subperiosteal, and soft tissue abscesses that may require surgical drainage. Follow-up MRI is useful in the evaluation of treatment failure, and also to assess for premature physeal fusion and related growth disturbance.

The specific bacterial pathogen responsible for osteomyelitis is not always identified. To minimize the risk for complications, empiric antibiotic therapy is often initiated before blood and/or bone/joint aspirate cultures are completed. Patients typically receive initial intravenous antibiotics followed by a long course of oral antibiotics. Surgical drainage is indicated for bone and/or soft tissue abscesses identified on MRI in the acute setting.

Subacute and Chronic Osteomyelitis

Subacute and chronic osteomyelitis may develop as a result of partial host response to contain an acute infection. The

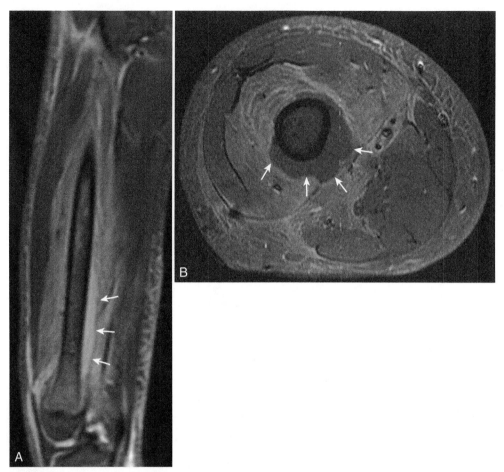

Figure 7.62 **Acute osteomyelitis in an 8-year-old boy. A,** Coronal fast spin-echo inversion-recovery and (**B**) axial T1 postcontrast images with fat saturation through the right femur show patchy abnormal increased signal throughout much of the femur, an extensive, nonenhancing subperiosteal abscess (*arrows*), and significant myositis and deep and superficial soft tissue edema.

distinction between the two is arbitrary. Clinical presentation is relatively mild in comparison with acute disease, consisting mainly of localized pain. Development of a Brodie abscess is characteristic of subacute disease. This typically forms in the metaphysis but may also be centered at the physis or epiphysis. On radiographs, a well-defined, central, or eccentric round or oval lucency is seen [**Fig. 7.61B**]. This may contain a small, dense bony sequestrum. On MRI, a characteristic target sign or multilayered appearance is seen. The center consists of pus, which is T2 hyperintense and does not enhance. A small, hypointense sequestrum may be present within this collection. Vascular granulation tissue surrounds the pus. This tissue is slightly hyperintense on T1-weighted images and intermediate to hyperintense on T2-weighted images, with avid enhancement after contrast administration. Sclerotic bone surrounds this granulation tissue and appears hypointense on all sequences [**Fig. 7.61C and D**]. Subperiosteal new bone formation and surrounding soft tissue swelling and edema may be seen in association with a Brodie abscess.

Subacute and chronic osteomyelitis are characterized by cortical and trabecular bone sclerosis. Affected bone is often thickened and may have a wavy, undulating contour [**Fig. 7.63A**]. *Sequestra* and *involucra* are also seen with subacute and chronic infection. A sequestrum is a necrotic bone fragment in the medullary cavity of a long bone, and an involucrum is a sheath of reactive bone that may form around a sequestrum. A *cloaca* may perforate an involucrum, forming a fistulous tract between the intramedullary abscess cavity and the extraosseous soft tissues

[**Fig. 7.63B**]. If this communicates with the skin, it is referred to as a *sinus tract.*

Radiographs will usually demonstrate bony changes related to subacute and chronic osteomyelitis. Although CT is not particularly useful in the imaging of acute osteomyelitis, it may be helpful in the setting of chronic disease. Sequestra, involucra, transcortical tracts, and overall bone quality are all well demonstrated by CT. MRI is useful in the detection of persistent infection and reactivation of disease, demonstrating the expected marrow and surrounding soft tissue changes.

Subacute and chronic disease often warrant surgical management as parenteral antibiotics alone will not penetrate a Brodie abscess or effectively treat the dead bone of a sequestrum, which may serve as a nidus for continued infection.

Septic Arthritis

Septic arthritis is a true medical and surgical emergency as delay in diagnosis can lead to destruction of a joint. In children, septic arthritis is most often secondary to osteomyelitis, with infection spreading from an adjacent metaphysis via transphyseal vessels to the intraarticular epiphysis. A joint may also become infected through hematogenous spread of organisms in the setting of sepsis. Direct inoculation from penetrating injury may occur, but is less commonly seen. The most common causative organism is *Staphylococcus aureus.* Infection is usually monoarticular with involvement of the large joints. The hip is most often affected in children, followed by the knee. Patients present clinically with

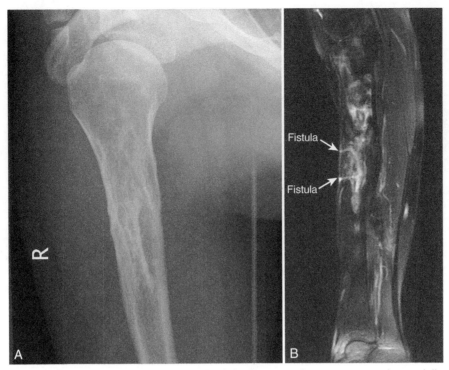

Figure 7.63 Chronic osteomyelitis. A, Radiograph of the humerus demonstrates patchy medullary sclerosis, cortical thickening, and remodeling in a region of chronic infection. **B,** Sagittal fast spin-echo inversion-recovery magnetic resonance image of the lower leg in a patient with a 3-month history of infection demonstrates fistulous tracts extending from areas of chronically infected marrow to the extraosseous soft tissues.

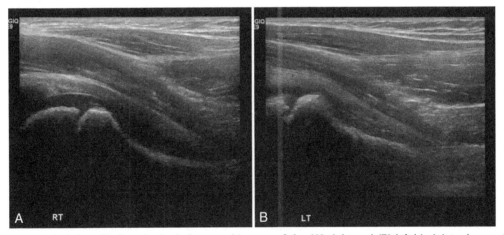

Figure 7.64 Hip joint effusion. Sagittal ultrasound images of the (**A**) right and (**B**) left hip joints demonstrate a moderate-sized right-sided effusion, with a normal-appearing joint on the left.

pain, limp, and refusal to bear weight. Fever may be present. Inflammatory markers are elevated, and the white blood cell count may be high.

Radiographs are usually obtained first. In the evaluation for septic hip, this is largely to exclude alternative causative factors such as a fracture or a bony lesion. In some cases of septic hip, asymmetric widening of the affected hip joint space may be seen. However, it is important to note that radiographs are not particularly sensitive for the presence of a hip joint effusion. When there is clinical concern for this, ultrasound is performed using a high-resolution linear transducer over the anterior aspect of the joint. A bilateral examination is done to allow direct comparison with the asymptomatic hip [**Fig. 7.64**]. If a joint effusion

is not seen, septic arthritis is excluded. If an effusion is seen, sonographic findings are nonspecific. A septic joint, transient synovitis, juvenile idiopathic arthritis (JIA), and a posttraumatic joint effusion may appear the same. Ultrasound guidance can be used for diagnostic joint aspiration when a hip joint effusion is present. The knee joint is most often sampled without the need for imaging guidance.

MRI is not typically performed for isolated septic arthritis, as joint aspiration is diagnostic. The appearance of a septic joint on MRI is nonspecific. A joint effusion, synovial thickening and hyperemia, and deep and superficial soft tissue edema may be seen, as with other entities such as transient synovitis and JIA. MRI may be pursued when there is concomitant

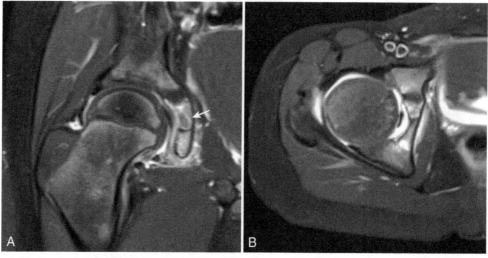

Figure 7.65 Septic arthritis with osteomyelitis. A, Coronal and (**B**) axial T1 postcontrast magnetic resonance images with fat saturation demonstrate abnormal enhancement of the acetabulum with a small intramedullary collection (*arrow*), synovitis, and deep soft tissue edema.

osteomyelitis, and evaluation of the bone marrow, subperiosteal space, and deep soft tissues is required [**Fig. 7.65**].

Septic arthritis is managed with emergent arthrotomy and washout, followed by a prolonged antibiotic course of 4 to 6 weeks. Complications include sepsis and osteonecrosis and/or chondrolysis at the affected joint.

Lyme Arthritis

Lyme disease is a systemic infection caused by the spirochete *Borrelia burgdorferi*, transmitted by deer ticks found in the New England area and Mid-Atlantic states. Arthritis is a late manifestation of Lyme disease, generally seen weeks to years after the initial infection. Approximately 25% of cases are seen in children younger than 15 years. Disease is usually monoarticular, and the knee is most frequently involved (80% of cases). Patients present clinically with pain, swelling, limp, and decreased range of motion.

Radiographs demonstrate a joint effusion [**Fig. 7.66A**]. MRI features of Lyme arthritis include a joint effusion, synovial thickening and hyperemia, myositis, and popliteal lymphadenopathy [**Fig. 7.66B** through **D**]. Juxta-articular marrow edema may also be seen. These features are nonspecific and overlap with those seen in septic and inflammatory arthritis. Lyme titers are usually obtained for diagnosis; however, results are not always available at the time of initial workup. Joint aspiration is often performed to help distinguish between Lyme and septic arthritis. Lyme arthritis is treated with a prolonged course of oral antibiotics, typically either doxycycline or amoxicillin.

Transient Synovitis

Transient (toxic) synovitis is a common, benign cause of childhood hip pain, thought to be secondary to a viral infection. It is a diagnosis of exclusion, as clinical presentation may overlap with that of septic hip and other more concerning entities. It is most often seen in children younger than 10 years of age and has a male preponderance. Patients typically present with pain and a limp, with a recent viral illness frequently reported. Radiographs are most often normal. Ultrasound demonstrates a joint effusion, which is a nonspecific finding as previously noted. If joint aspiration is performed, there will be no organisms in the aspirated fluid. Management is conservative, and symptoms typically resolve with rest.

ARTHRITIS/INFLAMMATORY DISORDERS

Juvenile Idiopathic Arthritis

JIA is the most frequent cause of chronic musculoskeletal pain in the pediatric population, and the most common chronic musculoskeletal disease of childhood. Age of onset is young, often between 1 and 3 years of age. Girls are affected twice as often as boys. Disease may be monoarticular or polyarticular, and typically involves the large joints. The knee is most frequently affected, followed by the ankle. Disease may also involve the hip, wrist, hand, elbow, cervical spine, and temporomandibular joints. Systemic manifestations are common, and may include fever, rash, iridocyclitis, pleuritis, pericarditis, anemia, fatigue, growth failure, and leukocytosis. In contradistinction to adult rheumatoid arthritis, the majority of cases are seronegative; thus diagnosis is typically made on clinical grounds.

JIA is characterized by an acute synovitis, with synovial proliferation and formation of a highly cellular, thick, redundant pannus in the joint space. This pannus erodes articular cartilage and subchondral bone. Inflammation may also involve the tendon sheaths and bursae. With significant chronic disease, joint instability, subluxation, and ankylosis may be seen. Although most cases of JIA are transient and self-limited, some children experience progressive disease, with up to 10% becoming severely disabled in adulthood.

Radiographic manifestations of disease are typically seen between 2 and 5 years after initial clinical presentation. The earliest abnormalities include soft tissue swelling, osteopenia, and joint effusions. Periosteal reaction may also be seen. With the erosion of articular cartilage and subchondral bone, joint space narrowing and marginal erosions are seen. The epiphyses may appear enlarged, as with other arthropathies characterized by hyperemia [**Fig. 7.67A**]. The femoral condyles and patella may appear "squared off." Alignment abnormalities of the fingers can be seen, including boutonniere and swan neck deformities. At the cervical spine, atlantoaxial subluxation, vertebral pseudosubluxation, and ankyloses are characteristic [**Fig. 7.67B**].

MRI is sensitive for the detection of active disease and is also used to monitor response to therapy and predict future articular destruction. The extent of synovial abnormality is well demonstrated, particularly with the administration of contrast material [**Fig. 7.67C**]. With prolonged synovial inflammation, characteristic "rice bodies" may be noted. These small intraarticular

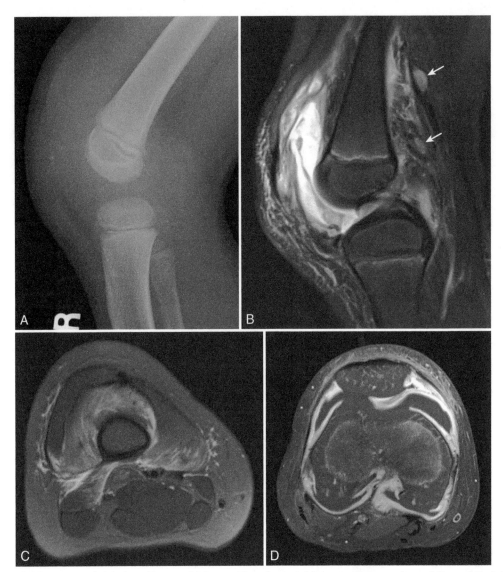

Figure 7.66 Lyme arthritis in a 5-year-old boy with a 2-week history of knee pain and fevers. A, Lateral radiograph of the knee demonstrates a large joint effusion. **B** through **D,** Sagittal T2, axial T2, and axial T1 postcontrast magnetic resonance images with fat saturation demonstrate a joint effusion, prominent popliteal lymph nodes (*arrows*), myositis, and significant synovitis.

nodules reflect detached fragments of hypertrophied synovium and demonstrate low signal intensity on T2-weighted sequences. Cartilage loss is well demonstrated on MRI. Ultrasound has been increasingly used in JIA to evaluate for joint effusions, synovial abnormality, and tenosynovitis.

Chronic Nonbacterial Osteomyelitis

Chronic nonbacterial osteomyelitis (CNO) is a nonpyogenic, inflammatory disorder of unknown cause seen in children and adolescents. The adult equivalent of CNO is SAPHO (synovitis, acne, pustulosis, hyperostosis, and osteitis). CNO is characterized by multifocal bony lesions commonly involving the lower extremities, spine, pelvis, clavicle, and mandible. In the long bones, metaphyseal lesions are most frequently seen. The disease course involves multiple exacerbations and remissions. There is an association with other inflammatory disorders including psoriasis and inflammatory bowel disease.

Patients present with pain localized to sites of involvement. Radiographs are obtained first, although bone lesions may be radiographically occult. On MRI, multifocal areas of marrow edema and enhancement are seen [**Fig. 7.68**]. Whole-body evaluation may be performed with bone scintigraphy or whole-body MRI. Diagnosis is typically confirmed with a bone biopsy. A causative organism is not isolated with this entity.

CNO is most often a self-limited entity, with no subsequent disability in adulthood. Several different therapies have been used for management of symptomatic disease, including nonsteroidal antiinflammatory drugs and corticosteroids.

Juvenile Dermatomyositis

Juvenile dermatomyositis (JDM) is the most common idiopathic inflammatory myopathy in the pediatric population. It is an autoimmune condition characterized by diffuse inflammation of striated muscle and skin. JDM typically presents between 2 and 15 years of age, and girls are affected more often than boys. Clinically, patients present with proximal muscle weakness, fatigue, and a rash involving the face and knuckles. Arthritis may be

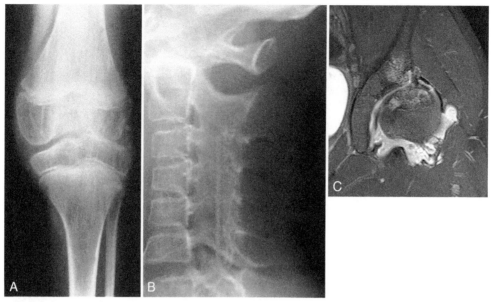

Figure 7.67 Juvenile idiopathic arthritis. A, Anteroposterior radiograph of the left knee shows epiphyseal overgrowth and widening of the intercondylar notch. **B,** Lateral radiograph of the cervical spine demonstrates bony fusion along the apophyseal joints. **C,** Coronal T1 postcontrast image with fat saturation through the left hip demonstrates extensive synovitis, evolving changes of avascular necrosis in the femoral head, and erosions and marrow edema in the acetabulum.

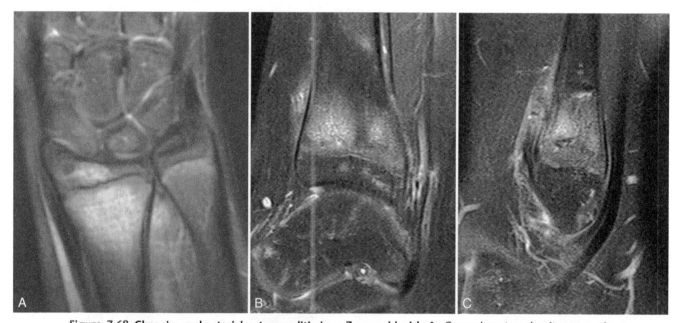

Figure 7.68 Chronic nonbacterial osteomyelitis in a 7-year-old girl. A, Coronal proton density magnetic resonance image of the right wrist with fat saturation shows abnormal increased signal in the metaphysis and epiphysis of the distal radius. **B** and **C,** Sagittal T1-weighted postcontrast images with fat saturation in the same patient show abnormal enhancement in the distal tibial and fibular metaphyses.

present, and vasculitis-like conditions such as skin and mucosal ulceration can be seen.

MRI is sensitive for the detection of acute disease. Diffuse, heterogeneous increased signal may be seen in the muscle, fascia, subcutaneous fat, and skin on fluid-sensitive sequences [Fig. 7.69]. Symmetric involvement is often seen in the appendicular skeleton. The thighs are typically affected first, followed by the upper arms. With chronic disease,

complications may be seen. These include dystrophic calcifications, muscle necrosis, and muscle atrophy with fatty replacement.

The clinical and imaging features of JDM are often sufficient for diagnosis. Muscle biopsy may be performed when the diagnosis is not clear. Treatment consists of high-dose oral corticosteroids and methotrexate. Clinical symptoms, muscle enzymes, and MRI are used to monitor response to therapy.

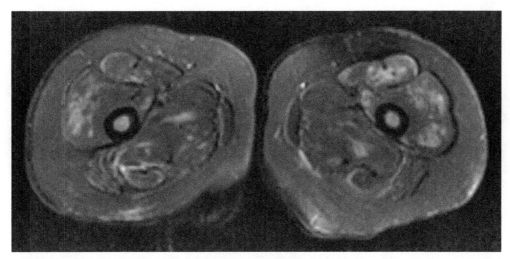

Figure 7.69 Juvenile dermatomyositis. Axial fast spin-echo inversion-recovery magnetic resonance image through both thighs demonstrates patchy increased fluid signal in the musculature bilaterally.

BENIGN MUSCULOSKELETAL TUMORS

Fibrous Bone Tumors

Fibrous Cortical Defect/Nonossifying Fibroma

Fibrous cortical defects (FCDs) and nonossifying fibromas (NOFs) are the most common benign bone lesions in children and adolescents. They occur in greater than one-third of patients, and are sometimes considered normal variants. These lesions are most often encountered between the ages of 4 and 12 years and are seen more frequently in boys. The two lesions are histologically identical, and are composed of fibroblasts, giant cells, and xanthoma cells. By convention, lesions smaller than 2 cm are considered FCDs, and those 2 cm or larger are classified as NOFs. These lesions are asymptomatic and discovered incidentally, except in the setting of a pathologic fracture. Multiple NOFs may be seen in patients with NF and Jaffe-Campanacci syndrome.

On radiography, an NOF is typically a multilobulated lucent lesion with a well-defined sclerotic margin [**Fig. 7.70**]. A "soap bubble" appearance is characteristic. Lesions are cortically based and most often are found in the metaphyses or metadiaphyses of long bones. The radiographic appearance of these lesions is characteristic and usually sufficient for diagnosis, with further imaging rarely necessary. NOFs and FCDs become progressively more sclerotic and "fill in" over time, ultimately undergoing involution.

Fibrous Dysplasia

Fibrous dysplasia is a relatively common fibroosseous lesion of bone. This lesion may be monostotic or polyostotic. Approximately 80% of cases are monostotic. Monostotic fibrous dysplasia is most often seen in adolescents and young adults, with females more frequently affected. The femur, ribs, and craniofacial bones are most often involved. Polyostotic fibrous dysplasia typically presents in the first decade of life. It is associated with McCune-Albright syndrome (unilateral polyostotic fibrous dysplasia, precocious puberty, and café-au-lait spots) and Mazabraud syndrome (polyostotic fibrous dysplasia and intramuscular myxomas).

Radiographically, fibrous dysplasia arises centrally or slightly eccentrically within the medullary cavity of the diaphysis or metadiaphysis of a long bone. The matrix may have the classic ground-glass appearance or may be relatively more lucent depending on the composition of the lesion. A well-defined margin is typically seen, which may be sclerotic or nonsclerotic.

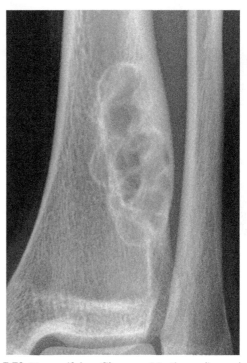

Figure 7.70 Nonossifying fibroma. Mortise radiograph of the left ankle demonstrates a lucent, expansile, bubbly-appearing lesion with a sclerotic rim along the lateral aspect of the distal tibial metadiaphysis.

Lesions are typically mildly expansile, with associated endosteal scalloping and cortical thinning [**Fig. 7.71**]. Angular deformity may result from weightbearing stress, as seen with the "shepherd's crook deformity" of the femur.

MRI is not usually necessary for diagnosis but may be performed when radiographic features are atypical. Fibrous dysplasia is most often hypointense on T1-weighted sequences and variable in signal intensity on T2-weighted sequences depending on lesion composition [**Fig. 7.71**]. A hypointense rim is typically noted on all sequences, and enhancement is seen which is most pronounced centrally.

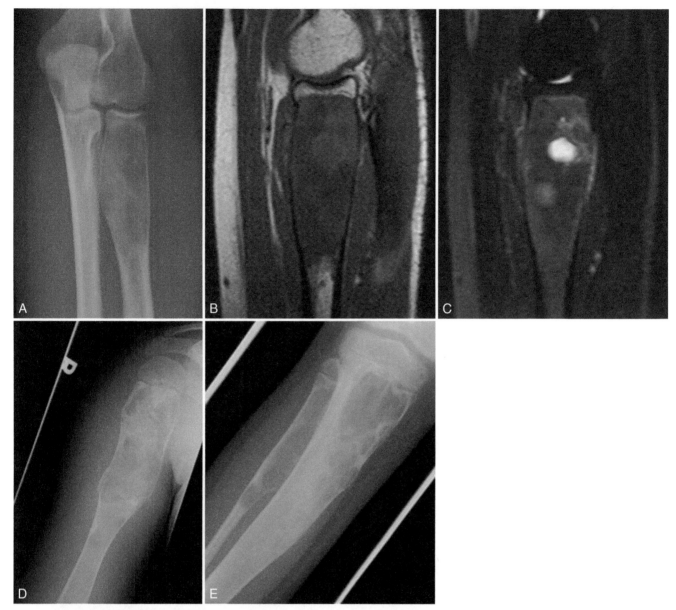

Figure 7.71 Fibrous dysplasia. A, Anteroposterior radiograph of the left elbow demonstrates a lucent, expansile lesion of the proximal radial metaphysis and metadiaphysis with the classic ground-glass matrix. **B,** Coronal T1-weighted magnetic resonance (MR) image shows low signal throughout the lesion with a well-defined, low-signal rim. **C,** Coronal fast spin-echo inversion-recovery MR image shows predominantly low signal intensity, with mild heterogeneity and a small focal fluid component noted. **D,** Radiograph of the right humerus and (**E**) radiograph of the right lower leg in a patient with McCune-Albright syndrome show polyostotic fibrous dysplasia in the humerus, tibia, and fibula, characteristically involving ipsilateral extremities.

Treatment for fibrous dysplasia is typically supportive. Surgical management may be indicated in cases of pathologic fracture or impending biomechanical failure. Sarcomatous transformation to osteosarcoma or fibrosarcoma can occur in rare circumstances. This is seen in approximately 0.5% of cases, with a higher incidence in the setting of polyostotic disease.

Osteofibrous Dysplasia

Osteofibrous dysplasia (OFD) is a rare, benign lesion that develops due to proliferation of fibroosseous tissue. It is histologically similar to fibrous dysplasia, although a distinguishing feature is the presence of active osteoblasts in OFD. This lesion most often affects younger children in the first decade of life. It is a cortically based lytic lesion classically seen in the diaphysis or metadiaphysis of the tibia. Patients typically present with prominent anterior bowing of the lower leg. Pathologic fracture is relatively common, and pseudoarthrosis may occur.

On radiographs, OFD appears as a lucent, unilocular or multilocular lesion expanding the anterior cortex of the tibia [**Fig. 7.72A**]. Larger lesions may extend posteriorly to replace the medullary cavity. The matrix of the lesion may be lucent or ground glass in character, and the margins are usually well-defined and often sclerotic. As indicated, associated anterior tibial bowing is common. On MRI, OFD is typically isointense on T1-weighted sequences and variably hyperintense on T2-weighted sequences, with enhancement after contrast administration [**Fig. 7.72B** and **C**].

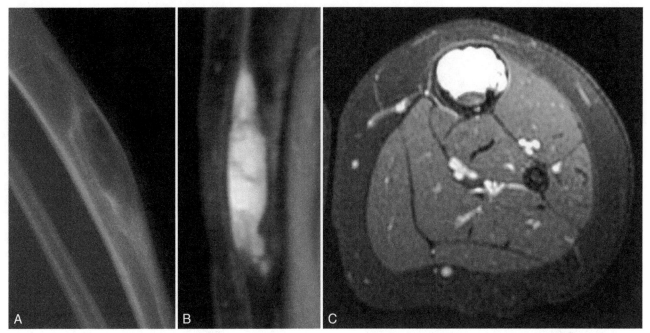

Figure 7.72 Osteofibrous dysplasia. A, Lateral radiograph of the lower leg shows a lucent, expansile lesion with a sclerotic rim along the anterior cortex of the tibia. Associated anterior tibial bowing is present. **B,** Sagittal fast spin-echo inversion-recovery magnetic resonance image shows heterogeneous T2 hyperintensity throughout the lesion. **C,** Axial T1-weighted postcontrast image with fat saturation shows fairly homogeneous, diffuse enhancement.

An important differential consideration is adamantinoma, a low-grade epithelial neoplasm that also occurs in the anterior cortex of the tibia [**Fig. 7.73**]. Although OFD is benign with no metastatic potential, adamantinoma can be locally aggressive and occasionally metastasizes, most often to the lungs. While OFD is typically seen in children younger than 10 years, adamantinoma usually occurs in young adults, with a mean age of 30 years. There is some overlap in the demographics and imaging features of these entities; thus biopsy is most often necessary.

Treatment for OFD is usually conservative. Intralesional treatment with curettage and bone graft packing is not successful, with a recurrence rate of virtually 100%. The only definitive treatment for this entity is intercalary resection of the involved bone. Reconstructive options are fairly aggressive for a benign lesion, and not without potential complications. Some data suggest that these lesions regress over time; thus watchful waiting and bracing to prevent pathologic fracture are most often the best course of action.

Langerhans Cell Histiocytosis

Langerhans cell histiocytosis (LCH) is a disease of unknown etiology characterized by abnormal proliferation of a histiocyte called a *Langerhans cell.* It encompasses a spectrum of disease ranging from a single, benign, self-limiting bony lesion to a fulminant, disseminated disorder involving multiple organ systems. Historically, three distinct forms of LCH have been described. Eosinophilic granuloma refers to localized skeletal or pulmonary disease presenting in children between 5 and 15 years of age. Hand-Schüller-Christian disease is characterized by the triad of osseous lesions, diabetes insipidus, and exophthalmos, typically presenting between 1 and 5 years of age. Letterer-Siwe disease is a fulminant form of LCH with osseous and solid organ involvement developing in infants younger than 6 months and associated with death 1 to 2 years after presentation. Generally speaking, disease confined to bone, whether monostotic or polyostotic, has a favorable prognosis, whereas

LCH with solid-organ involvement has a poor prognosis. LCH is most common in Caucasians, and there is a 2:1 male preponderance.

In 75% of cases of LCH, disease is confined to bone. Solitary bone lesions develop in the flat bones in 70% of cases, and in the diaphyses or metaphyses of the long bones in 30% of cases. The skull, vertebral column, pelvis, scapula, ribs, mandible, and femur are most often involved, and lesions are typically intramedullary. Multifocal lesions are seen in approximately 25% of cases, and a complete skeletal survey is indicated when LCH is a consideration. Patients with bone disease present with local pain and tenderness. Low-grade fever is sometimes present, and inflammatory markers may be elevated.

The imaging features of LCH vary based on disease activity. On radiographs, active lesions may have an aggressive appearance with a permeative matrix and wide zone of transition. Associated endosteal scalloping, cortical destruction, and periosteal new bone formation may be seen [**Fig. 7.74A** and **B**]. Inactive lesions demonstrate benign features, appearing lucent with well-defined, sclerotic margins and associated thick, mature periosteal new bone formation. Several distinctive features are noted on radiographs when LCH involves certain bones. In the skull, lesions have a "punched-out," geographic appearance with beveled borders caused by destruction of both the inner and outer tables of the calvarium. The "floating tooth" sign may be seen in the setting of a maxillary or mandibular lesion, with destruction of the root of the tooth. In the spine, "vertebra plana" is a nearly pathognomonic finding, with marked flattening of a single vertebral body.

During the active phase of disease, the MRI features of LCH are nonspecific, resembling those of other aggressive bone lesions including osteomyelitis, Ewing sarcoma, and lymphoma. An intramedullary lesion is seen, often with associated cortical destruction and an extraosseous soft tissue component. Active lesions are typically hypointense to isointense on T1-weighted sequences and hyperintense on T2-weighted sequences, with diffuse enhancement after contrast administration. Surrounding marrow edema and deep soft tissue edema

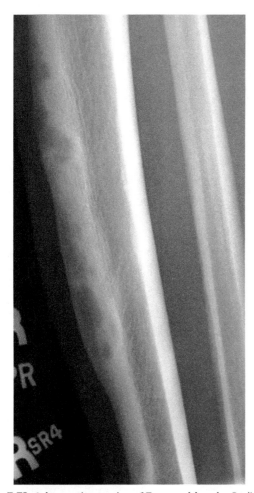

Figure 7.73 Adamantinoma in a 17-year-old male. Radiograph of the lower leg demonstrates a patchy, lucent lesion expanding the anterior cortex of the tibia. Biopsy of this lesion confirmed adamantinoma. Osteofibrous dysplasia was a differential diagnostic consideration based on imaging findings.

may be seen [**Fig. 7.74C and D**]. With inactive or healing lesions, there is usually hypointensity on both T1- and T2-weighted sequences.

Monostotic LCH is typically treated with intralesional steroid injection. In patients who require an open biopsy, curettage may be performed and is usually curative. For patients with polyostotic lesions, recurrent disease, and disseminated organ involvement, systemic treatment with chemotherapy is often required. Traditionally, radiographic skeletal surveys and bone scintigraphy have been used to identify and follow disease. More recently, whole-body MRI and PET scans have been used in this regard.

Cartilaginous Bone Tumors
Osteochondroma/Exostosis

An osteochondroma is thought to reflect a developmental defect related to focal abnormal bone growth in the setting of injury to the perichondrium. The lesion consists of a bony excrescence with an overlying cartilage cap. Solitary osteochondromas are seen in 1% of the population and are slightly more common in boys than in girls. An increased incidence is seen after trauma and in patients with a history of radiation therapy at a young age. Lesions are most often encountered in the metaphyses of long bones, most frequently at the knee. They may be sessile or pedunculated [**Fig. 7.75**]. Osteochondromas grow until the time

of skeletal maturity. Most are asymptomatic; however, complications may occur. These include pathologic fracture through a pedunculated lesion [**Fig. 7.75C**], pressure deformity of adjacent bones, impingement of adjacent myotendinous and neurovascular structures, and development of a reactive bursa overlying the lesion. Malignant transformation of a solitary osteochondroma to a chondrosarcoma is rare, occurring in less than 1% of patients.

Hereditary osteochondromatosis/multiple hereditary exostosis is associated with the development of multiple osteochondromas throughout the skeleton. An autosomal dominant pattern of inheritance is associated, although 10% of cases arise spontaneously. Most cases manifest by 10 years of age. The incidence of malignant transformation is somewhat higher than that seen with solitary osteochondromas, on the order of 5% to 25%. This is rare in childhood and typically occurs around 40 years of age. Focal pain is often associated.

Radiographs are typically sufficient for diagnosis without the need for additional imaging. The hallmark of an osteochondroma is continuity of the cortex and medullary cavity of the underlying bone into the lesion [**Fig. 7.75**]. MRI is most often pursued to assess the bony and soft tissue complications that may be associated with an osteochondroma. The lesion itself may be purely cartilaginous or may have some degree of ossification. The cartilage cap demonstrates hyperintensity on fluid and cartilage-sensitive sequences, with thin peripheral enhancement noted after contrast administration. In a benign lesion, the cap is typically less than or equal to 1.5 cm in thickness [**Fig. 7.75E**]. Increased thickness of the cartilage cap is seen in the setting of malignant transformation.

The majority of osteochondromas are simply observed with no treatment necessary. Surgical management is considered when symptoms are present related to fracture or soft tissue impingement.

Enchondroma

An enchondroma is a cartilaginous tumor that forms due to failure of normal endochondral ossification at the physis. Enchondromas are most commonly seen in the tubular bones of the hands and feet [**Fig. 7.76A**] and the metaphyses and metadiaphyses of the long bones. Approximately 80% of hand tumors in children are enchondromas, and lesions become more common with age.

Ollier disease/enchondromatosis is a nonheritable disorder characterized by the formation of multiple enchondromas in the metaphyses of the long bones, the short tubular bones, and the flat bones [**Fig. 7.76B**]. Disease is typically bilateral but asymmetric. Lesions may interfere with growth plate function, with resultant limb shortening and possibly angular deformity. Maffucci syndrome is a nonheritable disorder characterized by enchondromatosis and multiple soft tissue hemangiomas. Both Ollier disease and Maffucci syndrome are more common in boys than girls. Although isolated enchondromas most often present during the third and fourth decades of life, Ollier disease and Maffucci syndrome often present in infancy or early childhood. Malignant transformation of a solitary enchondroma is rare; however, it is more commonly seen with Ollier disease and Maffucci syndrome. Approximately 5% of patients with chondrosarcoma have Ollier disease. Patients with Maffucci syndrome have an increased risk for abdominal and central nervous system malignancies.

On radiography, enchondromas are lucent and expansile intramedullary lesions with thin, sclerotic margins, thinning of the overlying cortex, and endosteal scalloping. A cartilaginous "ring-and-arc" pattern may be seen in the matrix of the lesion [**Fig. 7.76A**]. On MRI, lesions follow the signal intensity of cartilage on all sequences, isointense to muscle on T1-weighted images and hyperintense on T2-weighted sequences. Peripheral

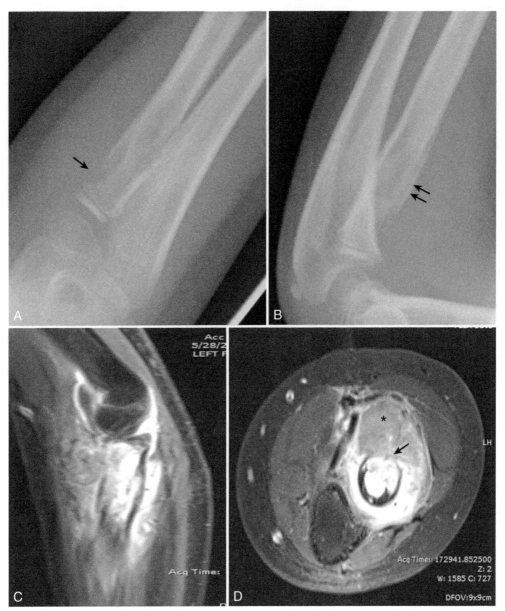

Figure 7.74 **Langerhans cell histiocytosis. A,** Anteroposterior and (**B**) lateral radiographs of the elbow show a permeative lesion in the proximal radius with cortical breakthrough (*arrow*) and subperiosteal new bone formation (*double arrows*). **C,** Sagittal and (**D**) axial T1-weighted postcontrast images with fat saturation show an enhancing intramedullary lesion with destruction of the cortex (*arrow*), an associated soft tissue component (*asterisk*), reactive synovitis, and deep soft tissue edema.

enhancement and central ring-and-arc enhancement may be seen. Surrounding marrow edema is typically absent.

Solitary enchondromas are typically managed nonoperatively. Imaging follow-up is not required unless a lesion becomes painful or a complication such as a pathologic fracture occurs.

Chondroblastoma

Chondroblastoma is an uncommon, benign cartilaginous tumor that most frequently presents in the second decade of life and affects boys more often than girls. It is an epiphyseal lesion and is most commonly seen in the proximal humerus, distal femur, and proximal tibia. It may also develop in epiphyseal equivalents, including the apophyses, the patella, and the carpal and tarsal bones. Extension to the adjacent metaphysis may be seen, and a striking associated inflammatory response is characteristic.

On radiographs, a lucent, well-defined, geographic lesion with sclerotic borders is seen eccentrically positioned within an epiphysis [**Fig. 7.77A**]. There may be endosteal erosion and cortical destruction. Periosteal reaction can be seen along the adjacent metaphysis. Chondroid calcification may be evident in the matrix of the lesion, although this is usually better seen on CT scan [**Fig. 7.77B**].

On MRI, a chondroblastoma may follow the signal intensity of cartilage, although signal characteristics are somewhat variable based on the extent of calcification within the lesion. A low signal rim is noted on all sequences. Local inflammatory change is well demonstrated and may include surrounding marrow and soft tissue edema, a joint effusion, and synovitis. An intralesional aneurysmal bone cyst (ABC) may develop in approximately 15% of cases, with characteristic fluid–fluid levels on MRI [**Fig. 7.77C** and **D**]. On radiographs, a chondroblastoma may appear similar to a Brodie abscess. MRI is particularly useful to distinguish these

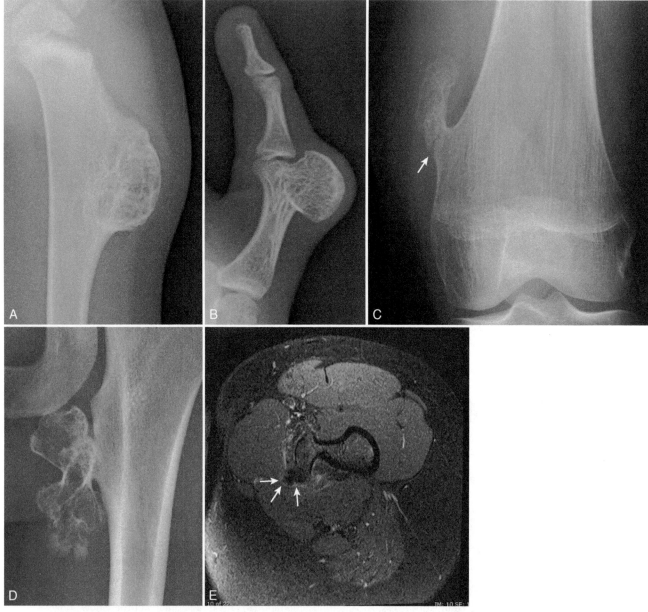

Figure 7.75 Osteochondroma. A, Anteroposterior radiograph of the humerus demonstrates a sessile osteochondroma arising from the metadiaphysis. **B,** Oblique radiograph of the fifth digit shows a pedunculated osteochondroma arising from the distal aspect of the proximal phalanx. **C,** Anteroposterior radiograph of the knee demonstrates a pedunculated osteochondroma at the distal femoral metadiaphysis, with a pathologic fracture at the base of the lesion (*arrow*). **D,** Anteroposterior radiograph of the left hip shows a prominent pedunculated osteochondroma arising from the lesser trochanter. **E,** Axial T1-weighted postcontrast image with fat saturation through the lesion depicted in (**D**) shows a very thin enhancing cartilage cap (*arrows*), compatible with benignity.

entities, as a chondroblastoma will demonstrate central enhancement while a fluid-filled abscess will not.

Chondroblastomas are treated with curettage and bone graft placement. The recurrence rate is 15% to 20% after operative management.

Osseous Tumors

Osteoid Osteoma/Osteoblastoma

Osteoid osteoma is a common benign tumor of bone most often seen in males in the second decade of life. The classic clinical presentation associated with this lesion is pain that is worse at night and relieved by aspirin or nonsteroidal antiinflammatory drugs. It is most often encountered in the femur and the tibia, usually in the diaphysis or metadiaphysis. The majority of lesions arise in the bony cortex, but they may also more rarely develop in the medullary cavity or periosteum. Lesions may be extraarticular or intraarticular. Lesions larger than 1.5 cm are referred to as osteoblastomas. Unlike osteoid osteomas, osteoblastomas have a predilection for the axial skeleton. These larger lesions have a relatively higher incidence of recurrence after local excision.

On radiography and CT scan, an intracortical nidus is seen which may be lucent or calcified. This is surrounded by periosteal reaction and bony proliferation [**Figs. 7.3A** and 7.78]. MRI findings may include demonstration of the nidus, associated marrow and soft tissue edema, and periosteal reaction. If

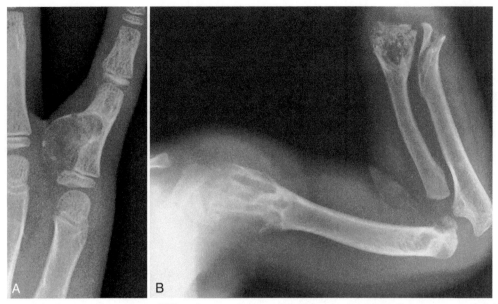

Figure 7.76 Solitary enchondroma/Ollier disease. A, Frontal radiograph of the fifth digit shows a well-defined, lucent, expansile lesion in the proximal phalanx, with a sclerotic rim and marked thinning of the overlying cortex. A characteristic "ring-and-arc" mineralization pattern is seen within the matrix of the lesion. **B,** Ollier disease, with enchondromas demonstrated in the proximal humeral, distal radial, and distal ulnar metaphyses.

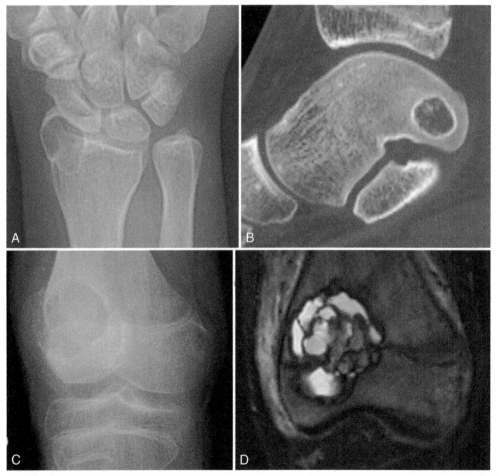

Figure 7.77 Chondroblastoma. A, Posteroanterior radiograph of the right wrist demonstrates a well-defined, lucent lesion with a sclerotic rim in the distal radial epiphysis. Faint calcification is noted in the matrix of the lesion. **B,** Sagittal reformatted computed tomography image of the ankle shows a chondroblastoma in the posterior talus, with characteristic "ring-and-arc" calcification. **C,** Oblique radiograph of the knee shows a well-circumscribed lucent lesion with a sclerotic rim in the distal femoral metaphysis and epiphysis. **D,** Coronal short tau inversion recovery magnetic resonance image of the lesion in (**C**) demonstrates a heterogeneous, multiloculated lesion of mixed signal intensity. At biopsy, a chondroblastoma with an intralesional aneurysmal bone cyst was confirmed.

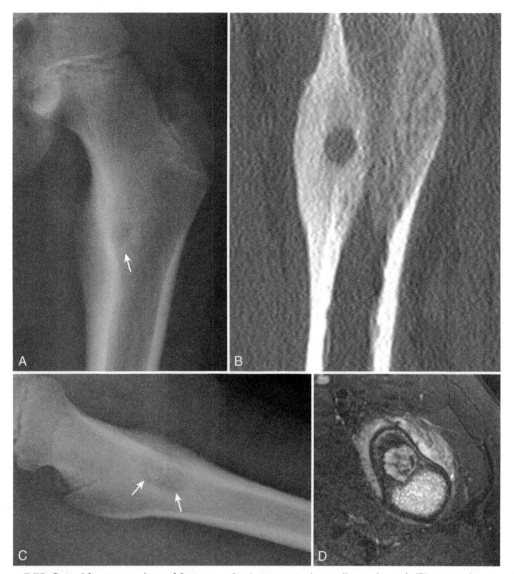

Figure 7.78 **Osteoid osteoma/osteoblastoma. A,** Anteroposterior radiograph and (**B**) coronal computed tomography reformatted image of the left hip show a small, well-defined, cortically based lucent lesion at the lesser trochanter with significant surrounding sclerosis (*arrow*), consistent with an osteoid osteoma. **C,** Frog-leg lateral image of the left hip in a different patient shows a larger, well-defined, cortically based lucent lesion with central sclerosis in the intertrochanteric region of the proximal femur (*arrows*). An osteoblastoma was confirmed at biopsy. **D,** Axial T2-weighted magnetic resonance image with fat saturation through the lesion in (**C**) demonstrates a heterogeneously high-signal lesion with a low-signal rim. There is adjacent marrow edema and deep soft tissue edema.

demonstrated, the nidus may be hypointense on T1-weighted images and hypointense or hyperintense on T2-weighted images, with enhancement after contrast administration. Notably, MRI is limited as a primary modality to investigate for osteoid osteoma. If a nidus is not demonstrated, other MR findings are nonspecific and may raise concern for various inflammatory and neoplastic processes [**Fig. 7.3B**]. Radiographic and CT correlation are important for definitive diagnosis of this entity.

Osteoid osteomas are most often treated with radiofrequency ablation. Osteoblastomas are more often managed by curettage or resection.

Cystic Bone Tumors

Unicameral Bone Cyst

A unicameral bone cyst (UBC) is a benign cystic lesion most commonly encountered in children 9 to 15 years of age. It is

more common in boys than in girls. This lesion develops centrally within the metaphysis of long bones, most commonly involving the proximal humerus, proximal femur, and proximal tibia. Pathologic fracture is common, as UBCs replace the normal architecture of bone.

On radiography, a radiolucent lesion with no internal matrix is seen centered in the medullary cavity. The cyst margin is well defined and usually sclerotic. The lesion may be expansile, with associated thinning of the bony cortex [**Figs. 7.26B**, **7.26C**, and **7.79**]. In the setting of a pathologic fracture, a "fallen fragment" sign may be seen, with a cortical fragment layering in the dependent portion of the cyst [**Fig. 7.79**]. MRI is not typically performed for a UBC provided patient age, lesion location, and radiographic features are consistent with this diagnosis. When radiographic features are atypical or symptoms cannot be explained by radiographic findings, MRI may be pursued. A simple cyst will follow fluid signal intensity on all sequences, appearing homogeneously

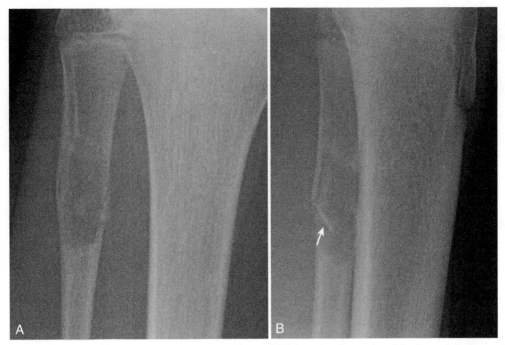

Figure 7.79 Unicameral bone cyst. A, Anteroposterior and (**B**) lateral radiographs of the lower leg demonstrate a well-defined, expansile lucent lesion with a sclerotic rim in the proximal fibular metadiaphysis. The bony cortex is thinned, and a pathologic fracture is present with a "fallen fragment" sign noted on the lateral image (*arrow*).

T2 hyperintense [**Fig. 7.26C**]. Thin rim enhancement is seen with contrast administration. With pathologic fracture, intralesional hemorrhage often occurs. T1 and T2 signal characteristics will vary, and fluid–fluid levels may be seen. With healing, there may be septations within the lesion, internal calcification, and enhancing granulation tissue. These features make it very challenging to distinguish a UBC from an ABC.

Most UBCs fill in with bone and involute over time. Larger lesions and those complicated by pathologic fracture are usually treated with curettage and bone grafting. Lesions may also be managed with aspiration and corticosteroid injection or sclerotherapy.

Aneurysmal Bone Cyst

An ABC may occur as a primary lesion or may occur as a secondary lesion concomitantly with numerous benign and malignant tumors. These include giant cell tumor (GCT), osteoblastoma, chondroblastoma, NOF, unicameral bone cyst, eosinophilic granuloma, fibrous dysplasia, and malignancies such as telangiectatic osteosarcoma [**Fig. 7.77C and D**]. ABCs are most common in the first three decades of life, with a mean age of presentation of 10 years. They are slightly more common in girls than in boys. The most common locations in the pediatric population are the femur, tibia, spine, humerus, and pelvis. Lesions are most commonly found in the metaphyses of long bones, eccentrically positioned within the medullary cavity. More rarely, lesions may be juxtacortical, interposed between the cortical surface and the periosteum.

On radiographs, a lucent, expansile lesion is seen which may appear multiloculated. The bony cortex is often thinned. Aggressive features can be demonstrated, including a relatively wide zone of transition and subperiosteal new bone formation [**Fig. 7.80A**]. On MRI, a well-circumscribed, multiloculated lesion is seen that is generally hypointense on T1-weighted sequences and hyperintense on T2-weighted sequences with multiple fluid–fluid levels reflecting layering blood products. With contrast administration, multiple enhancing septa are seen [**Fig. 7.80B**

and **C**]. This MR appearance is similar to that seen with a more aggressive telangiectatic osteosarcoma, and it is often difficult to distinguish these two entities by imaging. When the distinction cannot be made, biopsy is indicated before treatment.

ABCs are most often managed with curettage and bone grafting. Postoperative monitoring with imaging is important, as lesions recur in approximately 20% of cases.

Giant Cell Tumor/Osteoclastoma

GCT is a histologically benign tumor composed of multinucleated giant cells with osteoclastic activity. Despite benignity, there is a relatively high risk for local recurrence (approximately 25%), and distant metastases may rarely occur, most often to the lungs. The more common form of GCT occurs in skeletally mature individuals and develops in the epiphysis abutting the articular surface. A rarer form is seen in skeletally immature patients before physeal closure. In this population, GCT develops in the metaphysis adjacent to the physeal surface, eventually extending into the epiphysis. Lesions are commonly seen at the knee in the distal femur and proximal tibia.

On radiographs, a lucent, geographic lesion with nonsclerotic margins and a well-defined zone of transition is seen [**Fig. 7.81A**]. Endosteal scalloping, cortical disruption, and periosteal reaction may be present. On MRI, the appearance of a GCT is variable based on lesion composition. Cystic and solid elements may be present, and blood products may be identified. A thin, hypointense rim is often present [**Fig. 7.81B**].

GCT is typically treated with curettage extending beyond the margins of radiographic abnormality to limit the likelihood of recurrence, followed by packing with bone graft material or polymethylmethacrylate cement.

Synovial Metaplasia

Pigmented Villonodular Synovitis

PVNS is a benign disorder of synovial proliferation. This entity may involve synovial lined joints, bursae, and tendon sheaths.

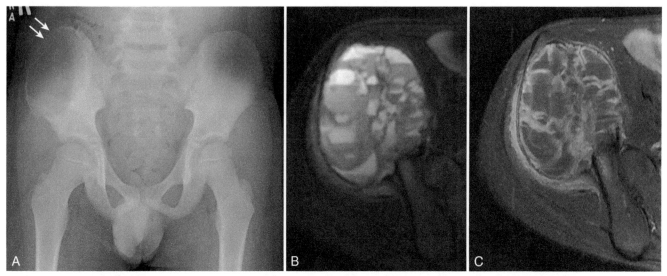

Figure 7.80 Aneurysmal bone cyst. A, Anteroposterior radiograph of the pelvis shows a large, expansile lucent lesion in the right iliac wing. A sclerotic border is seen medially. Laterally, the bony cortex is significantly thinned and focally disrupted (*arrows*). **B,** Axial T2-weighted magnetic resonance (MR) image with fat saturation shows a well-defined lesion with multiple fluid–fluid levels and a sclerotic rim. Surrounding marrow edema and deep soft tissue edema are noted. **C,** Axial T1-weighted MR image with fat saturation shows septal and rim enhancement.

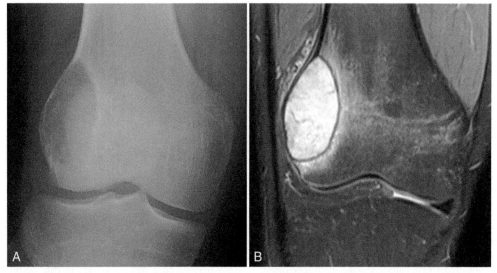

Figure 7.81 Giant cell tumor in a 17-year-old male. A, Anteroposterior radiograph of the knee demonstrates a well-defined, lucent lesion eccentrically positioned in the distal femoral metaphysis and epiphysis. The overlying cortex is thinned. **B,** Coronal proton density magnetic resonance image with fat saturation shows T2 hyperintensity throughout the lesion, a low-signal rim, and surrounding marrow and deep soft tissue edema.

The knee is most frequently involved, followed by the hip. PVNS is most common in the second and third decades of life, but it may be seen at any age. The involved synovium becomes thickened, redundant, and hypervascular, with villous and nodular proliferation. Disease may be localized and masslike, or alternatively more diffuse with involvement of the entire synovium. Invasion and destruction of surrounding soft tissue and bone may be seen. Histologically, PVNS is characterized by hemosiderin-laden, multinucleated giant cells, with hemosiderin also present in the surrounding soft tissues. This accounts for the pigmented appearance seen with PVNS.

On radiographs, soft tissue fullness may be noted at the involved joint or tendon. With more advanced disease, findings of secondary arthritis may be seen, including bony erosions and subchondral cysts. On MRI, there is diffuse and/or nodular thickening of the synovium. A joint effusion is often seen surrounding thick, frondlike synovial excrescences. Low signal intensity is typically seen on all imaging sequences, with blooming artifact on gradient echo imaging related to the presence of hemosiderin. Variable enhancement is seen with contrast administration [**Fig. 7.4**].

Definitive treatment for PVNS is synovectomy. Local recurrence rate is high, seen in up to 50% of cases.

Synovial Chondromatosis/Osteochondromatosis

Synovial chondromatosis/osteochondromatosis is a benign disorder of synovial metaplasia and proliferation. It is most often seen

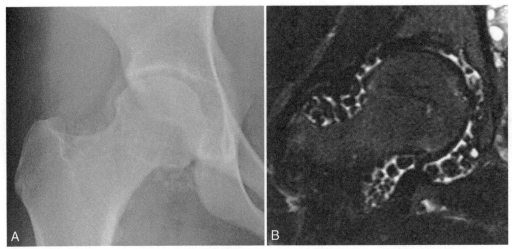

Figure 7.82 Synovial osteochondromatosis. A, Anteroposterior radiograph of the right hip shows numerous small bony fragments associated with the joint. **B,** Coronal short tau inversion recovery magnetic resonance image demonstrates a joint effusion with numerous intraarticular low-signal ossific densities. Secondary degenerative change is seen, with collar osteophytes noted.

in the third to fifth decades of life, and is less commonly encountered in the pediatric population in comparison with PVNS. With this entity, the synovium undergoes nodular proliferation, with fragmentation into the joint space. Intraarticular fragments of synovium may calcify or ossify. Disease is progressive, and joint destruction and secondary osteoarthritis may eventually be seen.

Although adults most often present with radiographically evident ossified loose bodies in the joint space, this is infrequently seen in the pediatric population [**Fig. 7.82A**]. In children the diagnosis is most often suggested on MRI with the presence of synovial abnormality and intraarticular loose bodies. MRI characteristics vary based on whether intraarticular fragments are calcified or ossified [**Fig. 7.82B**].

Synovial osteochondromatosis is managed with surgical synovectomy and removal of intraarticular loose bodies. Local recurrence of disease is seen in approximately 25% of cases.

MALIGNANT MUSCULOSKELETAL TUMORS

Bone Tumors

Osteosarcoma

Conventional osteosarcoma is the most common primary malignant bone tumor encountered in the pediatric population, accounting for nearly two-thirds of all malignant lesions. The peak incidence is between 15 and 25 years of age, and it is more common in males than in females. The metaphyses of the long bones are most frequently involved, and the majority of tumors are seen at the knee (distal femur, proximal tibia). The axial skeleton is rarely involved. Patients typically present with pain and swelling of the affected area. Although most cases arise in otherwise healthy children and young adults, predisposing factors include hereditary retinoblastoma and a history of radiation therapy.

Three subgroups of *conventional osteosarcoma* are described. The tumor may be primarily osteoblastic, chondroblastic, or fibroblastic, and the composition of the lesion will dictate its radiographic appearance [**Fig. 7.83A** through **D**]. Radiographs classically show a large, mixed lytic and sclerotic, aggressive-appearing lesion with a cloudlike matrix eccentrically positioned within the medullary cavity. Associated cortical destruction is common. Periosteal new bone formation with a spiculated, "sunburst" appearance is often seen. The periosteum may be elevated, with formation of a Codman triangle.

Radiographs are important in the initial evaluation of osteosarcoma, and are often more helpful than cross-sectional imaging in suggesting the specific diagnosis. MRI is necessary for staging and follow-up evaluation, revealing the extent of the tumor to best advantage. The full extent of marrow involvement and the presence of cortical destruction, transphyseal extension, intraarticular involvement, extraosseous soft tissue extension, and skip lesions are well demonstrated [**Fig. 7.83E** and **F**]. Sequences through the entire long bone are important for the detection of skip lesions, which may occur in up to 10% of cases. The tumor is typically isointense on T1-weighted images and variably hyperintense on T2-weighted sequences, with heterogeneous enhancement after contrast administration.

Metastatic disease is present in 10% to 20% of patients at the time of diagnosis. This primarily involves the lungs; thus chest CT is an essential component of the staging workup for osteosarcoma. Metastatic pulmonary nodules may calcify, and pleural-based metastases can be associated with pneumothorax, hemothorax, or malignant pleural effusions. Skeletal metastatic disease may occur but is less common.

Treatment most often consists of preoperative and/or postoperative chemotherapy, tumor resection with a limb-salvage procedure, and allograft reconstruction. The 5-year survival rate is greater than 75% in the absence of metastatic disease at diagnosis.

Other types of osteosarcoma, including telangiectatic osteosarcoma and the surface osteosarcomas, are much less common than the conventional form. *Telangiectatic osteosarcoma* is more frequent in males than in females, and most often develops in the second and third decades of life. It is most commonly seen in the metaphyses of the bones of the knee. This tumor is approximately 90% cystic, consisting of multiple cavities containing blood and necrotic tumor. On radiographs, the lesion is typically lytic and expansile. On MRI, it often appears identical to and may be indistinguishable from an ABC. Multiple fluid–fluid levels are seen throughout the lesion due to the presence of blood products of different ages. A distinguishing feature of telangiectatic osteosarcoma is enhancing soft tissue elements in the septations and periphery of the tumor. Biopsy is often necessary to differentiate these two entities. The prognosis of telangiectatic osteosarcoma is similar to that for the conventional form.

The surface osteosarcomas include parosteal and periosteal osteosarcoma. *Parosteal sarcoma* is more common in females than in males, and it typically develops after skeletal maturity. It

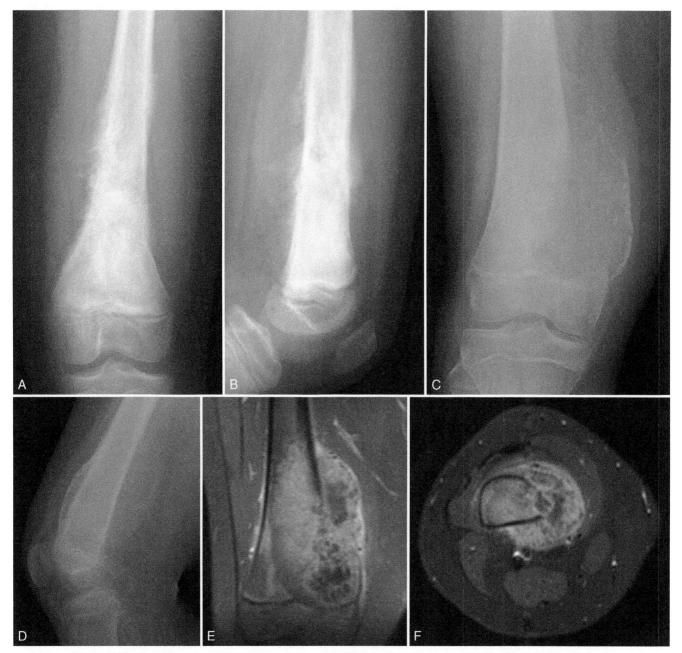

Figure 7.83 Osteosarcoma. A, Anteroposterior and (**B**) lateral radiographs of the distal femur show an aggressive-appearing, osteoblastic lesion of the distal femur. The classic "sunburst" pattern of subperiosteal new bone formation is seen, and a wide zone of transition is noted. **C,** Anteroposterior and (**D**) lateral radiographs of the distal femur in a different patient demonstrate an eccentrically positioned metaphyseal lesion with a relatively more lucent matrix. There is significant cortical destruction medially. **E,** Coronal and (**F**) axial T1-weighted postcontrast magnetic resonance images with fat saturation of the patient in (**C**) and (**D**) demonstrate a large, heterogeneously enhancing lesion with areas of central low signal which may reflect osteoid and/or necrosis. The lesion crosses the distal femoral physis, and a large soft tissue component is noted.

is a low-grade, osteoblastic tumor, most often seen as a lobulated, dense mass arising from the surface of a long bone [**Fig. 7.84**]. *Periosteal sarcoma* arises from the deep layers of the periosteum or outer layers of the bony cortex. It is a chondroblastic tumor which is of intermediate grade. It is typically diaphyseal or metadiaphyseal in location. Radiographs demonstrate an aggressive-appearing lesion with little to no matrix, and MRI reveals hyperintensity on fluid-sensitive sequences. Prognosis is less favorable than that for the parosteal form, but better than that associated with *conventional osteosarcoma.*

Ewing Sarcoma

Ewing sarcoma is an aggressive, small, round, blue cell tumor. It is the second most common malignant lesion of bone in the pediatric population. The peak incidence is somewhat younger than that for osteosarcoma, usually occurring between 10 and 20 years of age. It is more common in boys than in girls and is typically seen in Caucasians. The metadiaphyses and diaphyses of the long bones are most frequently involved, with lesions most often seen in the femur, tibia, and humerus. Flat bone

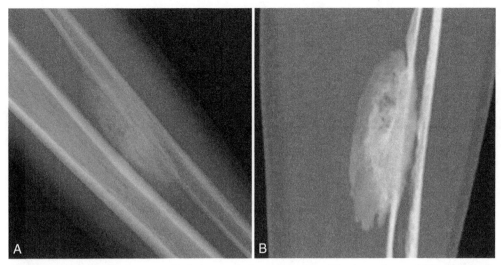

Figure 7.84 Parosteal osteosarcoma. A, Anteroposterior radiograph of the lower leg and (**B**) sagittal reformatted image from a computed tomography scan demonstrate a well-defined, sclerotic mass arising from the anteromedial aspect of the fibular shaft.

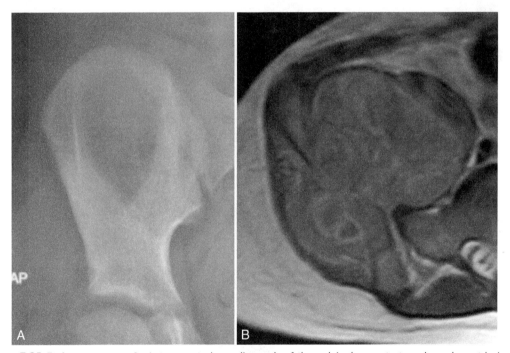

Figure 7.85 Ewing sarcoma. A, Anteroposterior radiograph of the pelvis demonstrates a large lucent lesion in the right iliac wing. A wide zone of transition is seen, particularly superiorly. **B,** Axial T1-weighted postcontrast magnetic resonance image shows a large, heterogeneously enhancing, dumbbell-shaped mass with a significant soft tissue component.

involvement is common, typically seen in the pelvis and ribs. Patients typically present with pain, fever, leukocytosis, and an elevated erythrocyte sedimentation rate.

Classic radiographic findings include an aggressive, lucent, permeative lesion with poorly defined margins and a wide zone of transition [**Fig. 7.85A**]. Areas of sclerosis may be present, correlating histologically with necrotic bone. Lamellated or "onion-skin" periosteal reaction is characteristic. MRI reveals a lesion which is typically isointense to muscle on T1-weighted images, with intermediate signal on T2-weighted images. Cortical permeation and destruction are often present, with a relatively large soft tissue component demonstrated [**Fig. 7.85B**].

Up to 25% of patients have metastatic disease at presentation, most often involving the lungs but possibly also involving local and regional lymph nodes and bone. Chest CT and bone scintigraphy are important in the diagnostic work up of Ewing sarcoma.

Treatment is multimodal, consisting of chemotherapy, radiation, and surgery. Surgical approaches are similar to those for osteosarcoma. The 5-year survival rate approaches 70% in the absence of metastatic disease at presentation.

There is a differential diagnosis for a permeative bone lesion in a child. This includes malignant tumors, nonmalignant but potentially aggressive tumors, and infection [**Box 7.2**].

Ewing sarcoma
Lymphoma/leukemia
Metastatic lesion—neuroblastoma
Langerhans cell histiocytosis
Osteomyelitis

Leukemia

Leukemia is the most common childhood malignancy, with acute lymphoblastic leukemia (ALL) comprising 80% of cases. The peak incidence of ALL is from 2 to 5 years of age. Patients may present with bone and joint pain, and tenderness and swelling of the extremities can be seen. Clinical presentation may mimic osteomyelitis or septic arthritis. Radiographs are abnormal in more than half of patients with leukemia. The most common finding is diffuse osteopenia. Characteristic "leukemic lines" may also be seen [**Fig. 7.86A** and **B**]. These are metaphyseal lucent

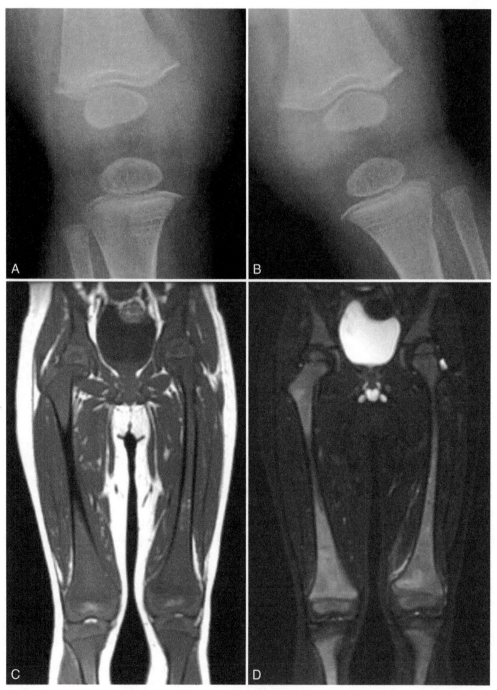

Figure 7.86 Leukemia. A and **B,** Anteroposterior radiographs of the bilateral knees in a child with acute lymphoblastic leukemia (ALL) demonstrate characteristic "leukemic lines" along the metaphyses. **C,** Coronal T1-weighted magnetic resonance (MR) image and (**D**) coronal T2-weighted MR image with fat saturation through the bilateral thighs in a different patient with ALL demonstrates changes related to marrow infiltration, with diffuse low signal on T1-weighted imaging and diffuse increased signal on T2-weighted imaging.

bands with variably sclerotic borders paralleling the physes, possibly reflecting stunted endochondral ossification in the setting of stress. MRI demonstrates leukemic infiltration of the marrow, with diffusely decreased signal intensity on T1-weighted images and increased signal intensity on fluid-sensitive sequences [**Fig. 7.86C and D**].

Lymphoma

Lymphoma in children may occur in two forms. Disseminated Hodgkin or non-Hodgkin lymphoma may secondarily involve the marrow, or alternatively, primary lymphoma of bone may be seen. With disseminated lymphoma, marrow involvement is typically multifocal, with a predilection for sites of hematopoietic marrow. Radiographically, this can be indistinguishable from leukemia. Fluorine-18-deoxyglucose-PET is sensitive for the detection of marrow involvement and is useful for following disease through treatment.

Primary lymphoma of bone is rare. It may be seen at any age but is not usually seen in children younger than 10 years of age and is most commonly encountered in the sixth decade of life. The diagnostic criteria include a pathologic diagnosis without evidence of nodal or distant disease within 6 months of presentation. On radiographs, a lytic lesion with a permeative matrix is typically seen [**Fig. 7.87A**]. On MRI, a discrete, well-marginated lesion is seen with marrow replacement. There may be cortical destruction, and a soft tissue component can be seen. Signal intensity on T1- and T2-weighted sequences is variable, and heterogeneous enhancement is typically seen [**Fig. 7.87B**].

Metastatic Disease

In children, metastatic disease to bone is rare relative to the adult population. The most common primary neoplasms that metastasize to bone are neuroblastoma, leukemia, and lymphoma. In a child younger than 3 years of age with an aggressive bony lesion, metastatic neuroblastoma is more likely than a primary malignancy.

Soft Tissue Tumors

Rhabdomyosarcoma

Rhabdomyosarcoma is the most common soft tissue sarcoma in the pediatric population. It most frequently occurs in the head and neck (40%), genitourinary tract (40%), and extremities (20%). Extremity tumors are associated with a less favorable prognosis. Rhabdomyosarcoma is the most common soft tissue tumor in children younger than 15 years, with two-thirds of cases presenting before 10 years of age. Signal characteristics on MRI are nonspecific, with T1 hypointensity, T2 hyperintensity, and heterogeneous enhancement with contrast administration [**Fig. 7.88**]. MRI is important for surgical planning, allowing the determination of single versus multiple compartment disease and the relationship of the tumor to neurovascular and bony structures. Management is surgical whenever possible, often with concomitant chemotherapy and/or radiation therapy. The 5-year survival rate approaches 70%.

Synovial Sarcoma

Synovial sarcoma is the second most common soft tissue sarcoma encountered in children after rhabdomyosarcoma. Approximately 30% of cases occur in patients younger than 20 years of age at presentation. The majority of lesions develop within 5 to 7 cm of a joint, with only a very small percentage being intraarticular. About 80% of lesions are seen in the extremities, with the lower extremities most commonly affected.

On MRI, a well-defined, lobulated lesion is seen within the deep soft tissues. This is typically isointense to muscle on T1-weighted sequences, with heterogeneous signal intensity on fluid-sensitive sequences. A "triple-signal pattern" is often described on T2-weighted imaging, with areas of hyperintensity, isointensity, and hypointensity. Cystic change and calcifications are sometimes seen, and fluid–fluid levels, hemorrhage, and fibrous elements may be noted [**Fig. 7.89**].

Notably, synovial sarcoma is a great mimic and may be mistaken for benign entities such as a ganglion cyst, synovial cyst,

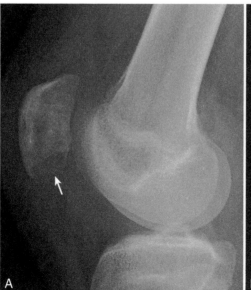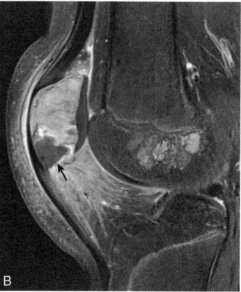

Figure 7.87 Lymphoma. A, Lateral radiograph of the knee demonstrates a permeative lesion in the patella, with cortical destruction at the inferior pole (*arrow*). **B,** Sagittal T1-weighted magnetic resonance image with fat saturation shows avid enhancement throughout the majority of the patella, with a focal of area of nonenhancement inferiorly reflecting necrosis (*arrow*). There is significant surrounding deep and superficial soft tissue edema and enhancement. An additional focus of disease is seen in the distal femoral epiphysis, appearing well-marginated with heterogeneous enhancement.

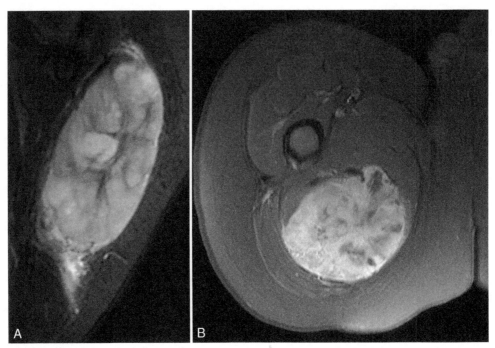

Figure 7.88 Rhabdomyosarcoma in a 2-year-old boy. A, Sagittal fast spin-echo inversion-recovery image through the thigh demonstrates a large, heterogeneously hyperintense, intramuscular soft tissue mass. **B,** Axial T1-weighted postcontrast image with fat saturation shows heterogeneous enhancement.

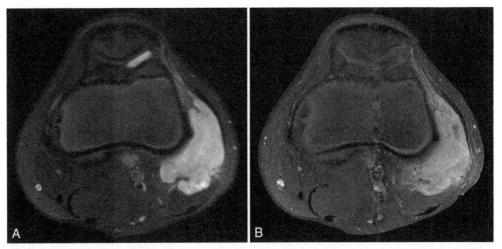

Figure 7.89 Synovial sarcoma in an 11-year-old girl. A, Axial T2-weighted magnetic resonance (MR) image with fat saturation through the left knee demonstrates a lobulated soft tissue mass interposed between the cortex of the distal femur and the iliotibial band and subcutaneous soft tissues. Heterogeneous T2 hyperintensity is noted. **B,** Axial T1-weighted MR image with fat saturation shows avid, mildly heterogeneous enhancement.

lymphatic malformation, or venous malformation. In considering these entities, it is imperative to search for characteristic features such as the "neck" extending toward a joint or tendon sheath in the setting of a ganglion cyst. When the diagnosis is not clear, biopsy should be considered. Synovial sarcoma is typically managed with surgical excision and radiation therapy.

TRAUMA

There are several unique features of the developing musculoskeletal system. These features dictate patterns of injury observed and unique aspects of the healing process in children. Pediatric bone is more porous and pliable than adult bone and can absorb relatively more force in the setting of trauma without sustaining

a fracture. The periosteum/perichondrium encasing developing bone is physiologically active and robust, and thicker and stronger than that associated with mature bone. This serves as a relative constraint to fracture displacement. For these reasons, incomplete fractures are common in the pediatric population. These include buckle/torus fractures, greenstick fractures involving a single side of the bony cortex, and plastic bowing injuries, with a bend in the bone but no obvious break across the cortex [**Fig. 7.90**].

The cartilaginous growth plate, or physis, is the weakest part of a long bone and is most susceptible to injury in the setting of trauma. The physis is the site of longitudinal bone growth by the process of endochondral ossification. It is composed of four layers of cartilage arranged in an organized fashion [see **Fig. 7.6**].

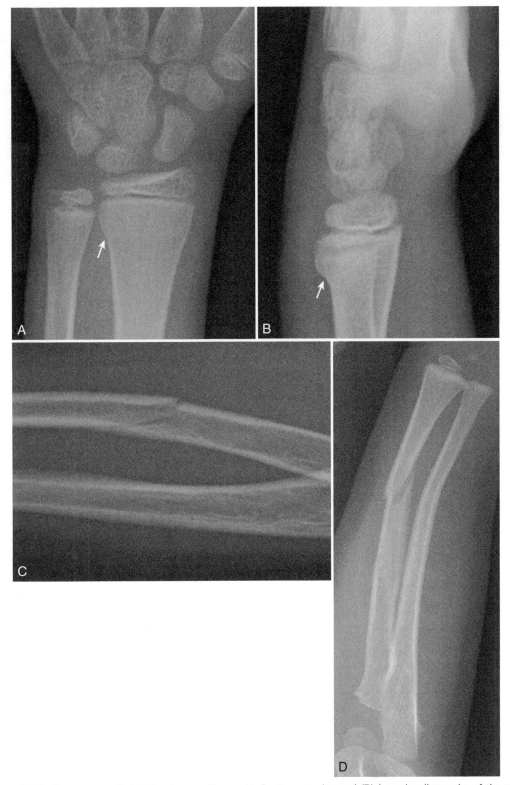

Figure 7.90 Common pediatric fracture patterns. A, Posteroanterior and (**B**) lateral radiographs of the wrist demonstrate a buckle fracture of the distal radial metaphysis (*arrows*). **C,** Radiograph of the forearm demonstrates a greenstick fracture of the radial shaft, with the fracture extending through a single cortex. **D,** Anteroposterior radiograph of the forearm shows an oblique fracture through the distal radial shaft, with plastic bowing deformity of the adjacent distal ulna.

**The Salter-Harris Classification
of Growth Plate Injuries**

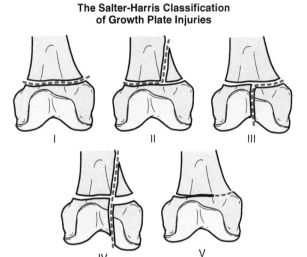

Figure 7.91 Illustration showing the Salter-Harris classification of growth plate injuries. A type I injury extends through the physis alone; a type II injury extends through the metaphysis and physis; a type III injury extends through the epiphysis and physis; a type IV injury extends through the metaphysis, physis, and epiphysis; and a type V injury obliterates the physis.

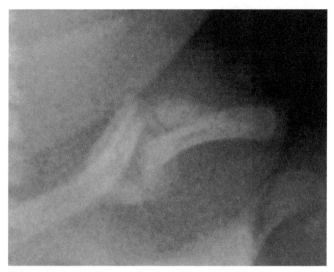

Figure 7.92 **Birth-related clavicle fracture.** Anteroposterior radiograph of the left clavicle in an infant demonstrates a mildly displaced fracture through the midshaft. Healing is evident, with subperiosteal new bone and callus formation noted.

The hypertrophic zone of the cartilage is relatively weakest, and is thus the site where fractures typically occur.

The Salter-Harris classification is commonly used to describe growth plate injuries [**Fig. 7.91**]. Injuries involving the physis carry the important risk of early fusion across the growth plate, sometimes with resultant growth disturbance and/or angular deformity. Salter-Harris type I and II injuries generally have an excellent result when treated appropriately. Type III and IV injuries more often require open reduction and/or internal fixation. Type V axial crush injuries rarely require operative management. Salter-Harris III, IV, and V fractures are most apt to result in growth disturbance.

Cartilaginous apophyses are located at tendinous insertion sites. They contribute to the ultimate shape of a bone, but not to longitudinal bone growth. Although tendinous and ligamentous injuries are common in the adult population, they are less commonly seen in children. These soft tissue structures are stronger and somewhat more lax in kids, and are relatively resistant to trauma. This accounts for the variety of apophyseal avulsion injuries commonly seen in the pediatric population, most often in older children and adolescents [see **Fig. 7.7**].

Most fractures in children heal completely without residual posttraumatic deformity. Pediatric fractures undergo robust repair and remodeling, and can often be managed less aggressively than their adult counterparts. Generally speaking, the younger the child, the more rapid the repair and the greater the potential for complete remodeling. Internal fixation is less often indicated, and complications such as nonunion are relatively less common.

Upper Extremity
Clavicle

Clavicle fractures are relatively common in the pediatric population. They are seen with some frequency in neonates due to traction on the shoulder as the infant passes through the birth canal [**Fig. 7.92**]. In older children (as in adults), they most often result from a fall on an outstretched hand. Fractures typically involve the midshaft of the clavicle, and displacement and/or angulation are common. In most cases, treatment is conservative. With minimal immobilization, most clavicle fractures heal

rapidly and completely. Surgical treatment is reserved for open fractures, severely displaced and/or foreshortened fractures, fractures in high-level athletes, and cases of delayed union or nonunion.

Humerus

Fractures of the proximal humerus are seen with some frequency in the pediatric population. Patterns of injury vary with age. In younger children, buckle fractures involving the proximal humeral metaphysis are most often seen. In older children, Salter-Harris II fractures are more common. Most proximal humeral fractures are managed conservatively, even in the setting of fairly significant displacement and/or angulation. Most fractures heal well and remodel completely without subsequent complications.

A pediatric-specific injury that deserves mention is chronic stress-related injury to the proximal humeral physis, so-called Little Leaguer's shoulder. As the name implies, this injury is seen in overhead throwing athletes. It is most often diagnosed in boys between 11 and 13 years of age. Repetitive microtrauma to the physis results from the large rotational torques involved in throwing. On radiographs, asymmetric physeal widening and irregularity are seen [**Fig. 7.93A**]. MRI is not typically needed for diagnosis; however, if pursued, it will show findings corresponding to those on radiographs, along with abnormal fluid signal along the metaphysis [**Fig. 7.93B**]. Treatment is conservative.

Elbow

The elbow is one of the more common sites of bony injury in children, and interpretation of elbow radiographs can be challenging. An appreciation of the subtle signs of occult osseous injury and an understanding of the complex developmental anatomy of the elbow are important for diagnostic accuracy. Knowledge of the most frequent injury patterns is important; a search for these should be routine in the interpretation of elbow radiographs.

Occult bony injury is suggested by the presence of a joint effusion on radiographs. On a 90-degree lateral view, an anterior fat pad is normally visible, while a posterior fat pad is not. In the

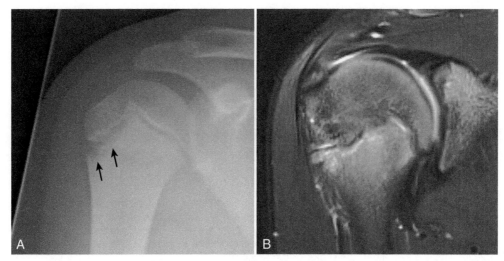

Figure 7.93 Little Leaguer's shoulder in a 12-year-old male baseball pitcher. A, Frontal image of the shoulder in a baseball pitcher demonstrates widening and irregularity of the lateral aspect of the proximal humeral physis (*arrows*). **B,** Coronal oblique T1-weighted magnetic resonance image with fat saturation shows similar findings, in addition to marrow edema in the metaphysis.

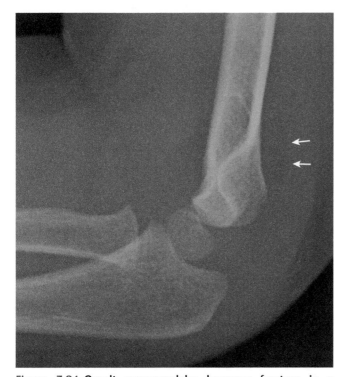

Figure 7.94 Occult supracondylar humerus fracture in a 3-year-old girl who fell on an outstretched upper extremity. Lateral radiograph of the elbow demonstrates a joint effusion. The anterior fat pad is lifted, and the posterior fat pad is visible (*arrows*). A fracture was not initially evident but was visible on follow-up radiographs.

setting of a joint effusion, the anterior fat pad is lifted, creating a "spinnaker sign," and the posterior fat pad becomes visible [**Fig. 7.94**]. The most common occult bony injury at the elbow in younger children is a nondisplaced supracondylar humerus fracture, while an occult radial head/neck fracture is more common in older children.

Alignment across the joint should be assessed on every radiographic series of the elbow. The *anterior humeral line* is evaluated on the 90-degree lateral view. This line is drawn along the

TABLE 7.1 Age of Appearance of the Elbow Ossification Centers

Ossification Center	Age
Capitellum	1–2 years
Radial head	3–4 years
Medial/internal epicondyle	5–6 years
Trochlea	7–8 years
Olecranon	9–10 years
Lateral/external epicondyle	11–12 years

On average, ossification centers appear 1 year earlier in girls.

anterior cortex of the humerus and should pass through the middle third of the capitellum [**Fig. 7.95A**]. If it does not, an angulated distal humerus fracture should be suspected. The *radiocapitellar line* should be assessed on all views of the elbow. This line is drawn along the center of the radial shaft and should intersect the capitellum on all views [**Fig. 7.95B**]. When it does not, radial head subluxation or dislocation is likely present.

The six ossification centers of the elbow appear in a predictable, orderly fashion as a child develops [**Fig. 7.96** and **Table 7.1**]. This order of ossification can be remembered with the acronym CRITOE, with the "I" and "E" standing for the internal (medial) and external (lateral) epicondyle, respectively. The ossification centers typically appear earlier in girls than in boys. This scheme is particularly important in the assessment for avulsion injuries involving the growth centers of the elbow. As an example, if a trochlear ossification center is present, the medial epicondyle should be seen in normal position. If it is not, a displaced avulsion injury is a concern. The medial epicondyle may be displaced, possibly trapped in an intraarticular position and not immediately apparent on radiographs.

The three most common pediatric elbow fractures are the supracondylar humerus fracture, lateral condyle fracture, and medial epicondyle fracture. Fractures involving the radial head/neck and the olecranon are also seen with some frequency.

Supracondylar humerus fractures account for approximately 65% of all elbow fractures encountered in the pediatric population. They are typically seen in the first decade of life. The

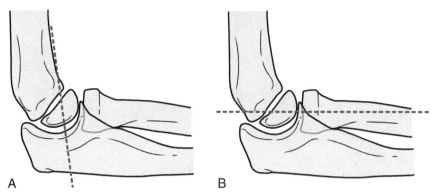

Figure 7.95 Illustration showing the anterior humeral and radiocapitellar lines, drawn to assess elbow alignment in the setting of injury. A, The anterior humeral line is drawn along the anterior cortex of the distal humerus on a 90-degree lateral radiograph. In a normal elbow, this line passes through the middle third of the capitellum. If it does not, an angulated fracture of the supracondylar humerus should be suspected. **B,** The radiocapitellar line is drawn along the center of the radial shaft. This line should intersect the capitellum on all radiographic views. When it does not, radial head subluxation or dislocation is likely present.

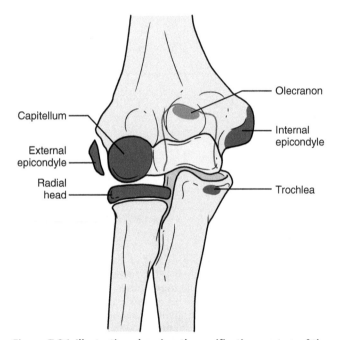

Figure 7.96 Illustration showing the ossification centers of the pediatric elbow. The mnemonic CRITOE is useful in remembering the order of appearance of the ossification centers: C = capitellum, R = radial head, I = internal epicondyle, T = trochlea, O = olecranon, E = external epicondyle.

mechanism is most often a fall on an outstretched hand with a hyperextension-rotation injury associated with valgus or varus stress. A fall from the monkey bars is often reported. Associated neurovascular injury may be seen in the acute setting.

Radiographs demonstrate a joint effusion, and the anterior humeral line may be disrupted. The Gartland classification system is typically used to describe supracondylar humerus fractures and guide management. A type I injury is nondisplaced or minimally displaced (<2 mm) with an intact anterior humeral line [see **Fig. 7.94**], and is typically treated by casting alone. A type II fracture is displaced (>2 mm) and angulated, with disruption of the anterior humeral line [**Fig. 7.97A**]. With a type III injury, complete displacement is seen, with no cortical continuity [**Fig. 7.97B**]. Types II and III are most often treated with

closed or open reduction and percutaneous pinning. In the setting of neurovascular compromise, immediate surgical intervention is indicated. Most supracondylar fractures are treated successfully with a low complication rate. Rarely, malunion may occur, or cubitus varus or valgus deformity may develop.

Lateral condyle fractures account for approximately 15% of all elbow fractures in children, and most often occur between 5 and 10 years of age. The mechanism is typically a fall on an outstretched hand with a varus stress at the elbow. The majority of lateral condyle fractures are Salter-Harris IV injuries, with involvement of the physis and extension to the articular surface. Fractures may be stable, with less than or equal to 2 mm displacement, or unstable, with greater than 2 mm displacement.

A lateral condyle fracture is often best profiled on an AP or internal oblique radiograph of the elbow, demonstrating the fracture pattern and maximum degree of displacement to best advantage [**Fig. 7.98**]. Stable fractures may be treated with a long arm cast. Unstable fractures with any degree of joint incongruity require surgical fixation. Outcomes associated with this injury have historically been worse than those associated with supracondylar humerus fractures. This is due to the frequency of missed diagnosis with this injury, the intraphyseal and intraarticular nature of the fracture, and the higher risk for complications which may include malunion/nonunion, physeal growth arrest, and osteoarthritis. For this reason, lateral condyle fractures are typically imaged weekly in the subacute phase to ensure maintained satisfactory alignment as healing progresses.

Medial epicondyle avulsion fractures are most often seen in children between 7 and 16 years of age, when the medial epicondyle ossification center is ossified but unfused. Traumatic avulsion of the medial epicondyle is relatively common in overhead throwing athletes, and it is included in the spectrum of injuries classified as "Little Leaguer's elbow." The mechanism of medial epicondyle avulsion is typically hyperextension with excess valgus stress at the elbow. Avulsion occurs because the physis and medial epicondyle are relatively weaker than the attached soft tissue structures, including the flexor-pronator mass and ulnar collateral ligament. Medial epicondyle avulsion may also occur in the setting of an elbow dislocation. Importantly, the avulsed medial epicondyle can displace into the joint space and remain entrapped despite elbow reduction. It is essential to search for and identify the avulsed fragment when it is not readily apparent.

The displaced medial epicondyle fracture fragment is usually best appreciated on an external oblique view of the elbow, but

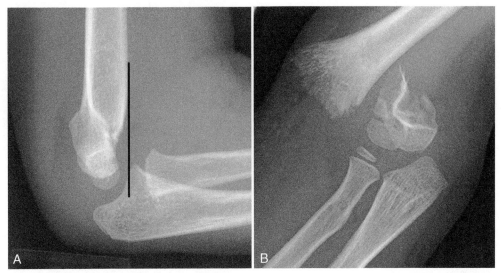

Figure 7.97 Supracondylar humerus fracture. A, Lateral radiograph of the elbow demonstrates a type II supracondylar humerus fracture, with disruption of the anterior humeral line (*black line*). A large joint effusion is noted. **B,** Anteroposterior radiograph of the elbow shows a type III supracondylar humerus fracture. There is no cortical continuity and significant displacement and overlap of fracture fragments.

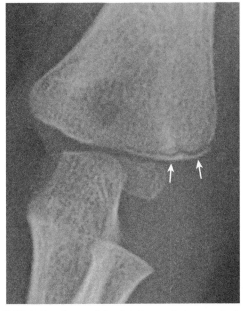

Figure 7.98 Lateral condyle fracture. Anteroposterior radiograph of the elbow shows a nondisplaced fracture through the lateral condyle of the distal humerus (*arrows*).

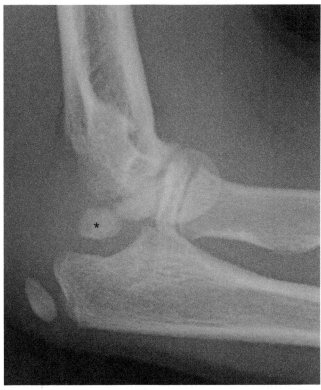

Figure 7.99 Radial head dislocation with medial epicondyle avulsion injury. Lateral radiograph of the elbow demonstrates radiocapitellar disruption. The medial epicondyle ossification center is avulsed, displaced inferiorly, and entrapped in the joint space (*asterisk*).

may also be appreciated on the AP view. If there is uncertainty about diagnosis, a view of the contralateral asymptomatic elbow may be useful for comparison [see **Fig. 7.1**]. A lateral radiograph is often helpful in the assessment for an intraarticular fragment, particularly in the setting of a radiocapitellar dislocation. Normally, the medial epicondyle ossification center projects over the posterior half of the distal humerus on a lateral view. In the setting of displacement, it may be encountered distal to the humerus or abnormally anterior in position within the joint space [**Fig. 7.99**]. CT scan may be helpful for further evaluation in the setting of a complex fracture-dislocation.

The majority of medial epicondyle fractures are managed nonoperatively. Surgical treatment is reserved for significantly displaced fractures (>4 mm), those associated with elbow instability, and those with an incarcerated intraarticular fragment.

Fractures of the proximal radius account for 5% of all pediatric elbow injuries. The mechanism is typically a fall on an outstretched hand with a valgus loading injury of the elbow. The radial neck (metaphysis) is most often involved, frequently with extension to the physis (Salter-Harris II injury) [**Fig. 7.100**]. It is important to note that a portion of the radial neck is

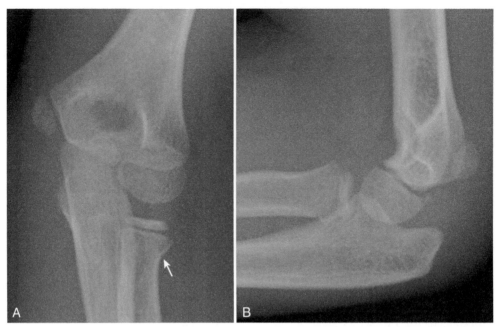

Figure 7.100 **Radial neck fracture. A,** Anteroposterior and (**B**) lateral radiographs of the elbow show a fracture at the radial neck with extension to the physis, compatible with a Salter-Harris II injury (*arrow*). A significant joint effusion is not seen.

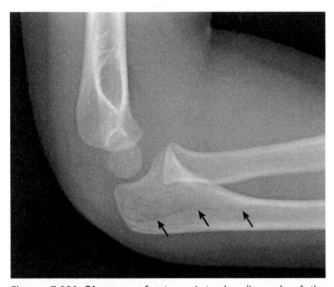

Figure 7.101 **Olecranon fracture.** Lateral radiograph of the elbow demonstrates a subtle, nondisplaced fracture through the olecranon (*arrows*).

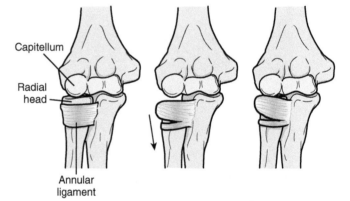

Figure 7.102 **Nursemaid's elbow.** Illustration depicting subluxation of the radial head inferior to the annular ligament, with interposition of the ligament to the radiocapitellar joint space. This entity is sometimes in the differential in the setting of upper extremity injury in a small child. Radiographs are negative, and serve only to exclude the presence of bony injury when the diagnosis is not clear.

extraarticular; thus a joint effusion and associated fat pad signs may be absent with this injury.

Fractures of the olecranon are relatively uncommon in children, accounting for less than 5% of all osseous injuries. They are most often seen in children between 5 and 10 years of age. The mechanism is typically a fall on an outstretched hand with the elbow in flexion or extension. Olecranon fractures are often nondisplaced and subtle radiographically [**Fig. 7.101**]; thus they should be included in the search pattern when bony injury at the elbow is suspected.

Nursemaid's elbow is not a radiologic diagnosis; however, it deserves mention as it is sometimes in the differential diagnosis for a small child presenting with a suspected upper extremity injury. This entity is most common in children between 2 and 5 years of age. It results when longitudinal traction is

applied to an extended arm. In a young child, the radial head can sublux in this setting, with interposition of the annular ligament to the radiocapitellar joint [**Fig. 7.102**]. The affected child presents with the arm abducted, the elbow in slight flexion, and the forearm pronated. Pain and tenderness are localized to the lateral aspect of the elbow. Radiographs are not routinely performed when classic clinical history and physical examination findings are present. Imaging is normal, and serves only to exclude the presence of a fracture. A nursemaid's elbow is nearly always successfully treated with a simple closed reduction maneuver involving flexion of the elbow with supination of the forearm.

Forearm/Wrist

Forearm fractures most commonly involve the distal radius and ulna, and usually result from a fall on an outstretched hand.

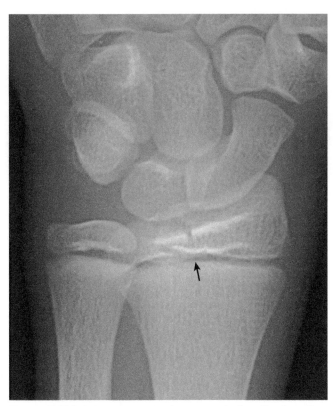

Figure 7.103 **Salter-Harris III fracture of the distal radius.** Radiograph of the wrist shows a nondisplaced fracture of the distal radial epiphysis (*arrow*), reaching the radiocarpal articular surface.

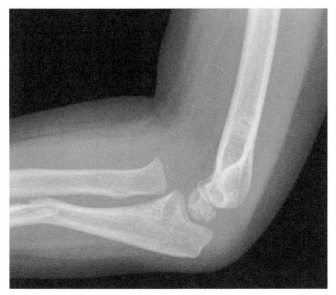

Figure 7.104 **Monteggia fracture-dislocation.** Lateral radiograph of the elbow demonstrates a fracture of the proximal ulnar shaft with anterior dislocation of the radial head.

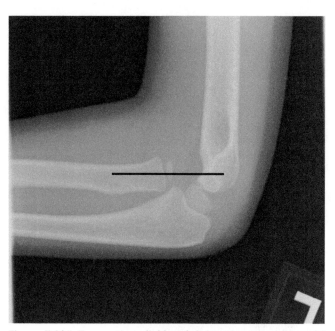

Figure 7.105 **Traumatic radial head dislocation in a 6-year-old boy who fell from a swing onto an outstretched hand.** Lateral radiograph of the elbow demonstrates anterior dislocation of the radial head with disruption of the radiocapitellar line (*black line*). This patient did not have a concomitant forearm fracture.

Buckle fractures through the metaphysis or metadiaphysis are very common. These injuries are most often seen along the dorsal cortex of the distal radius, and may be very subtle [see **Fig. 7.90A** and **B**]. A concomitant buckle fracture of the ulna may be present. Treatment is typically conservative, with a splint or short arm cast. Physeal fractures are also commonly seen at the distal radius [**Fig. 7.103**]. Salter-Harris II injuries are most frequent. Management involves closed reduction if displacement is present, followed by casting.

Fractures involving the radial and ulnar shafts usually occur together. Often a complete fracture is seen at one bone, with an incomplete fracture or plastic bowing deformity at the other [see **Fig. 7.90D**]. A forearm injury pattern seen with some frequency in the pediatric population is the Monteggia fracture-dislocation. This involves a proximal ulna fracture (or plastic deformation of the ulna) with subluxation or dislocation of the radial head [**Fig. 7.104**]. It is most commonly seen in children between 4 and 10 years of age. An isolated radial head dislocation is rarely seen in children in the setting of acute trauma [**Fig. 7.105**]. When the radial head is dislocated, it is important to image the entire forearm to evaluate for concomitant fracture. Similarly, the elbow should be included on forearm images, with one view at 90 degrees for complete assessment of alignment. A Monteggia fracture-dislocation is managed with closed or open reduction of the radial head with reduction of the ulna fracture. The ulna fracture may require fixation to maintain proper alignment, which is critical to maintenance of radial head reduction. The Galeazzi injury pattern, with fracture of the distal radius, disruption of the distal radioulnar joint, and dislocation of the distal ulna, is much less common in children [**Fig. 7.106**]. With Monteggia and Galeazzi injury patterns, it is helpful to remember that the bone that is relatively wider at the affected end of the forearm breaks, while the bone that is relatively narrower at the affected end of the forearm dislocates.

A chronic physeal stress injury may be seen at the distal radius in gymnasts, analogous to the chronic physeal stress injury at the proximal humerus in overhead throwing athletes discussed earlier (Little Leaguer's shoulder). This injury is referred to as gymnast's wrist. In gymnasts, the upper extremity is used as a weightbearing limb and may sustain up to twice the patient's body weight in this capacity. The radius is most affected by chronic stress in this setting, as it bears a disproportionate amount of the axial load (85%). Patients present with a relevant clinical history and pain over the dorsal aspect of the distal radial physis. Symptoms may be bilateral.

Radiographs show widening and irregularity of the distal radial physis. Metaphyseal lucency and sclerosis may be seen related to disrupted growth [**Fig. 7.107A and B**]. MRI is not always necessary for diagnosis; however, it may be useful when the diagnosis is uncertain, when response to therapy is atypical, or when complications such as physeal arrest or ulnar-carpal impaction syndrome are suspected. Physeal widening and irregularity will be seen, and increased signal may be noted along the metaphysis on fluid sensitive sequences [**Fig. 7.107C and D**]. Occasionally, foci of cartilaginous signal may extend from the physis into the metaphysis, reflecting disordered endochondral ossification. As with other chronic physeal stress injuries, management is conservative.

The scaphoid is the most frequently injured carpal bone in the pediatric population. Scaphoid fractures are most often seen in the second decade as skeletal maturation approaches. A transverse fracture through the scaphoid waist is most common, as in adults. In addition to standard radiographic views of the wrist, dedicated scaphoid views in ulnar deviation are helpful when a scaphoid fracture is suspected. CT or MRI may be pursued when there is concern for radiographically occult scaphoid injury. Most scaphoid fractures are managed successfully with closed treatment and immobilization. Complications include proximal pole avascular necrosis and nonunion.

Hand

Fractures involving the hand are fairly common in children. The most commonly encountered metacarpal fracture is the fifth metacarpal neck "boxer's fracture," typically seen in adolescents [**Fig. 7.108**]. Apex dorsolateral angulation across the fracture is common, with significant overlying soft tissue edema. Buckle fractures are often seen involving the digits. These usually occur at the base of a phalanx, with cortical irregularity best profiled along the dorsal cortex of the bone on a lateral view [**Fig. 7.109**]. Consecutive digits may be affected. These injuries may be challenging to identify because of their subtle nature and the degree of bony and soft tissue overlap often present on oblique and lateral radiographs of the hand. Salter-Harris fractures involving the digits are common. Salter-Harris II fractures are often seen, frequently involving the proximal phalanx of the thumb [**Fig. 7.110**]. Volar plate avulsion injuries are common at the base of the middle and distal phalanges. In children with open physes, these reflect Salter-Harris III injuries. "Mallet finger" may be seen in children, with an avulsion fracture at the dorsal aspect of the base of a distal phalanx, also reflecting a Salter-Harris III injury in a skeletally immature child. Fractures of the metacarpals and digits are most often managed conservatively with immobilization, with surgical treatment reserved for intraarticular injuries.

Pelvis/Hips

Acute fractures of the pelvic ring are relatively uncommon in children in comparison with the adult population. They are seen in the setting of high-energy trauma, such as pedestrian versus motor vehicle accidents, rear seat passenger motor vehicle accidents, and significant falls. Injuries in skeletally immature children differ from adult pelvic ring injuries in several ways. Younger children have a higher incidence of single-bone pelvic fractures than adults due to increased bony plasticity and flexibility within the sacroiliac joints and pubic symphysis. While anteroposterior compression injuries are most often seen in adults, lateral compression injuries are more common in children. Pelvic fractures in children are less often associated with hemorrhage than those in adults. This is due to smaller vessel size and a greater capacity for vasoconstriction in the setting of injury. In older children who are skeletally mature, pelvic ring and acetabular fractures follow adult injury patterns.

Apophyseal avulsion injuries are frequently seen involving the pelvis. As indicated previously, the apophysis is a relatively weak component of the musculoskeletal unit in a skeletally immature child. It is therefore most prone to injury, particularly

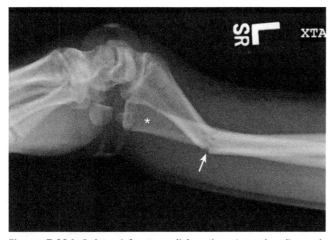

Figure 7.106 Galeazzi fracture-dislocation. Lateral radiograph of the wrist demonstrates a fracture of the distal radius (*arrow*) with volar dislocation of the distal ulna at the distal radioulnar joint (*asterisk*).

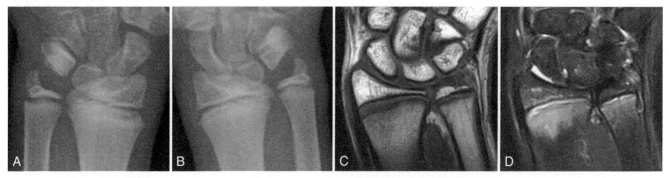

Figure 7.107 Gymnast's wrist. A and **B,** Posteroanterior radiographs of the bilateral wrists show widening and irregularity of the distal radial physis. Abnormal linear lucency is seen in the metaphyses, with surrounding sclerosis noted. Findings reflect disrupted growth at the physes. **C,** Coronal T1 and (**D**) coronal T2 magnetic resonance images with fat saturation show similar abnormality at the distal radial physis, along with abnormal increased fluid signal along the metaphysis.

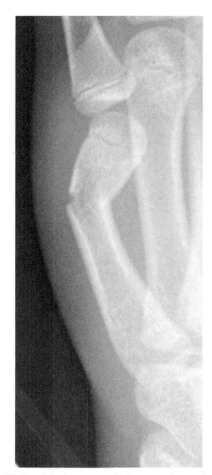

Figure 7.108 **Boxer's fracture.** Oblique radiograph of the fifth metacarpal shows a fracture through the distal diaphysis with apex dorsolateral angulation.

TABLE 7.2   Pelvic Apophyseal Avulsion Injuries

Site of Avulsion	Myotendinous Attachment
Iliac crest	Abdominal muscles
Anterior superior iliac spine	Sartorius
Anterior inferior iliac spine	Rectus femoris
Ischial tuberosity	Hamstrings
Lesser trochanter	Iliopsoas

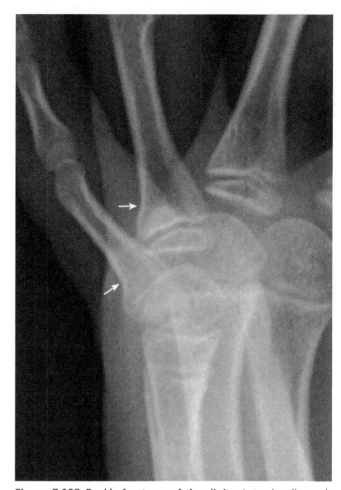

Figure 7.109 **Buckle fractures of the digits.** Lateral radiograph of the hand demonstrates buckle fractures along the dorsal aspect of the base of the proximal phalanges of the fourth and fifth digits (*arrows*). The third proximal phalanx has a normal, smooth cortical contour.

Apophyseal injuries are managed conservatively with rest from activity. Healing is typically well demonstrated on radiographs, with callous formation which may be exuberant.

Lower Extremity

Femur/Knee

Fractures of the distal femur are most often related to high-energy trauma such as motor vehicle accidents in younger children and sports injuries in older children and adolescents. Salter-Harris II fractures are commonly seen, with displacement in the coronal plane and widening and irregularity of the medial aspect of the physis. Nondisplaced, stable fractures are treated with immobilization, while displaced, unstable injuries require operative fixation.

The proximal tibial epiphysis and tubercle reflect a single entity that fuses to the proximal tibial metaphysis at approximately age 15 in girls and age 17 in boys. Any fracture involving the proximal tibial physis or tuberosity physeal equivalent is considered a Salter-Harris injury, and these injuries are often unstable [**Fig. 7.112A**]. Tibial plateau fractures may be depressed, and concomitant cartilage injury or internal derangement involving the menisci or other soft tissue structures of the knee may be present. Injuries to the region of the tibial tubercle may be associated with instability due to insertion of the extensor mechanism in this region. There is a relatively low threshold for

during periods of rapid growth. Avulsion injuries involving the apophyses of the pelvis are most often seen in adolescents, particularly those who participate in sports that involve sprinting, jumping, or kicking. Injuries involve disruption of the myotendinous unit from the apophysis, with classic patterns demonstrated in **Fig. 7.7** and listed in **Table 7.2**.

A spectrum of injuries may be seen. A true fracture will usually be evident on radiographs, with asymmetric apophyseal widening and/or irregularity [**Fig. 7.111A**], or possibly a displaced fracture fragment [**Fig. 7.111B**]. MRI demonstrates similar findings, in addition to edema within the apophysis and surrounding bone marrow and signal abnormality within the associated myotendinous unit and other deep soft tissue structures [**Fig. 7.111C**]. MRI should always be interpreted in conjunction with radiographs in this clinical setting, as MR findings alone may suggest the possibility of a more aggressive process than isolated musculoskeletal injury.

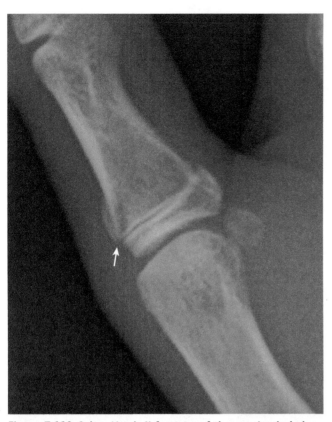

Figure 7.110 **Salter-Harris II fracture of the proximal phalanx of the thumb.** Radiograph of the thumb shows a subtle lucency extending through the metaphysis at the base of the proximal phalanx, reaching the physis (*arrow*).

surgical management of injury involving the proximal tibial epiphysis and/or tubercle in children [**Fig. 7.112B**].

Fractures of the patella are relatively infrequent in skeletally immature individuals. Patellar sleeve fractures are most often seen. On radiographs, a small linear or curvilinear avulsed fragment is seen at the inferior patellar pole [**Fig. 7.113A**]. MRI is not typically needed for diagnosis, but if obtained reveals edema in the avulsed fragment and the parent bone, superior aspect of Hoffa's fat pad, and prepatellar soft tissues [**Fig. 7.113B**].

Osgood-Schlatter disease is an overuse injury related to repeated trauma with chronic avulsive change at the patellar tendon insertion site at the tibial tubercle. It is most often seen in adolescents, and boys are affected more often than girls (3 : 1). In 30% of patients, disease is bilateral. The diagnosis is made clinically in a patient presenting with tenderness over the tibial tubercle. Radiographs may support the diagnosis. Fragmentation of the tibial tubercle is seen, along with soft tissue changes that may include thickening and indistinctness of the distal patellar tendon at its insertion and surrounding soft tissue edema [**Fig. 7.114A**]. MRI is not necessary for diagnosis, but may be indicated to exclude other pathology. Marrow edema is seen in the fragmented tibial tuberosity, the distal patellar tendon appears thickened and edematous, and edema may be seen in Hoffa's fat pad and in the deep soft tissues overlying the patellar tendon [**Fig. 7.114B**]. Management is conservative with rest.

Sinding-Larsen-Johansson disease is an equivalent injury affecting the inferior patellar pole. Adolescent boys are most frequently affected, and disease is often bilateral. Radiographs demonstrate fragmentation of the inferior patellar pole, with well-corticated ossicles of varying size [**Fig. 7.115A**]. On MRI, marrow edema is seen within the fragmented ossicles, and proximal patellar thickening and edema may be seen [**Fig. 7.115B**]. Jumper's knee is notably a distinct entity seen in skeletally

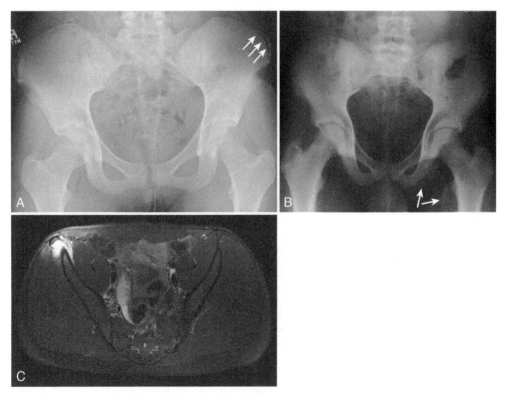

Figure 7.111 **Pelvic apophyseal avulsion injuries. A,** Anteroposterior radiograph of the pelvis demonstrates asymmetric widening of the iliac crest apophysis on the left (*arrows*). **B,** Anteroposterior radiograph of the pelvis shows comminuted avulsion injury at the left ischial apophysis, with distraction of avulsed fracture fragments (*arrowheads*). **C,** Axial T2-weighted magnetic resonance image with fat saturation through the pelvis demonstrates apophyseal avulsion injury at the right anterior superior iliac spine. There is significant edema in the widened apophysis and also in the surrounding deep soft tissues.

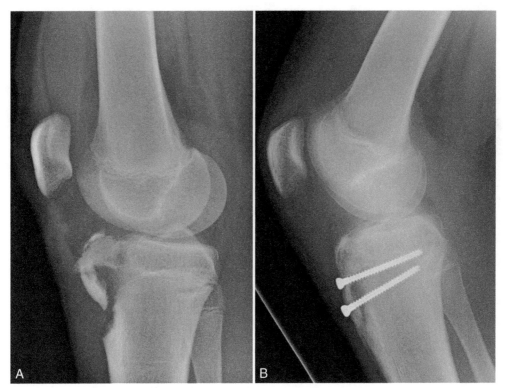

Figure 7.112 **Tibial tubercle/epiphyseal fracture. A,** Lateral radiograph of the knee demonstrates a comminuted fracture through the tibial tubercle and proximal tibial epiphysis with extension to the femorotibial articular surface. There is a large joint effusion and significant overlying soft tissue edema. **B,** Anatomic alignment is restored after open reduction and internal fixation.

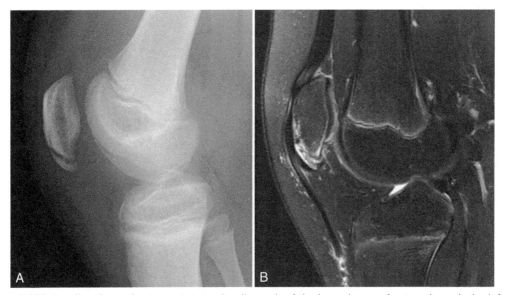

Figure 7.113 **Patellar sleeve fracture. A,** Lateral radiograph of the knee shows a fracture through the inferior patellar pole, with edema in Hoffa's fat pad and the overlying soft tissues. **B,** Sagittal T2-weighted magnetic resonance image with fat saturation shows edema in the fracture fragment and parent bone. There is abnormal increased signal in the distal quadriceps tendon and proximal patellar tendon, and also in the surrounding deep soft tissues.

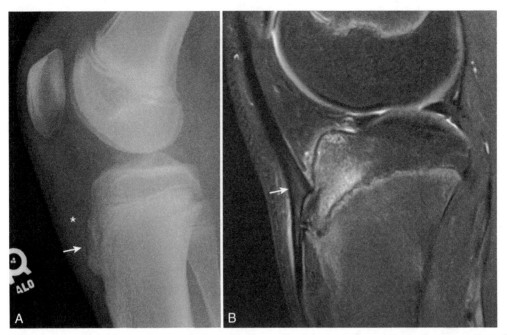

Figure 7.114 Osgood-Schlatter disease. A, Lateral radiograph of the knee demonstrates fragmentation of the tibial tubercle (*arrow*), thickening of the distal patellar tendon (*asterisk*), and soft tissue stranding in Hoffa's fat pad. **B,** Sagittal T2-weighted magnetic resonance image with fat saturation shows edema in the fragmented tubercle, extending into the proximal tibial epiphysis. There is abnormal increased signal in the thickened distal patellar tendon (*arrow*), the deep infrapatellar recess, and the overlying soft tissues.

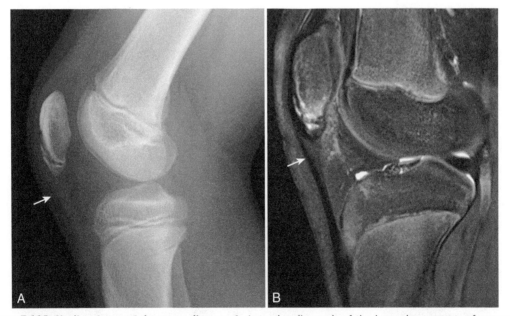

Figure 7.115 Sinding-Larsen-Johansson disease. A, Lateral radiograph of the knee demonstrates fragmentation of the inferior patellar pole, thickening of the proximal patellar tendon (*arrow*), and soft-tissue stranding within Hoffa's fat pad. **B,** Sagittal T2-weighted magnetic resonance image with fat saturation shows marrow edema in the fragmented inferior patella, abnormal increased signal in the thickened proximal patellar tendon (*arrow*), and edema within Hoffa's fat pad.

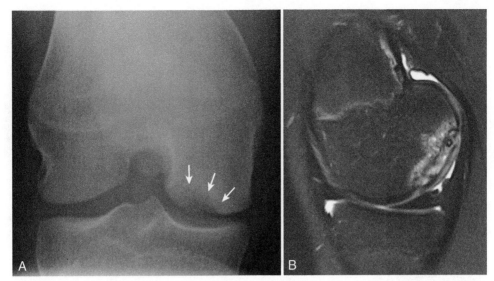

Figure 7.116 **Osteochondritis dissecans. A,** Notch view of the right knee demonstrates a focal crescentic lucency along the posterior surface of the lateral aspect of the medial femoral condyle (*arrows*). **B,** Sagittal T2-weighted magnetic resonance image with fat saturation shows heterogeneous high signal within the lesion and surrounding marrow edema and cystic change. There is irregularity of the overlying cartilage. This lesion was treated surgically as there was concern for instability.

mature individuals, and characterized by an isolated proximal patellar tendon tear. Like Osgood-Schlatter disease, Sinding-Larsen-Johansson disease is treated conservatively with rest.

Osteochondral injuries involving the knee may be acute or chronic in nature. Acute injuries may involve cartilage alone or both cartilage and the underlying bone. Chronic osteochondral injury is referred to as OCD. In children this most frequently involves the lateral aspect of the medial femoral condyle of the knee, but may also be seen elsewhere at the knee, at the capitellum of the elbow, and at the medial talar dome of the ankle.

Radiography is obtained first in the evaluation of osteochondral lesions. Subchondral fragmentation may be seen, or a crescentic lucency may be demonstrated [**Fig. 7.116A**]. On MRI, acute cartilage injury is classified as partial thickness, full thickness, or delaminating. OCD lesions are characterized as stable or unstable [**Fig. 7.116B**]. In children, the majority of lesions are stable. Features of instability include fluid undercutting the lesion, peripheral cystic change, an overlying cartilage defect, and the presence of intraarticular loose bodies.

Stable OCD lesions are treated conservatively, while unstable lesions often require surgical management. This most often involves arthroscopic drilling or microfracture to improve blood supply and healing, with removal of intraarticular loose bodies.

Lower Leg/Ankle

Toddler's fractures involving the lower extremity are very common. These injuries are most often seen in young children between 9 months and 3 years of age who are beginning to cruise, walk, and run. They are somewhat analogous to stress injuries in athletes, as they occur due to new/increased stress on normal bone. A single specific incident of trauma is typically not reported. Instead, the presentation is often more insidious, with limp or refusal to bear weight.

The injury pattern most commonly seen is a nondisplaced, oblique or spiral fracture through the mid to distal tibial shaft [**Fig. 7.117A**]. Oblique views of the lower leg are sometimes helpful as an adjunct to standard views to assess for this often subtle injury. When clinical suspicion for fracture is high but

radiographs are negative, follow-up imaging in 10 to 14 days is often useful to assess for fracture healing [**Fig. 7.117B**]. Toddler's fractures of the tibia are usually treated successfully in a long leg cast, and complications are rare.

With less frequency, toddler's fractures may involve the fibula, cuboid, and calcaneus. When the bones of the foot are involved, fractures often present and are most radiographically evident in a healing phase. A linear band of sclerosis may be seen within the affected bone [**Fig. 7.118**].

Transitional fractures of the ankle include the juvenile Tillaux and triplane fractures. These injuries are seen in the early teenage years when the distal tibial physis is nearing the time of fusion or partially fused. The posteromedial and central portions of the physis fuse first, in a focal region referred to as "Kump's bump." The anterolateral aspect of the physis fuses last, and remains relatively vulnerable to injury for a longer period. This accounts for the characteristic patterns of fracture seen at the distal tibia in this patient population.

The juvenile Tillaux fracture is a Salter-Harris III injury involving the distal tibial physis and epiphysis. The mechanism of injury is typically forced external rotation, with anterolateral avulsion of the distal tibial epiphysis and associated injury to the anterior tibiofibular ligament. There is a fracture in the axial plane through the physis, and a fracture in the sagittal plane through the epiphysis [**Fig. 7.119**]. The vertical fracture lucency through the epiphysis is often well profiled on an AP radiograph of the ankle, and is seen lateral to Kump's bump. The major concern with Tillaux fractures is involvement of the tibiotalar articular surface. It is important to assess the fracture gap in this location and evaluate the degree of incongruity or step-off present. Significant displacement without proper management may lead to degenerative disease at the ankle joint. CT should be pursued when the fracture and joint involvement cannot be adequately assessed on radiographs. Nondisplaced fractures can be treated with immobilization, while displacement greater than 2 mm requires surgical fixation at the level of the epiphysis.

Similar to the Tillaux fracture, the triplane fracture involves a sagittal fracture through the epiphysis and an axial fracture through the physis. A third fracture plane is seen, typically a

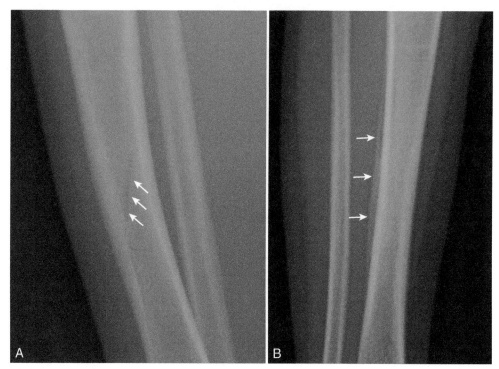

Figure 7.117 Toddler's fracture of the tibia in a 2-year-old girl presenting with a limp and no history of trauma. A, Lateral radiograph of the lower leg shows a subtle, nondisplaced, oblique fracture through the tibial shaft (*arrows*). **B,** Anteroposterior radiograph obtained 10 days later shows healing, with subperiosteal new bone formation along the tibial shaft (*arrows*).

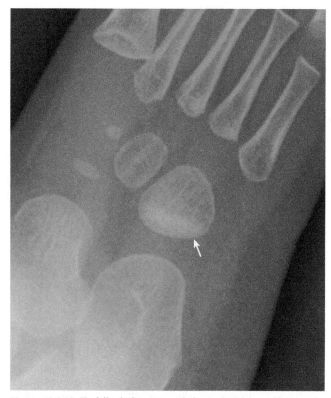

Figure 7.118 Toddler's fracture of the cuboid in a 23-month-old boy with refusal to bear weight and no trauma history. Oblique radiograph of the foot demonstrates a linear band of sclerosis within the proximal cuboid, consistent with a healing stress fracture (*arrow*).

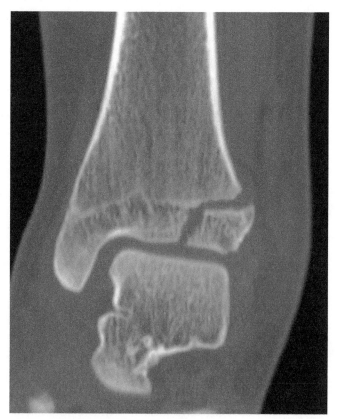

Figure 7.119 Tillaux fracture. Coronal reformatted computed tomography image through the left ankle in a patient with nearly fused physes shows a fracture extending through the lateral aspect of the distal tibial epiphysis and physis.

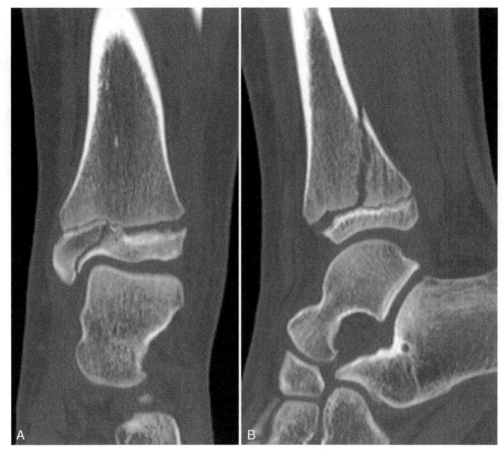

Figure 7.120 Triplane fracture. A, Coronal and (**B**) sagittal reformatted computed tomography images demonstrate a fracture that extends through the epiphysis in the sagittal plane, the physis in the axial plane, and the metaphysis in the coronal plane.

coronal fracture through the distal tibial metaphysis [**Fig. 7.120**]. As with the Tillaux fracture, this injury is typically well-seen on radiographs. CT may be helpful for mapping of the fracture planes and complete assessment of displacement at the articular surface. Fractures with greater than 2 mm displacement require surgical management, with fixation of both the epiphyseal and metaphyseal fracture components.

Foot

Fractures of the foot most often involve the midfoot and forefoot in children, with hindfoot injuries less commonly encountered. Metatarsal fractures are seen with some frequency. In younger children, the first metatarsal is most commonly injured, while in older children, injury to the fifth metatarsal is most often seen.

A "bunk bed fracture" is a buckle fracture of the first metatarsal base, typically seen in young children between 3 and 6 years of age [**Fig. 7.121**]. As the name implies, this injury is often related to a fall or jump from a height onto a hard surface, with the majority of the child's weight placed on the first metatarsal. Associated ligamentous injury at the first tarsometatarsal joint is common. Treatment is conservative with immobilization.

Approximately 40% of all metatarsal fractures involve the fifth metatarsal, with several fracture patterns described. The most common fifth metatarsal fracture in children is an apophyseal avulsion injury. The mechanism of injury is typically forced flexion and inversion. This injury is often difficult to distinguish from a normal apophysis, which may have a highly varied appearance with some degree of irregularity and

even distraction from the parent bone [see **Fig. 7.13**]. Assessment for overlying soft tissue edema is important, and correlation with clinical history and physical examination findings is helpful. Apophyseal injuries are treated conservatively with immobilization.

An adult-type Jones fracture may also be seen in the pediatric population in the setting of inversion injury. A transverse fracture is seen extending through the base of the fifth metatarsal approximately 1.5 cm distal to the tip of the metatarsal tuberosity, reaching the intermetatarsal facet. These injuries may be unstable with a predisposition to delayed union or nonunion. Thus surgical management is more common.

Fractures of the toes are fairly frequent in children, often sustained when an object falls directly onto the foot. Buckle fractures are common in younger children and may affect consecutive digits. Salter-Harris fractures are more commonly seen in older children. A specific Salter-Harris injury worthy of mention is the "stubbed toe fracture." This injury involves a Salter-Harris I or II fracture of the distal phalanx of the great toe, with concomitant injury to the overlying nail bed [**Fig. 7.122**]. The nail bed is very closely apposed to the physis of the distal phalanx; thus nail bed injury may result in contamination of the physis and the potential development of osteomyelitis. This injury is considered an open fracture; thus surgical debridement is most often performed, and prophylactic antibiotics are typically administered.

Nondisplaced phalangeal fractures usually heal well with only buddy taping required. Displaced fractures may require reduction and possibly surgical management with K-wire fixation.

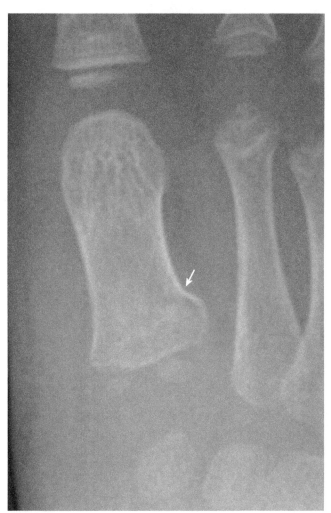

Figure 7.121 **First metatarsal/"bunk bed fracture."** Anteroposterior radiograph of the foot demonstrates a buckle fracture at the first metatarsal base (*arrow*).

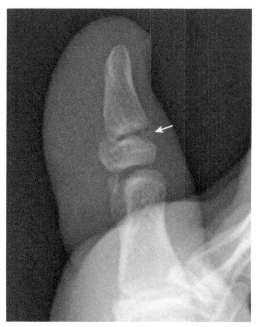

Figure 7.122 **Stubbed toe fracture.** Lateral radiograph of the great toe demonstrates a Salter-Harris II fracture of the distal phalanx, immediately subjacent to the nail bed (*arrow*).

Child Abuse

It is estimated that 1.5 million children per year in the United States suffer some form of abuse or neglect, and that more than 1500 children die annually as a result of child abuse. Boys and girls are equally affected, and the overwhelming majority of victims are infants and young children. Infants younger than 1 year of age are most often affected and account for most fatalities as a result of abuse. Imaging plays a very important role in the diagnosis of child abuse, as radiologic findings are positive in about two-thirds of cases.

In the evaluation for possible child abuse, the radiologist must consider whether the provided mechanism of injury and imaging findings are consistent with the developmental stage of the infant or child and the timing of injury reported. An understanding of patterns of fracture healing is important, in addition to the expected timetable for fracture healing at various patient ages.

A radiographic skeletal survey is performed in all cases of suspected abuse in children younger than 2 years. Additional views may be added to the initial survey as indicated for further evaluation of potentially concerning findings. A high-detail imaging system is typically used for infants younger than 12 months. A follow-up survey is often performed 2 weeks after initial evaluation. This allows for detection of additional fractures, dating of injuries, and differentiation of fractures from normal developmental variants. Beyond 2 years of age, the radiographic skeletal survey is of lower yield. Fractures are less common and less often occult, and the bony injury patterns highly specific for abuse are no longer seen. A survey may occasionally be indicated in this older age group based on clinical presentation.

The radiographic findings of abuse vary in specificity. A highly specific injury pattern for child abuse is the classic metaphyseal lesion seen in infants [**Fig. 7.123A**]. This injury most often results from the forceful pulling of an extremity. The fracture extends through the relatively weak primary spongiosa of the metaphysis of a long bone. This appears as a "corner fracture" when viewed tangentially and as a "bucket-handle fracture" when viewed obliquely. Another injury highly specific for abuse is the posterior rib fracture occurring near the costovertebral junction, thought to occur when an adult squeezes an infant's thorax. Several consecutive rib fractures may result [**Fig. 7.123B**]. These are often subtle and best seen in a healing phase. Fractures of the scapula, sternum, and spinous processes are also highly specific for abuse [**Fig. 7.123C**]. A skeletal survey may reveal the presence of multiple fractures of different ages. In the absence of an underlying condition with a predisposition for fractures, this pattern is also highly specific for abuse.

In the setting of suspected head trauma, CT or MRI may be performed. CT scan of the abdomen and pelvis is indicated when clinical history, physical examination, and/or laboratory findings suggest possible traumatic intraabdominal injury.

If imaging findings are positive or suspicious, it is the radiologist's legal obligation to report findings as consistent with or concerning for child abuse. Cases of suspected abuse are managed by a multidisciplinary team which typically includes primary care pediatricians and/or emergency department physicians, radiologists, and dedicated child protection specialists.

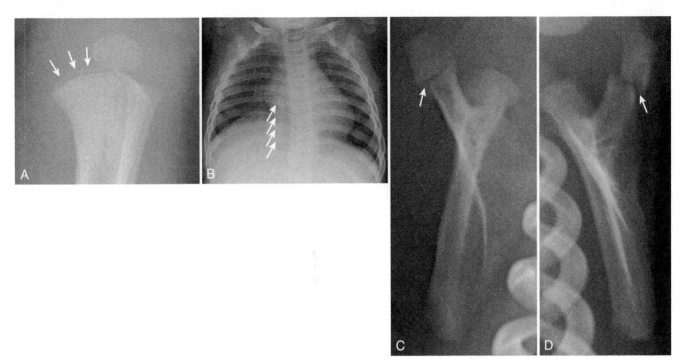

Figure 7.123 Child abuse. A, Radiograph of the proximal lower leg in a 23-day-old infant with fussiness and suspected lower extremity pain reveals a classic metaphyseal lesion of the proximal tibia with a bucket-handle configuration (*arrows*). **B,** Chest radiograph in a 12-month-old boy presenting with constipation reveals multiple consecutive rib fractures, seen posteriorly near the costovertebral junctions (*arrows*). Fractures are healing, with callous formation evident. The patient had several additional rib head fractures better profiled on other views obtained as part of a complete skeletal survey. **C** and **D,** Radiographic views of the bilateral scapulae reveal minimally displaced fractures of the acromion processes (*arrows*) in an infant with multiple fractures of different ages on skeletal survey.

SUGGESTED READINGS

Bedoya MA, Jaramillo D, Chauvin NA. Overuse injuries in children. *Top Magn Reson Imaging*. 2015;24:67-81.

Cleveland Clinic Children's Hospital. Pediatric Radiology. Available from: <https://www.cchs.net/onlinelearning/cometvs10/pedrad/default.htm>; Published 2012.

Coley BD. *Caffey's Pediatric Diagnostic Imaging*. 12th ed. Philadelphia, PA: Saunders; 2013.

D'Alessandro MP. PediatricRadiology.com: A pediatric radiology and pediatric imaging digital library. Available from: <http://www.pediatricradiology.com>.

Duncan AW. Normal variants—an approach. In: Carty H, Brunelle F, Stringer D, et al., eds. *Imaging Children*. 2nd ed. Philadelphia, PA: Elsevier; 2005.

Herman KJ, Kleinman PK. *Pediatric and Adolescent Musculoskeletal MRI*. New York, NY: Springer; 1995.

Ho-Fun VM, Jaimes C, Jaramillo D. Magnetic resonance imaging assessment of sports-related musculoskeletal injury in children: Current techniques and clinical applications. *Semin Roentgenol*. 2012;47:171-181.

Jarrett DY, Matheney T, Kleinman PK. Imaging SCFE: Diagnosis, treatment and complications. *Pediatr Radiol*. 2013;43(suppl 1):S71-S82.

Kan JH, Hernanz-Schulman M, Damon BM, et al. MRI features of three paediatric intra-articular synovial lesions: A comparative study. *Clin Radiol*. 2008;63:805-812.

Keats TE, Anderson MW. *Atlas of Normal Roentgen Variants That May Simulate Disease*. Philadelphia, PA: Elsevier/Saunders; 2013.

Khanna G, Sato TS, Ferguson P. Imaging of chronic recurrent multifocal osteomyelitis. *Radiographics*. 2009;29:1159-1177.

Kleinman PK. *Diagnostic Imaging of Child Abuse*. 3rd ed. Cambridge, UK: Cambridge University Press; 2015.

Laor T. MR imaging of soft tissue tumors and tumor-like lesions. *Pediatr Radiol*. 2004;34:24-37.

Laor T, Jaramillo D. MR imaging insights into skeletal maturation: What is normal? *Radiology*. 2009;250:28-38.

Laor T, Zbojniewicz AM, Eismann EA, et al. Juvenile osteochondritis dissecans: Is it a growth disturbance of the secondary physis of the epiphysis? *AJR Am J Roentgenol*. 2012;199:1121-1128.

Swischuk L, Hernandez JA. Frequently missed fractures in children (value of comparative views). *Emerg Radiol*. 2004;11:22-28.

Zbojniewicz AM, Laor T. Focal periphyseal edema (FOPE) zone on MRI of the adolescent knee: A potentially painful manifestation of physiologic physeal fusion? *AJR Am J Roentgenol*. 2011;197:998-1004.

Zbojniewicz AM, Laor T. Imaging of osteochondritis dissecans. *Clin Sports Med*. 2014;33:221-250.

Chapter 8
Brain Imaging

Micheál Anthony Breen and Richard L. Robertson

IMAGING THE PEDIATRIC BRAIN

The central nervous system (CNS) consists of the skull, brain, spine, and spinal cord. Imaging the brain in children differs from imaging adult patients in many respects. Ultrasound, a modality rarely used in adult neuroradiology, plays a central role in imaging the brain in fetal life and infancy. Similar to adult neuroradiology, magnetic resonance imaging (MRI) is now the most widely used modality to image the brain in older children. In addition, MRI is of particular benefit in pediatric patients given a lack of ionizing radiation. Also, many advanced MRI techniques have important and unique applications in pediatric practice. Computed tomography (CT) continues to play an important role in the rapid evaluation of acute trauma and evaluation of the bony calvarium, but its use for other indications in pediatric patients has diminished as pediatric imagers, clinicians, and families strive to reduce exposure to ionizing radiation in children. Positron emission tomography (PET) allows functional imaging based on glucose metabolism, and the growing use of PET-CT and PET-MRI allows the coregistration of metabolic and structural information, which is especially important in epilepsy imaging. The use of catheter angiography for diagnostic purposes has certainly diminished with advances in noninvasive CT and magnetic resonance angiography (MRA) techniques, but catheter angiography maintains a unique role in diagnostic imaging, and the number of types of catheter-based interventions in pediatric neuroradiology continues to increase.

Radiography

Skull radiographs lack both sensitivity and specificity for most clinical indications and carry a not insignificant radiation dose. Their use has fallen with the increased utilization of cross-sectional imaging. Skull radiographs have a limited role in the evaluation of trauma or suspected skull fracture where, in general, if imaging is deemed clinically appropriate, CT is preferred. However, skull radiographs continue to be included in skeletal surveys performed for suspected child abuse. The use of radiographs in the evaluation of craniosynostosis has largely been superseded by CT. The use of skull radiographs is no longer considered routine in the evaluation of a palpable head lump, with most practitioners preferring the use of ultrasound and/or CT-MRI.

Ultrasound

Ultrasound is the primary modality used for imaging the fetal and neonatal brain. Screening fetal ultrasound can detect many structural brain anomalies in utero, which can be further assessed with more detailed ultrasound scanning and/or fetal MRI.

After birth, the open anterior and posterior fontanels provide acoustic windows that allow exquisite depiction of the infant brain by ultrasound. Neonatal head ultrasound was first performed in the 1970s, but the image quality has improved immensely in recent years with the development of better high-frequency transducers with smaller footprints. Head ultrasound is now the most commonly used neuroimaging modality in neonates.

Advantages of ultrasound include accessibility, portability, rapid image acquisition (obviating the need for sedation), and low cost. The use of head ultrasound is particularly important when imaging critically unwell newborns. Ultrasound can be performed portably in the neonatal intensive care unit providing important real-time diagnostic information, which is especially important with neonates who are too unstable to be transferred or for neonates receiving extracorporeal membrane oxygenation. Ultrasound can be used to screen for congenital anomalies, hydrocephalus, intracranial hemorrhage, periventricular leukomalacia, and other abnormalities. Disadvantages of ultrasound are its limited sensitivity for ischemia (especially in the early stages of ischemic injury) and sometimes limited views of the peripheral structures and posterior fossa.

American College of Radiology guidelines for a standard head ultrasound consist of a series of sagittal, parasagittal, and coronal grayscale images acquired through the anterior fontanel. Ultrasound is operator dependent, and it is important to adjust time gain compensation (TGC) curves and to use multiple focal zones to optimize the imaging during acquisition. A combination of vector, curved, and linear array transducers can be used to produce diagnostic images of both superficial and deeper structures. Color and spectral Doppler can be performed to assess the circle of Willis, the cortical veins and venous sinuses, and suspected vascular anomalies such as vein of Galen malformations. Supplemental images of the posterior fossa can be acquired via the mastoid fontanel, and imaging of the craniocervical junction can be achieved by using the "foramen magnum view," which involves scanning below the occipital protuberance. In addition to static images, real-time cine sweeps can be useful. Head ultrasound becomes progressively more technically challenging as the anterior fontanel closes, and it is rarely of diagnostic quality in children older than 9 months.

Magnetic Resonance Imaging

For the majority of clinical indications in most children, MRI is the modality of choice when imaging of the brain is required. MRI has many advantages over other modalities including excellent soft tissue resolution, excellent spatial resolution, multiplanar imaging acquisition, and very importantly in pediatric patients it does not involve the use of ionizing radiation. One of the main disadvantages of MRI is the longer time required to obtain a diagnostic study compared with other modalities. MRI is also very susceptible to imaging artefact related to patient motion. For these reasons, pediatric MRI studies are often performed using sedation or general anesthesia. In general, neonates and infants younger than 6 months do not require sedation. An infant who is recently fed, swaddled, warmed, and has hearing protection in place will often tolerate a lengthy MRI examination without sedation. Between the ages of 6 months and 4 years, it is usually necessary for children to be sedated for MRI. Between the ages of 4 and 6 years, many, but not all, children can cooperate with an MRI examination. Most children older than 6 years will cooperate with MRI without sedation. Child life specialists and distraction techniques such as the use of video goggles and an entertaining movie can be invaluable in achieving a diagnostic study without sedation.

The individual sequences chosen for an MRI protocol vary depending on the clinical indication, the age of the patient, and the individual scanner. In general, an MRI of brain includes sagittal T1-weighted imaging, axial and coronal T2-weighted imaging, axial T2 fluid attenuation inversion recovery (FLAIR), and axial diffusion-weighted imaging (DWI). A brain MRI does not always require the administration of a paramagnetic contrast agent such as gadolinium; however, postcontrast imaging can be used, in particular for the identification and characterization of primary and metastatic brain tumors and leptomeningeal disease, intracranial infections, demyelination, and neurocutaneous disorders. Administration of gadolinium can also allow the assessment of cerebral perfusion using dynamic susceptibility contrast MRI techniques.

DWI uses gradient sequences to generate images based on differences in the rate of diffusion of water molecules. The rate of diffusion, or apparent diffusion coefficient (ADC), is higher for free water (eg, cerebrospinal fluid [CSF]) than for macromolecular-bound water (eg, gray matter and white matter). DWI is very sensitive to primary or secondary derangements of cellular energy metabolism such as hypoxia and ischemia, hypoglycemia, inborn errors of metabolism disorders, viral encephalitis, and status epilepticus. These changes are manifest as reduced ADC (ie, high intensity on DWI and low intensity on ADC maps). Acute diffusion restriction can be seen within minutes of injury and much earlier than on conventional imaging sequences. Current clinical applications of DWI include the assessment of brain maturation, the evaluation of ischemia, and the characterization of tumors. Diffusion tensor imaging (DTI) is a technique whereby characterization of the magnitude, anisotropy, and orientation of the diffusion tensor allows the creation of three-dimensional (3D) tractographic maps of the white matter; these can be invaluable when planning surgery for pediatric patients.

Gradient recalled echo (GRE) sequences can be used to generate susceptibility-weighted images (SWI); the signal void caused by magnetic susceptibility artefact may be the only evidence of old hemorrhage and can be especially useful in the investigation of traumatic brain injury (TBI) and concussion.

Two-dimensional and 3D time-of-flight (TOF) MRA techniques use flow compensation gradients and permit the creation of superb maximal intensity projection angiograms and venograms based on flow relating signal without the need for administration of intravenous contrast.

CSF flow dynamics are often of particular interest in pediatric patients, for example, in the setting of hydrocephalus, Chiari malformation, or evaluating response to treatments such as endoscopic third ventriculostomy (ETV). Phase-contrast techniques can provide both quantitative and qualitative information regarding CSF flow. Qualitative information can be obtained from the more widely used steady-state free procession techniques (eg, constructive interference in steady state (CISS), fast imaging with steady-state precession (FISP), steady state free precession (SSFP)).

Arterial spin labeling is an MRI technique that uses a radiofrequency pulse to magnetically "tag" arterial blood water before it enters the tissue of interest. Using a delay between tagging and image acquisition allows quantitative and qualitative measurement of tissue perfusion. This technique can be used in ischemic injury, epilepsy, moyamoya, and tumor evaluation. It is especially important in pediatric patients because the CT perfusion techniques widely used in adult practice are associated with a high radiation dose.

Proton (hydrogen) magnetic resonance spectroscopy (MRS) allows noninvasive assessment of cellular metabolism, and this is especially important when evaluating newborns with hypoxic ischemic encephalopathy, children with suspected neurometabolic disorders, and children with brain tumors. MRS can provide quantitative information regarding cellular metabolites before the detection of morphological changes by MRI or other imaging modalities. The proton MR spectrum in normal tissue is characterized by at least three peaks. The dominant peak corresponds to *N*-acetyl aspartate (NAA), which is a marker of neuronal integrity/density. The peak associated with creatine and phosphocreatine represents cellular energy metabolism, and the peak associated with choline represents cell membrane synthesis. A lactate peak is not seen in the normal spectrum, but a characteristic lactate doublet can be demonstrated with inflammation, infarction, and some tumors.

Blood oxygen level–dependent contrast imaging uses the $T2^*$ effect of deoxyhemoglobin to identify focal areas of increased perfusion in the brain during the performance of specific tasks. This functional MRI (fMRI) technique has been shown to localize the motor strip, speech center, and memory centers. fMRI is an area of intense ongoing research, but it has yet to translate into widespread clinical practice.

Computed Tomography

Modern, multidetector CT scanners permit rapid, high-resolution imaging acquisition in the axial plane and creation of isotropic, multiplanar, reformatted images, or 3D reconstructions using a variety of soft tissue, bone, vascular, and other algorithms. The speed of acquisition is one of the main advantages of CT, particularly in the setting of trauma where prompt diagnosis is critically important. CT is sensitive at depicting skull fractures, pneumocephalus, acute intraaxial or extraaxial hemorrhage, and herniation. Another indication where CT is preferred to other modalities is the evaluation of children with craniofacial anomalies or craniosynostosis.

The benefits of CT need to be weighed against the risks related to the use of ionizing radiation. When performing CT in pediatric patients, it is important to collimate appropriately to the area of interest and use child- and indication-appropriate parameters with reduced kilovoltage (kV) and milliamperesecond (mAs). The increased use of more rapid iterative reconstruction techniques on modern clinical scanners has allowed further reductions in radiation dose.

It is especially important to reduce lifetime radiation exposure in children with chronic health conditions who may undergo many diagnostic imaging investigations in their lifetime. In the past, many children with ventriculoperitoneal shunts received a large number of CT examinations for the evaluation of suspected shunt malfunction. Many centers now use a truncated MR protocol consisting of a rapidly acquired axial steady-state free procession sequence to screen for signs of shunt malfunction in preference to performing a head CT. If a rapid MRI is not available in this setting, a lower-dose CT may suffice to evaluate the size of the ventricles.

Contrast-enhanced CTA can provide exquisite vascular imaging. A tight bolus of contrast (3 mL/kg body weight up to a total dose of 120 mL) should be administered through a large-bore intravenous catheter to achieve a good-quality CTA. Adverse reactions to contrast are rare in pediatric patients; asthma and previous reactions to contrast medium are risk factors for acute reaction. Advantages of CTA over MRA include more rapid acquisition and better spatial resolution, but given the high

TABLE 8.1 Malformations of Cortical Development

Disorders of Proliferation	Disorders of Migration	Disorders of Organization
• Microlissencephaly • Hemimegalencephaly • Focal cortical dysplasia	• Type II (classic) lissencephaly • Type II (cobblestone) lissencephaly • Gray matter heterotopias	• Polymicrogyria • Schizencephaly

radiation dose involved, the technique is less used in pediatric patients than in adults.

Positron Emission Tomography

PET imaging is based on the detection of photons related to the decay of injected radiotracers. 18-Fluorodeoyglucose (FDG), which is a marker for glucose metabolism, is the most widely used tracer in current clinical practice. Interictal FDG-PET studies may show hypometabolism corresponding with an epileptogenic focus which may not be apparent on conventional imaging. Coregistration with CT or MRI can improve the presurgical workup in patients with intractable seizures. Currently, FDG-PET has a limited part in the evaluation of pediatric brain tumors, but there is ongoing research with newer tracers such as labeled amino acids, which may be able to provide information regarding presence or absence of tumor, grade of tumor, and treatment response and distinguish between tumor recurrence and radiation necrosis in the future.

CONGENITAL MALFORMATIONS OF BRAIN DEVELOPMENT

Malformations of brain development may be due to a variety of causes, including genetic abnormalities, infections, toxins, and ischemia. Recent advances in genetics, molecular biology, and imaging have resulted in an improved understanding of the pathogenesis and manifestations of many malformations of the CNS. As our knowledge of malformations has improved, the classification of the various malformations has evolved. In the paragraphs that follow, we will be referencing the classification scheme updated by Barkovich and colleagues in 2012 (see Suggested Readings for more details).

Malformations of Cortical Development

The cerebral cortex is the outermost layer of gray matter that covers the cerebrum. Histologically it is divided into six layers, each with a characteristic distribution of neuronal cell types and connections with other cortical and subcortical regions. Embryologically, the cortical neuronal cells originate as progenitor cells in the periventricular germinal matrix. These progenitor cells differentiate into neurons and glial cells. The neurons start to proliferate around the seventh week of gestation and begin their migration from the periventricular zone to the surface of the brain along radially oriented glial fibers around the eighth week. After migration, there is progressive organization of the cortex with refinement of connectivity between neurons as development proceeds. Disruption of any of the normal developmental processes can result in a malformation of the cortex. Although the phenotype of many malformations is determined by multiple errors along the pathway of normal development, the malformations are currently classified based on the earliest process that is interrupted: proliferation, migration, or organization [**Table 8.1**]. Note that in this classification system, the term *cortical dysplasia* is a specific entity and the term should not be used in a general fashion to describe other malformations of cortical development.

Disorders of Neuronal Proliferation

Microlissencephaly. Microlissencephaly is used to describe children with severe microcephaly, a simplified sulcal pattern, and a thickened cortex. Different causative factors have been implicated including cytomegalovirus (CMV) infection and mutations of the *RELN* gene. Children with microlissencephaly tend to present with seizures and profound developmental delay.

Hemimegalencephaly. Hemimegalencephaly refers to **hamartomatous overgrowth** of all or part of a cerebral hemisphere. Hemimegalencephaly refers to a heterogeneous group of conditions and may occur in isolation or in association with hemihypertrophy and neurocutaneous disorders. In some cases, there is a familial predisposition.

Children with hemimegalencephaly may present with macrocephaly, hemiplegia, seizure disorder, and developmental delay. MRI reveals diffuse enlargement of an entire cerebral hemisphere or a specific lobe of the brain [**Fig. 8.1**]. Other anomalies such as polymicrogyria (PMG), lissencephaly, or gray matter heterotopia may be present. The ipsilateral lateral ventricle tends to be enlarged. In patients with intractable seizures, anatomic or functional hemispherectomy may be performed. Surgery may be contraindicated if there are contralateral malformations. Therefore a careful assessment of the contralateral "normal" hemisphere is especially important when reviewing MRI studies in these patients.

Focal Cortical Dysplasias. Focal cortical dysplasias (FCD) are not associated with a single, known genetic abnormality and most likely arise because of mutations in a number of different genes. Histologically, FCD is divided into three main categories based on cortical delamination, disruption of cell architecture, cell composition, and any associated destructive brain lesions. The most common clinical presentation of children with FCD is medication-refractory, focal epilepsy.

Identification of FCD on MRI can be challenging. High-resolution T1, T2, and FLAIR images need to be scrutinized carefully for subtle cortical thickening with or without T1 shortening, abnormal gyration with an indistinct interface between the cortex and subcortical white matter, and the presence of adjacent white matter signal abnormality [**Fig. 8.2**]. The *transmantle sign* has been described in type II FCD and refers to T2 prolongation (hyperintensity) within the subcortical white matter underlying the cortical abnormality extending to the ventricle. The signal abnormality is due to the presence of balloon cells and ectopic neurons along the radial glial pathway. Because MR delineation of a lesion for resection strongly correlates with surgical outcome, identification of FCD is critically important in patients, with intractable epilepsy being considered for operative intervention. FCD can be clinically occult and is occasionally seen on MRIs performed for an indication other than seizure. The differential diagnosis for an FCD on MRI often includes low-grade neoplasm. Follow-up imaging to assess stability of the lesion may help differentiate FCD, which should not change over time, from a slowly growing neoplasm.

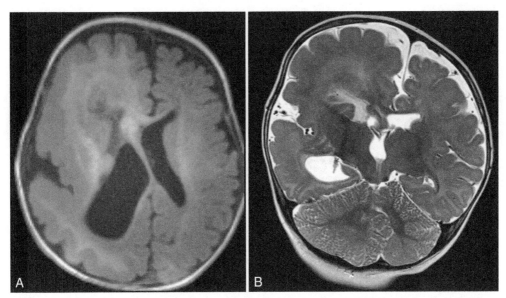

Figure 8.1 Hemimegalencephaly. Four-month-old with seizures. **A,** Axial T1-weighted and (**B**) coronal T2-weighted magnetic resonance images demonstrate diffuse enlargement of right cerebral and cerebellar hemispheres and right lateral ventricle. Note associated band heterotopia.

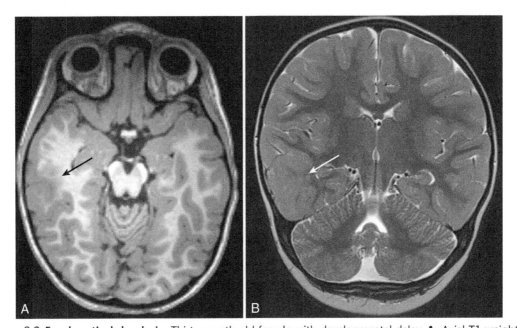

Figure 8.2 Focal cortical dysplasia. Thirty-month-old female with developmental delay. **A,** Axial T1-weighted and (**B**) coronal T2-weighted images show a focal area of cortical thickening and blurring of the gray-white matter junction along the lateral aspect of the right temporal lobe (*arrows*).

Disorders of Neuronal Migration

Lissencephaly. Lissencephaly means "smooth brain" and is characterized by reduced gyral and sulcal development. It is also referred to as the *agyria-pachygyria complex.* Agyria is defined as absence of the gyri in association with a thickened cortex; pachygyria is defined as the presence of a few broad, flat gyri. Lissencephaly encompasses a number of heterogeneous disorders that can be grouped into two major types: type 1 (classic) lissencephaly and type 2 (cobblestone lissencephaly).

Type 1 (classic) lissencephaly occurs in 1 in 500,000 live births and is caused by *disruption* of neuronal migration between the 10th and 14th weeks of gestation. Up to 70% of patients with type 1 lissencephaly have mutations of either *LIS1* or doublecortin (*DCX*) gene. LIS1 type 1 lissencephaly includes the

Miller-Dieker syndrome and results from a de novo mutation in 80% of affected children. DCX has an X-linked pattern of inheritance. Males with the *DCX* mutation have lissencephaly, whereas heterozygous females have subcortical laminar heterotopia referred to as "band heterotopia."

Children with type 1 lissencephaly are typically hypotonic at birth with a normal or small head circumference. They subsequently experience development of seizures, hypertonia, and hyperreflexia. On imaging, type 1 lissencephaly consists of a diffusely thickened and abnormally smooth cerebral cortex. *Band heterotopia* or "double cortex" is characterized by a layer of incompletely migrated neurons and more normally gyrated appearance of the outer cortex [**Fig. 8.3**]. The clinical phenotype tends to be much less severe in band heterotopia.

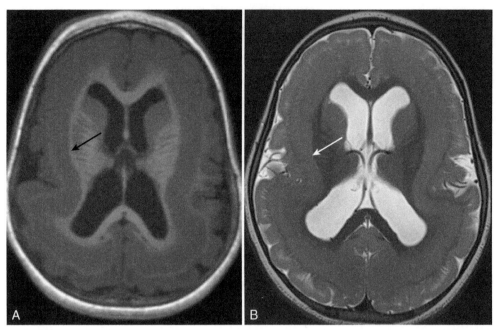

Figure 8.3 **Band heterotopia.** Two-year-old girl with developmental delay and seizures. (**A**) Axial T1-weighted and (**B**) axial T2-weighted images show thick band of gray matter heterotopia (*arrows*) with diminished overlying sulcal-gyral formation.

Type 2 (cobblestone) lissencephaly occurs because of *excessive neuronal migration.* It represents a heterogeneous group of disorders characterized by morphological abnormalities in the brain and merosin-negative or merosin-deficient congenital muscular dystrophy including Fukuyama disease, muscle-eye-brain disease, and Walker-Warburg syndrome. A combination of clinical findings, elevated serum creatine kinase levels, brain imaging, muscle and skin biopsy, and molecular genetic testing helps make the specific diagnosis. The imaging appearance on MRI can vary from mild pachygyria and a lack of normal sulcation to a highly abnormal, "cobblestone" appearance to the cortex, particularly anteriorly [**Fig. 8.4**]. Because of overmigration of neurons, the CSF spaces surrounding the brain are typically reduced. The reduction in CSF surrounding the brain can be one of the earliest signs of cobblestone lissencephaly on fetal MR. Abnormalities can also be seen in the brainstem and in the cerebellum, and occipital cephalocele may be present in Walker-Warburg syndrome.

Gray Matter Heterotopia. Gray matter heterotopia are focal collections of gray matter that arise because of interruption of normal neuronal migration. Heterotopia can be seen in isolation or in association with other anomalies. They can be subdivided into three groups: periventricular/subependymal, focal subcortical, and leptomeningeal; periventricular heterotopia are the most common. The majority of cases are sporadic. An X-linked dominant filamin-1 gene mutation is associated with extensive periventricular heterotopia and is seen mostly in girls. Heterotopia may cause seizures; with seizures usually more severe in children with multiple heterotopia. On all imaging modalities, heterotopia appear as nodules with the same imaging features as gray matter [**Fig. 8.5**]. fMRI and blood oxygenation level–dependent imaging can demonstrate activation in epileptogenic heterotopia. Contrast enhancement should not be present.

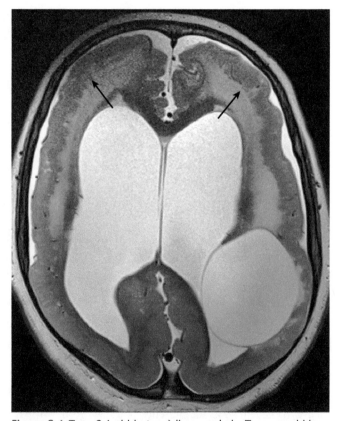

Figure 8.4 Type 2 (cobblestone) lissencephaly. Ten-year-old boy. Axial T2-weighted magnetic resonance imaging shows diffuse cobblestone appearance of the cortex with irregular inner cortical margin (*arrows*), ventriculomegaly, and left parietotemporal cyst.

Disorders of Neuronal Organization

Polymicrogyria. PMG occurs because of disruption of late neuronal migration and cortical organization. It results in

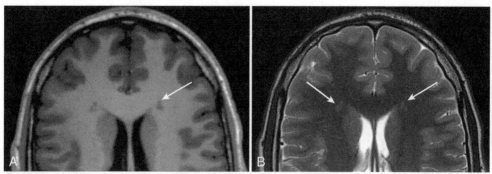

Figure 8.5 Gray matter heterotopia. Seventeen-year-old with intractable complex partial seizures. **A,** Axial T1-weighted and (**B**) axial T2-weighted imaging demonstrate periventricular gray matter heterotopia adjacent to the frontal horn of the lateral ventricle bilaterally (*arrows*).

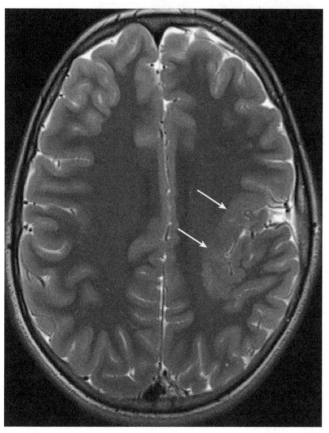

Figure 8.6 Peri-Sylvian polymicrogyria. Ten-year-old boy with intractable epilepsy. Axial T2-weighted image demonstrates abnormal orientation of the left Sylvian fissure and small, irregularly marginated peri-Sylvian gyri (*arrows*).

abnormalities in the deeper cortical cell layers and the formation of small and overly convoluted gyri. PMG can be unilateral or bilateral and focal or diffuse. The *peri-Sylvian region* is the most commonly involved [**Fig. 8.6**]. Patients can present with developmental delay, focal neurological signs/symptoms, or seizures depending on the cortical area involved. PMG can be sporadic and isolated, associated with other genetic syndromes or related to CMV infection or cerebral ischemia.

The most constant feature of PMG is *cortical thickening.* High-resolution imaging better depicts the small abnormal gyri and bumpy contour. A volumetric acquisition with multiplanar evaluation is often helpful to diagnose subtle irregularities of the

gray-white matter junction, which may be the only evidence of PMG. In unmyelinated areas, the abnormal cortex may appear thin and bumpy, as opposed to myelinated areas where it can appear thicker and relatively smooth. Perisylvian PMG is often accompanied by an abnormally vertical orientation of the Sylvian fissure [see **Fig. 8.8**]. The abnormality of the Sylvian fissure may be one of the first clues to the presence of PMG on fetal MR. Subtle cases of PMG may be difficult to diagnose in the neonate because of the high water content in the inner cell layers of the cortex, and follow-up imaging later in infancy may be required to detect or confirm PMG.

Schizencephaly. Schizencephaly refers to *congenital clefts* in the cerebral hemisphere extending from the ventricular ependyma to the pia mater overlying the cerebral cortex. Schizencephaly is a disorder of neuronal organization and the clefts are lined with heterotopic gray matter, usually PMG. This is in contrast with *porencephaly,* which is a cystic lesion lined by white matter that occurs secondary to an encephaloclastic insult such as trauma or infarction.

The incidence of schizencephaly is estimated at 1.5 in 100,000 live births. Patients may be asymptomatic but usually present with seizures or developmental delay.

MRI is the imaging modality of choice. The lips (margins) of the cleft may be in apposition (closed-lip) or separated (open-lip). Closed-lip schizencephaly produces a nipple-like outpouching at the ependymal surface [**Fig. 8.7**]. In open-lip schizencephaly, the CSF cleft can be seen extending from ventricular ependyma to the cortical surface. Schizencephaly may be associated with absence of the septum pellucidum and small optic nerves in patients with septooptic dysplasia (SOD).

Abnormalities of Ventral Induction

Holoprosencephaly

Holoprosencephaly (HPE) is the most common congenital anomaly affecting the ventral forebrain. *Incomplete cleavage* of the forebrain, *absence of the interhemispheric falx,* and *fusion of the central gray nuclei* characterize HPE. Abnormalities of the corpus callosum are usually present in all but the most subtle forms. Because the corpus callosum normally forms in an anterior-to-posterior direction, most callosal dysgenesis is accompanied by deficiencies in the posterior portions of the corpus callosum, but in HPE, the callosal anomalies are more often seen in the anterior portion of the commissure. In HPE, a failure of hemispheric cleavage occurs during the fifth and sixth weeks of gestation. HPE occurs in 1 in 250 embryos and in 1 in 8300 to 16,000 live births. It is associated with facial anomalies including cyclopia, ethmocephaly, cebocephaly, and hypotelorism. A central "megaincisor" may be present. The more severe the facial anomalies, the more severe the brain anomalies are likely to be,

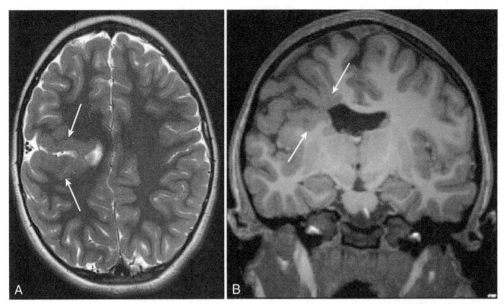

Figure 8.7 Schizencephaly. Six-year-old girl with intractable partial seizures. **A,** Axial T2-weighted and (**B**) coronal T1-weighted images of a cerebrospinal fluid–filled cleft surrounded by abnormal gray matter (*arrows*).

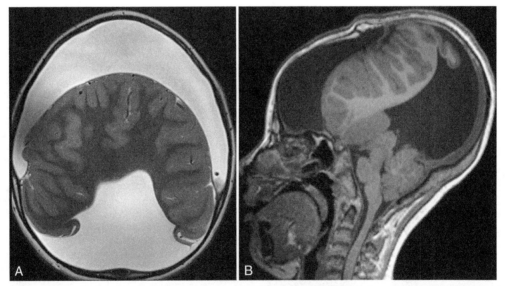

Figure 8.8 Alobar holoprosencephaly. Six-year-old with developmental delay. **A,** Axial T2-weighted and (**B**) sagittal T1-weighted images demonstrate fusion of the cerebrum across midline with absence of the corpus callosum, interhemispheric fissure and falx cerebri, and a monoventricle with dorsal cyst.

leading to the statement that, in HPE, the "face predicts the brain."

In the most severe form, known as *alobar HPE,* there is complete fusion of the cerebral hemispheres, with absence of the falx, corpus callosum, and septum pellucidum. A rudimentary monoventricle is present, which is often in communication with a dorsal cyst [**Fig. 8.8**].

In *semilobar HPE,* the posterior parts of the interhemispheric fissure and falx are present with fusion of hypoplastic frontal lobes. The globus pallidi may be hypoplastic or absent, and the caudate nuclei and thalami are fused. The hippocampus is usually present but often dysplastic. A dorsal cyst may be present. Facial anomalies are less severe than in the alobar form [**Fig. 8.9**].

In an unusual *middle hemispheric variant* of HPE, also known as syntelencephaly, the hemispheres are cleaved

anteriorly and posteriorly but fused in the posterior frontal region. Syntelencephaly is not associated with craniofacial anomalies. Unlike other forms of HPE which have been linked to abnormalities in the sonic hedgehog gene, the interhemispheric variant has been linked to abnormalities in the *ZIC2* gene.

A milder form, *lobar HPE,* is characterized by hypoplasia of the frontal poles with agenesis of the septum pellucidum. The posterior frontal, parietal, and occipital lobes are normally formed. The splenium and body of the corpus callosum are present. Usually very mild or no facial anomalies are associated with lobar HPE [**Fig. 8.10**].

Septooptic Dysplasia

SOD was originally described by de Morsier in 1956 as hypoplasia of the optic nerves and absence of the septum pellucidum.

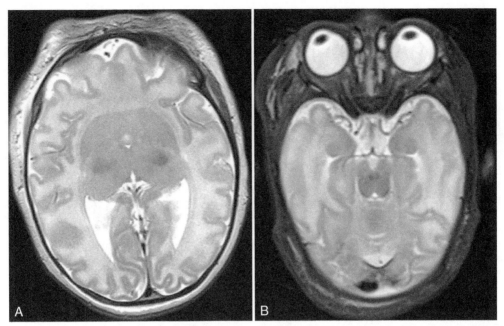

Figure 8.9 Semilobar holoprosencephaly. One-day-old. **A,** Axial T2-weighted image shows fusion of the inferior frontal lobes and absence of the anterior part of the interhemispheric fissure (present more posteriorly). **B,** Axial T2-weighted image more inferiorly shows hypotelorism.

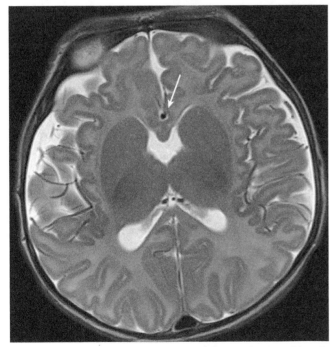

Figure 8.10 Lobar holoprosencephaly. Fifty-eight-day-old male infant with cleft palate. Axial T2-weighted image shows partial absence of the septal leaflets, an enlarged massa intermedia, and azygous anterior cerebral artery (*arrow*).

It is now used to describe any combination of *optic nerve hypoplasia, pituitary hypoplasia, and midline ventral cerebral abnormalities* and is often considered a mild form of HPE. Two-thirds of patients have hypothalamic-pituitary dysfunction. The incidence is estimated at 1 in 50,000 live births. A number of different genetic mechanisms have been implicated.

Absence of the septal leaflets results in downward displacement of the fornices into the third ventricle. The posterior

pituitary gland may be ectopic or absent, and the infundibulum may be interrupted. The optic nerves and chiasm show varying degrees of hypoplasia [**Fig. 8.11**]. SOD is often associated with *schizencephaly.*

Anomalies of Corpus Callosum

The corpus callosum is the largest of the telencephalic commissures. Agenesis or partial absence of the corpus callosum is one of the most common congenital CNS anomalies with an incidence of 1 in 4000.

The development of the corpus callosum occurs between the 12th and 20th weeks of gestation. The genu is the first portion to form with development continuing posteriorly along the body to the splenium. The rostrum is the last portion to be formed. *Agenesis* is used to describe a primary failure to form the corpus callosum [**Fig. 8.12**]. In agenesis, other interhemispheric commissures, such as the anterior commissure, are usually enlarged. Complete or partial agenesis should be distinguished from secondary callosal destruction that may be caused by toxic, ischemic, or traumatic insults.

In complete callosal agenesis, the lateral ventricles have a characteristic parallel orientation with dilatation of the trigones and occipital horns (*colpocephaly*), which has also been described as the "race-car sign" on axial imaging with the dilated occipital horns resembling the rear tires of an open-wheel car [**Fig. 8.13**]. Axons that fail to cross the midline course along the medial aspect of the lateral ventricle forming the longitudinally oriented *Probst bundles,* which can be elegantly illustrated as anteroposterior tracts on DTI and as dark, densely myelinated structures along the medial wall of the lateral ventricles on T2-weighted imaging [**Fig. 8.14**]. Callosal agenesis is often associated with an interhemispheric cyst and a high riding third ventricle. On sagittal imaging, there is absence of the cingulate gyrus with a radial orientation of the sulci over the mesial surface of the frontal lobes.

Callosal agenesis may be isolated or associated with a multitude of other malformations including Chiari II malformation, aqueductal stenosis, and anomalies of cortical, cerebellar, and brainstem development. *Aicardi syndrome* is a rare X-linked

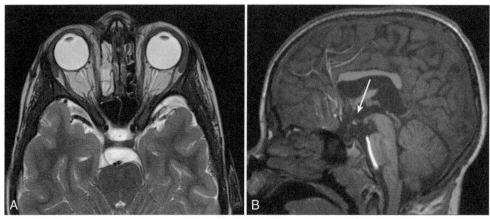

Figure 8.11 Septooptic dysplasia. Seven-year-old boy with blindness, growth hormone deficiency, central hypothyroidism, central adrenal insufficiency, and hypoglycemia. **A,** Axial T2-weighted image shows bilateral optic nerve hypoplasia. **B,** Midline sagittal T1-weighted image shows agenesis of the genu and rostrum of the corpus callosum, hypoplasia of the pituitary, and ectopic posterior pituitary bright spot (*arrow*).

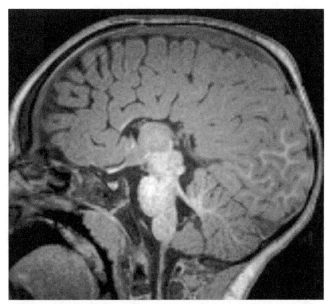

Figure 8.12 Agenesis of the corpus callosum. Fourteen-month-old girl. Sagittal T1-weighted image shows complete absence of the corpus callosum and absence of the cingulate gyrus posteriorly with gyri extending to the roof of the third ventricle.

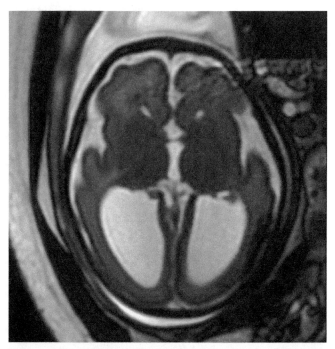

Figure 8.13 Colpocephaly. Thirty-week gestation fetus with T2-weighted fetal magnetic resonance showing complete agenesis of the corpus callosum and marked dilatation of the trigones and occipital horns of the lateral ventricles.

dominant condition that occurs in females who present with seizures and developmental delay. Imaging findings in Aicardi syndrome include callosal agenesis, interhemispheric neuroepithelial cysts, gray matter heterotopia, PMG, cerebellar malformation, spinal anomalies, chorioretinal lacunae, and coloboma [**Fig. 8.15**].

Partial callosal agenesis is usually characterized by absence of the splenium and dorsal body with preservation of the genu and rostral body. Diffuse callosal hypoplasia and segmental callosal hypoplasia refer to global and focal thinning of the callosum, respectively.

Intracranial lipomas indicate abnormal brain development and are usually associated with hypoplasia of the adjacent brain. *Pericallosal lipomas* are usually associated with partial absence or formational anomalies of the corpus callosum. Lipomas follow the signal intensity of fat on all MRI sequences, that is, hyperintense on T1, hypointense on fat-saturated sequences, and high

signal but hypointense relative to CSF on T2 [**Fig. 8.16**]. Similarly, they are hyperechoic on fetal/cranial ultrasound and exhibit negative Hounsfield units on CT.

Hindbrain Anomalies

Recent advances in correlation of imaging phenotype with genetics and developmental biology have led to improved understanding and classification of posterior fossa anomalies. A detailed consideration of the hindbrain anomalies is beyond the scope of this text; however, some of the more common anomalies will be considered.

A fundamental principle of understanding hindbrain malformations is that the brainstem and cerebellar development are

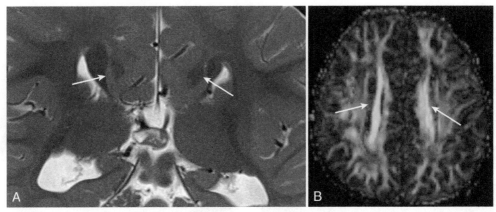

Figure 8.14 Probst bundles. A, Coronal T2-weighted image demonstrates Probst bundles running along the medial aspect of the lateral ventricles (*arrows*). Probst bundles are displayed as green anteroposterior tracts on (**B**) axial diffusion tensor imaging image (*arrows*).

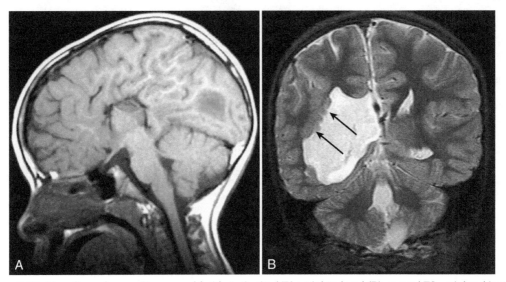

Figure 8.15 Aicardi syndrome. Five-year-old girl. **A,** Sagittal T1-weighted and (**B**) coronal T2-weighted images demonstrating agenesis of the corpus callosum, right temporal cortical malformation, and right subependymal gray matter heterotopia (*arrows*).

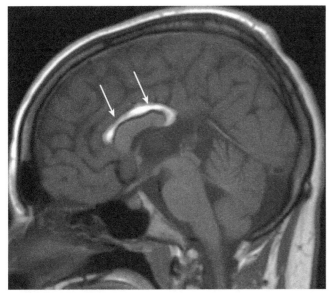

Figure 8.16 Pericallosal lipoma. Fifteen-year-old boy. Sagittal T1-weighted image shows dysmorphic corpus callosum and T1 hyperintense pericallosal lipoma (*arrows*).

interrelated, and that abnormalities in one are typically associated with abnormalities in the other. Postformational destructive processes should be suspected when only the cerebellum or brainstem is abnormal.

Malformation of the Cerebellar Vermis

A variety of disorders may be associated with complete or partial absence of the cerebellar vermis. These include entities such as Joubert syndrome, *Dandy-Walker spectrum* anomalies, and rhombencephalosynapsis.

Joubert syndrome. Joubert syndrome is a hindbrain malformation with underdevelopment of the cerebellar vermis. Symptoms include hyperpnea, hypotonia, abnormal eye movements, ataxia, and developmental delay. On imaging, the cerebellar vermis is extremely underdeveloped or completely absent, the cerebellar hemispheres are apposed to one another in the midline, and there is enlargement of the superior cerebellar peduncles ("molar tooth sign") [**Fig. 8.17**]. Cleft lip and palate may also be present.

Rhombencephalosynapsis. Rhombencephalosynapsis is a rare disorder in which the cerebellar vermis does not form

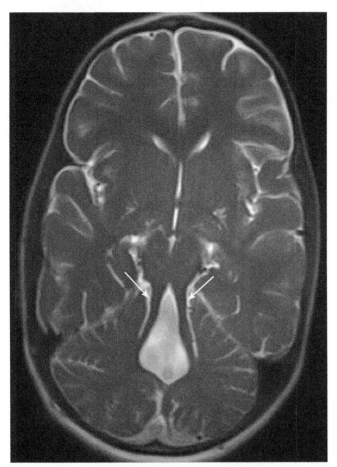

Figure 8.17 Joubert syndrome. Nine-year-old boy. Axial T2-weighted image demonstrates vermian hypoplasia and enlargement of the superior cerebellar peduncles "molar tooth sign" (*arrows*).

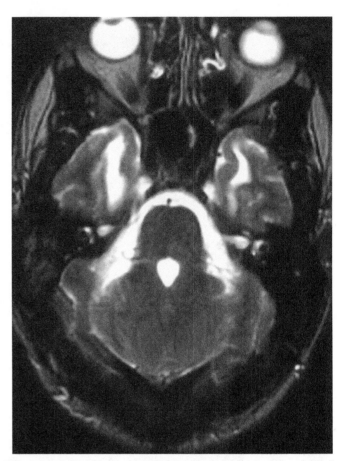

Figure 8.18 Rhombencephalosynapsis. Axial T2-weighted image shows absence of the cerebellar vermis, a triangular-shaped fourth ventricle, and fusion of the cerebellar hemispheres across the midline.

and there is fusion of the cerebellar hemispheres across the midline producing a diamond-shaped fourth ventricle [**Fig. 8.18**]. Associated supratentorial anomalies including hypoplasia of the corpus callosum, optic nerves, and agenesis of the posterior lobe of the pituitary gland may be present.

Dandy-Walker spectrum. Classification of the Dandy-Walker spectrum anomalies continues to be controversial. The term *Dandy-Walker spectrum* may variably be used to encompass a number of anomalies including the classic Dandy-Walker malformation, the Dandy-Walker variant (less dilatation of the fourth ventricle and less enlargement of the posterior fossa), retrocerebellar arachnoid cysts, Blake pouch cysts (ballooning of the superior medullary velum into the cisterna magna), and mega cisterna magna. The classic Dandy-Walker malformation consists of an enlarged posterior fossa, elevated torcular Herophili, severe hypoplasia or agenesis of the cerebellar vermis, and a dilated, cystic-appearing fourth ventricle [**Fig. 8.19**]. These anomalies are seen in approximately 1 in 30,000 live births. A number of different gene and modes of inheritance have been implicated.

Other anomalies associated with Dandy-Walker spectrum include hydrocephalus (70–90%), callosal abnormalities (30%), PMG or gray matter heterotopias (5–10%), and occipital encephaloceles in up to 16%. Clinical presentation varies depending on the severity of the abnormality. Eighty percent of patients with classic Dandy-Walker malformation present in the first year of life with symptoms secondary to hydrocephalus.

Abnormalities of Dorsal Induction

Chiari Malformations

Anomalies of the cervicomedullary junction are commonly known as Chiari malformations, after Hans Chiari who described the original three cervicomedullary malformations in 1891.

Chiari I Malformation. The Chiari I malformation is defined as caudal extension of the cerebellar tonsils below the level of the foramen magnum [**Fig. 8.20**]. The most common type of Chiari I malformation is related to a congenitally small, bony posterior fossa. Chiari I can also develop in patients with premature closure of the sutures as seen in Crouzon syndrome and Pfeiffer syndrome, and in some infants with ventriculoperitoneal shunts for hydrocephalus. Children with a Chiari I malformation may be asymptomatic or present with irritability (in younger children), headaches, lower cranial nerve palsies, or dissociated extremity anesthesia secondary to syringohydromyelia.

Potentially significant tonsillar descent in Chiari I should be distinguished from milder tonsillar ectopia, which is likely an incidental, clinically silent finding. Although the imaging findings distinguishing "Chiari I" from "tonsillar ectopia" historically focused on the extent of tonsillar ectopia present, clinical symptoms are related to the degree of obstruction of CSF flow at the foramen magnum, and surgical decompression is directed at relieving the obstruction. In Chiari I malformation, the tonsils extend to a variable degree (typically >6 mm), have a "pointed" configuration, and obstruct the flow of CSF at the foramen

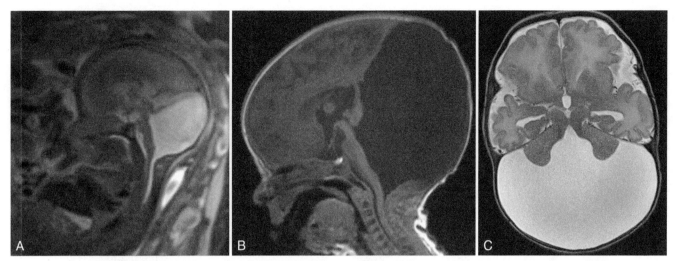

Figure 8.19 Dandy-Walker malformation. A, Fetal and neonatal (**B, C**) magnetic resonance images demonstrate an enlarged posterior fossa with a retrocerebellar cerebrospinal fluid collection, severe vermian hypoplasia with splaying of hypoplastic cerebellar hemispheres.

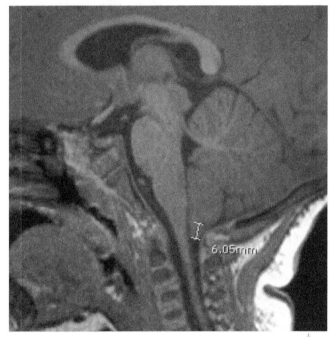

Figure 8.20 Chiari I malformation. Ten-month-old with intermittent apnea. Sagittal T1-weighted image demonstrates "pointed" cerebellar tonsils extending 6 mm below the plane of the foramen magnum.

magnum. Clinically asymptomatic tonsillar ectopia may occur when the tonsils extend into the upper cervical canal, retain a rounded configuration, and do not significantly impede CSF flow. Hydromyelia is present in 20% of patients with a Chiari I malformation. The hydromyelic cavity usually, although not exclusively, involves the cervical spinal cord and extends a variable distance into the thoracic spinal cord. Hydromyelia produces a typical, partially "septated" appearance that serves to differentiate it from syringomyelia [**Fig. 8.21**]. The demonstration of hydromyelia in the spinal cord should prompt evaluation of the cervicomedullary junction for the Chiari I malformation that will usually be present.

Chiari II Malformation. The Chiari II malformation is a complex malformation of the hindbrain and skull that occurs in association with an open neural tube defect. This pathogenesis of Chiari II malformations remains controversial, but the anomaly arises in combination with different genetic polymorphisms and in association with environmental factors, including deficient maternal folate intake and abnormalities of folate metabolism. It is relatively common with an incidence of approximately 1 in 1000 live births. Almost all patients with a Chiari II malformation have a myelomeningocele. The hindbrain abnormalities are thought to occur secondary to the failure of closure of the posterior neuropore. This leads to a pressure gradient between the intracranial (higher pressure) and intraspinal (lower pressure spaces) with resultant inferior herniation of the developing structures of the posterior cranial fossa. Most of the hindbrain findings can be thought of as resulting from a normal-sized cerebellum developing in a small posterior fossa with a low-lying tentorium [**Fig. 8.22**].

Features commonly seen in Chiari II include hydrocephalus, dysplastic tentorium, a small, bony posterior fossa, and a characteristic skull dysplasia known as *Lückenschädel skull.* Lückenschädel skull results from mesodermal dysplasia, which gives rise to the characteristic scalloped appearance. These dysplastic foci ossify and normalize by 6 months of age.

Other stigmata of Chiari II malformation include inferior displacement and elongation of the brainstem, kinking of the cervicomedullary junction, upward cerebellar herniation, an enlarged massa intermedia, elongated cranial nerves, tectal beaking, and callosal hypogenesis. Approximately 50% of patients have syringohydromyelia. Many patients have small-appearing gyri with shallow sulci in the posterior and medial aspects of the cerebral hemispheres; this pattern is known as stenogyria. Subependymal heterotopia are often present along the trigones of the lateral ventricles.

Chiari II malformations are being more frequently diagnosed antenatally. The classic antenatal sonographic appearance includes the **lemon sign** (which describes an indentation of the frontal bone) and the **banana sign** (which describes the appearance of the cerebellum tightly wrapped around the brainstem with obliteration of the cisterna magna). Fetal MRI can add diagnostic information regarding the intracranial abnormalities [**Fig. 8.23**].

Early neonatal repair of the myelomeningocele and shunting of hydrocephalus has been the standard management of children

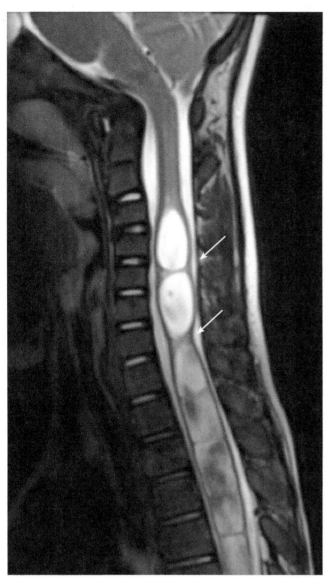

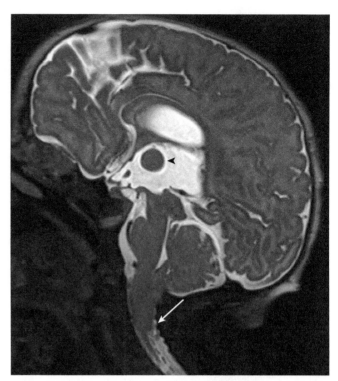

Figure 8.22 Chiari II malformation. Ten-day-old neonate. Sagittal T2-weighted image after repair of myelomeningocele demonstrates small posterior fossa, herniation of the cerebellum to the level of C4 (*arrow*), and enlarged massa intermedia (*arrowhead*).

Figure 8.21 Chiari I malformation with hydromyelia. Sagittal T2-weighted image shows inferior displacement of the cerebellar tonsils and marked dilatation of the central canal of the spinal cord with septations (*arrows*) typical of hydromyelia with Chiari I.

born with Chiari II. Prenatal surgical repair of the myelomeningocele is now being performed at some centers and has been reported to reduce hydrocephalus, reduce requirement for postnatal ventriculoperitoneal shunt placement, and improve motor outcomes at 30 months. The long-term impact on neurocognitive development of fetal repair of the myelomeningocele has not yet been established.

Chiari III malformation was originally used to describe herniation of posterior fossa contents through a low occipital calvarial defect or high cervical spinal dysraphism. Chiari III malformations are rare.

Anencephaly and Cephalocele

Anencephaly. Complete failure of early closure of the cephalic end of the neural tube results in anencephaly in which the forebrain, skull, and scalp are absent. It is associated with raised maternal serum alpha-fetoprotein. It is easily detected on antenatal ultrasound [**Fig. 8.24**]. In the first trimester, neural tissue is still present; however, the normal head contour is absent and crown rump length is less than expected. As the pregnancy continues, neural tube superior to the orbits dissolves and the absent calvarium becomes more apparent. MRI is not required for diagnosis. Anencephaly is invariably lethal within a few days of delivery.

Cephalocele. A cephalocele refers to herniation of CNS tissue through a defect in the skull. Most cephaloceles are midline in location. They are classified according to their contents and the location of the skull defect. A herniation containing CSF lined by meninges is referred to as a *meningocele*. A *meningoencephalocele* contains CSF and brain tissue, and a *meningoencephalocystocele* contains CSF, brain, and ventricle [**Figs. 8.25** and **8.26**].

Occipital cephaloceles are the most common. Additional anomalies can be seen in up to 50% of cases including aneuploidy, Dandy-Walker spectrum, and Meckel-Gruber syndrome. Occipital encephaloceles often contain dysplastic occipital or cerebellar tissue, and anomalies of the adjacent dural venous sinuses are common.

Frontal and frontoethmoidal encephaloceles are more common in Asian populations. These may present with hypertelorism or a glabellar mass [**Fig. 8.27**]. Failure of closure at the foramen cecum may result in a nasofrontal cephalocele, dermoid-epidermoid, or nasal "glioma" (isolated ectopic, dysplastic brain tissue) [**Fig. 8.28**]. Rare sphenoidal cephaloceles can result in a nasopharyngeal mass.

Cephaloceles can be seen on prenatal ultrasound or fetal MR; they may appear cystic or solid depending on their contents. In postnatal patients, MRI is the best modality for delineating the composition of the contents and intracranial relationships. Thin-section CT with multiplanar reformats can be used for more accurate assessment of the osseous anatomy.

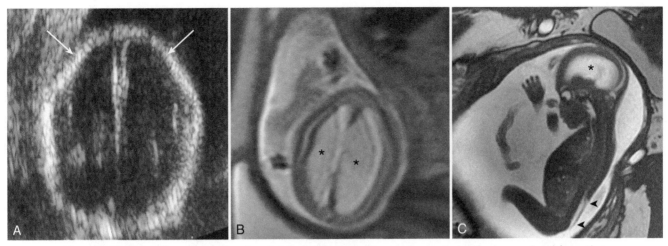

Figure 8.23 Chiari II malformation in a fetus. A, Ultrasound image demonstrates the lemon sign (elongation of the frontal bones) (*arrows*). **B,** Axial and (**C**) sagittal fetal magnetic resonance images demonstrate ventriculomegaly (*asterisks*), small posterior fossa, herniation of the hindbrain, and thoracolumbar neural tube defect (*arrowheads*).

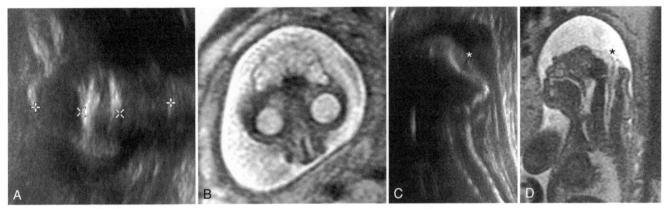

Figure 8.24 Anencephaly. A, Coronal and (**C**) sagittal fetal ultrasound and correlative magnetic resonance (**B, D**) images demonstrating a "frog-eye" appearance (axial views) caused by absent cranium and bulging orbits. Sagittal views confirm absence of the cranium (*asterisks*).

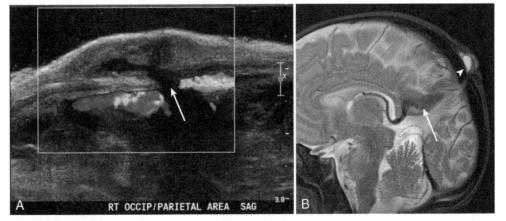

Figure 8.25 Atretic parietal cephalocele. Twelve-day-old girl noted to have raised skin lesion over the occiput at birth. **A,** Sagittal ultrasound shows soft tissue thickening surrounding a cystic scalp lesion associated with underlying skull defect (*arrow*). **B,** Sagittal T2-weighted magnetic resonance images confirm the presence of an atretic parietal cephalocele (*arrowhead*) with a partially demonstrated persistent falcine sinus (*arrow*) coursing anteriorly toward the tectum.

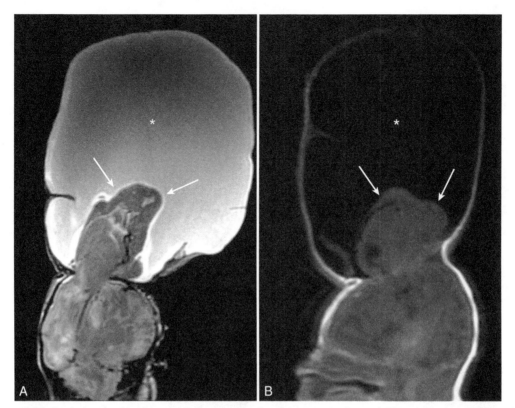

Figure 8.26 Cephalocele. Newborn with frontoparietal scalp mass. **A,** Coronal T2-weighted and (**B**) sagittal T1-weighted magnetic resonance images demonstrate a large calvarial defect containing a large cerebrospinal fluid (*asterisk*) and brain (*arrows*).

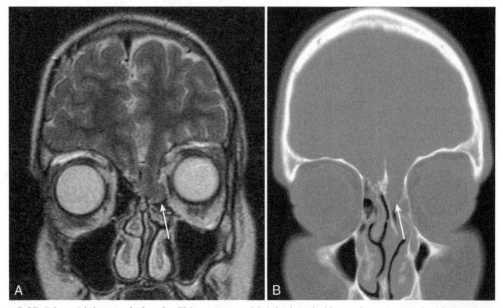

Figure 8.27 Ethmoidal encephalocele. Thirteen-year-old right-handed boy who presented with pneumococcal meningoencephalitis. **A,** Coronal T2-weighted magnetic resonance image and (**B**) coronal computed tomography image demonstrate a cribriform plate defect and herniation of the left gyrus rectus (*arrows*) into the ethmoid sinuses.

Hydranencephaly

Hydranencephaly is a condition in which most of the cerebral hemispheres are damaged, liquefied, and resorbed in utero, resulting in replacement with a membranous sac containing CSF and the remnants of the cerebral cortex and white matter [**Fig. 8.29**]. It can occur secondary to a variety of destructive causative factors including bilateral occlusion of the supraclinoid segment of the internal carotid artery (ICA), diffuse hypoxic-ischemic necrosis, necrotizing vasculitis caused by intrauterine infection, and thromboplastic emboli originating in a deceased co-twin.

Craniosynostosis. Craniosynostosis is the term applied to the premature fusion of a calvarial suture. It can affect the whole or part of a suture and can involve a single or multiple sutures.

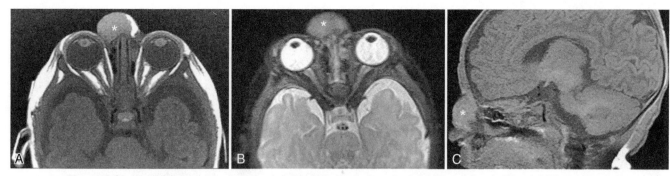

Figure 8.28 Nasal glioma. Newborn male with glabellar lesion. **A,** Axial T1-weighted, (**B**) axial T2-weighted, and (**C**) sagittal postcontrast T1-weighted images demonstrate a well-defined, nonenhancing mass (*asterisk*) at the nasal root which is isointense to brain parenchyma on all imaging sequences.

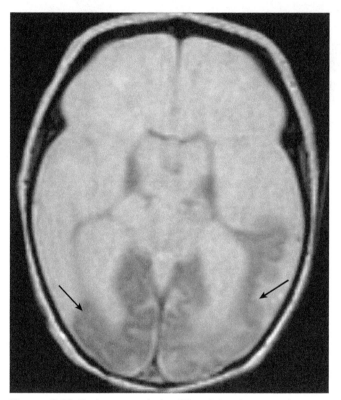

Figure 8.29 Hydranencephaly. T2-weighted magnetic resonance image of a neonate demonstrating a fluid-filled cranium and near-total absence of the brain parenchyma except for the occipital lobes (*arrows*) in keeping with bilateral occlusion of the supraclinoid segment of the internal carotid artery (ICA).

Failure of growth at the closed sutures causes increased growth along open sutures and resultant craniofacial abnormality [**Table 8.2**]. Craniosynostosis can be either primary, caused by abnormal suture fusion, or secondary, caused by a failure of brain growth. Isolated single-suture synostosis does not restrict brain development and is usually only of cosmetic importance.

Primary craniosynostosis is relatively common with an estimated incidence of 1 in 2000 to 2500 live births. Most cases of craniosynostosis are isolated, but 15% are syndromic and associated with other developmental abnormalities.

Embryologically, the cranial vault is derived from the mesodermal neurocranium. The ossification centers begin to ossify around the 13th gestational week. By the 18th gestational week, the borders of the mineralizing bones have approached each other and begun to form the nonossified sutures. The presence of nonossified sutures and open fontanels at term allows overlap and deformation of the skull bones during parturition. The sutures permit further remodeling during rapid phases of brain and skull growth during the first few years of life.

Sutures normally close from back to front and from lateral to medial. The metopic suture is the exception; it closes from the glabella to the anterior fontanelle and is the first to close (9–11 months). The fontanels normally close by the second year of life. The coronal, lambdoid, and sagittal sutures may remain open until the fourth decade of life.

Sagittal synostosis is the most common isolated synostosis. It is four times more common in males than in females. It clinically manifests as a long, narrow head shape with sagittal ridging, restricted growth the parietotemporal regions, frontal bossing, and occipital protrusion. The long, narrow skull has been described as *scaphocephalic,* which means "boat-shaped" [**Fig. 8.30**].

Unicoronal synostosis is the second most common form of craniosynostosis. Two-thirds of affected patients are female. The clinical features include a flattened ipsilateral forehead, a flattened ipsilateral occipital area, the "harlequin eye" deformity (caused by superior displacement of the ipsilateral orbital roof and lesser sphenoid wing), ipsilateral temporal bulging and cheek protrusion, contralateral forehead bossing, and deviation of the nose to the contralateral side [**Fig. 8.31**].

Bicoronal synostosis causes a short, wide head that can be described as *brachycephalic.* There is depression of the supraorbital rims with bitemporal and upper forehead bulging. In bicoronal synostosis, the frontosphenoidal and frontozygomatic sutures are typically fused as well.

Bilambdoid synostosis causes a shallow posterior fossa and towering skull known as *turricephaly.* In a more severe form when bicoronal and bilambdoid synostoses are combined, the skull can adopt a characteristic towering and narrow shape, with bulging temporal areas and shallow orbits known as cloverleaf or *Kleeblattschädel skull.*

Metopic synostosis, when it occurs before the age of 6 months, is associated with a triangular wedding of the forehead (*trigonocephaly*), hypotelorism, narrow anterior cranial fossa, hypoplasia of the ethmoids, and a metopic ridge. After 6 months of age, premature closure of the metopic suture is associated with minimal deformity.

More than 180 described syndromes are associated with craniosynostosis. The management of syndromic craniosynostosis is complicated by associated skull base, facial, and brain abnormalities. Children with one of the syndromic craniosynostoses are at risk for raised intracranial pressure (ICP), hydrocephalus, optic atrophy, cleft palate, respiratory problems, and hearing disorders [**Table 8.3**]. The most common of the syndromic causes of craniosynostosis affect the coronal sutures. Bicoronal

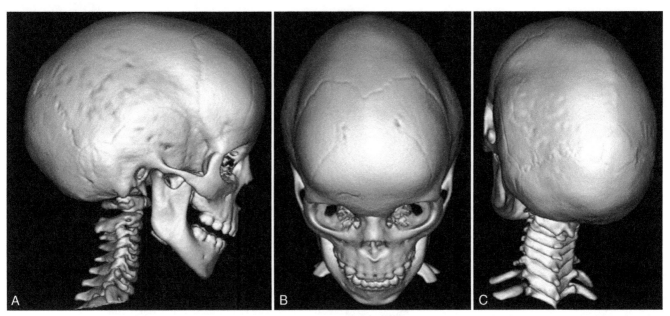

Figure 8.30 Sagittal synostosis. Three-dimensional reconstructed computed tomography demonstrating a (**A**) long, boat-shaped skull (scaphocephaly), (**B**) frontal bossing, and (**C**) midsagittal osseous ridging in a 3-year-old male with sagittal synostosis.

TABLE 8.2 Craniosynostosis

Suture	Calvarial Configuration	Descriptive Terms
Sagittal	• Long, narrow head	Scaphocephaly
Bicoronal	• Short, wide head • Hypertelorism • Small anterior fossa	Brachycephaly
Metopic	• Triangular wedging of forehead • Keel-shaped head	Trigonocephaly
Bilambdoid	• Shallow posterior fossa, • Prominent bregma	Turricephaly
Unicoronal	• Unilateral frontal flattening • Uptilting of orbit (harlequin eye) • Nasal deviation	Plagiocephaly
Bicoronal and bilambdoid	• Unilateral posterior flattening	Cloverleaf or Kleeblattschädel skull
All sutures	• Small, round head	Microcephaly

TABLE 8.3 Syndromic Craniosynostosis

Syndrome	Gene Affected	Clinical Findings
Apert syndrome	*FGFR2*	Bicoronal craniosynostosis, midface hypoplasia, hypertelorism, exorbitism, complex syndactyly
Crouzon syndrome	*FGFR2*	Bicoronal craniosynostosis, midface hypoplasia, hypertelorism, exorbitism
Pfeiffer syndrome	*FGFR1* or *FGFR2*	Multiple craniosynostoses, midface hypoplasia, hypertelorism, severe exorbitism, broad thumbs, broad hallux, soft tissue syndactyly
Muenke syndrome	*FGFR3*	Coronal synostosis, thimblelike middle phalanges, carpal/tarsal coalition, sensorineural hearing loss

synostosis may be associated with hydrocephalus, most often caused by jugular foraminal stenosis and venous hypertension.

Apert syndrome (also known as type I acrocephalosyndactyly) is an autosomal dominant condition that results from mutations of the *FGFR2* gene. It is characterized by bicoronal craniosynostosis, midface hypoplasia, hypertelorism, exorbitism, and severe complex syndactyly of fingers and toes [**Fig. 8.32**].

Crouzon syndrome is also due to mutations of the *FGFR2* gene. Crouzon syndrome has similar calvarial deformities, facial anomalies, and exorbitism but is not associated with hand and foot abnormalities.

Pfeiffer syndrome (also known as type V acrocephalosyndactyly) can occur because of mutations in *FGFR1* or *FGFR2*. It is characterized by craniosynostosis affecting multiple sutures, midfacial hypoplasia, severe exorbitism, and hypertelorism. The clinical findings in the periphery include broad and medially deviated great toes, broad thumbs, and soft-tissue syndactyly.

Muenke syndrome is caused by a mutation in the *FGFR3* gene and is strongly associated with coronal synostosis. The hands and feet are often affected but with mild abnormalities such as thimble-like middle phalanges, carpal or tarsal coalition, and coned epiphyses that may not be clinically significant. All

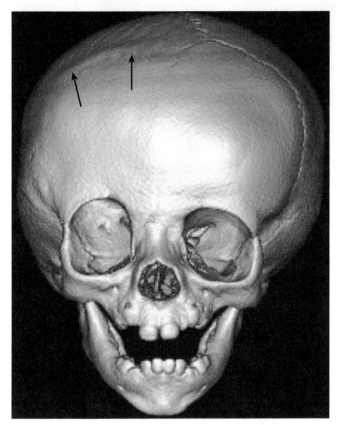

Figure 8.31 Unicoronal synostosis. Three-dimensional reconstructed computed tomography demonstrating right coronal synostosis (*arrows*) with resultant harlequin deformity of the right orbit.

patients with Muenke syndrome should be tested for sensorineural hearing loss, but only a few are actually affected.

Imaging plays an important role in confirming the diagnosis and management of craniosynostosis, evaluating the extent of involvement, which is difficult with clinical examination alone. CT is the primary imaging modality used to evaluate the sutures. The closed suture is demonstrated by bone bridging across the suture, loss of architecture, or ridging. A very-low-dose technique can be used when the primary concern is osseous anatomy, and 3D reconstructions can depict the abnormalities exquisitely and are critical for operative planning.

Imaging can also help differentiate lambdoid craniosynostosis from positional plagiocephaly, which is an abnormal skull shape caused by infant positioning and not by premature fusion of the sutures [**Fig. 8.33**]. There has been an increase in occipital plagiocephaly over the past two decades because of "back to back" campaigns encouraging that infants sleep in the supine position to reduce the risk for sudden infant death syndrome. In positional plagiocephaly, in addition to the lambdoid sutures being open, the ear on the flattened side is "pushed" forward; but in lambdoid synostosis, the ipsilateral ear is "pulled" posteriorly toward the fused suture.

In complex cases, dedicated magnetic resonance venography (MRV) or computed tomographic venography (CTV) imaging may be performed preoperatively to assess for associated dural venous sinus anomalies. In bicoronal synostosis with jugular foraminal stenosis, enlarged transosseous emissary veins (sinus pericranii) may be present. MRI may be required if there is a need to assess for underlying parenchymal abnormalities inadequately imaged using the low-dose CT technique.

Surgical intervention is unique to each type of synostosis. Surgery may be undertaken to correct cosmetic deformity in single-suture synostosis or may be required to permit normal brain growth or prevent complications such as raised ICP in multisutural synostosis.

NEUROCUTANEOUS SYNDROMES

The phakomatoses are a collection of hereditary disorders that are characterized by hamartomas and other congenital malformations involving structures arising from the ectoderm such as the nervous system, skin, retina and globe. The phakomatoses are

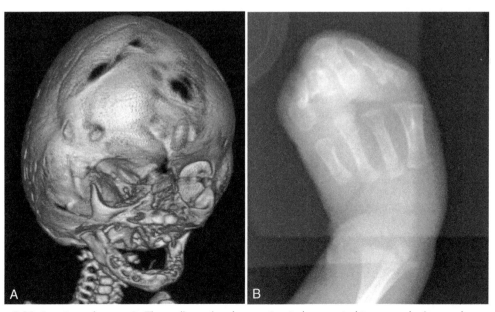

Figure 8.32 Apert syndrome. A, Three-dimensional reconstructed computed tomography image demonstrating turribrachycephalic skull with craniosynostosis involving the sagittal and bilateral coronal sutures and midfacial hypoplasia. **B,** Hand radiograph demonstrates the classic soft tissue and part osseous syndactyly.

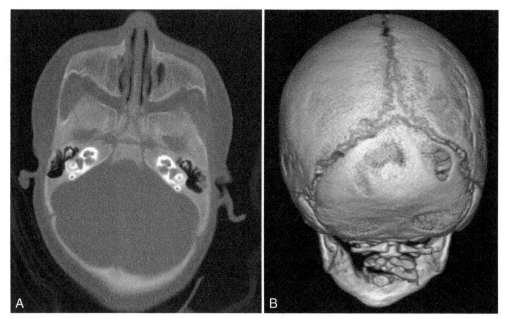

Figure 8.33 Positional plagiocephaly. Three-month-old female referred with concern for synostosis. **A,** Low-dose axial computed tomography with (**B**) reconstruction shows patent lambdoid sutures, flattening of the right parietooccipital region, and anterior positioning of the right pinna consistent with positional plagiocephaly.

also referred to as neurocutaneous disorders because of their involvement of both skin and neural tissues. Some of the more common phakomatoses include neurofibromatosis, tuberous sclerosis complex (TSC), Sturge-Weber disease, von Hippel-Lindau disease (VHL), and ataxia-telangiectasia.

Neurofibromatosis

Neurofibromatosis has multiple subtypes. The two most common are types I and II.

Neurofibromatosis Type 1

Neurofibromatosis type 1 (NF-1) is one of the most common autosomal dominant conditions that affect the CNS. It was first described by von Recklinghausen in 1885. Its incidence is estimated at 1 in 2000 to 3000 live births. The *NF1* gene has been mapped to chromosome 17q11.2 and produces a cytoplasmic protein called *neurofibromin*. In the CNS, this protein is mainly expressed in neurons, Schwann cells, oligodendrocytes, and astrocytes.

The phenotypic expression of *NF1* is variable. A diagnosis requires two or more of the following clinical criteria: (1) six or more café-au-lait spots, (2) two or more neurofibromas *or* one or more plexiform neurofibromas, (3) axillary freckling, (4) optic pathway glioma (OPG), (5) two or more Lisch nodules of the iris, (6) distinctive bone dysplasia or thinning of long-bone cortex, and (7) first-degree relative with NF-1 [**Box 8.1**].

Café-au-lait spots are the earliest manifestation of NF-1 to develop and are present in more than 95% of patients. Axillary freckling develops in approximately two-thirds of patients. Cutaneous neurofibromas and Lisch nodules increase in number throughout life. Cognitive impairment occurs in up to 50% of patients.

Ninety percent of children with NF-1 have *characteristic multiple T2/FLAIR hyperintense lesions* that can be found in the brainstem, cerebellar white matter, basal ganglia, thalamus, internal capsule, and occasionally the corona radiata [**Fig. 8.34**]. These were previously referred to as "unidentified bright objects" or "NF-1 spots." It is now known that these foci represent focal areas of myelin vacuolization. These lesions regress late in the

---

BOX 8.1   Criteria for Diagnosis of Neurofibromatosis Type 1

Diagnosis requires two or more of the following criteria:
1. Six or more café-au-lait spots
2. Two or more neurofibromas *or* one or more plexiform neurofibromas
3. Axillary freckling
4. OPG
5. Two or more Lisch nodules of the iris
6. Distinctive bone dysplasia or thinning of long-bone cortex
7. First-degree relative with NF-1

---

first decade of life and are rarely seen after the age of 20 years. Features that help to distinguish these lesions from astrocytomas include their characteristic location, isointensity or slight hyperintensity on T1-weighted sequences, and lack of enhancement. Although NF-1 spots do not have mass effect, the brain may be slightly malformed locally, especially in the brainstem and middle cerebellar peduncle. This deformity and signal abnormality may lead to the erroneous diagnosis of brainstem glioma if other clinical or imaging stigmata of NF-1 are not recognized.

The most important primary CNS abnormality seen in NF-1 is *OPG,* which occurs in 15% to 20% of patients. OPGs tend to occur before the age of 7 years and can involve a single optic nerve, both nerves, the chiasm, and posterior optic pathways [**Fig. 8.35**]. OPG in patients with NF-1 tends to have a more indolent course than sporadic OPG. Some optic pathway tumors in NF-1 even spontaneously involute with time. Most OPGs seen in NF-1 are histologically low-grade pilocytic astrocytomas. The optic nerves are often tortuous in NF-1, even in the absence of OPG. Optic pathway tumors may be either nonenhancing or may enhance avidly. Astrocytomas in locations other than the optic pathway are also more common in NF-1 than in the general population. Apart from OPGs, cranial nerve tumors are rare in NF-1 in contrast with neurofibromatosis type 2 (NF-2).

Macrocephaly and enlargement of the corpus callosum can also be seen in NF-1. Up to 6% of patients with NF-1 have

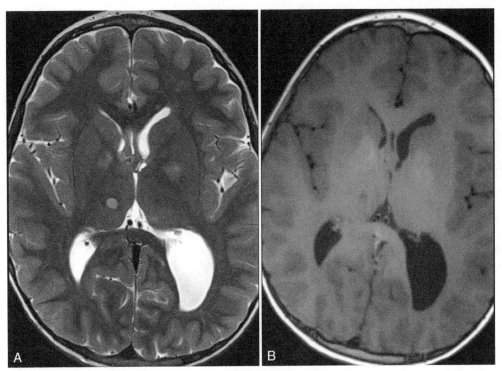

Figure 8.34 Neurofibromatosis type 1 (NF-1) vacuolization. Eight-year-old with NF-1. **A,** Axial T2 and **(B)** axial T1 postcontrast images show multiple rounded T2 hyperintensities in the deep gray matter with no enhancement postcontrast.

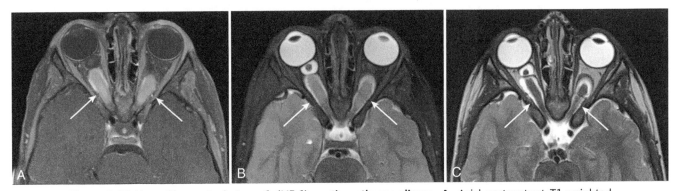

Figure 8.35 Neurofibromatosis type 1 (NF-1), optic pathway glioma. A, Axial postcontrast T1-weighted fat-suppressed and **(B)** axial T2-weighted images show diffuse enlargement of the optic nerves *(arrows)* bilaterally consistent with optic pathway glioma. **C,** Axial T2-weighted magnetic resonance imaging after 9 months of chemotherapy with vincristine and carboplatin shows a reduction in the size of the tumor.

cerebral vascular dysplasia. This most commonly consists of intimal and smooth muscle proliferation causing multifocal stenosis and occlusion of the internal carotid terminus and proximal middle cerebral artery (MCA) and anterior cerebral artery (ACA). This results in a moyamoya vasculopathy pattern with proximal steno-occlusive change and prominent lenticulostriate and thalamoperforate or collaterals in many such patients [**Fig. 8.36**]. The vasculopathy may occur even without a history of radiation for suprasellar glioma in children with NF-1.

Calvarial and orbital abnormalities are seen in NF-1, with the classic lesion being *sphenoid wing dysplasia* [**Fig. 8.37**]. Craniofacial neurofibromas and plexiform neurofibromas can secondarily cause intracranial complications. Neurofibromas are characterized on MRI by central T2 hypointensity giving rise to the "target sign." Plexiform neurofibromas are larger, more extensive, and tend to be more heterogeneous in signal intensity.

Spinal manifestations of NF-1 include scoliosis, intramedullary tumors, dural ectasia, lateral meningocele, and nerve root neurofibromas.

Neurofibromatosis Type 2

NF-2 is a separate and distinct disease from NF-1. The NF-2 gene maps to chromosome 22q12 and produces a protein called merlin or schwannomin. NF-2 is autosomal dominant but much less prevalent than NF-1, with an estimated incidence of 1 in 50,000. Fifty percent of cases are sporadic. Manifestations of NF-2 are extremely uncommon in children. The major clinical feature of NF-2 is the presence of bilateral vestibular (CN VIII) schwannomas in nearly all patients. Other manifestations can be remembered using the mnemonic *MISME* (*m*ultiple *i*nherited schwannomas, *m*eningiomas and *e*pendymomas) [**Fig. 8.38**].

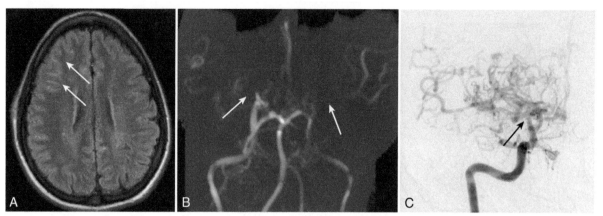

Figure 8.36 Neurofibromatosis type 1 (NF-1) vasculopathy (moyamoya syndrome). Eight-year-old with NF-1 and headaches. **A,** Axial fluid attenuation inversion recovery demonstrates the classic "ivy sign" consisting of high signal intensity in the sulci (*arrows*) caused by slow flow in leptomeningeal vessels. **B,** Frontal view of three-dimensional time-of-flight magnetic resonance angiography shows diminished flow-related enhancement in the proximal portions of the middle (*arrows*) and anterior cerebral arteries bilaterally. **C,** Frontal view of a right internal carotid artery angiogram demonstrates occlusion of the internal carotid artery terminus (*arrow*) with numerous basal collaterals, the "puff of smoke," reconstituting the middle cerebral artery branches.

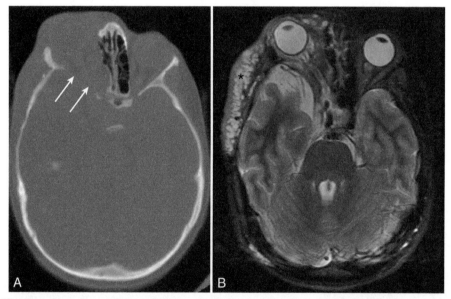

Figure 8.37 Neurofibromatosis type 1 (NF-1), sphenoid wing dysplasia, and facial plexiform neurofibroma. **A,** Axial computed tomography and (**B**) axial T2-weighted magnetic resonance image demonstrate right sphenoid wing dysplasia (*arrows*) and extensive right facial plexiform neurofibroma (*asterisk*).

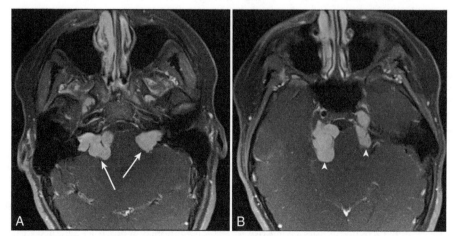

Figure 8.38 Neurofibromatosis type 2 (NF-2), multiple schwannomas. Axial postcontrast fat-saturated T1-weighted images show numerous enhancing schwannomas involving many cranial nerves (CNs) including (**A**) CN VIII bilaterally (*arrows*) and (**B**) CN V bilaterally (*arrowheads*).

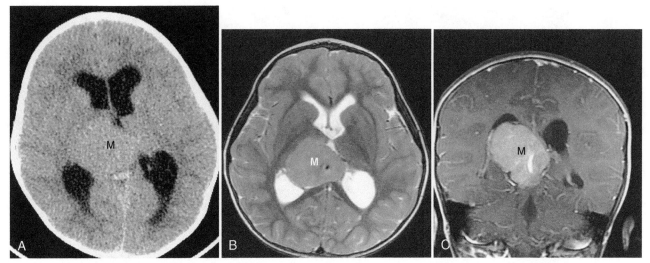

Figure 8.39 Neurofibromatosis type 2 (NF-2), meningioma. Meningioma (*M*) on (**A**) axial computed tomography scan and (**B**) axial T2-weighted magnetic resonance (MR) image. Enhancement can be seen on a (**C**) coronal gadolinium-enhanced MR image.

Simplistically, NF-2 can be thought of as involving tissues that surround neural structures, whereas NF-1 typically affects the neural structures directly.

Schwannomas are derived from the Schwann cells that form the myelin sheaths around the axons of nerves. Most vestibular schwannomas have an intracanalicular component that often results in widening of the porus acusticus and the "trumpeted" internal auditory meatus sign. Extracanalicular growth into the cerebellopontine angle can give rise to the "ice-cream cone" sign. On MRI, although their signal characteristics vary based on cellular composition, schwannomas tend to be isointense or slightly hypointense on T1, heterogeneously hyperintense on T2, and show avid contrast enhancement. Lesions containing predominantly Antoni A cells tend to be lower signal intensity on T2-weighted MR than lesions containing predominantly Antoni B cells. However, tumors with Antoni B cells are more likely to undergo intratumoral hemorrhage. Other cranial nerves can be affected by schwannomas in NF-2, most commonly the trigeminal (V) and occulomotor (III) nerves.

Meningioma is a rare tumor in young patients and, when present, should raise suspicion for NF-2. An intraventricular location of meningioma occurs more commonly in children than in adults. Childhood meningiomas are often large, grow rapidly, and have a higher rate of malignant degeneration than is typical of meningioma in adults. Meningiomas are isodense to hyperdense on precontrast CT, and the solid components show diffuse enhancement postcontrast. On MRI, they are typically isointense to gray matter on T1, hyperintense on T2/FLAIR, and enhance avidly postcontrast. Two-thirds show reactive thickening of the adjacent dura giving rise to the "dural tail" sign; however, this is not specific for meningioma [**Fig. 8.39**].

Spinal tumors affect up to 75% of patients with NF-2 and include paraspinal nerve sheath tumors, intraspinal meningiomas, and intramedullary tumors (predominantly ependymomas). Syringohydromyelia has also been described in NF-2.

Tuberous Sclerosis Complex

TSC, also known as *Bourneville disease,* is an autosomal dominant condition that is characterized by multiorgan hamartomas. Incidence is estimated at 1 in 6000 live births. Two-thirds of cases are sporadic. Two separate genes have been implicated: the *TSC1* gene, which maps to chromosome 9q34 and codes for a protein called *hamartin*; and the *TSC2* gene, which maps to chromosome 16p13.3 and codes for a protein called *tuberin.*

TABLE 8.4 Revised Criteria for Diagnosis of Tuberous Sclerosis Complex

Major features	• Facial angiofibromas or forehead plaque • Nontraumatic ungual or periungual fibroma • Hypomelanotic macules (more than three) • Shagreen patch (connective tissue nevus) • Multiple retinal nodular hamartomas • Cortical tubera • Subependymal nodule • Subependymal giant cell astrocytoma • Cardiac rhabdomyoma, single or multiple • Lymphangiomyomatosis • Renal angiomyolipoma
Minor features	• Multiple randomly distributed pits in dental enamel • Hamartomatous rectal polyps • Bone cysts • Cerebral white matter migration lines • Gingival fibromas • Nonrenal hamartoma • Retinal achromic patch • "Confetti" skin lesions • Multiple renal cysts
Definite TSC	Either two major features or one major feature with two minor features
Probable TSC	One major feature and one minor feature
Possible TSC	Either one major feature or two or more minor features

TSC, tuberous sclerosis complex.

These proteins combine in vivo to form a heterodimer that functions as a tumor suppressor by inhibiting the mammalian target of rapamycin (mTOR) kinase pathway. Increased activation of mTOR in TSC leads to disorganized cell overgrowth and abnormal cell differentiation.

The classic clinical triad associated with TSC consists of intellectual impairment, seizures, and adenoma sebaceum (a nodular red-brown facial rash originating in the nasolabial folds). However, it is now known that all these findings exist in less than one-third of patients. Half of patients with TSC have normal intelligence and one-fourth do not have seizures. Autism occurs with certain forms of the syndrome. More sophisticated criteria for establishing a diagnosis of TSC are listed above [**Table 8.4**].

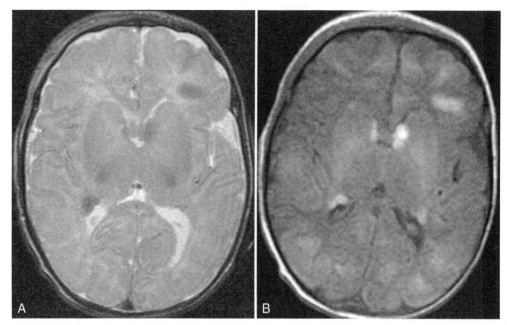

Figure 8.40 Tuberous sclerosis (infant). Five-day-old with multiple rhabdomyomas. **A,** Axial T2-weighted and (**B**) axial T1-weighted magnetic resonance images demonstrating cortical tubers and subependymal nodules consistent with tuberous sclerosis. Note that the tubers and nodules show T2 shortening (hypointensity) and T1 shortening (hyperintensity) relative to unmyelinated white matter.

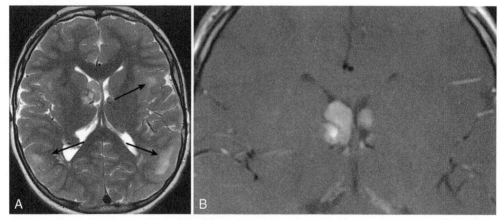

Figure 8.41 Tuberous sclerosis (juvenile). Ten-year-old boy with tuberous sclerosis. **A,** Axial T2-weighted image shows multiple cortical tubers (*arrows*) with broad gyri and subependymal nodules. Note that in contrast with the neonate, the subcortical white matter is hyperintense on T2-weighted images relative to myelinated white matter. **B,** Postcontrast T1-weighted image demonstrates typical enhancement of the subependymal nodules.

The most common presenting symptoms in children with TSC are infantile spasms or myoclonic seizures in early childhood. These can evolve into generalized epilepsy, partial epilepsy, or a mixture of both. Neuroimaging plays a critical role in the diagnosis of TSC [**Figs. 8.40** and **8.41**]. Characteristic abnormalities are present in more than 95% of patients. The CNS abnormalities are present from before birth, in contrast with the skin and systemic malformations, which may form much later in childhood.

The most common intracranial lesion in TSC is the *subependymal hamartoma* (nodule). These are histologically different from cortical hamartomas (tubers) and exhibit different imaging characteristics. On ultrasound, subependymal hamartomas appear as echogenic masses. The appearance on CT and MRI is variable. Calcification of subependymal hamartomas increases

with age, increasing their conspicuity on CT. On MRI, subependymal nodules tend to be isointense to brain if unmineralized and show T1 and T2 shortening if mineralized. Subependymal nodules show variable enhancement; the pattern and degree of enhancement are not of any clinical significance.

Subependymal giant cell astrocytoma (SEGA) refers to any subependymal nodule that shows a progressive increase in size; these can occur anywhere along the ependyma, but most are situated near the foramen of Monro. The incidence rate of SEGA in patients with TSC is 5% to 10%. Histologically, they are indistinguishable from subependymal hamartomas. Children with SEGA can present with fatigue, lack of appetite, headache, visual field defects, or behavioral issues caused by hydrocephalus. Increasing size on serial examinations, rather than absolute size or inherent signal characteristics, and the typical location are the most reliable criteria for diagnosing SEGA. Treatment usually consists of surgical excision.

Cortical and subcortical *tubers/hamartomas* are seen in up to 90% of TSC patients. These hamartomas appear as enlarged, atypically shaped gyri on imaging studies. Affected patients may have one to dozens of tubers. They are more common supratentorially but may involve the cerebellum. Calcification of cortical tubers increases with age. In infants, cortical tubers may be seen as focal areas of increased echogenicity on ultrasound. On MRI, cortical tubers have an imaging appearance similar to type II (balloon cell) cortical dysplasia. They appear hyperintense relative to unmyelinated white matter on T1 and hypointense on T2. In older children, tubers have a hypointense central component on T1 and are high signal on T2 and FLAIR. Tubers show increased diffusivity. They usually do not enhance. Tubers show normal/slightly elevated choline and slightly diminished NAA, in contrast with most malignancies, which show marked elevation of choline and marked depression of NAA. In children with refractory epilepsy, combining MRI, interictal FDG-PET, and ictal single-photo emission CT with electroencephalographic findings can help identify potential tubers for epilepsy surgery.

Various white matter abnormalities can be seen in TSC; these are most commonly seen as radial bands spanning the entire cerebral mantle from cortex to ependymal surface. Nodular and ill-defined white matter lesions may also be seen. About 10% to 15% of patients with TSC have parenchymal cysts. There is a slightly increased risk for cerebral aneurysm in children with TSC.

Sturge-Weber Syndrome

Sturge-Weber Syndrome (SWS) (also known as *encephalotrigeminal angiomatosis*) is a sporadic condition that is characterized by vascular anomalies involving the face, orbit, and leptomeninges. Patients often have hemiparesis, seizures, and intellectual disability. The facial vascular anomaly manifests as a port wine stain (nevus flammeus), usually in the V1 distribution, and is a capillary malformation. Children with SWS typically have normal early development before occurrence of infantile spasms and seizures around 1 year of life. Seizures become progressively more refractive to medication with increasing hemiparesis and hemianopsia.

The primary intracranial abnormality in SWS is a leptomeningeal capillary-venular malformation associated with abnormal

development of the cortical veins. The other intracranial manifestations are thought to be secondary to this anomaly. Because the cortical veins are not normally formed, collateral venous pathways develop. The medullary (parenchymal) veins are increased in size. The ipsilateral choroid plexus becomes engorged. The brain underneath the malformation is subject to chronic venous hypertension and ischemia, and eventually atrophies and develops laminar calcification. The calvarium becomes thickened on the side of the anomaly because of lack of growth of the brain and possibly increased flow to the capillary malformation of the skin.

The underlying pathology in the leptomeningeal malformation in SWS is not fully understood. One theory suggests that the vascular anomaly represents the persistence of primordial sinusoidal vascular channels that are present between the fourth and eighth weeks of gestation. A second theory is that the superficial venous drainage never develops with secondary dilatation of the capillaries and small veins.

On CT and radiographs, the cortical calcifications give rise to a characteristic "tram-track" gyral pattern, although these are often not present at birth. Contrast-enhanced MRI better demonstrates the full extent of the meningeal vascular anomaly as prominent leptomeningeal enhancement, filling the cortical sulci in the affected area [**Fig. 8.42**]. Early in life, only subtle volume loss in the brain underlying the malformation may be present on noncontrast imaging. Contrast administration may be critical to making the diagnosis early in infancy. Dynamic MRI perfusion studies show that the brain under the vascular anomaly is hypoperfused. MRS of the affected brain shows elevated choline, reduced NAA, and slightly elevated lactate.

Von Hippel-Lindau Syndrome

VHL is an autosomal dominant disorder that is characterized by cerebellar and spinal cord hemangioblastomas, retinal angiomas, renal cell carcinomas, endolymphatic sac tumors, pheochromocytomas, hepatic and renal angiomas, and pancreatic, renal, hepatic, and epididymal cysts. VHL affects 1 in 40,000 individuals; it has a high expression with variable penetrance. Classically it results from inactivation of the tumor suppressor VHL gene located on chromosome 3p25-p26. VHL is diagnosed in patients with more than one CNS hemangioblastoma, those with one CNS hemangioblastoma and one visceral manifestation, or in patients with one manifestation and a family history of VHL.

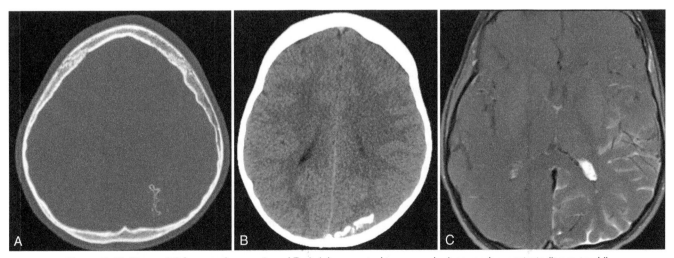

Figure 8.42 Sturge-Weber syndrome. A and **B,** Axial computed tomography images demonstrate "tram-track" gyral calcification in left parietooccipital region. **C,** Axial postcontrast T1-weighted fat-suppressed image demonstrates enhancement in the leptomeningeal capillary-venular malformation and enlargement of the ipsilateral choroid plexus.

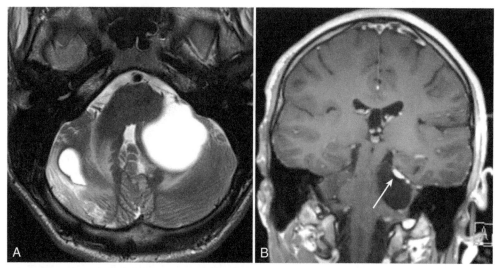

Figure 8.43 **Von-Hippel Lindau (VHL).** Seventeen-year-old male with VHL with multiple hemangioblastomas. **A,** T2-weighted and (**B**) postcontrast T1-weighted images show cystic lesions in the cerebellum. The dominant left cerebellar lesion is associated with an enhancing mural nodule (*arrow*).

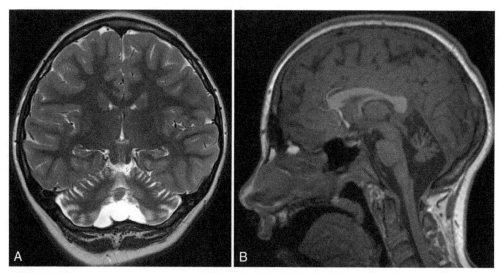

Figure 8.44 **Ataxia telangiectasia.** Seven-year-old girl with ataxia telangiectasia. **A,** Coronal T2-weighted and (**B**) sagittal T1-weighted images show hypoplasia of the cerebellar hemispheres and inferior vermis.

Hemangioblastomas may develop in childhood, adolescence, or early adulthood. Fifty percent are found in the spinal cord, 38% in the cerebellum, 10% in the brainstem, and 2% in the cerebrum. Hemangioblastomas typically consist of a well-circumscribed cyst with a solid enhancing mural nodule. Occasionally, especially when small, hemangioblastomas are entirely solid. In the spinal cord, extensive edema may surround the tumor. Calcification is not typical. On MRI, the solid nodule tends to be hypointense to isointense on T1 and hyperintense on T2 with avid contrast enhancement. Curvilinear areas of signal void may be seen within the nodule. Surgical resection is usually curative; preoperative embolization is performed in some larger lesions [**Fig. 8.43**].

Ataxia-Telangiectasia

Ataxia-telangiectasia is an autosomal recessive disorder characterized by cerebellar degeneration, vasculopathy, immunodeficiency, premature aging, predisposition to cancer, and increased sensitivity to ionizing radiation. The incidence is estimated at 1 in 40,000 live births. The involved gene, *ATM,* maps to chromosome 11q22-23 and encodes a nuclear protein kinase involved in DNA repair. Children typically present with cerebellar ataxia when the child starts to walk before showing progressive severe neurologic decline.

The major abnormalities seen on imaging are cerebellar atrophy and dilatation of the fourth ventricle [**Fig. 8.44**]. Intra-axial hemorrhage can be seen secondary to rupture of parenchymal telangiectasias. Cerebral infarcts can result from emboli shunted through pulmonary telangiectasias. Parenchymal telangiectasias may be apparent on postcontrast imaging. Because of the increased sensitivity to the effects of ionizing radiation, imaging of the CNS should be performed with ultrasound or MR whenever possible in these children, with CT and angiography reserved for specific indications that cannot be addressed through other imaging studies.

HYDROCEPHALUS

Hydrocephalus occurs when there is an excess of CSF associated with an increase in ICP. It is characterized by increased size of the ventricles and progressive compression of brain tissue. It is important to differentiate hydrocephalus that is associated with raised ICP from other causes of ventriculomegaly such as ex vacuo dilatation caused by white matter volume loss and dysmorphic ventriculomegaly that results from malformation of the brain.

Cerebrospinal Fluid Production and Circulation

The precise timing of the onset of CSF formation is not clear; however, circulation of CSF from the ventricles to the subarachnoid spaces begins around the 9th to 10th week of gestation. The choroid plexus produces approximately 60% of CSF. The rate of CSF production by choroid plexus in adults is approximately 500 mL per 24 hours. The site of CSF absorption is a controversial topic. In adults and older children the arachnoid granulations play a major role. However, these granulations do not form until closure of the fontanels, and in infants it appears that most CSF absorption occurs through the venous system. Consequently, venous hypertension is a potential cause of hydrocephalus.

Historically, the total volume of CSF was estimated at 40 to 60 mL in infants, 60 to 100 mL in children, and approximately 150 mL in adults. Volumetric MRI studies have suggested that these values underestimate the true volume of CSF present.

CSF flow dynamics are complex. In the intracranial compartment, each atrial systole results in an increase in the volume of intracranial blood. Because the skull is a confined space, and fluid is noncompressible, CSF is forced out through the foramen magnum after arterial systole and returns during diastole. CSF flow is readily demonstrable on cine MR studies.

Causes of Hydrocephalus

Hydrocephalus is most often due to impaired resorption of CSF, although there are rare causes of overproduction of CSF including choroid plexus papilloma (CPP) and choroid plexus hyperplasia. Any condition that obstructs the free passage of CSF, either within or outside of the ventricles, can result in hydrocephalus [**Fig. 8.45**]. Historically when the obstruction occurred within the ventricles it was termed *noncommunicating* hydrocephalus, and when the site of obstruction occurred outside of the ventricles it was termed *communicating*. Because both communicating and noncommunicating hydrocephalus are due to obstruction, the terms are not that helpful and should probably be avoided. Instead, the site of suspected obstruction should be reported. Impaired CSF resorption can occur because of both congenital and acquired conditions [**Table 8.5**].

Imaging of Hydrocephalus

Ventriculomegaly caused by increased pressure should be distinguished from ventriculomegaly caused by lack of brain growth or abnormal brain malformation. Imaging is frequently insufficient in isolation to make this determination, and correlation with head growth is essential at understanding the significance of ventriculomegaly. For example, the finding of mildly prominent ventricles in a 6-month-old child may reflect normal development or may be a sign of hydrocephalus. If the growth chart shows the head circumference following expected growth percentiles, then the imaging finding is likely normal, whereas if the head circumference is crossing growth curve lines, there may be cause for concern.

Ultrasound is the primary imaging modality for detecting and monitoring hydrocephalus in the fetus. Fetal MRI plays a secondary role in monitoring and assessing for an underlying cause.

Until about 2 years of age, hydrocephalus is almost always associated with progressive head enlargement (macrocephaly). Other clinical signs of raised ICP in infancy include engorged scalp veins, sutural diastasis, and bulging fontanels.

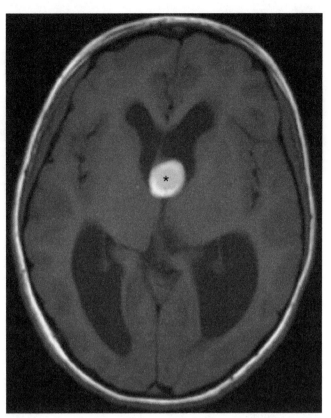

Figure 8.45 Hydrocephalus secondary to colloid cyst. Sixteen-year-old girl with vomiting. Axial T1 demonstrates intrinsic T1 shortening related to proteinaceous content in the colloid cyst (*asterisk*), which is obstructing the foramina of Monro, producing enlargement of the lateral ventricles.

TABLE 8.5   Causes of Childhood Hydrocephalus

Congenital causes of hydrocephalus	• Chiari II malformation • Aqueductal stenosis • Congenital cysts • Encephaloceles • Craniosynostosis • Skull base abnormalities • Foraminal atresia • Vein of Galen malformations
Acquired causes of hydrocephalus	• Posthemorrhagic • Postinfection • Tumors • Venous sinus thrombosis

In older children, the classic clinical triad of *headache, vomiting, and lethargy* is commonly present. Children with chronic hydrocephalus caused by an obstructing tumor often present with persistent morning headaches and intermittent vomiting. Papilledema may be present, as well as hypothalamic-pituitary dysfunction secondary to mass effect from the enlargement of the anterior recesses of the third ventricle.

MRI is the ideal modality to assess for the presence of hydrocephalus, evaluate for an underlying cause, and monitor its consequences. Ultrasound is a useful modality in fetal cases and in infancy when imaging can be performed using the open fontanels as an acoustic window. In practice, CT is often used in the emergency setting. Advantages of CT include its widespread availability and rapid speed of image acquisition; however, the risks of ionizing radiation, particularly in children and those who require frequent imaging because of the presence of a ventricular shunt, need to be considered.

Raised intraventricular pressure can force CSF to cross the ependyma and result in periventricular interstitial edema. This is most elegantly depicted as periventricular white matter hyperintensity on axial MRI FLAIR sequences. It manifests as periventricular low attenuation on CT.

In evaluating patients with ventriculomegaly, an attempt should be made to define the site of obstruction. If there is

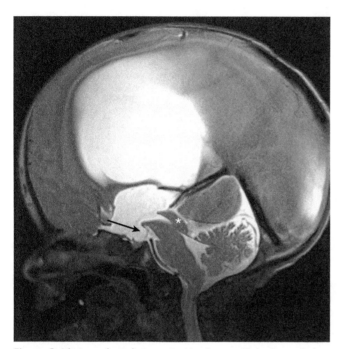

Figure 8.46 Aqueductal stenosis. Newborn with hydrocephalus. Midline sagittal T2-weighted image shows marked narrowing of cerebral aqueduct with elevation of the tectum (*asterisk*) and no evidence of a flow void through the aqueduct consistent with stenosis. Note marked enlargement of the lateral ventricles and depression of the floor of the third ventricle (*arrow*) indicating that the ventricle is dilated.

disproportionate enlargement of a portion of a lateral ventricle, an intraventricular cyst or web may be present. Dilated lateral ventricles with a normal-sized third and fourth ventricle point to obstruction at the foramen of Monro. If the third ventricle is dilated as well, the obstruction is likely at the level of the aqueduct [**Fig. 8.46**]. Aqueductal obstruction may occur from a posterior third ventricular mass such as a pineal tumor, tectal tumor, or aqueductal stenosis due to a web. Stenosis of the aqueduct is usually associated with elevation of the tectum and may be caused by prior hemorrhage or infection in addition to congenital causes. A dilated fourth ventricle suggests obstruction at the outlets of the fourth ventricle or around the surface of the brain. High-resolution T2-weighted imaging may be required to demonstrate webs within the CSF, and T2-weighted GRE imaging is helpful for demonstrating evidence of prior hemorrhage as a cause of obstruction.

Rapid increases in ventricular size and ICP can result in downward herniation of the mesial temporal structures along the free edge of the tentorium. The resultant compression of the midbrain, the aqueduct, basal cisterns, and circle of Willis can lead to ischemia and infarction. The posterior cerebral arteries are particularly vulnerable to compression as they pass around the midbrain. Compression of the venous sinuses and cortical veins against the inner table of the skull reduces venous outflow and causes further increases in ICP. Increased pressure in the posterior fossa can cause upward or downward herniation. Occlusion of the foramen magnum can result in a rapid, tamponade-like rise in ICP [**Fig. 8.47**]. Eventually, perfusion pressure cannot overcome the ICP, leading to intracranial circulatory arrest.

Treatment of Hydrocephalus

The traditional treatment of hydrocephalus has been with the placement of an *intraventricular shunt* that decreases ICP by providing an alternative drainage pathway for CSF. The proximal part of the catheter can be inserted via a frontal, parietal, temporal, or occipital approach. This segment is connected to a valve and distal catheter that in the majority of cases drains CSF into the peritoneal cavity. The pleural space, central veins, right atrium, and the gallbladder can also be used if there is a contraindication to placement of the catheter in the peritoneum.

Hemorrhage secondary to insertion of the intracranial portion of the shunt occurs in 1% of patients. Hemorrhage is more common after removal of an old shunt. Seizures can occur after

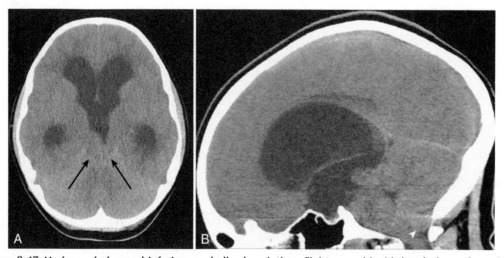

Figure 8.47 Hydrocephalus and inferior cerebellar herniation. Eight-year-old with headache and vomiting. **A,** Axial and (**B**) sagittal reconstructed computed tomography images show marked ventriculomegaly, diffuse sulcal effacement, attenuation of the quadrigeminal cistern (*arrows*), and inferior cerebellar tonsillar herniation (*arrowhead*).

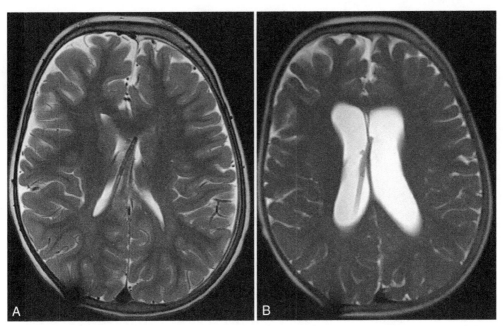

Figure 8.48 Shunt malfunction. Six-year-old girl with ventriculoperitoneal shunt presenting with increasing lethargy. **A,** Axial T2-weighted image demonstrates her baseline. **B,** Axial T2-weighted image in the setting of new symptoms reveals an increase in the size of the ventricles consistent with shunt malfunction.

shunt placement and are more common with frontal approach catheters.

After the immediate postoperative period, the two most common reasons for shunt malfunction are mechanical failure and shunt infection.

Mechanical shunt failure is the most common cause of shunt malfunction. Obstruction can occur at the proximal end secondary to occlusion by brain parenchyma, choroid plexus, or tumor [**Fig. 8.48**]. Disconnection can occur at any point along the course of the catheter but is most common at the junction of the valve and distal catheter and at sites of increased mobility such as the neck. The formation of a pseudocyst around the tip of the distal catheter in the peritoneal cavity is the most common distal cause of mechanical failure.

Shunt infection is the second most common cause of shunt failure and is seen in 5% to 10% of cases of shunt malfunction. Most shunt infections present within 2 months of shunt placement. Shunt infection can also result from abdominal surgical procedures.

The diagnosis of shunt malfunction is primarily based on clinical evaluation. Imaging studies include a "shunt series" of radiographs of the entire shunt catheter. These radiographs need to be interrogated carefully for evidence of discontinuity or migration of the catheter.

In cases of suspected shunt malfunction, imaging of the head is performed to assess for changes in the size and shape of the ventricles. Traditionally this was performed in the acute setting using CT; however, fast MRI sequences allow rapid assessment of ventricular size without the risks of ionizing radiation associated with CT. Head imaging needs to be evaluated for the position of the intracranial portion of the catheter and any change in the size or shape of the ventricles compared with prior studies. In general, an increase in ventricular size is concerning for shunt malfunction; however, some shunted children show little, if any, increase in ventricular size with malfunction or raised ICP. Seventy percent of children with mechanical obstruction will show an increase in ventricular size compared with 30% of children with shunt infection. In the absence of prior CNS imaging studies, the significance of a given ventricular size may be difficult to determine given the wide variation in baseline

ventricular size among patients with shunts. In addition to assessing ventricular size, brain imaging should also be reviewed for abnormal fluid collections along the course of the shunt, within the scalp, or in the subdural space that may indicate shunt catheter obstruction or disconnection.

Some patients exhibit markedly collapsed ventricles after shunting. The term *slit ventricle syndrome* should be used only in cases where there is clinical evidence of overshunting (such as chronic headache or neurologic symptoms) or other evidence such as calvarial thickening.

Given the frequent complications seen with shunts, there has been renewed interest in endoscopic treatments for hydrocephalus. Endoscopic third ventriculostomy (ETV) is one of the most commonly used techniques, with success rates of up to 60% to 70% for hydrocephalus caused by intraventricular obstruction. ETV involves the use of an endoscope to perforate the floor of the third ventricle anterior to the mammillary bodies forming a drainage pathway between the third ventricle and the basal cisterns. Successful ETV requires that the site of obstruction be within the ventricles rather than over the surface of the brain because the goal is to provide a means of bypassing the obstruction.

Endoscopic treatment of hydrocephalus is characterized by a much slower and less dramatic reduction in the size of the ventricles, taking weeks to months as opposed to days after shunt catheter placement. MRI is the modality of choice for follow-up in these patients. Confirmation of patency of the third ventriculostomy is indicated on midline sagittal high-resolution T2-weighted sequences by a signal void across the defect in the floor of the third ventricle [**Fig. 8.49**]. Phase-contrast MR flow studies can also be used to provide evidence of CSF flow across the ventriculostomy site.

Extraaxial Fluid Collections in Infancy

In evaluating children with prominent extraaxial spaces, it is important to differentiate between enlargement of the subarachnoid space, which may be either normal or pathologic, and abnormal fluid within the subdural space.

Some infants, especially in families where one or both parents have large heads, may have benign prominence of the CSF

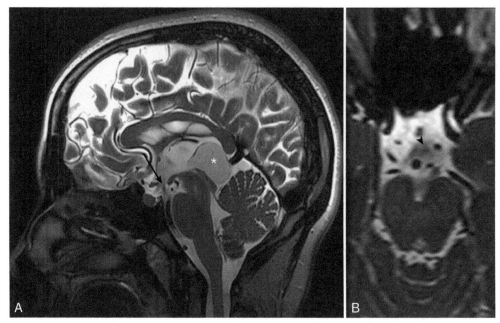

Figure 8.49 Patent endoscopic third ventriculostomy. Fifteen-year-old with hydrocephalus caused by pineal cyst. **A,** Sagittal T2-weighted image shows a defect in the floor of the third ventricle (*arrow*) with a signal void indicating patency of the third ventriculostomy. **B,** Axial T2-weighted image confirms a signal void extending into the suprasellar cistern (*arrowhead*). Note the large pineal cyst (*asterisk*) compressing the aqueduct.

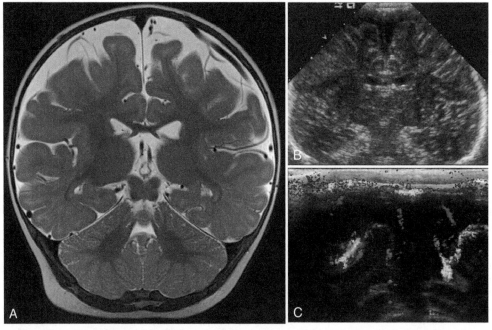

Figure 8.50 Benign extraaxial fluid collections of infancy. Four-month-old girl with increased head circumference. **A,** magnetic resonance imaging and (**B and C**) ultrasound demonstrate symmetric prominent extraaxial fluid spaces. Note that the cortical veins course through the enlarged subarachnoid space and are not compressed against the parenchyma by the fluid as occurs with subdural collections.

spaces. In this situation, there is mild prominence of the ventricles and extraaxial CSF spaces. Although macrocrania may be present, the head size should track along normal growth curves. This is in contrast with infants with prominent CSF spaces caused by external hydrocephalus in whom the head circumference crosses growth curves over time. Infants with benign prominence of the CSF spaces most often come to attention between the ages of 2 and 6 months. Their head circumference is above the 95th percentile and stabilizes along a curve paralleling the

95th percentile until about 18 to 24 months of age when the prominence of the extraaxial spaces decreases.

Distinguishing between excess CSF in the subarachnoid space and abnormal fluid in the subdural space is especially important in the setting of suspected abusive head trauma. With either benign CSF prominence or extraventricular obstructive hydrocephalus, on ultrasound and MRI, cortical veins course through the enlarged subarachnoid space and lie close to the inner table of the skull [**Fig. 8.50**]. Conversely, if the subdural space is enlarged secondary to hematoma or fluid, the cortical veins are displaced medially toward the cerebral cortex. Whether enlargement of the CSF spaces predisposes the child to the subdural bleeding with minor trauma is the subject of considerable controversy and is an issue frequently raised in cases of suspected abusive head trauma.

INFLAMMATORY

Intracranial infection, caused by bacterial, viral, fungal, or parasitic organisms, can manifest as encephalitis, cerebritis, or meningitis. Encephalitis refers to diffuse inflammation of the brain parenchyma; cerebritis refers to a more focal parenchymal infection. Meningitis refers to inflammation of the pia, arachnoid, and dural membranes. Complications of infection include abscess and empyema.

MRI is the best imaging modality to evaluate intracranial infection and in particular to search for complications such as empyema, vasculitis, and ischemia. Postcontrast T1-weighted sequences are useful in assessing fluid collections and meningeal enhancement. DWI may help localize abscesses in the epidural or subdural space. MRV and postcontrast GRE T1-weighted sequences can be used to determine whether the infection has been complicated by the development of venous sinus thrombosis. CT can be used to assess for hydrocephalus and cerebral edema if MRI is unavailable in the time frame required for management. CT is superior to MRI in the depiction of osseous erosion and destruction in osteomyelitis, although MRI is more sensitive for early signs of bone infection, such as marrow edema and enhancement.

Bacterial Infections

Meningitis

Bacterial meningitis is the most common cause of pediatric CNS infection. Bacterial meningitis can be secondary to hematogenous spread of infection, direct trauma, extension from adjacent sinus, or mastoid disease. It may also occur as a congenital infection or be acquired during parturition.

In neonates, the most common causes of bacterial meningitis are group B *Streptococcus* and *Escherichia coli.* In children older than 1 month, the most common causative organisms are *Haemophilus influenza* type B, *Streptococcus pneumonia, Neisseria meningitides,* and *Escherichia coli.* The use of a vaccine for *Haemophilus influenza* type B has greatly decreased the incidence of this infection of the CNS in children.

The diagnosis of bacterial meningitis can be made without imaging, and indeed imaging can be negative early in the clinical course. However, imaging plays a role when the diagnosis is unclear or when persistent symptoms despite treatment raise concern for complications [**Fig. 8.51**]. Complications of bacterial meningitis include cerebritis, abscess, empyema, hydrocephalus, venous thrombosis, infarction, ventriculitis, mycotic aneurysms, and sensorineural hearing loss. Cranial ultrasound can be a useful tool to screen for complications of meningitis in neonates [**Fig. 8.52**]. In older children, MRI is the imaging modality of choice.

Cerebritis and Abscess

It is important to differentiate between focal cerebritis, which in general will respond to intravenous antibiotics, and a cerebral abscess, which in general will require surgical drainage. Cerebritis manifests as patchy hypoattenuation on CT, with corresponding T1 hypointensity and high signal on T2/T2-weighted FLAIR MRI. Mild mass effect may be present. Patchy enhancement may be evident on postcontrast imaging. A cerebral abscess is a circumscribed, fluid-filled structure with a peripheral rim that is typically T1 hyperintense and T2 hypointense. The medial wall of an abscess is usually thinner than the lateral wall. The rim of an abscess shows enhancement postcontrast. The necrotic central portion of an abscess shows low diffusivity on DWI in contrast with the increased diffusion present in regions of necrosis in tumors [**Fig. 8.53**]. MRS of abscesses is notable for the presence of amino acid and lactate peaks.

Epidural abscesses or subdural empyemas are most commonly seen as complications of sinusitis and mastoiditis. These collections can be small and may exhibit various degrees of mass effect. They show low diffusivity and rim enhancement on MRI [**Fig. 8.54**].

Superficial or deep cortical venous or dural venous sinus thrombosis can complicate CNS infections. Enlargement of or abnormal signal within a cortical vein or dural sinus should prompt formal evaluation with MRV or postcontrast T1-weighted

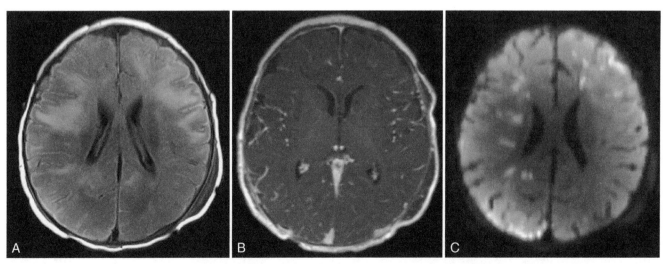

Figure 8.51 Bacterial meningitis. Six-month-old girl with streptococcal meningitis. **A,** Axial T2 fluid attenuation inversion recovery demonstrates extensive white matter edema and abnormal signal within the sulci. **B,** Axial postcontrast T1-weighted image shows diffuse leptomeningeal enhancement. **C,** Axial diffusion-weighted imaging demonstrates multiple periventricular foci of decreased diffusion, likely caused by medullary venous infarction.

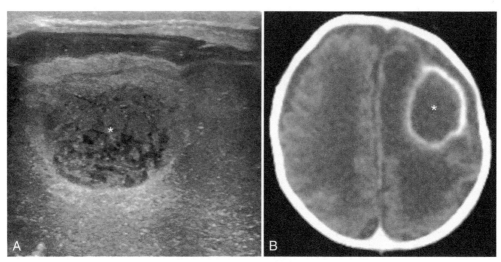

Figure 8.52 Cerebral abscess. Two-month-old infant (born at 26 weeks' gestation). **A,** Ultrasound demonstrates a well-circumscribed, mixed echogenicity mass (*asterisk*) in left frontal lobe with surrounding hyperechogenicity in the white and gray matter. **B,** Axial contrast-enhanced computed tomography demonstrates a ring-enhancing mass (*asterisk*) in the left frontal lobe.

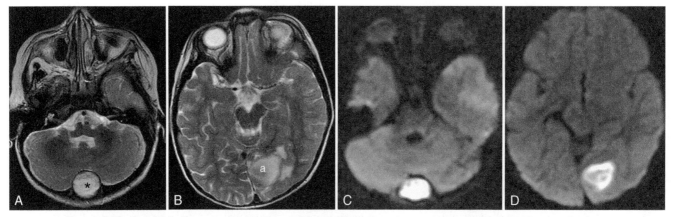

Figure 8.53 Cerebral abscess complicating a dermoid cyst. Twenty-seven-month-old girl with posterior fossa dermoid cyst and fever. **A** and **B,** Axial T2-weighted images show a midline posterior fossa dermoid cyst (*asterisk*) and adjacent abscess in the left occipital lobe (*a*). **C** and **D,** Axial diffusion-weighted images demonstrated decreased diffusion in the midline dermoid cyst and the occipital lobe abscess.

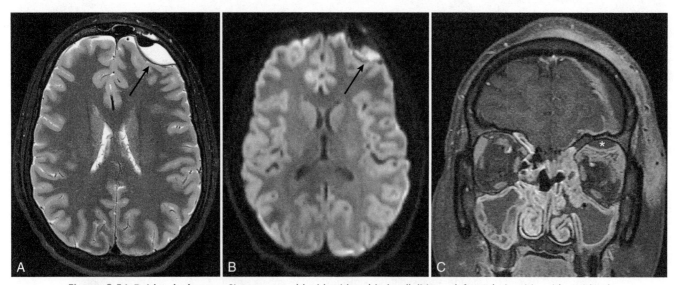

Figure 8.54 Epidural abscess. Sixteen-year-old girl with orbital cellulitis and frontal sinusitis with epidural abscess. **A,** Axial T2-weighted image shows left frontal epidural fluid and gas collection (*arrows*). **B,** Diffusion-weighted image demonstrates decreased diffusion within the fluid indicating pus (*arrows*). **C,** Postcontrast T1-weighted image shows left orbital enhancement/cellulitis, subperiosteal abscess (*asterisk*), and extensive paranasal sinus disease.

volumetric GRE imaging to evaluate venous patency. Venous sinus thrombosis can result in infarction and hemorrhage [**Fig. 8.55**].

Tuberculosis Infections

CNS infection secondary to *Mycobacterium tuberculosis* is clinically and radiologically very different from pyogenic infection. Hematogenous dissemination of the tuberculous bacilli produces tuberculomas (caseating granulomas) in the meninges, at the gray-white matter junction, in the spinal cord, and rarely in the choroid plexus. Rupture of these tuberculomas with resultant discharge of bacilli into the CSF or subarachnoid space causes granulomatous meningitis. Tuberculous meningitis is typically most severe in the basal cisterns and can present with cranial nerve palsies or obstructive hydrocephalus secondary to occlusion of the fourth ventricular exit foramina.

Marked subarachnoid and cisternal enhancement is often present on postcontrast MRI sequences. Tuberculomas, which are most commonly seen at the gray-white matter, are hyperintense on T1-weighted MRI, hypointense on T2-weighted MRI, and enhance uniformly or peripherally when larger. A tubercu-

lous abscess is rare and may be differentiated from bacterial abscess by the presence of increased diffusivity within the cavity [**Fig. 8.56**].

Lyme disease is a multisystem disorder arising from infection with the tick-borne *Borrelia burgdorferi* spirochete. It involves the CNS in 20% of patients and may manifest as lymphocytic meningitis, meningoencephalitis, or cranial neuropathy. MRI may show T2 hyperintense white matter lesions throughout the cerebrum, cerebellum, brainstem, and basal ganglia that may or may not enhance with contrast. Postcontrast MRI may also show leptomeningeal or cranial nerve enhancement [**Fig. 8.57**].

Viral Infections

Congenital and neonatal CNS infections are most commonly related to the TORCH organisms (*t*oxoplasmosis, *o*ther, *r*ubella, *c*ytomegalovirus, and *h*erpes simplex virus type 2 [HSV-2]/*h*uman immunodeficiency virus type 1 [HIV-1]). Toxoplasmosis, rubella, CMV, and HIV-1 are transmitted via the placenta, whereas HSV-2 and bacterial infections are acquired during parturition.

CMV is the most common of the TORCH infections and occurs in 1% of all live births. Clinical signs of CMV infection

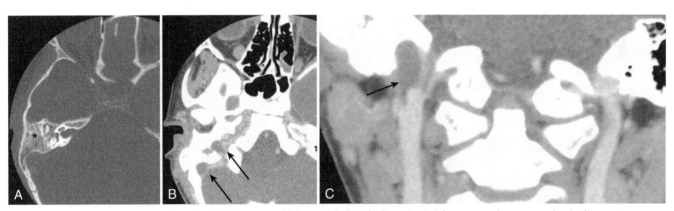

Figure 8.55 Sinus thrombosis. Five-year-old boy with headaches. **A,** Axial computed tomography in bone window reveals coalescent right otomastoiditis (*asterisk*) and in (**B**) soft tissue window, thrombus within the dominant right internal jugular vein and sigmoid sinus (*arrows*). **C,** Coronal reformatted image confirms clot within the proximal right internal jugular vein (*arrow*).

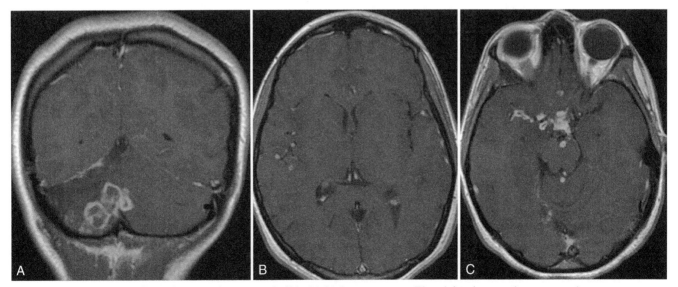

Figure 8.56 Tuberculous meningoencephalitis. Multiple postcontrast T1-weighted magnetic resonance images demonstrate (**A**) right cerebellar parenchymal abscesses, (**B**) nodular leptomeningeal enhancement in the right Sylvian fissure, and (**C**) enhancement in the basal cisterns.

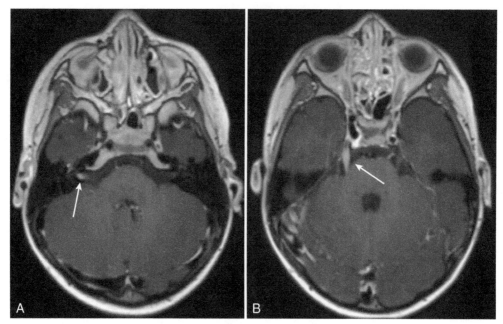

Figure 8.57 Lyme disease. Six-year-old girl with right facial paralysis. Postcontrast T1 images show (**A**) enhancement of cranial nerve VII within the Internal auditory canal (IAC) (*arrow*) and (**B**) right trigeminal nerve (*arrow*). Enzyme-linked immunosorbent assay and Western blot analysis were positive for Lyme disease.

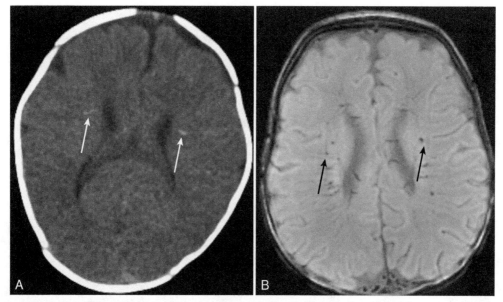

Figure 8.58 Cytomegalovirus. Four-week-old with irritability. Periventricular calcifications seen on (**A**) computed tomography (CT) (*arrows*) and (**B**) susceptibility-weighted imaging (SWI) (*arrows*). Note that SWI is sometimes more sensitive than CT for the demonstration of mineralization, showing many more foci.

include microcephaly, hearing impairment, seizures, chorioretinitis, developmental delay, and hepatosplenomegaly. Cranial ultrasound in affected patients often shows mineralizing vasculopathy of the basal ganglia. Manifestations depend on the gestational age at which the infection is acquired. Infection during the first and second trimester may result in cortical malformations including PMG, lissencephaly, and gray matter heterotopia. Central, periventricular calcification, ventriculomegaly, gliosis, hypomyelination, and cysts are associated with later fetal infection [**Fig. 8.58**].

Toxoplasmosis is far less common than CMV. It is a parasitic infection (*Toxoplasma gondii*) that is associated with maternal

ingestion of undercooked pork or beef. Clinically toxoplasmosis produces seizures, developmental delay, and chorioretinitis. The severity depends on the timing of fetal infection. Imaging characteristically shows diffuse calcifications (as opposed to the periventricular calcification in CMV). Cortical malformations are less common with toxoplasmosis than in CMV [**Fig. 8.59**].

Neonatal *herpes* infection occurs secondary to passage through an HSV-2 colonized birth canal during vaginal delivery. Neonatal HSV-2 infection occurs in 1 in 10,000 live births. Infected children present between 2 and 4 weeks of life with seizures, meningoencephalitis, lethargy, and fever. HSV-2 infection can proceed to profound CNS destruction. Imaging is

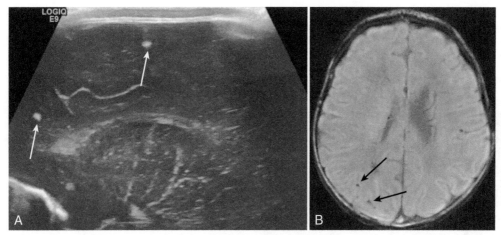

Figure 8.59 Toxoplasmosis. Six-day-old girl tested positive for toxoplasmosis on newborn screen. **A,** Multiple punctate echogenic foci on head ultrasound (*arrows*) and (**B**) susceptibility artifact on susceptibility-weighted imaging (SWI) (*arrows*). Note that the calcifications in toxoplasmosis are more likely subcortical as opposed to the central periventricular calcifications of cytomegalovirus (see Fig. 8.58).

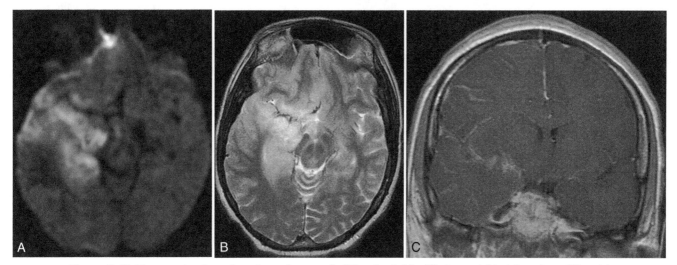

Figure 8.60 Herpes simplex virus type 1 encephalitis. A, Axial diffusion-weighted imaging, (**B**) axial T2-weighted, and (**C**) coronal T1 postcontrast show signal abnormality, decreased diffusion, and associated mass effect involving the right temporal lobe, right thalamus, right basal ganglia, right insula, and right frontal lobe with overlying leptomeningeal enhancement.

typified by cerebral edema, infarction, encephalomalacia, and hypomyelination. Restricted diffusion on DWI is the earliest imaging sign of herpetic parenchymal destruction. Unlike reactivation encephalitis caused by HSV-1, which tends to involve the temporal and frontal lobes, the encephalitis caused by HSV-2 does not demonstrate a regional predilection.

In older children, primary viral CNS infection typically results in encephalitis or meningoencephalitis. In general, acute viral infection results in parenchymal edema, which manifests as T2/FLAIR hyperintensity on MRI [**Fig. 8.60**].

HSV-1 CNS infection (as opposed to the prenatally acquired HSV-2) is most commonly due to reactivation of a latent orofacial herpes infection. Early symptoms include fever, malaise, and lethargy. This can progress to seizure, hemiparesis, and impaired consciousness. Because the virus is within the branches of the trigeminal nerve that supply the meninges of the temporal lobe and subfrontal region, these areas are preferentially involved with the resulting encephalitis. Imaging is typified by unilateral or bilateral mesial temporal lobe changes with restricted diffusion on DWI being the earliest imaging sign. Leptomeningeal

enhancement and calcifications may also be seen. Cortical petechial hemorrhage and necrosis are common.

Acute disseminated encephalomyelitis (ADEM) is a parainfectious demyelinating disorder that affects both brain and spinal cord after vaccination or viral infection. Clinically, ADEM may cause seizures, lethargy, or focal neurologic deficit. ADEM responds to steroids and complete recovery is common. ADEM is characterized by multifocal T2/FLAIR white matter hyperintensities in the cerebrum, brainstem, cerebellum, and spinal cord. Occasionally lesions may be seen within deep gray matter structures, most often the thalami. Enhancement of demyelinating lesions in ADEM is variable but can be very marked. Although the imaging appearance is nonspecific and can be confused with infectious and other demyelinating conditions, the lesions often appear to "cup" the base of a gyrus [**Fig. 8.61**].

Subacute sclerosing panencephalitis occurs as a reactivation of the measles virus years after the original infection. It is characterized by cortical and basal ganglia signal abnormalities on MRI. There tends to be no associated enhancement or mass effect.

Rasmussen encephalitis is a chronic, focal encephalitis that may be viral, postviral, or autoimmune. It causes intractable focal epilepsy in children. It is characterized by unilateral progressive regional atrophy most often in the frontal and temporal lobe. Hemispherectomy may be required for seizure control [**Fig. 8.62**].

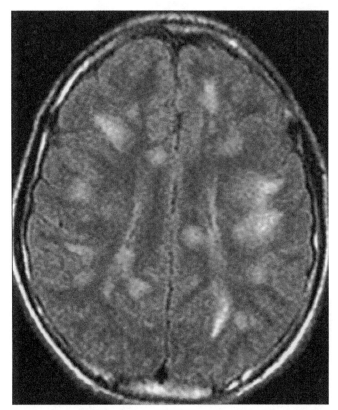

Figure 8.61 Acute disseminated encephalomyelitis (ADEM). Three-year-old with mental status changes. Axial fluid attenuation inversion recovery image demonstrates white matter lesions with typical "fuzzy" margins of ADEM.

CENTRAL NERVOUS SYSTEM NEOPLASMS

Brain tumor is the most common type of solid-organ malignancy in children and the most common cause of death due to solid neoplasm in children. Tumor location tends to vary with the age of the patient. Tumors in the first year of life occur with relatively equal frequency in the infratentorial and supratentorial compartments. After 1 year of age, an infratentorial location is more common.

Supratentorial Tumors

Astrocytoma

Astrocytomas are primary glial cell tumors and are the most common brain tumor in children. They are divided into low-grade (World Health Organization [WHO] grades I-II) and high-grade (WHO grades III-IV) tumors. Prognosis typically depends on both the histology and the location of the tumor.

Pilocytic astrocytomas are grade 1 tumors and make up 20% to 30% of all pediatric CNS tumors. They tend to occur in patients younger than 20 years and can be found both above and below the tentorium. The most common locations are the optic pathway, hypothalamus, cerebellum, and brainstem, although occasionally pilocytic astrocytoma occurs within the cerebral hemispheres. Hemispheric tumors tend to be similar in imaging characteristics to pilocytic astrocytomas elsewhere in the brain and are typically well-circumscribed masses with low signal on T1-weighted imaging and high signal on T2-weighted imaging because of their high water content. Contrast enhancement is often avid due to the lack of a normal blood barrier [**Fig. 8.63**]. Increased ADC values help to differentiate pilocytic astrocytoma from higher-grade lesions. An unusual MR spectroscopic feature of pilocytic astrocytoma is the presence of lactate in the tumor, which is otherwise only present in high-grade neoplasms. Gross total resection of pilocytic astrocytomas is usually curative.

High-grade gliomas account for 20% of all gliomas in children and most often occur in the cerebral hemispheres or in the pons. They are less well defined on CT and MRI than lower-grade lesions. They often show intralesional hemorrhage and marked local mass effect. Occasionally, however, hemispheric tumors are predominantly cystic and can mimic the appearance of a low-grade pilocytic astrocytoma. Enhancement of high-grade

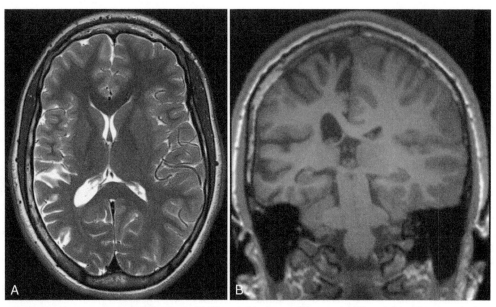

Figure 8.62 Rasmussen encephalitis. A, Axial T2-weighted and (**B**) coronal T1-weighted images demonstrate extensive right hemispheric atrophy.

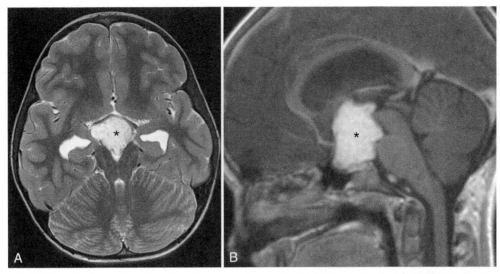

Figure 8.63 Hypothalamic juvenile pilocytic astrocytoma. A, Axial T2-weighted and (**B**) postcontrast sagittal T1-weighted images show an avidly enhancing suprasellar mass (*asterisks*) that compresses the third ventricle and abuts the vessels of the circle of Willis.

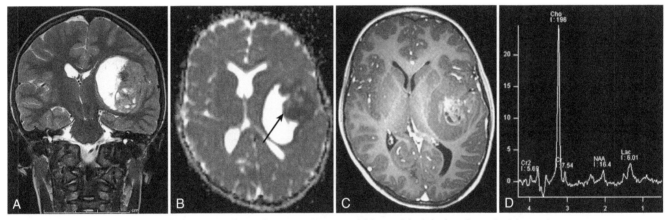

Figure 8.64 Primitive neuroectodermal tumor. Six-year-old boy with right hemiparesis. Magnetic resonance (MR) reveals a heterogeneous cystic/solid mass lesion centered at the level of the left insula. Note low signal on (**A**) coronal T2-weighted image and decreased diffusion in the solid portion of the mass (*arrow*) on the (**B**) apparent diffusion coefficient map and associated enhancement on (**C**) postcontrast T1. **D,** MR spectroscopy in the solid portion of the lesion demonstrates a markedly elevated choline, reduced *N*-acetyl aspartate, and a small amount of lactate consistent with a high-grade tumor.

tumors tends to be irregular with areas of nonenhancing necrosis. Treatment consists of surgical resection if possible, combined with adjuvant radiotherapy and chemotherapy. The 5-year progression-free survival rate for high-grade gliomas in children is about 30%.

Supratentorial Primitive Neuroectodermal Tumor

Supratentorial primitive neuroectodermal tumors (PNET) are rare tumors that are most common in the first decade of life and often come to clinical attention in the first year of life. Histologically these are high-grade embryonal tumors, which are composed of undifferentiated neuroepithelial cells (WHO grade IV). The characteristic imaging appearance is of a large, well-circumscribed, heterogeneous hemispheric mass with variable surrounding edema [**Fig. 8.64**]. Calcification is present in 50% to 70% of cases. Intratumoral hemorrhage may occur. The solid components tend to enhance heterogeneously and show restricted diffusion on MRI. Treatment consists of surgical resection, chemotherapy, and craniospinal radiation. In general,

supratentorial PNETs have a poor prognosis with a 5-year survival rate of 30% to 35%.

Dysembryoplastic Neuroepithelial Tumor

Dysembryoplastic neuroepithelial tumor (DNT) is a pathologically benign tumor of the cerebral cortex that frequently is associated with histologic evidence of cortical dysplasia at its margin. DNT is a frequent cause of seizures in childhood or young adulthood. Sixty percent of DNTs are found in the temporal lobe. DNTs have heterogeneous imaging appearances, but the majority are well-demarcated, lobulated cortical masses that are hypodense to white matter on CT. They are usually hypointense on T1-weighted and hyperintense on T2-weighted MR sequences [**Fig. 8.65**]. DNT often exhibits a multicystic or "bubbly" appearance. Calcifications are present in one-third of cases. Peripherally located and slow-growing tumors, DNTs may be associated with remodeling of the inner table of the calvarium. Twenty to 30% of DNTs show enhancement, which may be nodular, patchy, or ringlike. Surgical resection of

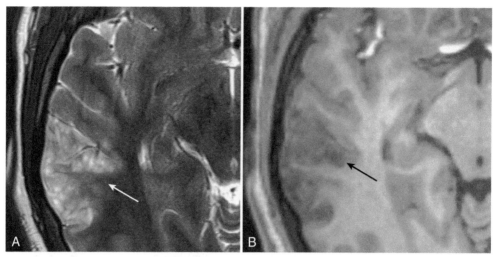

Figure 8.65 Dysembryoplastic neuroepithelial tumor (DNT). Fifteen-year-old boy presented with first-time seizure. **A,** Axial T2-weighted and (**B**) postcontrast T1-weighted images show a hyperintense ("soap bubble"), nonenhancing superficial mass (*arrows*) in the posterolateral right temporal lobe. Although there is no enhancement of this lesion, a minority of DNTs do show some enhancement.

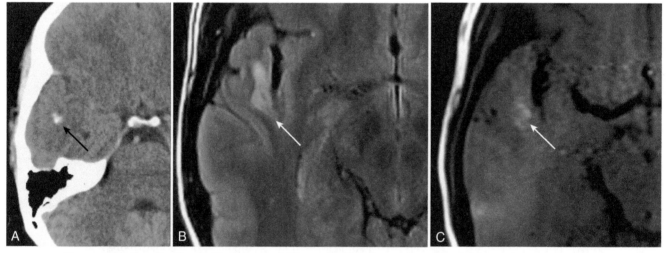

Figure 8.66 Ganglioglioma. Twelve-year-old boy with first-time seizure. **A,** Axial unenhanced computed tomography demonstrates a right temporal calcification (*arrow*). **B,** Axial T2-weighted image shows a cortical-based lesion (*arrow*) with faint T1 shortening (*arrow*) on (**C**) T1-weighted magnetic resonance.

symptomatic lesions is usually curative, but local recurrence is occasionally seen.

Ganglioglioma

Ganglioglioma is most often a low-grade tumor composed of both neuronal and glial elements. The glial elements determine the biological behavior of the lesions, and higher-grade lesions do occur. The tumors tend to be cortical in location and are frequently associated with seizures, especially when occurring in the temporal lobe. Ganglioglioma is generally a well-circumscribed tumor with variable MR signal characteristics [**Fig. 8.66**]. Approximately one-third of the tumors calcify and one-third of tumors are cystic. Contrast enhancement is variable.

Choroid Plexus Tumors

Choroid plexus papilloma (CPP) is a benign neoplasm that accounts for 85% of choroid plexus tumors. In children, CPP typically occurs in the trigone of the lateral ventricle as opposed

to adults where the tumor is more common in the fourth ventricle. On CT CPP tends to be lobulated, hyperdense, and may have punctate calcification. On MRI, the tumor is hypointense on T1, hyperintense on T2, and enhances homogenously [**Fig. 8.67**]. Choroid plexus carcinoma (CPC) is a malignant tumor originating from the choroid plexus and is characterized by a more heterogeneous appearance than CPP on both CT and MRI and invasion into, or edema within, the adjacent brain parenchyma [**Fig. 8.68**]. However, the more aggressive imaging features may be absent in CPC, and the tumor may mimic benign CPP on imaging. Intracranial or intraspinal leptomeningeal metastases may occur with both CPP and CPC. CPP has an excellent prognosis after surgical resection. CPC is treated with resection, chemotherapy, and radiotherapy with 5-year survival rates of approximately 40%.

Pineal Region Tumors

Tumors arising in the pineal region represent 3% to 8% of all pediatric brain tumors. Pineal tumors frequently present with

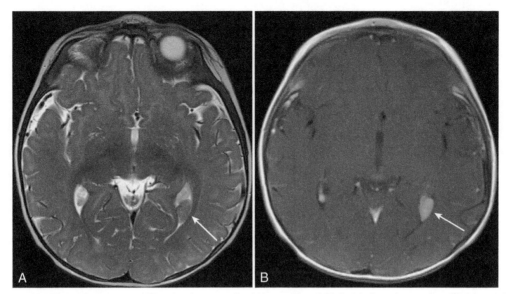

Figure 8.67 Choroid plexus papilloma. Nine-month-old boy with mild left-sided weakness. **A,** Axial T2-weighted and (**B**) axial T1-weighted postcontrast images show an enhancing mass (*arrows*) within the occipital horn of the left lateral ventricle. Surgical resection confirmed choroid plexus papilloma.

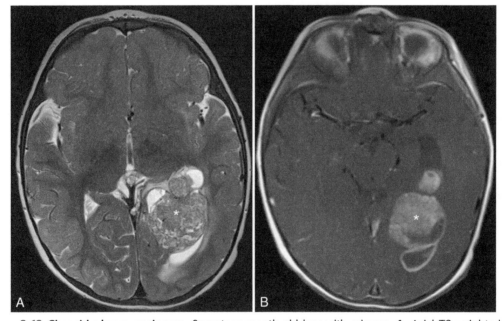

Figure 8.68 Choroid plexus carcinoma. Seventeen-month-old boy with seizures. **A,** Axial T2-weighted and (**B**) axial T1-weighted postcontrast images demonstrate a large mixed solid/cystic heterogeneously enhancing mass (*asterisks*) within the occipital horn of the left lateral ventricle with surrounding edema. Surgical resection confirmed choroid plexus carcinoma.

obstructive hydrocephalus caused by compression of the cerebral aqueduct. The most common tumors arising in the pineal region are germ cell tumors, of which 65% are pure germinomas. There is a 10:1 male preponderance in germinoma. Germinoma is hyperdense on CT, is isointense to gray matter on all MR sequences, and enhances avidly [**Fig. 8.69**]. Germinoma can grow anteriorly into the floor of the third ventricle. Synchronous lesions may be present along the pituitary infundibulum. Leptomeningeal dissemination is seen in up to 36% of patients with germinoma. Response to radiotherapy tends to be excellent.

Teratomas are the most common nongerminomatous germ cell tumor in the pineal region. They are heterogeneous on all imaging modalities that contain fat, cysts, and calcification [**Fig. 8.70**]. Pineal parenchymal tumors such as pineoblastoma

and pineocytoma are much less common in children than germ cell tumors but do occur occasionally in adolescents.

Pineal cysts are a common incidental finding on imaging studies of the brain; their incidence increases in the second and third decades. If the cysts are less than 1 cm and do not have any atypical features, then they do not warrant further imaging follow-up.

Sellar and Parasellar Tumors

Craniopharyngioma

Craniopharyngioma is a histologically benign, but locally aggressive low-grade tumor that arises from ectodermal remnants of Rathke pouch in the sellar and parasellar region.

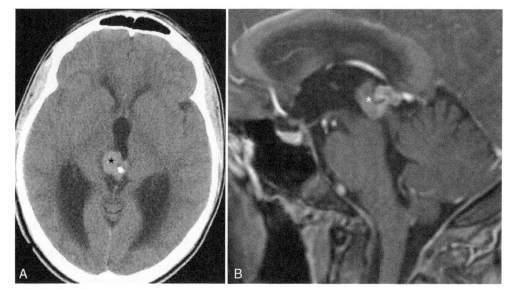

Figure 8.69 Pineal germinoma. Seventeen-year-old boy with 2 weeks of headache. **A,** Axial unenhanced computed tomography demonstrates acute hydrocephalus caused by a mass (*asterisk*) in the pineal region with focal calcification. **B,** Sagittal T1 postcontrast shows heterogenous enhancement of the mass which obstructs the cerebral aqueduct. The lesion was resected, and pathology confirmed germinoma.

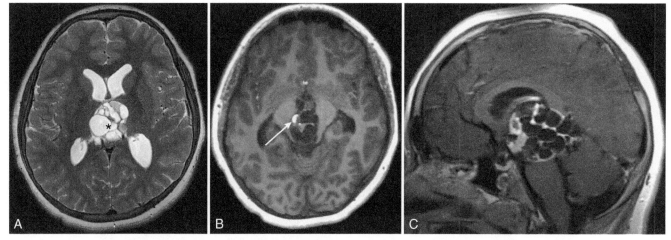

Figure 8.70 Pineal teratoma. Twelve-year-old boy with headaches and double vision. **A,** Axial T2-weighted image shows a multilocular predominantly cystic mass (*asterisk*) in the pineal region. **B,** Axial T1-weighted precontrast reveals punctate foci of intrinsic T1 shortening (*arrow*) indicating fat. **C,** Sagittal T1 postcontrast shows enhancing septations. Biopsy revealed teratoma.

Craniopharyngioma accounts for 3% to 10% of all pediatric CNS tumors. Craniopharyngioma has a bimodal incidence, peaking in the first and fifth decades of life. Clinically craniopharyngioma may be associated with short stature.

The imaging appearance of craniopharyngioma is characterized by a mixed cystic and solid appearance [**Fig. 8.71**]. Ninety percent of craniopharyngiomas exhibit calcification on CT. On T1-weighted MRI, focal areas of increased signal can indicate increased protein content within the cysts or intracystic hemorrhage. Surgical resection is the treatment of choice, although complete resection may not be achievable because of adherence of the tumor to vascular structures at the base of the tumor. The development of aneurysmal dilatation of involved vessels is a recognized late complication of surgery, presumably related to damage of the adventitia of the vessel at the time of operation. Radiotherapy plays a role in treatment as well. Recurrence-free 5-year survival is close to 87% but declines to less than 50% with subtotal resection.

Rathke Cleft Cyst

Rathke cleft cyst, like craniopharyngioma, results from remnants of Rathke pouch present embryologically. Rathke cleft cyst usually originates within the sella but may extend into the suprasellar cistern. Like craniopharyngioma, the cyst often has high signal on T1-weighted imaging, but the cyst tends to be smaller than the cysts of craniopharyngioma. Unlike craniopharyngioma, calcification and cyst wall enhancement are not present in Rathke cleft cyst.

Chiasmatic/Optic Pathway/Hypothalamic Gliomas

Optic pathway glioma (OPG) makes up 15% of supratentorial tumors. Patients most often present with impaired vision. Bilateral OPGs are considered pathognomonic for NF-1. Overall, 20% to 50% of all OPGs occur in patients with NF-1. The tumor may involve the optic nerves, chiasm, optic tracts, geniculate bodies, or optic radiations.

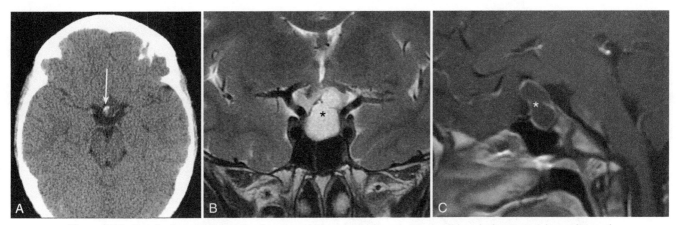

Figure 8.71 Craniopharyngioma. Twelve-year-old boy with altered vision and headache. **A,** Axial unenhanced computed tomography shows hypoattenuating mass with focal calcification (*arrow*) in the suprasellar region. **B,** Coronal T2-weighted and (**C**) sagittal postcontrast T1-weighted images demonstrate a predominantly cystic, rim-enhancing mass (*asterisks*) filling the sella and extending into the suprasellar cistern. The lesion was resected and confirmed to be craniopharyngioma.

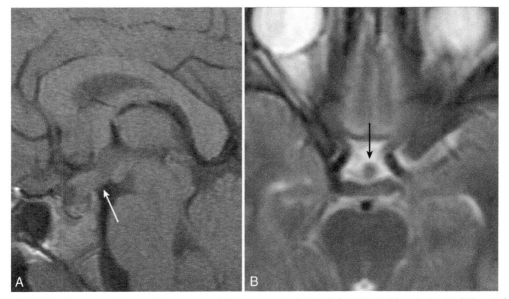

Figure 8.72 Pituitary germinoma. Seven-year-old boy presented with diabetes insipidus. **A,** Sagittal T1-weighted and (**B**) axial T2-weighted magnetic resonance images show thickening of the infundibulum (*arrows*) and absence of the posterior pituitary bright spot.

OPG is isointense to hypointense on T1-weighted sequences and of mixed signal intensity on T2-weighted imaging. Most, but not all, tumors enhance with contrast. Cysts may develop during treatment and may wax and wane over time. Cysts are usually not a cause for a change in therapy or intervention unless they produce significant symptoms because of mass effect.

The clinical course of OPG varies widely. Tumors can be extremely slow growing or aggressive. Metastases are uncommon with hypothalamic pilocytic astrocytomas but may occur in children younger than 2 years with hypothalamic pilocytic or pilomyxoid astrocytomas. Treatment is based on clinical symptoms. A combination of surgery and adjuvant therapy is frequently used.

Germinoma. Germinoma is an occasional cause of central diabetes insipidus due to infiltration of the pituitary infundibulum by tumor. As with pineal region germinoma, there is a strong male predominance. Most often in suprasellar germinoma, the infundibulum is thickened or shows an obvious mass

[**Fig. 8.72**]. The normal posterior pituitary bright spot is absent when the stalk is invaded by tumor. Occasionally the only indication of abnormality is absence of the posterior bright spot in a patient with central diabetes insipidus. These patients should be monitored with serial imaging studies as thickening of the stalk may occur slowly over time. Synchronous lesions in the pineal region or leptomeningeal spread of tumor should be carefully looked for. Germinoma tends to be very responsive to radiotherapy.

Hypothalamic Hamartoma

Although nonneoplastic, hypothalamic hamartoma produces a masslike lesion in the hypothalamus and may cause gelastic seizures (sudden onset of inappropriate laughter) or precocious puberty. The hamartomas tend to closely follow the signal intensity of gray matter on all MR sequences and should not enhance [**Fig. 8.73**]. Associated absence of the olfactory bulbs should suggest a diagnosis of Kallmann syndrome.

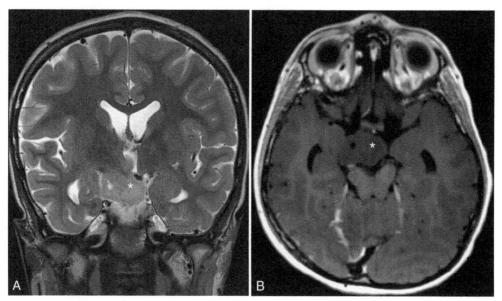

Figure 8.73 Hypothalamic hamartoma. Six-year-old boy with intractable seizures. **A,** Axial T2- and (**B**) axial T1-weighted postcontrast demonstrate nonenhancing mass (*asterisks*) involving the hypothalamus with extension inferiorly to fill the suprasellar cistern and prepontine cistern and third ventricle. The mass is close in signal to normal gray matter on all sequences.

Pituitary Adenoma

Pituitary adenoma is uncommon in children, although it occasionally occurs in adolescents. As with adenoma in adults, microadenomas may be hormonally active, the most common being lesions producing prolactin. On imaging, adenomas vary in size but are typically less enhancing than surrounding pituitary tissue. Intralesional hemorrhage rarely occurs but may produce symptoms of pituitary apoplexy.

Posterior Fossa Tumors

Medulloblastoma

Medulloblastoma is the most common posterior fossa tumor in childhood and accounts for 30% to 40% of all posterior fossa tumors and approximately 15% to 20% of all pediatric brain tumors. Medulloblastoma is the most common brain tumor in children between the ages of 6 and 11. Medulloblastoma is highly malignant consisting of very primitive, undifferentiated, small, round cells. All subtypes are classified as WHO grade IV tumors.

In children medulloblastoma tends to arise within the inferior vermis and grow into the fourth ventricle resulting in obstructive hydrocephalus [**Fig. 8.74**]. Medulloblastoma is classically *hyperdense* on CT. On MRI the appearance can vary, but the tumor is typically mildly hypointense relative to brain on T2-weighted imaging. The tumor may show homogenous enhancement, heterogeneous enhancement, or no enhancement after contrast. Calcifications are seen in approximately 20%, and cysts or necrotic areas occur in up to 50%. Medulloblastoma usually shows *restricted diffusion* relative to the brain parenchyma. MRS reveals an aggressive spectral pattern with an elevated choline peak and a markedly reduced NAA peak. MRS may also show an *elevated taurine peak.*

CSF dissemination occurs in 25% to 30% at the time of diagnosis in medulloblastoma. Postcontrast MRI of the brain and spine is the most sensitive imaging for metastases. The treatment of medulloblastoma consists of surgery, radiotherapy, and chemotherapy. Poor prognostic indicators are a lack of complete surgical resection, expression of the c-erbB-2 (*HER2/neu*) oncogene, and the presence of CSF metastases at the time of diagnosis. Patients with nonmetastatic, *HER2*-negative tumors that are

completely resected have 5-year survival rates approaching 100%. Those with incompletely resected tumors with *HER2* expression and metastases at diagnosis have a 5-year survival rate of 24%.

Cerebellar Astrocytoma

Cerebellar astrocytoma is the second most common tumor of the posterior fossa after medulloblastoma. Forty percent of all astrocytomas arise in the cerebellum, and 70% are juvenile pilocytic astrocytomas (JPAs). JPAs can occur in the vermis or cerebellar hemisphere. Lateral tumors tend to be more common in younger children. JPAs may be cystic, solid, or solid with a necrotic center. Cystic lesions frequently have a solid "mural" nodule arising in the cyst wall. Surrounding edema is highly variable. Cerebellar astrocytomas have varying appearances on CT and MRI. In the cystic type, the mural nodule tends to show intense enhancement postcontrast [**Fig. 8.75**]. JPAs tend to have increased diffusivity [**Fig. 8.76**]. Patients with cystic JPAs have an excellent prognosis. Tumors that are solid or in which gross total excision is not achieved carry a more guarded prognosis.

Atypical Teratoid Rhabdoid Tumor

Atypical teratoid rhabdoid tumor (ATRT) is a highly malignant tumor that tends to occur in the first 3 years of life and accounts for 2% of all pediatric tumors. The majority of tumors arise at the cerebellopontine angle but may also develop in the spine, pineal, and suprasellar regions. Their imaging appearance in the posterior fossa is similar to that of medulloblastoma, but the possibility of an ATRT must be strongly considered when an aggressive tumor is seen in younger children or when there is significant intratumoral hemorrhage [**Fig. 8.77**]. ATRT historically has had a very poor prognosis with survival rates between 2 weeks and 11 months, although there has been some improvement in survival rates in recent years.

Ependymoma

Infratentorial ependymoma comprises 8% to 13% of all posterior fossa tumors in children. Ependymoma has a bimodal incidence

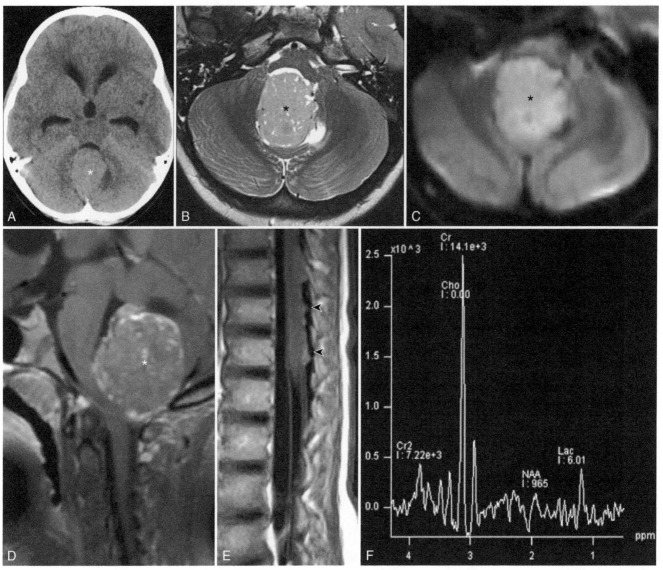

Figure 8.74 **Medulloblastoma.** Eight-year-old boy with 6-week history of headache and vomiting. **A,** Computed tomography demonstrates hyperdense posterior fossa mass (*asterisk*) centered in the fourth ventricle. **B,** Axial T2-weighted, (**C**) diffusion-weighted, and (**D**) postcontrast T1-weighted images show a heterogeneous mass (*asterisks*) which is hypointense to gray matter on T2 and has decreased diffusion and heterogenous enhancement. **E,** Postcontrast T1-weighted image of the spine shows leptomeningeal spread of disease (*arrowheads*). **F,** Proton magnetic resonance spectroscopy demonstrates a high-grade tumor spectrum with very elevated choline, low *N*-acetyl aspartate, and lactate.

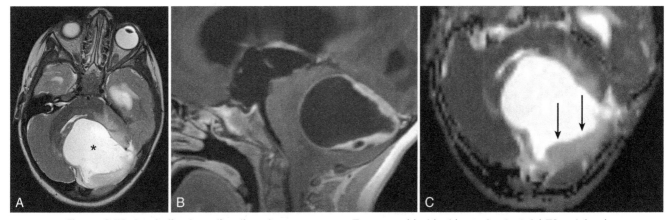

Figure 8.75 **Cerebellar juvenile pilocytic astrocytoma.** Two-year-old girl with ataxia. **A,** Axial T2-weighted image shows a large predominantly cystic mass (*asterisk*). **B,** Sagittal T1-weighted image shows intense enhancement within the peripheral solid portion of the mass. **C,** Axial apparent diffusion coefficient (ADC) map from diffusion-weighted imaging reveals high diffusivity within the cyst and slightly elevated ADC within the solid tissue rim (*arrows*).

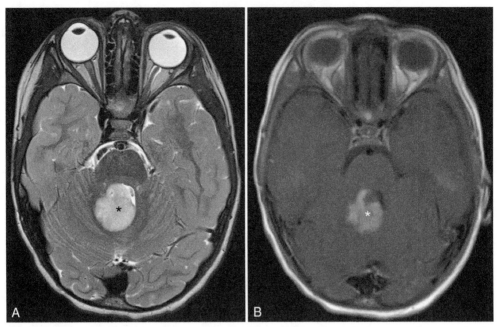

Figure 8.76 Cerebellar astrocytoma. Two-year-old boy with leftward head tilt. **A,** Axial T2-weighted image shows a solid, mildly hyperintense mass (*asterisk*) with enhancement on (**B**) postcontrast T1-weighted imaging.

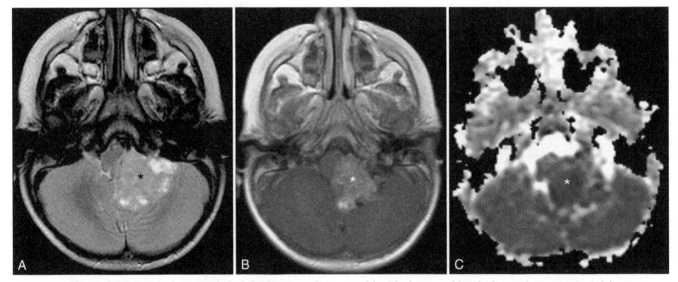

Figure 8.77 Atypical teratoid rhabdoid tumor. One-year-old with decreased level of consciousness. **A,** Axial T2 and (**B**) axial T1 postcontrast show enhancing tumor (*asterisk*) centered in the left cerebellopontine angle. **C,** Apparent diffusion coefficient map reveals low diffusivity within the mass because of the dense cellularity of the lesion.

with peaks between the ages of 1 and 5 years and in the fourth decade of life. Posterior fossa ependymomas arise from the ependymal lining in the medullary portion of the fourth ventricle. They characteristically do not directly invade the medulla but grow out of the foramina of Luschka and Magendie into the cerebellopontine angles and cisternal spaces surrounding the brainstem and cervicomedullary junction.

Ependymomas tend to be isointense to gray matter on CT. Up to 50% contain foci of calcification. On MRI they tend to be hypointense on T1- and isointense on T2-weighted sequences with heterogeneous enhancement [**Fig. 8.78**]. Heterogeneity within the tumor, in addition to the pattern of growth through the fourth ventricular outlet foramina, is particularly suggestive

of ependymoma. Prognosis is related to the extent of surgical resection; complete surgical resection is associated with a 3-year survival rate of more than 80%.

Brainstem Glioma

Brainstem gliomas account for 15% of all pediatric CNS tumors and 30% of infratentorial tumors. Brainstem gliomas are subdivided based on anatomic location into tectal, pontine, and cervicomedullary lesions, each having a predilection for a tumor of different predominant histology and biological behavior.

Tectal tumors are generally very benign, slowly growing tumors and are associated with a favorable prognosis. Tectal

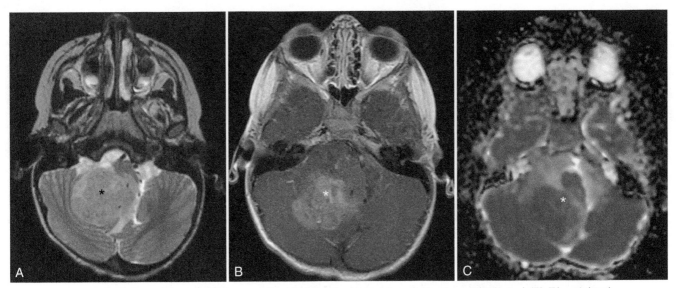

Figure 8.78 Ependymoma. Thirty-month-old girl with progressive ataxia. **A,** Axial T2- and (**B**) T1-weighted images demonstrate an inferior fourth ventricular mass (*asterisks*) with heterogeneous enhancement extending through the right foramen of Luschka. **C,** Diffusion is not significantly decreased relative to normal brain parenchyma.

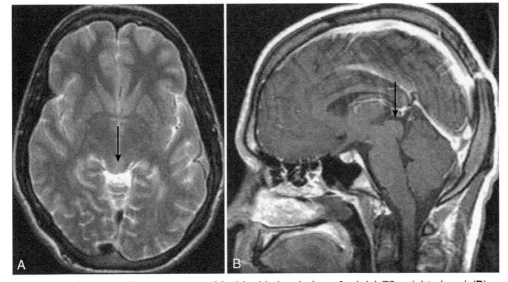

Figure 8.79 Tectal glioma. Seventeen-year-old girl with headaches. **A,** Axial T2-weighted and (**B**) sagittal postcontrast T1-weighted images show a nonenhancing mass expanding the tectum (*arrow*).

gliomas cause hydrocephalus secondary to aqueductal obstruction. The hydrocephalus is usually treated with ventricular shunting or a third ventriculostomy. Tectal gliomas tend not to increase in size and rarely require any additional surgery, chemotherapy, or radiotherapy [**Fig. 8.79**].

The pons is the most common location of tumors arising in the brainstem. The classic clinical presentation of a pontine glioma is a child with new cranial nerve palsies (especially cranial nerve VI) and pyramidal tract and cerebellar signs. Pontine gliomas are most often diffusely infiltrative, aggressive tumors and are associated with a poor prognosis. Pontine glioma expands the pons, filling the prepontine cistern. Extension into the middle cerebellar peduncle is frequent, as is rostral and caudal extension within the brainstem. Pontine glioma is hypoattenuating on CT, hypointense on T1, and hyperintense on T2 and FLAIR sequences [**Fig. 8.80**]. Enhancement and necrosis are most often present during treatment and are not typically evident at presentation. The diagnosis of pontine glioma portends an extremely poor prognosis with a 2-year survival rate of only 7%. Focal pontine glioma has a better prognosis but is much less common than the diffusely infiltrating tumor.

Cervicomedullary glioma is most often a pilocytic astrocytoma. The tumor tends to arise at the cervicomedullary junction and grow caudally into the spinal cord and rostrally to the pontomedullary junction [**Fig. 8.81**]. Crossing fibers at the pontomedullary junction restrict further rostral growth, and the tumor then grows dorsally into the fourth ventricle producing an "ice cream cone" appearance on MRI. As with pilocytic astrocytoma elsewhere, the cervicomedullary astrocytoma is characterized by a high water content and absent blood–brain barrier, producing marked hyperintensity on T2-weighted MR sequences and avid contrast enhancement.

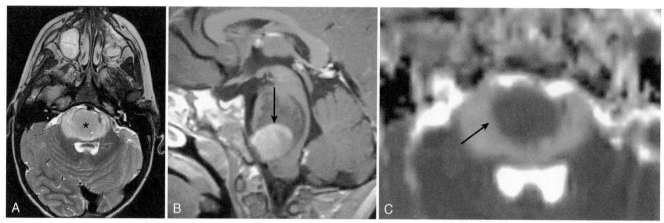

Figure 8.80 Pontine glioma. Two-year-old boy with left-sided weakness. **A,** Axial T2-weighted imaging shows an expansile mass (*asterisk*) centered within the pons. **B,** Sagittal postcontrast T1-weighted image shows enhancement (*arrow*) within the inferior portion of the mass. Note that enhancement at presentation occurs in only a minority of pontine gliomas and is more commonly seen after treatment. **C,** The nodular component situated inferiorly shows restricted diffusion (*arrow*) on apparent diffusion coefficient map.

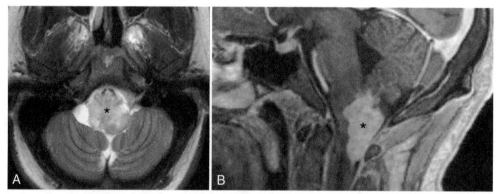

Figure 8.81 Cervicomedullary glioma. Nineteen-year-old male who underwent magnetic resonance imaging of brain to evaluate a concussion and was incidentally found to have a mass at the cervicomedullary junction. **A,** Axial T2-weighted and (**B**) sagittal postcontrast T1-weighted imaging show an enhancing mass at the posterior aspect of the cervicomedullary junction (*asterisk*). The lesion was pathologically confirmed to be a low-grade glioma.

VASCULAR DISEASE

Stroke

Stroke is defined as a neurological deficit lasting longer than 24 hours. It can result from ischemia or hemorrhage. Stroke is among the top 10 causes of death in childhood. The predisposing factors for stroke in children differ considerably from the causes of stroke in adults [**Table 8.6**].

Fetal and Neonatal Stroke

In utero or perinatal stroke may be detected on fetal imaging or later in childhood when a focal neurological deficit or developmental delay becomes evident. There are maternal, placental, and fetal risk factors for stroke, but none is identified in 50% of patients. Intraparenchymal hemorrhage, cavitation, and ventriculomegaly are the most common findings on antenatal imaging. Antenatally discovered strokes are most frequently due to periventricular hemorrhagic venous infarction, although focal arterial ischemic strokes and global ischemic brain injury may also occur.

Focal neonatal stroke should be differentiated from diffuse hypoxic-ischemic injury. Neonatal arterial ischemic stroke leads to focal ischemic necrosis in an arterial distribution, most commonly in the territory of the MCA and most often on the left side. These infarctions are most likely embolic in origin. Neonatal arterial ischemic stroke is associated with congenital heart disease, coagulopathies, dehydration, and sepsis. Clinical presentation is often nonspecific and includes seizures. Cranial ultrasound can be negative in the acute setting. Decreased diffusion in an arterial territory on diffusion-weighted MRI is the earliest imaging finding for ischemic infarction.

Risk factors for venous stroke in the newborn include dehydration, sepsis, asphyxia, maternal diabetes, and thrombophilia. Presentation is nonspecific and may consist of lethargy, seizures, or evidence for raised ICP. CT may show hyperdense clot in the involved vein or dural venous sinus or acute parenchymal hemorrhage. MRI is the best modality for confirming the diagnosis and extent of the injury.

Childhood Stroke

The incidence of stroke in children beyond the first month of life is estimated at 2.4 per 100,000 patients. Pathologies that can result in arterial ischemic stroke include thromboembolic disease (from intracranial or extracranial vessels, congenital heart disease, or cardiac procedures), arteriopathy (including moyamoya disease, sickle cell disease (SCD), and vasculitis), and hypercoagulable states (such as protein C or S deficiency). An underlying cause is found in less than half of cases. Dehydration, otitis media, and sinusitis are the major risk factors for venous stroke in childhood.

CT is often the first imaging study performed in childhood stroke, although its sensitivity is limited in the acute setting. A hyperdense artery corresponding with acute intravascular thrombus may occasionally be demonstrated [**Fig. 8.82**]. Over the next few hours and days, there is progressive loss of gray-white matter differentiation, sulcal effacement, and hypoattenuation seen in the involved territory. Encephalomalacia and volume loss take months to become apparent on CT.

TABLE 8.6 Causes of Pediatric Stroke

Cardiac	• Congenital heart disease • Valvular heart disease • Cardiac neoplasm • Myocarditis • Cardiac surgery
Cerebral vasculopathy	• Central nervous system infection • Congenital vascular anomalies • Collagen vascular diseases • Primary angiitis • Trauma • Arterial dissection
Coagulopathies	• Protein C or S deficiency • Antithrombin III deficiency • Anticardiolipin antibodies • Lupus anticoagulant • Polycythemia and hyperviscosity syndromes
Moyamoya vasculopathy	• Idiopathic • Secondary/associated (sickle cell disease, neurofibromatosis type 1, suprasellar radiation)
Metabolic diseases	• Fabry disease • Hyperhomocysteinemia • Ehlers-Danlos type IV
Venous/Sinus thrombosis	• Infection • Dehydration • Hypercoagulable states • Chemotherapy • Iatrogenic

Hemorrhagic conversion of arterial ischemic strokes in children is rare.

In venous stroke, as in the neonate, CT may show hyperdense clot within the involved vein or dural venous sinus. Parenchymal hemorrhage is more common with veno-occlusive infarctions than in arterial causes of infarction in children [**Fig. 8.83**].

MRI has significantly better sensitivity and specificity than CT for acute arterial stroke in the hours after onset. DWI is the most sensitive sequence in the hyperacute phase with restricted diffusion evident within minutes of onset. Within 6 to 12 hours, the infarct will develop T2 hyperintensity. On T1-weighted imaging, a ribbon of high signal can be seen within days to weeks and represents cortical laminar necrosis. Hemorrhagic transformation is well seen on GRE or SWI but is much less common in children than in adults. MRA and MRV can be used to image the arterial and venous systems, respectively. CTA and CTV may be required for clarification or better delineation of findings on MRA and MRV in some patients.

Moyamoya Vasculopathy

Moyamoya vasculopathy refers to an angiographic abnormality characterized by steno-occlusive changes in the internal carotid artery terminus accompanied by the development of stereotypical basal and leptomeningeal collaterals. The prominent basal collaterals are responsible for the name *moyamoya,* which is a Japanese term loosely translated into English as "something hazy hanging in the air like a puff of smoke" [**Fig. 8.84**]. It should be remembered that moyamoya is a descriptive term and does not imply a specific cause. The moyamoya pattern may be produced by idiopathic disease (more common in patients of Asian ancestry) or may be associated with other conditions such as NF-1, Posterior fossa brain malformations, hemangiomas, arterial anomalies, cardiac anomalies and coarctation of the aorta, eye and endocrine abnormalities, and sternal cleft (PHACES) syndrome, Down syndrome, or SCD and after suprasellar radiation. Infarctions may be either within the white matter of the vascular border zones or cortically based.

Sickle Cell Disease

SCD increases the risk for childhood stroke 200 to 400 times. The rigid, sickle-shaped erythrocytes can lead to vascular occlusion,

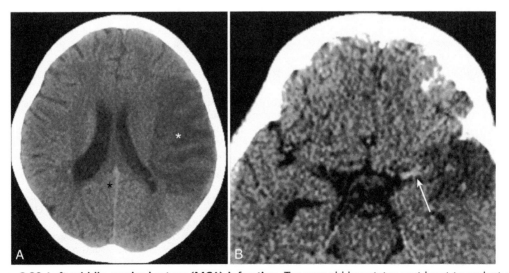

Figure 8.82 Left middle cerebral artery (MCA) infarction. Ten-year-old boy status post heart transplant and extracorporeal membrane oxygenation with new right-sided weakness. **A** and **B,** Axial unenhanced computed tomography images show swelling and loss of gray-white matter differentiation in the left MCA territory in keeping with a subacute infarction (*asterisk*) with hyperdense thrombus in the left MCA (*arrow*).

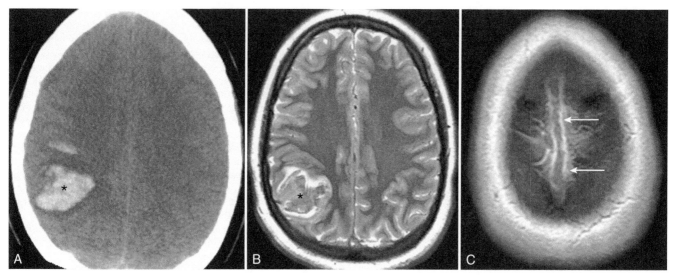

Figure 8.83 Venous infarction. Seventeen-year-old with headaches. **A,** Axial unenhanced computed tomography reveals a right peri-Rolandic hemorrhage (*asterisk*). **B,** Axial T2-weighted image shows hemorrhage (*asterisk*) with surrounding edema. **C,** Postcontrast T1-weighted image demonstrates a lack of enhancement within the superior sagittal sinus (*arrows*) indicating thrombosis of the sinus and cortical veins as a cause of the parenchymal hemorrhagic venous infarction.

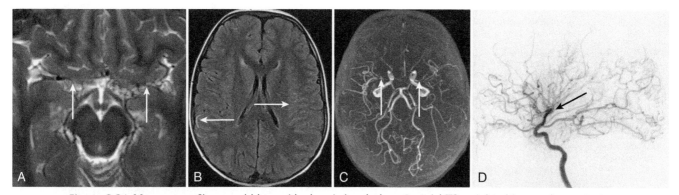

Figure 8.84 Moyamoya. Six-year-old boy with chronic headaches. **A,** Axial T2-weighted image demonstrates absence of the normal signal voids in the middle cerebral arteries (*arrows*) with small surrounding collaterals. **B,** Axial fluid attenuation inversion recovery shows high signal in the sulci (*arrows*) caused by slow flow in leptomeningeal vessels ("ivy sign"). **C,** Three-dimensional time-of-flight magnetic resonance angiography shows decreased flow enhancement in the middle cerebral arteries (*arrows*) and anterior cerebral arteries. **D,** Lateral view of left internal carotid angiogram shows severe stenosis of the Internal carotid artery (ICA) terminus (*arrow*), faint basal, moyamoya collaterals, delayed filling of the middle cerebral artery branches, and absence of filling of the anterior cerebral artery.

or the abnormal erythrocytes may adhere to the intracranial arterial walls, damaging the intima and resulting in progressive, multifocal arterial fibrosis and stenosis. This arteriopathy has a predilection for the terminal portions of the internal carotid arteries and is one of the leading causes of moyamoya vasculopathy.

Children with SCD should be screened every 6 months with transcranial Doppler ultrasound. Abnormally elevated peak systolic velocity (>200 cm/s) in the terminal ICA and proximal MCA is an indication for initiation of recurring blood transfusions which may reduce the risk of stroke by up to 92%.

On imaging, acute infarction in patients with SCD is often superimposed on a background of chronic multifocal atrophic changes. MRA demonstrates the steno-occlusive arterial disease and the presence of multiple tiny collaterals from the lenticulostriate and thalamoperforators. It is important to remember that the sickle cells and anemia in SCD both result in an increase in turbulence in blood flow at vessel bifurcations and that this

turbulence may result in artifactual loss of signal on MRA simulating steno-occlusive change. The presence of artifactual signal loss is more problematic with longer echo times used in some MRA protocols.

Hypoxic-Ischemic Encephalopathy

Generalized asphyxia in a term neonate results in neonatal **hypoxic-ischemic encephalopathy (HIE)**. The pattern of the injury is variable and depends on the severity and duration of the inciting ischemia and secondary reperfusion injury. The central highly metabolic structures, including those which are actively myelinating, are the most vulnerable to an abrupt interruption in blood supply. In particular the ventral lateral thalami, dorsolateral lentiform nuclei, posterior midbrain, vermis, hippocampi, lateral geniculate nuclei, perirolandic cerebral cortex, and optic radiations are especially susceptible. In cases with a more prolonged, but less profound ischemia, compensatory shunting offers the metabolically active areas relative protection at the expense of the cerebral cortex and white matter resulting in vascular watershed zone injuries.

Ultrasound and CT are both insensitive in detecting early ischemic changes. MRI provides more sensitive and specific imaging in infants with suspected hypoxic-ischemic brain injury. Imaging in the first 72 hours may underestimate the extent of the injury because HIE is often associated with evolving injury over the first few days. HIE involving the deep gray matter nuclei [**Fig. 8.85**] or cerebral cortex [**Fig. 8.86**] demonstrates characteristic abnormal hyperintensity on T2-weighted imaging associated with decreased diffusion. The injury is usually symmetric, which may make detection difficult for those unfamiliar with the normal pattern of myelination in the neonate. MRS typically demonstrates an elevated lactate and diminished NAA in HIE. Recently infants with suspected HIE have begun to be treated with hypothermia. The use of hypothermia may result in the MRI being normal or the changes typical of HIE being delayed in their appearance on imaging.

White Matter Injury of Prematurity/ Periventricular Leukomalacia

White matter injury of prematurity is the result of complex hemodynamic interactions and other inciting or potentiating factors, such as amnionitis, affecting infants born before about 35 weeks' gestational age. The term *periventricular leukomalacia* has fallen out of favor because periventricular leukomalacia is more specifically associated with hypoperfusion in immature vascular territories. The forces producing periventricular white matter injury are now known to be more complex and the term *white matter injury of prematurity* is consequently preferred. Ultrasound imaging of vulnerable infants may show increased echoes in the periventricular white matter in the acute setting. MRI is often normal or only subtly abnormal in the acute setting because of the relatively long T2 of unmyelinated white matter in the periventricular region normally present in premature infants. DTI may show a decrease in white matter connectivity. There are occasional reports of decreased diffusion in the white matter early in the injury. Chronically, white matter injury of

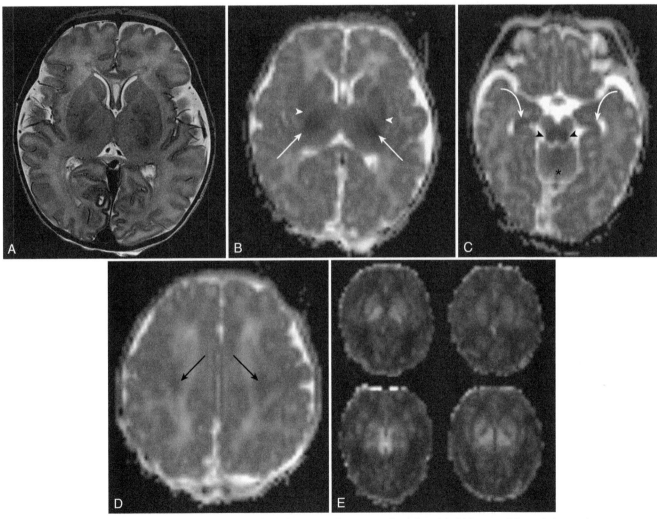

Figure 8.85 Hypoxic-ischemic encephalopathy, central pattern. One-day-old girl born at 37 weeks' gestation via emergency cesarean section with APGAR scores of 0 at 0 and 10 minutes. **A,** Axial T2 shows very subtle abnormal high signal in the ventral lateral thalami. (**B–D**) ADC maps show conspicuous diffusion restriction in the ventral lateral thalami (*white arrows*), posterior putamina (*white arrowheads*), corona radiata (*black arrows*), dorsal brainstem (*black arrowheads*), cerebellar vermis (*asterisk*), and hippocampi (*curved white arrows*) in keeping with an extensive central pattern of injury secondary to hypoxia/ischemia. These areas show corresponding hyperperfusion on arterial spin labeling perfusion study (**E**) caused by hyperemic reperfusion.

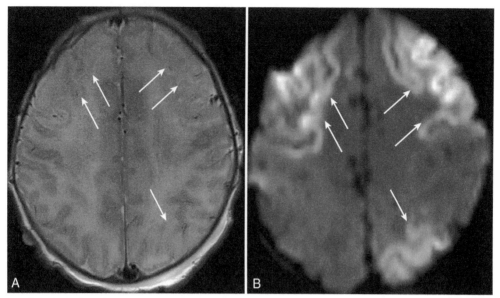

Figure 8.86 Hypoxic-ischemic encephalopathy, cortical pattern. Term infant with perinatal depression. **A,** Axial T2 and (**B**) axial diffusion-weighted images show cortical infarctions (*arrows*) in the frontal lobes bilaterally and in the left parietal lobe. The distribution of the infarctions is largely in the vascular border zone territories.

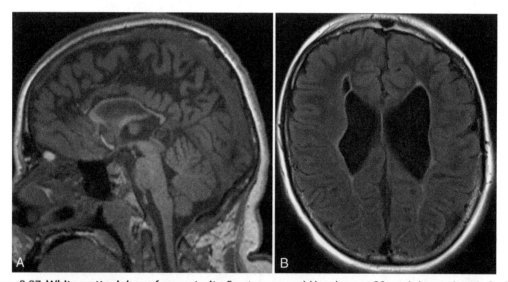

Figure 8.87 White matter injury of prematurity. Fourteen-year-old boy born at 33 weeks' gestation. **A,** Sagittal T1-weighted image shows marked thinning of the corpus callosum. **B,** Axial fluid attenuation inversion recovery demonstrates bilateral white matter volume loss, periventricular white matter signal abnormality, and ex vacuo prominence of lateral ventricles which have irregular margins.

prematurity has a typical appearance with reduced periventricular white matter volume, especially in the periatrial regions, irregular margins of the lateral ventricles, periventricular white matter signal abnormalities, and thinning of the corpus callosum [**Fig. 8.87**]. Periventricular cysts, which used to be relatively common, are much less frequently present now due to advances in perinatal care in the preterm infant.

Germinal Matrix Hemorrhage

The germinal matrix is formed early during embryogenesis and is a transient area of glial and neuronal differentiation and proliferation. From here cells migrate peripherally to form the developing brain. It is densely cellular and highly vascular. The blood

vessels of the germinal matrix are thin walled and predisposed to hemorrhage.

During the end of the second trimester, the germinal matrix starts to involute. At 32 weeks it is only present at the caudothalamic groove. By 36 weeks' gestation the germinal matrix has essentially disappeared and hemorrhage is very unlikely to occur beyond this age.

Germinal matrix hemorrhage is also referred to as hemorrhagic brain injury of prematurity. It is identified in 67% of infants born prematurely at 28 to 32 weeks. Germinal matrix hemorrhage is classified into four grades, depending on the extent of hemorrhage seen at time of diagnosis [**Fig. 8.88** and **Table 8.7**].

Grades 1 and 2 have low morbidity and mortality, whereas grades 3 and 4 have higher mortality rates and substantial risk

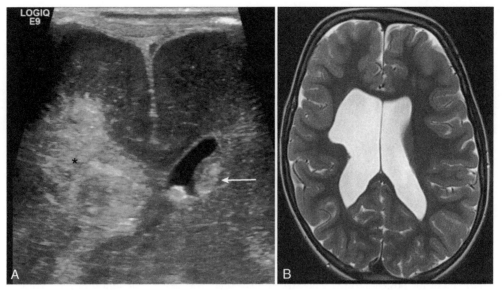

Figure 8.88 Germinal matrix hemorrhage. Two-day-old male infant, born at 26 weeks' gestation. **A,** Coronal ultrasound shows hydrocephalus secondary to bilateral germinal matrix hemorrhage; grade 4 on the right with periventricular hemorrhagic venous infarction (*asterisk*) and grade 1 on the left (increased echogenicity confined to the caudothalamic groove) (*arrow*). **B,** T2-weighted magnetic resonance demonstrates chronic ex vacuo dilatation of the lateral ventricle caused by prior periventricular hemorrhagic venous infarction.

TABLE 8.7 Classification of Germinal Matrix Hemorrhage

Grade	Definition
1	Hemorrhage confined to the germinal matrix
2	Intraventricular hemorrhage without ventriculomegaly
3	Intraventricular hemorrhage with ventriculomegaly
4	Parenchymal hemorrhage (related to venous infarction)

for poor neurodevelopment outcomes among survivors. If hydrocephalus is present, CSF diversion may be necessary. In grade IV hemorrhage the venous infarction results in atrophy and porencephalic cysts in the posterior frontal/anterior parietal region.

Vascular Anomalies

Vascular anomalies are congenital disorders of vascular development that may come to clinical attention only months to years after birth. Intracranial vascular anomalies are subdivided based on their vascular composition and hemodynamics.

High-Flow Vascular Anomalies

High-flow vascular anomalies occur when an abnormal communication between an artery and vein bypasses the normal capillary network. In *arteriovenous fistula (AVF)* the supplying artery communicates directly with a draining vein via a macroscopic connection. In *arteriovenous malformation (AVM)* the supplying artery communicates with the draining vein via a nidus of abnormal vessels. AVF and AVM are further classified into dural, subarachnoid (vein of Galen), pial, and parenchymal lesions based on their anatomic location.

The clinical presentation of high-flow lesions is variable and includes high-output cardiac failure, venous hypertension, and/ or steal phenomenon producing cerebral ischemia, seizures, and hydrocephalus.

Dural high-flow anomalies often present in the prenatal or neonatal period as a cause of congestive heart failure. Arterial supply to these lesions is from meningeal arteries with drainage into the dural venous sinuses [**Fig. 8.89**].

Vein of Galen malformations (VOGMs) consist of an abnormal arteriovenous communication from a primitive choroidal arterial arcade to an aneurysmally dilated *median vein of the prosencephalon* (the embryological precursor to a normal vein of Galen). VOGMs with numerous high-flow shunts may result in congestive cardiac failure in the fetus or neonate. VOGMs with lower flow or fewer shunts often become symptomatic only later in infancy when hydrocephalus or cerebral ischemia develops because of chronic venous hypertension [**Fig. 8.90**].

Pial AVF/AVM consists of an abnormal communication between a branch of the anterior, middle, or posterior cerebral artery and a cortical vein along the surface of the brain. Because the cortical vein is unsupported, it becomes dilated. As a result hemorrhage from the varix is common.

Parenchymal high-flow AVM is similar to its counterpart in adults. The lesion is composed of abnormal connections between arteries and veins coursing through the brain substance. Symptoms are most often related to the anatomic location of the anomaly, and high-output cardiac failure is rare. Venous flow may be into either the superficial or the deep venous system.

Imaging of high-flow lesions is directed toward delineating and characterizing the abnormality and demonstrating any complications. Ultrasound or MRI of dural AVF and AVM demonstrates an off-midline vascular mass with enlarged meningeal arteries. VOGMs are depicted as midline vascular masses with increased flow on Doppler ultrasound evaluation. Pial AVF/AVMs commonly cause hemorrhage and show a massively dilated superficial vein on imaging. Parenchymal AVMs are recognized as a tangle of abnormal vessels within the brain substance. Treatment of high-flow lesions depends on the type and location of the lesion. Certain anomalies are amenable to endovascular treatment, whereas others require surgery, radiation therapy, or multimodal treatment [**Fig. 8.91**].

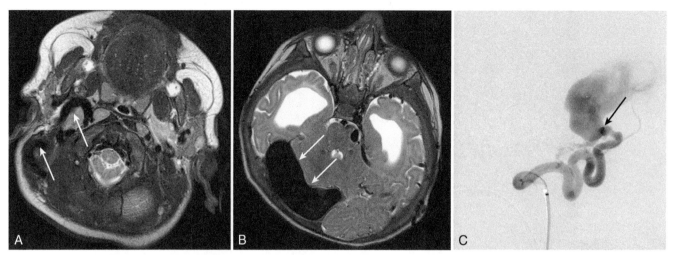

Figure 8.89 Dural arteriovenous fistula. Five-month-old infant with increasing head circumference and bruit. **A,** Axial T2-weighted image below the skull base shows an enlarged occipital artery (*arrows*). **B,** Axial T2-weighted image throughout the posterior fossa demonstrates marked enlargement of the right transverse sinus (*arrows*). **C,** Lateral view of a selective right occipital artery angiogram shows a fistula (*arrow*) between the occipital artery and the junction of the transverse and sigmoid sinus.

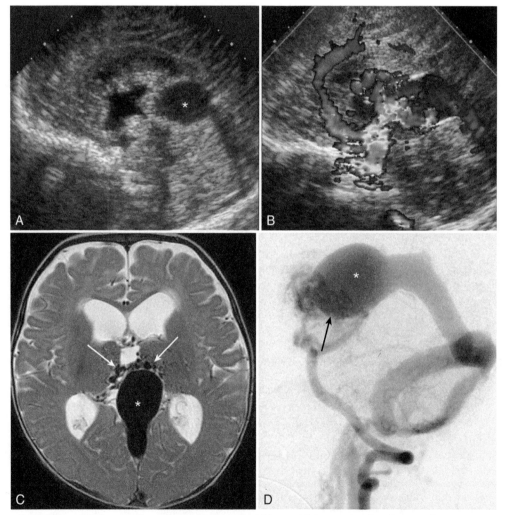

Figure 8.90 Vein of Galen malformation. Six-month-old boy with increasing head circumference. **A,** Sagittal grayscale ultrasound shows an anechoic mass posterior to the tectum (*asterisk*). **B,** Sagittal color Doppler image confirms that the mass is highly vascular. **C,** Axial T2-weighted magnetic resonance image shows a signal void in the median prosencephalic vein (*asterisk*) and signal voids of the arteriovenous malformation (*arrows*) along the anterior surface of the varix. **D,** Lateral view of a left vertebral artery angiogram confirms a vascular nidus (*arrow*) adjacent to the varix of the median prosencephalic vein (*asterisk*).

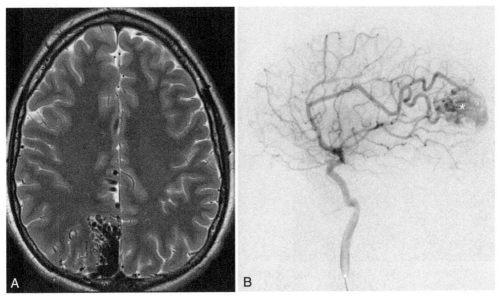

Figure 8.91 Parenchymal arteriovenous malformation (AVM). Sixteen-year-old boy with 1-year history of headache presented for magnetic resonance imaging (MRI) after first seizure. **A,** Axial T2-weighted MRI demonstrates tangle of abnormal low voids consistent with right parietal parasagittal AVM. **B,** Catheter angiogram demonstrates dominant feeders from the right pericallosal artery and right parieto-occipital branches of the right posterior cerebral artery (PCA).

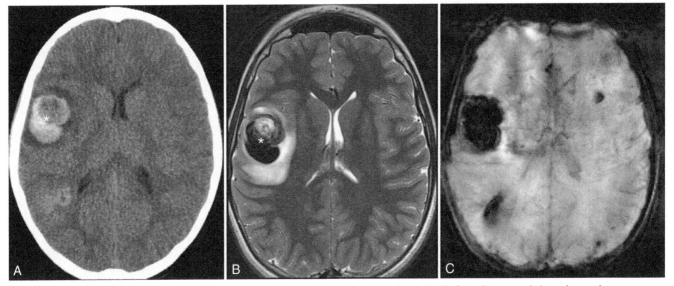

Figure 8.92 Cavernomas. Thirteen-year-old boy with acute headache, left-sided weakness, and slurred speech. **A,** Axial unenhanced computed tomography shows hemorrhage (*asterisk*) in right frontal lobe with rim of low attenuation and local mass effect. **B,** Axial T2 magnetic resonance image reveals a corresponding focus of low signal (*asterisk*) surrounded by vasogenic edema. **C,** Susceptibility-weighted image demonstrates multiple foci of susceptibility artifact bilaterally consistent with multiple cavernous malformations.

Low-Flow Vascular Anomalies

Low-flow vascular anomalies consist of malformed, endothelial-lined, blood-filled vascular structures and include capillary telangiectasias, cavernomas, and developmental venous anomalies (DVAs).

Capillary telangiectasias consist of dilated capillaries. Telangiectasias are most commonly found in the pontine tegmentum and are usually clinically silent, discovered incidentally as subtle foci of T2 hyperintensity without mass effect but with subtle enhancement postcontrast.

Cavernomas are localized endothelial-lined spaces with collections of venous blood. They may be single or multiple.

Occasionally cavernomas are familial. Cavernomas can be asymptomatic or produce symptoms because of hemorrhage or mass effect. On imaging they are characterized as areas of signal void and susceptibility artifact on GRE or SWI. A rim of low signal can be seen on T1- and T2-weighted sequences because of hemosiderin deposition [**Fig. 8.92**].

DVAs are abnormal veins that drain normal brain parenchyma. They are usually asymptomatic but can produce hemorrhage, particularly if associated with a cavernoma. On contrast-enhanced CT or MRI, DVAs produce a cluster of enhancing medullary veins radially arranged around a dilated colleting vein (known as the "caput medusa" sign) [**Fig. 8.93**].

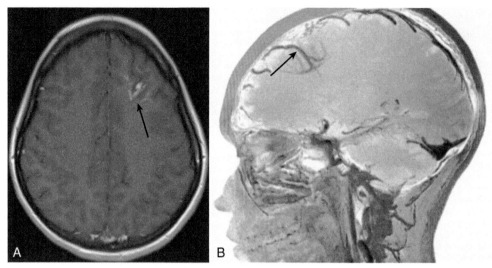

Figure 8.93 **Developmental venous anomaly.** Thirteen-year-old girl with headache. **A,** Axial postcontrast T1-weighted magnetic resonance imaging demonstrates a cluster of enhancing medullary veins (*arrow*) surrounding a more dilated collecting vein in the left frontal lobe shown in (**B**) sagittal reconstruction (*arrow*) consistent with a developmental venous anomaly.

Aneurysms

Intracranial aneurysms are less common in children than in adults. Pediatric aneurysms are more likely to be *fusiform,* involve the *posterior* circulation, and be *larger* at time of presentation compared with aneurysms in adults. In children symptoms from mass effect due to the aneurysm are as common as subarachnoid hemorrhage (SAH) from aneurysm rupture. Twenty-five percent of pediatric aneurysms are associated with underlying conditions such as collagen vascular disease, polycystic kidney disease, SCD, moyamoya syndrome, or intracranial infection. The typical "berry" aneurysms seen in adults are distinctly unusual in children.

CT is often the first study performed in suspected aneurysm. Subarachnoid, intraventricular, or parenchymal hemorrhage may be seen on an unenhanced scan. A giant aneurysm may be seen as a hyperattenuating mass in close proximity to a vessel. CTA with multiplanar and 3D reformatting may be used to delineate the relationship of an aneurysm to the native vessel, measure the neck of the aneurysm, and assess for thrombus and collateral vessels, all of which are important in treatment planning. MRA has less spatial resolution and can be limited by flow artifacts but is favored for follow-up and screening because of absence of ionizing radiation. Catheter angiography remains the gold standard for diagnostic planning and in many cases allows for endovascular treatment of the aneurysm.

TRAUMA AND NONACCIDENTAL INJURIES

Head trauma and resulting TBI is the most common cause of morbidity and mortality in children. There are approximately 475,000 cases of TBI in infants, children, and adolescents in the United States each year. Half of these cases occur in children younger than 5 years. Head trauma alone or in combination with other injuries is responsible for half of all deaths in children 1 to 14 years old.

Overall, motor vehicle accidents are the most common cause of TBI in children. In children younger than 2 years, accidental falls, the infant being dropped, and abusive trauma, also known as inflicted trauma/child abuse/nonaccidental trauma, are common causes.

In general, the initial evaluation of significant head trauma in pediatric patients is performed with CT. CT is widely available and can be performed quickly and safely even in unstable patients. The limitations of CT include limited information on nonhemorrhagic parenchymal injury, beam-hardening artifacts (particularly at the base of skull and in the posterior fossa), and the use of ionizing radiation in a vulnerable population.

MRI plays a secondary role in the evaluation of acute trauma but offers a number of advantages over CT including improved sensitivity and specificity for parenchymal, nonhemorrhagic brain injury. MRI is particularly useful in the subacute and chronic stages of TBI but may also be used in the acute setting to help guide management decisions and as a source of important supplemental information in patients with abusive head trauma. Advanced MRI techniques such as MRS, arterial spin labeling, and magnetoencephalography can provide useful additional information in select circumstances.

Skull Fractures

Falls and motor vehicle accidents account for the majority of skull fractures in children. In infants, skull fractures may be linear, depressed, diastatic, compound, "ping-pong" (the calvarial equivalent of a buckle fracture) [**Fig. 8.94**], or penetrating.

Linear fractures usually heal without complication. Diastatic fractures involve the sutures, typically the lambdoid in infants and children [**Fig. 8.95**]. A fracture is depressed when a fragment is displaced inward by at least the thickness of the skull. Depressed fractures often require surgical correction.

Depressed fractures are classified as compound when an overlying scalp laceration is present and penetrating when associated with a dural tear. Compound fractures can be complicated by CSF leak and infection. Herniation of the pia and arachnoid into the fracture line can result in a leptomeningeal cyst. CSF pulsations within the cyst can give rise to the classic "growing fracture" sign.

Fractures involving the skull base carry an increased risk for vascular and cranial nerve injury.

Cerebral Injury

Contusion

A brain contusion is bruising of the brain parenchyma. It typically involves the cortex with varying involvement of the white matter. Brain contusions are more common in children than in

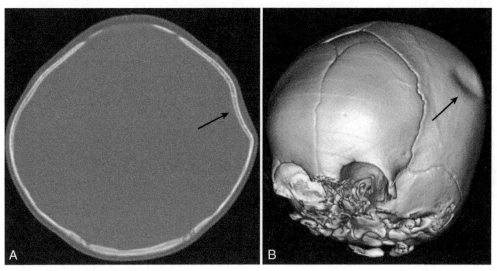

Figure 8.94 **Ping-pong fracture.** Eight-month-old with fall onto hardwood floor. **A,** Axial and (**B**) three-dimensional surface reconstruction of unenhanced computed tomography show depression (*arrow*) of the left parietal bone without cortical break.

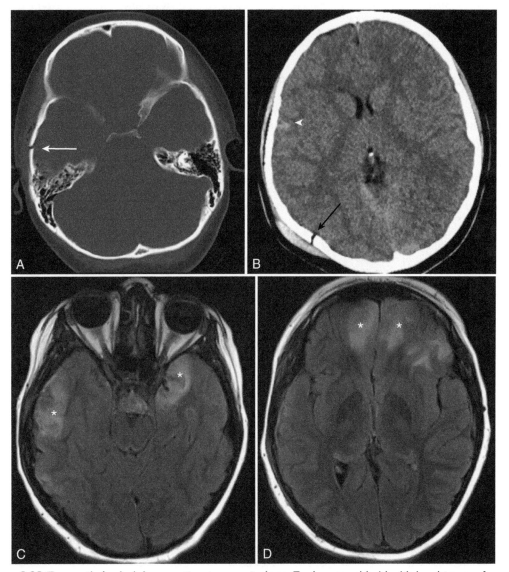

Figure 8.95 **Traumatic brain injury, contrecoup contusions.** Twelve-year-old girl with head trauma from fall off of a golf cart. **A** and **B,** Axial unenhanced computed tomography images demonstrate a comminuted fracture of the right squamosal temporal bone (*white arrow*), diastasis of the right lambdoid suture (*black arrow*) with overlying hematoma, and subarachnoid hemorrhage (*white arrowhead*). **C** and **D,** Axial T2 FLAIR images demonstrate extensive parenchymal contusions both at the site of impact and contrecoup in the anterior frontal lobes (*asterisks*).

adults. Brain contusions can occur because of shearing in acceleration/deceleration injuries (these are most commonly located in the anterior temporal and orbitofrontal regions). Direct trauma can result in contusions at the site of impact (*coup*) and diagonally opposition (*contrecoup*) [**Fig. 8.95**]. Contusions can occur adjacent to the falx cerebri, tentorium, and foramen magnum in cases of herniation. Approximately 50% of brain contusions are hemorrhagic.

CT depicts contusions as focal areas of hypoattenuation and reduced gray-white matter contrast in nonhemorrhagic contusion. Microhemorrhagic foci are seen as punctate areas of increased attenuation along the cortex. Coalescence into larger, hyperattenuating focal parenchymal hematoma is associated with poor neurologic outcome.

MRI is more sensitive than CT for demonstrating brain contusion. In the first 24 hours, DWI is the most sensitive sequence. After 1 to 2 days, the contusions will appear hyperintense on T2- and FLAIR-weighted images with areas of microhemorrhage or coalescent hematoma appearing hypointense on GRE or SWI.

A laceration of the brain parenchyma consists of a focal tear extending from the cortex into the white matter. Lacerations are more commonly seen in penetrating or perforating injury. The inferior frontal and anterior temporal lobes are the most common location.

Diffuse Axonal Injury, Diffuse Cerebral Edema, and Hypoperfusion Injuries

Diffuse axonal injury (DAI) is the most common cause of neurological and cognitive disability after TBI. DAI is associated with rapid acceleration and/or deceleration, a combination of angular and rotational forces causing indirect shearing injuries of the white matter. There tends to be an immediate severe impairment of consciousness at the time of injury.

The most common locations involved with DAI are the subcortical white matter, the posterior body and splenium of the corpus callosum, the dorsolateral midbrain, and upper pons. In the most severe cases, the internal and external capsules, basal ganglia, thalami, and cerebellum are also involved.

Clinical findings are often disproportionate to imaging findings. CT is normal in 20% to 50% of cases of DAI. Signs of DAI on CT include multiple, bilateral foci of increased or decreased attenuation less than 1 cm, oriented along the white matter tracts. MRI is more sensitive than CT and may depict multiple small ovoid foci that are hypointense on T1, hyperintense on T2 and FLAIR, and show abnormal signal on DWI [**Fig. 8.96**].

Diffuse brain swelling occurs in 21% of pediatric head trauma and is much more common than in adults with brain trauma. When young children sustain a head injury, the immature vasoregulatory system responds with vasodilation and increased cerebral blood flow that can result in diffuse cortical swelling and edema. The characteristic findings of diffuse edema on CT include generalized loss of cerebral gray-white matter differentiation; diffuse hypoattenuation of the cerebral parenchyma and effacement of the sulci, basal cisterns, and ventricles. The reduced cerebral attenuation can cause circulating blood or the cerebellum to appear hyperdense, resulting in the "pseudo-SAH" and "white cerebellar" signs, respectively [**Fig. 8.97**].

Progressive cerebral edema and raised ICP can result in transtentorial, subfalcine and tonsillar herniation, and death in children with severe head injury.

Hypoperfusion injury can also be seen in pediatric head trauma and can be caused by hypotension or shock. Markedly elevated raised ICP can also result in hypoperfusion of the brain. Hypoperfusion results in a loss of gray-white matter differentiation on CT and restricted diffusion and cortical edema on MRI.

Subdural Hematoma

Subdural hematomas are more common in infants than in older children and adults. Subdural hematomas arise from tearing of the bridging veins that traverse the inner layer of the dura and the arachnoid membrane. In infants, subdural hematomas are bilateral in 80% to 85% of cases.

The majority of subdural hematomas, beyond those caused by parturition, in children younger than 2 years occur from abusive head trauma. Other signs of child abuse include additional injuries, a history inconsistent with the severity or type of injury, interhemispheric subdural hematoma, and retinal hemorrhages.

Other causative factors of subdural hematoma include accidental trauma, shunt placement, or intracranial hypotension related to overshunting. Although it is controversial, there does appear to be an increased risk for development of subdural hematomas in children with prominent subarachnoid spaces.

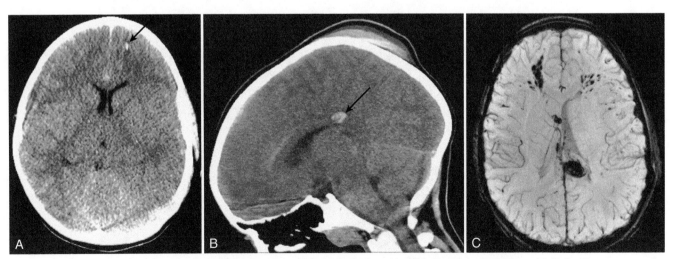

Figure 8.96 Diffuse axonal injury. Seven-year-old girl with closed head injury from a motor vehicle accident. **A,** Axial unenhanced computed tomography shows a subcortical hemorrhage from shear injury in the left frontal lobe (*arrow*). **B,** Sagittal reformat demonstrates acute hemorrhage in the posterior body/splenium of corpus callosum (*arrow*). **C,** Axial susceptibility-weighted imaging from magnetic resonance imaging performed 7 days later shows extensive foci of susceptibility artifact indicating multifocal parenchymal hemorrhage.

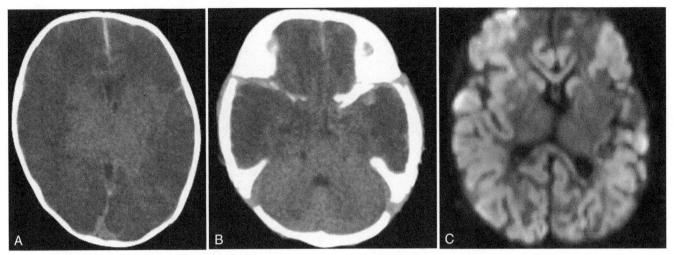

Figure 8.97 **Abusive head trauma.** Four-month-old with seizures, facial ecchymoses, and retinal hemorrhages. **A** and **B,** axial unenhanced computed tomography images demonstrating extensive cortical edema, the "white cerebellum" sign of diffuse cerebral edema (cerebral hypoattenuation and preservation of cerebellar density) and effacement of the sulci, ventricles, and basal cisterns. **C,** Diffusion-weighted image confirms extensive injury throughout the cortex.

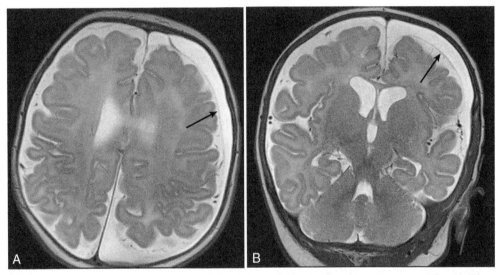

Figure 8.98 **Subdural fluid.** Two-month-old who sustained abusive head trauma. **A,** Axial and (**B**) coronal T2-weighted images demonstrating moderate-sized left and small right subdural fluid collections. A thin hypointense line representing the arachnoid membrane (*arrow*) separates the subdural fluid from the cerebrospinal fluid in the subarachnoid space. Note that the cortical veins are displaced medially as opposed to their position in benign extraaxial fluid collections of infancy depicted in Fig. 8.50.

Younger children can be asymptomatic or present insidiously with vomiting, poor feeding, lethargy, or present with increasing head circumference or fullness of the fontanelle. Older children tend to present with more classical signs of raised ICP including headache, altered consciousness, increased blood pressure, asymmetric pupils, and hemiparesis.

Subdural hematomas are most commonly found over the frontal, parietal, and temporal lobes. Subdural hematomas cross sutures but do not cross the falx or tentorium; this is the most important distinguishing feature from epidural hematomas. Subdural hematomas are classically crescenteric in morphology, but this configuration is not uniformly present [**Fig. 8.98**].

The appearance of subdural hematomas on CT depends on the contents of the subdural collection. Hyperacute hematomas consisting of nonclotted blood may be isodense to the dural sinuses. Within a few hours, an acute subdural hematoma is usually hyperattenuating due to blood clotting; however, there may be mixing in the acute phase because of active bleeding, clot retraction, or presence of CSF within the collection (hematohygroma) altering the density of the subdural, either uniformly or in a heterogeneous manner. Within 1 to 3 weeks, the attenuation of a subdural hematoma tends to decrease and becomes similar to brain parenchyma. After 2 to 3 weeks, the attenuation may reduce to that of CSF.

MRI is more sensitive for detection of small subdural hematomas. As on CT, the appearance of a subdural hematoma varies depending on its contents. CSF in the subdural space will tend to follow CSF signal within the ventricles, but T1 shortening can occur because of the admixture blood or protein. Hemorrhage causes variable signal intensity depending on the state of the blood products present. There is a temptation in inflicted trauma cases to use CT density or MR signal characteristics of parenchymal hematomas to date the age of subdural hematomas. This practice should be avoided because dating of subdural collections by imaging is often imprecise. Extreme care should be used in reporting mixed density/intensity subdural collections. Mixed density/intensity collections may occur when CSF leaks into the subdural space, when clotted and unclotted blood is present, or when there has been rebleeding into a preexisting subdural collection. Interpreting all mixed density/intensity subdural collections as "acute on chronic" bleeding does not take into account other potential causes and often has medicolegal implications.

A subdural hygroma is a collection of CSF in the subdural space due to laceration of the arachnoid. Subdural hygroma can occur independently or in combination with acute hemorrhage after trauma. Subdural hygromas are hypodense on CT and follow CSF signal characteristics on all MR sequences.

Epidural Hematoma

Epidural hematomas are uncommon in infants but become progressively more common with age. In younger children, venous epidural hematomas are more common than the classic arterial epidural hematomas seen in older children and adults. Tearing of a dural venous sinus or an emissary or diploic vein are the most common causes of venous epidural hematomas. In neonates, epidural venous hemorrhages are most common in the posterior fossa.

An epidural hematoma is limited by the periosteal attachments and does not cross calvarial sutures; however, they can cross over the falx and tentorium. This is the most important distinguishing feature from a subdural hematoma but can occur only when the hematoma is near these structures. Classically, epidural hematomas have a biconvex or lentiform shape, but this shape is not always present, particularly in children and in hematomas in the posterior fossa.

An acute epidural hematoma is typically hyperattenuating on CT due to the presence of acute blood clot. Mixed attenuation can represent active bleeding, a dural tear with mixed CSF and hemorrhage, or clot retraction [**Fig. 8.99**]. An epidural hematoma will progress to isodensity and hypodensity in the subacute and chronic phases, respectively.

The evolution of epidural hematomas on MRI is related to the state of blood products it contains. Hyperacute blood has similar signal to fluid. The signal of acute hemorrhage is largely related to the presence of deoxyhemoglobin and is generally isointense to hypointense on both T1- and T2-weighted imaging. Gradually intracellular methemoglobin results in T1 and T2 shortening within the hemorrhage and as the blood ages further, the cells lyse and the methemoglobin becomes extracellular resulting in T2 prolongation (hyperintensity).

Subarachnoid Hemorrhage

Traumatic SAH is usually due to laceration of the pia-arachnoid vessels and is often associated with intraparenchymal injury. SAH is present in up to 25% of closed head injuries in children. In patients with large SAH without parenchymal injury or extra-axial hemorrhage, an underlying aneurysm or arteriovenous malformation should be considered.

Traumatic intraventricular hemorrhage can occur because of tearing of the subependymal veins or result from ventricular extension of subarachnoid or parenchymal hemorrhage.

CT of SAH shows increased attenuation within the sulci, layering along the interhemispheric fissure, or tentorium. CT shows increased attenuation in a dependent location within the ventricles with intraventricular hemorrhage. MRI is more sensitive than CT for small amounts of SAH. SAH is hyperintense on FLAIR sequences and hypointense on GRE and SWI sequences.

Abusive Head Trauma

Five children die in the United States every day as a result of abuse and neglect. Head injury after inflicted, "nonaccidental" trauma is one of the leading causes of mortality in infants and young children. Injuries include skull fractures, retinal hemorrhage, intracranial hemorrhage, and brain parenchymal injuries including contusions, edema, ischemia, and infarction.

The clinical presentation on abusive head trauma can be nonspecific; infants may present with irritability or lethargy without external stigmata of injury. Imaging findings may provide the first indication of inflicted brain injury. Injuries inconsistent with the history provided and evidence for injuries of varying ages should raise suspicion for abusive injury. A multidisciplinary approach to the clinical circumstances is important. Communication with the referring physician,

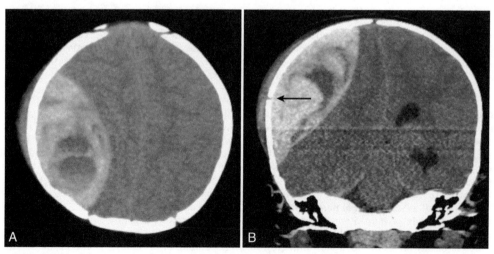

Figure 8.99 Epidural hematoma. Four-month-old male boy with vomiting and right scalp swelling the day after a fall. **A,** Axial and (**B**) coronal unenhanced computed tomography images demonstrate a large right frontoparietal biconvex epidural hematoma underlying a linear skull fracture (*arrow*) and causing mass effect on the right cerebral hemisphere. The mixed attenuation suggests the possibility of active bleeding into the collection.

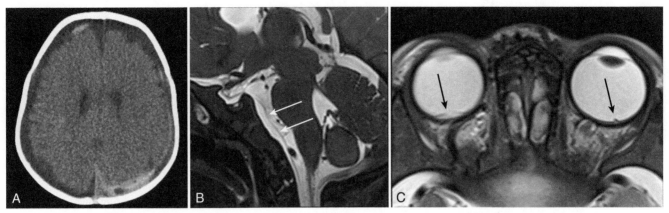

Figure 8.100 Abusive head trauma. Six-month-old infant found unresponsive. **A,** Axial computed tomography shows bilateral mixed density subdural fluid collections and loss of gray matter-white matter contrast. **B,** Sagittal heavily T2-weighted magnetic resonance imaging (MRI) shows retroclival subdural hematoma (*arrows*). **C,** Axial T2-weighted MRI shows irregularity and thickening of the retina bilaterally (*arrows*) corresponding with retinal hemorrhages noted clinically.

correlation with clinical history, and further imaging if necessary are vitally important.

Subdural hemorrhages, secondary to rotational forces on the head that tear the bridging veins, are more common in inflicted head injury than are epidural hemorrhages. The density on CT or intensity on MR of a subdural hemorrhage can vary because of dilution from mixing CSF in a dural tear or an aging hematoma. The key to differentiating a fluid density subdural hematoma from prominent subarachnoid spaces is the medial displacement of bridging veins when a hematoma is present [see **Fig. 8.98**]. The presence of a retroclival subdural hematoma may be a subtle but important finding suggesting abusive head injury [**Fig. 8.100**]. Cervical spine MR may sometimes show edema within the cervical soft tissues in cases of suspected abusive injury.

Death from abuse is often due to a parenchymal brain injury. Hypoxic ischemic injury and edema are more commonly seen than parenchymal contusions or DAI. MRI is more sensitive than CT for delineating the full extent of a parenchymal injury.

METABOLIC BRAIN DISORDERS

A large number of inherited genetic mutations cause alterations in enzyme production, protein expression, and mitochondrial expression that manifest as disorders of brain metabolism and structure. Children with inherited metabolic brain disorders tend to present with nonspecific symptoms such as hypotonia, seizures, loss of developmental milestones, and unexplained developmental delay. These metabolic disorders have varied clinical phenotypes but tend to be characterized by an unrelenting progressive course.

The imaging appearance of metabolic brain disorders varies widely, although many disorders exhibit a characteristic pattern on imaging at some point in their course. Some of the more common imaging findings are progressive changes over time, progressive demyelination, symmetric involvement of the white matter tracts, and pervasive, symmetric involvement of white and gray matter.

Traditionally, the diagnosis of inherited metabolic disorders was made using clinical findings, analysis of blood and urine samples, and tissue biopsy. Localizing the sites of primary involvement on MRI and the use of advanced imaging techniques such as DWI and MRS helps narrow the differential diagnosis and identify candidate conditions for genetic testing. Indications for performing such advanced imaging techniques include developmental regression, progressive impairment, feeding difficulties, consanguinity, sibling with known metabolic diagnosis/similar

phenotype, family history of developmental delay, multiple organ involvement, and delayed or progressive demyelination on conventional MR sequences.

A large number of metabolic disorders exist, but most of them are rare. They can be classified according to predominant CNS site of involvement on MRI [**Table 8.8**] or by the underlying metabolic defect. A final diagnosis cannot be made in up to 60% of cases.

An in-depth discussion of inherited metabolic disorders is beyond the scope of this text; however, some of the more common disorders and some conditions with more distinctive imaging appearances and a few in which there are effective therapeutic interventions available will be presented.

Disorders That Primarily Affect White Matter (Leukodystrophies)
Metachromatic Leukodystrophy

Metachromatic leukodystrophy (MLD) is the most common leukodystrophy with an incidence of approximately 1 in 100,000. It arises from mutations of the arylsulfatase A (*ARSA*) gene located on chromosome 22q13 that results in CNS and systemic accumulation of sulfatides. The age of presentation is variable. The most common late infantile form presents insidiously in the second year of life with gait disturbance, ataxia, speech disturbance, and hypotonia. Death usually occurs within 4 years after progressive neurological decline. The typical appearance on MRI is of confluent, periventricular T2/FLAIR hyperintensity. Radial stripes can be seen extending from the ventricles to the cortex due to relative sparing of perivenular myelin; this striped appearance creates the so-called tigroid sign [**Fig. 8.101**]. No contrast enhancement is seen in MLD. Areas of abnormal myelin may show restricted diffusion on DWI. MRS shows decreased NAA and elevated myo-inositol.

Krabbe Disease

Krabbe disease is caused by a deficiency of the lysosomal enzyme galactocerebroside β-galactosidase. There are infantile, late infantile, and adult forms. Infants usually present between the ages of 3 and 6 months with extreme irritability. If CT is performed early in the disease, characteristic faint hyperdensity may be seen in the thalami. On MRI, patchy bilateral T2 hyperintensity is seen in the thalami and basal ganglia early in the disease [**Fig. 8.102**]. The distribution of abnormalities is reminiscent of the sites of involvement with hypoxic-ischemic brain injury but

TABLE 8.8 Metabolic Brain Disorders

Area Primarily Affected	Disorders	Imaging Findings
Cortical gray matter	• Lysosomal disorders • Mucopolysaccharidoses • Mucolipidosis	• Cortical atrophy • Ventriculomegaly • Secondary white matter changes
Deep gray matter	• Mitochondrial disorders • Organic and aminoacidopathies • Pantothenate kinase–associated neurodegeneration • Juvenile Huntington disease • Krabbe disease • Wilson disease • Fahr disease • Cockayne syndrome	• Abnormal signal intensities in the basal ganglia or thalami • Deep gray matter mineralization • Third or lateral ventriculomegaly
White matter	• Lysosomal disorders • Peroxisomal disorders • Pelizaeus-Merzbacher disease • Canavan disease • Alexander disease • Cockayne syndrome	• Superficial involvement of the subcortical arcuate U fibers • Deep involvement of deep white matter fibers • Secondary gray matter changes occur late
White matter and cortical gray matter	• Lysosomal disorders • Mitochondrial disorders	
White matter and deep gray matter	• Leigh syndrome • MELAS syndrome • Wilson disease • Cockayne syndrome • Krabbe disease • Canavan disease • Maple syrup urine disease	

MELAS, mitochondrial encephalomyopathy with lactic acidosis and stroke.

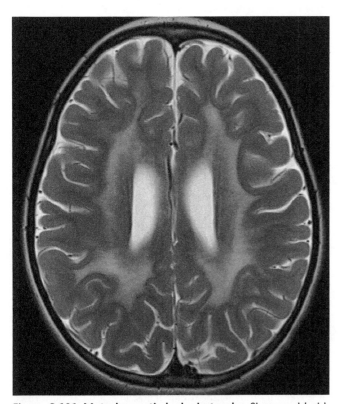

Figure 8.101 Metachromatic leukodystrophy. Six-year-old girl. Axial T2-weighted imaging shows T2 periventricular prolongation with relative sparing of perivenular myelin resulting in the "tigroid sign" of radial hypointense stripes.

occurs in infants without a history of significant perinatal ischemia. The initial findings progress and become more confluent and diffuse over time. *Optic nerve enlargement* is seen in Krabbe disease and is somewhat distinctive for this condition. MRS shows reduced NAA, elevated choline, and may show elevated lactate.

Classic X-Linked Adrenal Leukodystrophy

Classic X-linked adrenal leukodystrophy is the result of a mutation of the *ABCD1* gene found on chromosome Xq28. This gene codes for a peroxisomal membrane protein, and the mutation results in the excessive accumulation of very long chain fatty acids. There are various forms, but the classic childhood presentation consists of behavioral difficulties, gait disturbance, and visual/hearing problems in boys aged between 5 and 10 years. *Adrenal involvement* may manifest with skin bronzing, nausea and vomiting, and fatigue. The clinical course is progressive, with death usually occurring within 3 years. On imaging, 80% of patients have *posterior predominant* white matter demyelination, which typically begins in a peritrigonal distribution. The edge of the involved area may show enhancement on postcontrast imaging [**Fig. 8.103**]. MRS shows reduced NAA, increased choline, glutamine, and glutamate, and increased lactate.

Maple Syrup Urine Disease

Maple syrup urine disease is a rare metabolic disorder; however, it differs from many others in that in presents in the *first few days of life* and can be successfully managed with careful dietary restriction. It is caused by mutations that result in an inability to decarboxylate the branched-chain amino acids. Affected infants present in the first few days of life with poor feeding, vomiting, ketoacidosis, seizures, and lethargy. The sweet smell

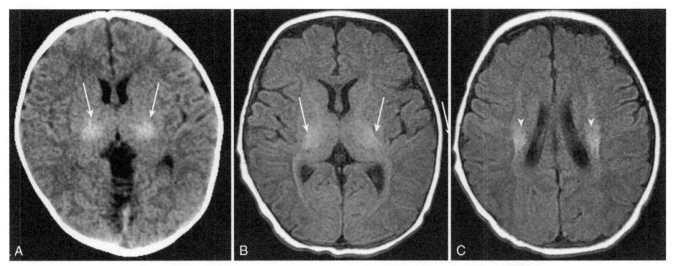

Figure 8.102 **Krabbe disease.** Seventy-nine-day-old girl with neurological decline. **A,** Axial unenhanced computed tomography shows hyperdensity in the thalami (*arrows*). **B** and **C,** Axial T1-weighted images show hyperintensity in the thalami (*arrows*) and corona radiata (*arrowheads*).

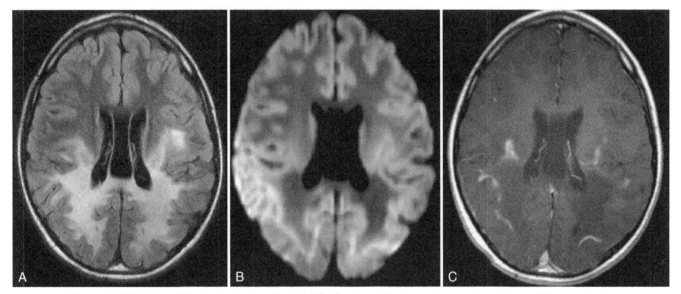

Figure 8.103 **Adrenal leukodystrophy. A,** Axial fluid attenuation inversion recovery shows diffuse posterior predominant white matter hyperintensity associated with a leading edge of (**B**) restricted diffusion and (**C**) enhancement postcontrast.

of ketoacids in the urine gives the disorder its name. Cranial ultrasound may show symmetrically increased echogenicity of the periventricular white matter. MRI typically shows profound localized *edema involving the areas that are myelinated/myelinating at time of birth* (deep cerebellar white matter, dorsal brainstem, cerebral peduncles, posterior limb of the internal capsule). The involved areas show restricted diffusion on DWI. MRS may show a broad peak at 0.9 ppm corresponding with the accumulation of branched-chain amino acids [**Fig. 8.104**].

Disorders That Primarily Involve Gray Matter

Pantothenate Kinase–Associated Neuropathy

Pantothenate kinase–associated neuropathy is also known as neurodegeneration with brain iron accumulation 1 and was formerly known as Hallervorden-Spatz disease. It causes progressive gait impairment, choreoathetotic movements, dysarthria, and mental deterioration caused by iron deposition in the globus

pallidus and zona reticulata of the substantia nigra. MRI shows T2 hypointensity in the globus pallidus bilaterally with central foci of T2 hyperintensity caused by pallidal destruction and gliosis creating the distinctive "eye of the tiger" sign [**Fig. 8.105**]. There is restricted diffusion in the globus pallidus on DWI. MRS shows decreased NAA and increased myo-inositol.

Disorders That Affect Both Gray and White Matter

Canavan Disease

Canavan disease, also known as spongiform leukodystrophy, is an autosomal recessive disorder caused by a deficiency of aspartoacylase that leads to accumulation of NAA in the brain and *N*-acetyl aspartic aciduria. Patients with Canavan disease usually present in the first few months of life with profound hypotonia. They show progressive neurological deterioration and often experience macrocrania and seizures. Death usually

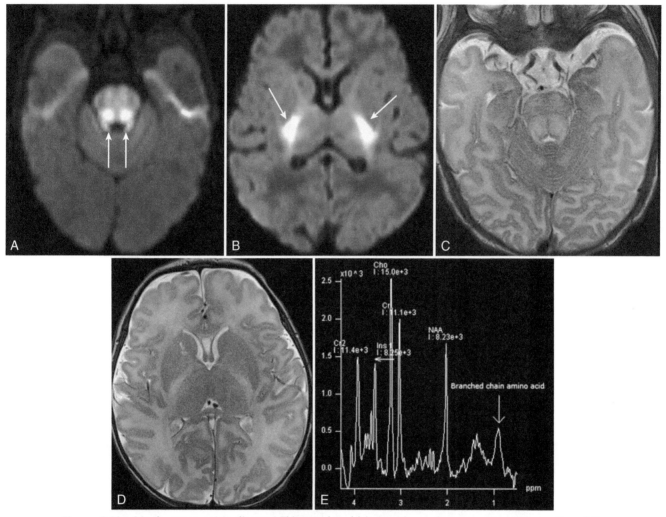

Figure 8.104 Maple syrup urine disease. Thirteen-day-old boy with maple syrup urine disease. **A** and **B**, Diffusion-weighted images show decreased diffusion in the brainstem and posterior limb of internal capsule (*arrows*) caused by intramyelinic edema. **C** and **D**, T2-weighted images show hypomyelination indicated by hyperintensity in regions corresponding to the diffusion abnormalities. **E**, Proton magnetic resonance spectroscopy demonstrates abnormal peak at 0.9 ppm representing elevated branched-chain amino acids.

occurs within 5 years. MRI shows diffuse, confluent cerebral white matter hyperintensity that preferentially *involves the subcortical U fibers early* in the disease in contrast with Krabbe disease and MLD, which begin in the deep white matter initially sparing the subcortical U fibers. The affected white matter shows restricted diffusion. MRS reveals elevations of the NAA peak; MRS abnormalities may predate the T2 abnormalities [**Fig. 8.106**].

Alexander Disease

Alexander disease, which is also known as fibrinoid leukodystrophy, is caused by mutations that cause dysfunction of the glial fibrillary acid protein. There are three broad clinical phenotypes: infantile onset, juvenile onset, and adolescent onset. Infantile-onset Alexander disease has a rapidly fatal course. The other two forms are more slowly progressive. MRI characteristically shows *anterior-predominant* T2 hyperintensity [**Fig. 8.107**]. A periventricular rim of high T1 signal and low T2 signal has been described as the periventricular "garland." With disease progression, T2 hyperintensity can also be seen in the basal ganglia, thalami, and brainstem. Contrast enhancement is sometimes seen in the involved areas. MRS shows marked reduction of NAA and elevated myo-inositol, choline, and lactate.

Mucopolysaccharidoses

The mucopolysaccharidoses result from specific lysosomal enzyme deficiencies resulting in excessive accumulation of mucopolysaccharides. There is typically a mixture of skeletal, hepatic, cardiac, ocular, and CNS involvement; *Hurler syndrome* and *Morquio syndrome* are two of the most well-known disorders with characteristic imaging findings. CNS involvement is often partly secondary to skeletal abnormalities at the skull base. Imaging may demonstrate macrocrania, calvarial thickening, meningeal thickening, megalencephaly, white matter degeneration, volume loss, and hydrocephalus. Prominent perivascular spaces may be present. A J-shaped sella is often seen [**Fig. 8.108**].

Mitochondrial Encephalomyopathy With Lactic Acidosis and Stroke

Mitochondrial encephalomyopathy with lactic acidosis and stroke (MELAS) refers to a group of disorders that occurs secondary to deletions of mitochondrial DNA. Patients present with headaches, nausea, and vomiting and permanent or reversible strokelike events. The onset of symptoms is usually in the second decade of life. Imaging during acute episodes shows T1

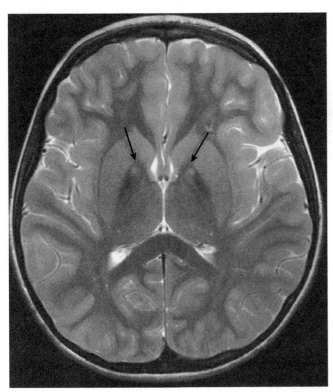

Figure 8.105 Pantothenate kinase–associated neuropathy. Six-year-old with ataxia. T2-weighted magnetic resonance imaging shows T2 hypointensity in the globus pallidus bilaterally with central foci of T2 hyperintensity (*arrows*) caused by pallidal destruction and gliosis creating the distinctive "eye of the tiger" sign. The patient was subsequently shown to have pantothenate kinase–associated neuropathy.

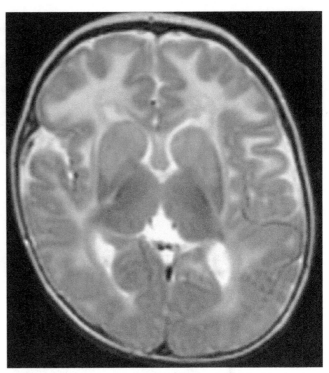

Figure 8.107 Alexander disease. Five-month-old with developmental delay and seizures. Axial T2-weighted image demonstrates the characteristic anterior-predominant white matter T2 hyperintensity of Alexander disease. T2 hyperintensity can also be seen in the basal ganglia.

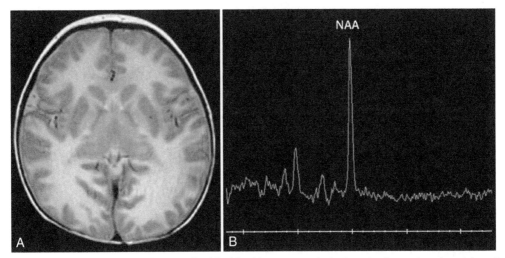

Figure 8.106 Canavan disease. Six-month-old girl with macrocephaly, hypotonia, and motor delay. **A,** T2-weighted magnetic resonance (MR) reveals diffuse white matter signal abnormalities. **B,** Proton MR spectroscopy demonstrates a markedly elevated *N*-acetyl aspartate peak on MR spectroscopy in keeping with subsequently confirmed Canavan disease.

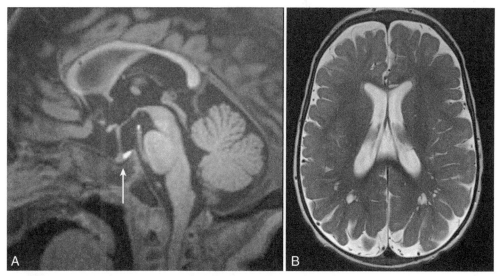

Figure 8.108 Hurler syndrome. Six-year old girl diagnosed with deficiency in alpha-L-iduronidase enzyme (Hurler syndrome) at the age of 2 years when she was noted to have developmental delay. **A,** Midline sagittal T1 demonstrates J-shaped sella (*arrow*). **B,** Axial T2 demonstrates white matter degeneration with prominent perivascular spaces and volume loss.

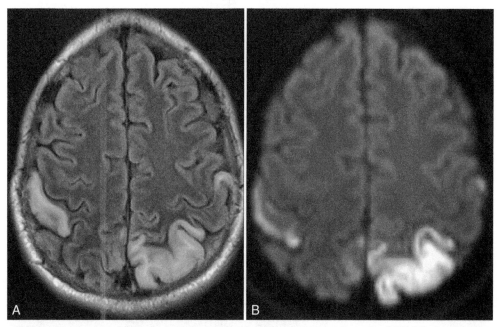

Figure 8.109 Mitochondrial encephalomyopathy with lactic acidosis and stroke (MELAS). Fourteen-year-old boy with known MELAS with altered mental status. (**A**) Axial fluid attenuation inversion recovery demonstrates bilateral cortical signal abnormalities. **B,** Diffusion-weighted image shows decreased diffusion within the lesions.

hypointensity and T2/FLAIR hyperintensity in the involved areas of the brain, typically the *occipital and parietal* cortices and subcortical white matter [**Fig. 8.109**]. In MELAS, cortical lesions often cross arterial boundaries in contrast with embolic or thrombotic infarcts. The imaging findings may be transient and resolve completely or can proceed to atrophy. MRS shows high lactate in the involved areas.

Zellweger Syndrome

Zellweger, or cerebrohepatorenal, syndrome is a peroxisomal disorder. Most patients have mutations that reduce the activity in 1 of more than 10 identified *PEX* genes which are involved in the biogenesis of peroxisomes. Patients usually do not survive beyond 1 year of age. Imaging classically shows PMG, white matter hypomyelination, and periventricular germinolytic cysts [**Fig. 8.110**].

Pelizaeus-Merzbacher Disease

Pelizaeus-Merzbacher is a rare, X-linked, recessive leukodystrophy that occurs in 1 in 500,000 male children and is characterized by an inability to form myelin. The condition is due to mutations in the *PLP1* gene that is required for production of Proteolipid 1 protein. Affected children usually present with hypotonia, nystagmus, and delayed motor development. Imaging shows a diffuse absence of normal myelination [**Fig. 8.111**].

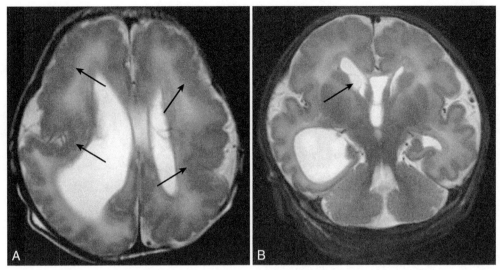

Figure 8.110 Zellweger syndrome. Two-day-old full-term infant with Zellweger syndrome. **A,** Axial T2-weighted image shows extensive bilateral polymicrogyria (*arrows*) and abnormal white matter. **B,** Coronal T2-weighted image demonstrates a germinolytic cyst in the caudothalamic regions (*arrow*).

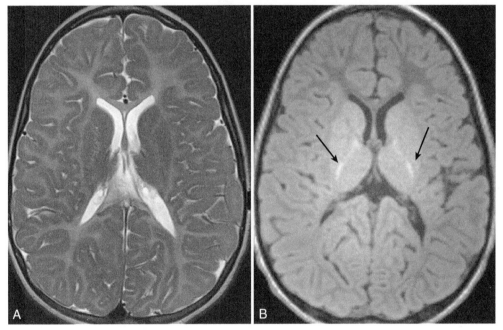

Figure 8.111 Pelizaeus-Merzbacher disease. Twenty-seven-month-old boy with Pelizaeus-Merzbacher disease. **A,** Axial T2-weighted image shows diffuse absence of myelination as depicted by abnormal hyperintense white matter. **B,** Axial T1-weighted image shows minimal hyperintensity caused by myelination in the posterior limb of the internal capsule (*arrows*).

Miscellaneous

Mesial Temporal Sclerosis

Seizures and seizure disorders are a significant cause of morbidity in children and a frequent reason for obtaining neuroimaging. Many entities described in the earlier sections, in particular malformations of cortical development, tumors, infection, and metabolic abnormalities can present with seizures. For patients with intractable epilepsy refractory to medication, neuroimaging plays an important role in identifying patients with localization-related forms that may benefit from surgical resection. Mesial temporal sclerosis (MTS) is the most common localization-related form of epilepsy, particularly in older children and adults. The exact underlying pathophysiology of MTS is unclear, and there

is ongoing debate whether temporal lobe epilepsy results in MTS or vice versa. There is some evidence that MTS may be related to febrile seizures in infancy, although this is disputed.

Pathologically, MTS is characterized by neuronal loss and gliosis of the hippocampus and adjacent structures; the hippocampal body is the most commonly affected site. High-resolution coronal T2-weighted MRI is the sequence of choice for identifying MTS. The hallmarks of MTS on MRI are atrophy of the hippocampus and ipsilateral fornix, loss of normal architecture/gray white matter differentiation, and dilatation of the adjacent temporal horn or choroidal fissure [**Fig. 8.112**]. ^{18}F-FDG PET may show interictal hypometabolism in the epileptogenic focus, whereas ictal single-photon emission CT may show hypermetabolism.

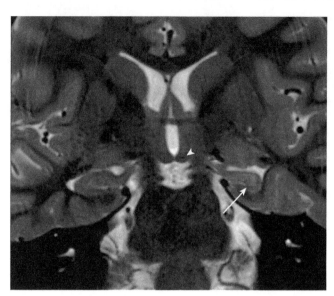

Figure 8.112 Mesial temporal sclerosis. Eleven-year-old boy with medically intractable seizures. Coronal T2-weighted imaging through the mesial temporal lobes shows volume loss, mild T2 prolongation, and loss of the normal interdigitations of the left hippocampus (*white arrow*). The left mamillary body is smaller than the right (*white arrowhead*).

SUGGESTED READINGS

Adamsbaum C, Barr M. Imaging in abusive head trauma: an in-depth look at current issues. *Pediatr Radiol.* 2014;44(suppl 4):S535-S536.

Barkovich AJ, Guerrini R, Kuzniecky RI, et al. A developmental and genetic classification for malformations of cortical development: update 2012. *Brain.* 2012;135:1348-1369.

Barkovich AJ, Millen KJ, Dobyns WB. A developmental and genetic classification for midbrain-hindbrain malformations. *Brain.* 2009;132(Pt 12):3199-3230.

Barkovich AJ, Raybaud CA. Neuroimaging in disorders of cortical development. *Neuroimaging Clin N Am.* 2004;14:231-254, viii.

Barkovich AJ, Raybaud C, eds. *Pediatric Neuroimaging.* 5th ed. Philadelphia, PA: Lippincott Williams & Wilkins; 2011.

Barnes P, Krasnokutsky M. Imaging of the central nervous system in suspected or alleged nonaccidental injury, including the mimics. *Top Magn Reson Imaging.* 2007;18:53-74.

Lowe L, Bailey Z. State-of-the-art cranial sonography: part 1, modern techniques and image interpretation. *AJR Am J Roentgenol.* 2011;196:1028-1033.

Lowe L, Bailey Z. State-of-the-art cranial sonography: part 2, pitfalls and variants. *AJR Am J Roentgenol.* 2011;196:1034-1039.

Osborn A. *Osborn's Brain: Imaging, Pathology, and Anatomy.* Salt Lake City, UT: Amirsys; 2012.

Panigrahy A, Blüml S. Neuroimaging of pediatric brain tumors: from basic to advanced magnetic resonance imaging (MRI). *J Child Neurol.* 2009;24: 1343-1365.

Sivaganesan A, Krishnamurthy R, Sahni D, et al. Neuroimaging of ventriculoperitoneal shunt complications in children. *Pediatr Radiol.* 2012;42:1029-1046.

Yang E, Prabhu SP. Imaging manifestations of the leukodystrophies, inherited disorders of white matter. *Radiol Clin North Am.* 2014;52:279-319.

Yousem DM, Grossman RI. *Neuroradiology: The Requisites.* 3rd ed. Philadelphia, PA: Mosby; 2010.

Chapter 9
Spine Imaging

Thangamadhan Bosemani and Thierry A. G. M. Huisman

The spinal cord is an integral part of the neural axis or central nervous system. Disease entities in the brain or spinal cord may have a direct or indirect influence on each other. Imaging of the pediatric spine differs from that in adults in terms of relevant anatomy and associated pathology. An accurate imaging evaluation requires familiarity with the wide differential diagnosis of pediatric spinal disease. Spinal disease in children includes common processes, such as infection, trauma, and neoplasia. Developmental abnormalities of the spine require a thorough understanding of spinal embryology. A complete evaluation of the spine should include the bones of the spinal column, spinal canal, covering meningeal layers, and the spinal cord itself. The imaging technique of choice may differ depending on the age of the patient and the entity being evaluated. In this chapter, we will discuss the imaging techniques, embryology and development, and radiologic findings of developmental abnormalities and various spinal diseases in children.

IMAGING TECHNIQUES

Plain Films

Conventional radiography (CR) is the initial modality of choice for evaluation of the osseous structures of the spine after trauma, scoliosis, atlantoaxial (AA) instability, and formation/segmental anomalies. Frontal and lateral projections of the spine are typically obtained. However, depending on the indication, further views or follow-up imaging may be required. For instance, scoliosis often requires serial CR examinations to monitor evolution of the curvature. The scoliosis curvature may be influenced by patient posture—that is, sitting, standing, lying supine or bending. CR is often the initial modality for the evaluation of back pain in children and may be used to screen for congenital, traumatic, neoplastic and infectious causes of pain. Back pain with scoliosis is considered a red flag for the presence of underlying spinal pathology in children. Hence back pain with scoliosis should be investigated with a thorough clinical history, physical examination, laboratory tests, and neuroimaging including magnetic resonance imaging (MRI). Increasingly, concern over radiation exposure in children has resulted in the substitution of MRI for CR and computed tomography (CT) for the evaluation of scoliosis, formation/ segmentation anomalies and craniocervical junction (CCJ) instability. CR, however, remains an important imaging tool of the spine but must be used according to the "as low as reasonably achievable" (ALARA) principle.

Ultrasound

Ultrasound is a portable, bed-side, readily available, and radiation-free technique that is extremely helpful in the evaluation of neonates and young infants. The most common indication in the neonate is closed spinal dysraphism, which includes lesions such as dorsal dermal sinus tracts. Images are obtained in the longitudinal and transverse planes using a linear 5- to 12-MHz transducer with the patient lying prone. Dynamic real-time images can be acquired to assess movement of the lumbosacral nerve roots if there is a question of spinal cord tethering. Counting down from the 12th rib and counting up from the sacral elements will determine the vertebral level. If the vertebral level is unclear, CR may be helpful for correlation with markers. Color or power Doppler ultrasound may be used as an adjunct to characterize soft tissue masses on the skin or within the spinal canal.

Magnetic Resonance Imaging

MRI represents the modality of choice for imaging of the spine and the spinal canal contents. The strengths of conventional MRI include its unique contrast resolution, multiplanar capability, and high-resolution isotropic three-dimensional (3D) acquisitions. Diffusion tensor imaging is an advanced MRI technique that allows for studying the white matter tracts in vivo. Diffusion tensor imaging may be used when there is a suspicion of spinal cord ischemia or infarction. In addition, functional imaging, for example, of cerebrospinal fluid (CSF) flow can be measured.

The conventional MRI protocol includes sagittal T1- and T2-weighted images plus axial T2-weighted images of the entire spine (as one or more series) from the posterior fossa through the coccyx. The sequences can be performed with and without fat saturation. Fat saturation is helpful to confirm bone marrow edema or for assessment of intraspinal fatty lesions (eg, lipoma). In addition, axial T1-weighted images may be added to evaluate for filar thickening, extent of a dermal sinus, and a tethering mass (eg, lipoma) or subacute hemorrhage. Coronal T2-weighted images assist in evaluating for spinal column anomalies (eg, hemivertebra in congenital scoliosis), split-cord malformations (eg, diastematomyelia), and renal anomalies. Sagittal short tau inversion recovery (STIR) images are helpful in the evaluation of ligamentous injury after trauma and the presence of marrow edema in infectious processes. T1-weighted acquisitions after intravenous gadolinium administration, both with and without fat saturation, in sagittal and axial planes, enhance the ability of MRI to evaluate inflammation and tumor, whether intramedullary, intradural, or extradural.

MRI is the imaging modality of choice for evaluating the bone marrow, intervertebral disks, and extradural soft tissues. Bone marrow signal intensity in children is age dependent due to its varying content of hematopoietic and fatty marrow. T1 signal intensity of hematopoietic marrow is equal to or slightly higher than muscle but less than fat. Diffuse marrow involvement in systemic disease (leukemia) with marrow replacement or localized bone marrow edema (traumatic/inflammatory) is best evaluated with T1-weighted images without fat suppression and T2-weighted images with fat suppression. For evaluation of extradural traumatic, inflammatory, or neoplastic processes (eg, ligamentous injury, disk herniation, osteomyelitis, sarcoma), sagittal T1-weighted images are performed, followed by sagittal fat-suppression T2-weighted or STIR images. Additional gadolinium-enhanced sagittal and axial fat-suppression T1-weighted images are necessary for evaluating neoplastic and inflammatory processes, as well as for assessing recurrent disk protrusion (nonenhancing) from scar (enhancing) after disk surgery. These techniques allow for the complete assessment of marrow, bony, and paraspinal soft tissue involvement and extent, as well as for spinal cord, cauda equina, or nerve root compression. Gadolinium enhancement is also necessary in the assessment of intramedullary tumors (eg, astrocytoma, ependymoma, and ganglioglioma) and intradural tumors (eg, neurofibroma and schwannoma), and for neoplastic leptomeningeal seeding (eg, medulloblastoma and germ cell tumors).

Sagittal and axial T2-weighted MRI may also be done in flexion and extension (with patient cooperation or physician supervision) to assess craniocervical instability or fixation (eg, craniocervical anomalies). Sagittal T2-weighted or STIR imaging, along with axial T2-weighted imaging and postcontrast T1-weighted imaging, is helpful to evaluate for intramedullary inflammation or degeneration, including the assessment of spinal cord atrophy. A combination of sagittal and coronal T1- and T2-weighted imaging plus axial T2-weighted imaging is performed for screening of patients with suspected spinal vascular malformation.

Additional pulse sequences may be helpful in certain circumstances. For example, hemorrhage is best demonstrated using gradient recalled echo (GRE) techniques (eg, MEDIC—a fast T2-weighted two-dimensional spoiled GRE multiecho sequence), which can be positive as early as 3 hours after trauma. High-resolution sequences (eg, a heavily T2-weighted high-resolution isotropic 3D-constructive interference in steady state [CISS] or 3D-T1 magnetization-prepared rapid gradient-echo (MPRAGE), a fast GRE sequence with fat saturation, with multiplanar reconstruction (MPR) may be helpful in the evaluation of sinus tracts, CSF leaks, or pseudomeningocele. Functional assessment of CSF movement can be achieved by using "velocity-encoded imaging" which may be useful in planning posterior fossa decompression in Chiari I malformation.

Computed Tomography

Computed tomography (CT) imaging of the spine is typically performed without the administration of intravenous contrast. Axial images are obtained followed by coronal and sagittal MPR in bone and soft tissue kernels. CT is replacing CR and becoming the standard for the emergency evaluation of spine trauma. However, due to the relatively greater radiation exposure with CT compared to CR, CT should be restricted for use to areas in question on CR or to assess for additional injury when there is evidence of osseous trauma or ligamentous injury on CR. CT continues to be the choice for assessment of localized bony abnormalities, particularly when the level is precisely defined clinically or by plain film, single-photon emission computed tomography (SPECT), or MRI (eg, diastematomyelia, spondylolysis, spinal stenosis, spondylitis, bone tumor—ie, osteoid osteoma or aneurysmal bone cyst). Axial sections with two-dimensional reformatting (coronal, sagittal, or oblique) and/or 3D reconstructions are often important in the preoperative evaluation of spine trauma, craniocervical anomalies, and congenital scoliosis, as well as for the postoperative assessment of instrumentation and fusion. CT may also be obtained (with patient cooperation or physician supervision) with the spine in flexion and extension or with right and left head turning, to evaluate for translational craniocervical instability or rotatory atlanto-axial (AA) instability or fixation, respectively. CT myelography is rarely needed except when MRI is contraindicated or spinal instrumentation does not allow adequate MRI quality. It may also assist in the more precise delineation of nerve root or other intradural lesions (eg, cysts). A water-soluble, low-osmolar, nonionic contrast material specifically approved for

myelography is used because of its low toxicity and infrequent side effects. These techniques are best used in a limited and selective manner and using ALARA guidelines to minimize radiation exposure.

Radionuclide Imaging

Radionuclide imaging plays an important role in the evaluation of children with suspected infection. In vitro radiolabeling of leukocytes with ^{111}In-oxyquinoline or ^{99m}Tc-HMPAO (hexamethylpropyleneamine oxime) may be helpful to localize bacterial infection. Bone scintigraphy with ^{99m}Tc-labeled diphosphonates (^{99m}Tc-methyl diphosphonate) and single-photon emission CT (SPECT) is frequently helpful for evaluating children with lesions of the spinal column (eg, osteoid osteoma and metastases). Fluorine 18-fluorodeoxyglucose positron emission tomography (PET) is used for infection and tumor imaging. PET (including PET-CT) is also used in the assessment of treatment response or tumor progression in childhood neoplasia.

EMBRYOLOGY AND NORMAL DEVELOPMENT

The normal development of the spinal canal and its contents involves four principal processes: (1) gastrulation with development of the notochord, (2) primary neurulation with ganglion development, (3) segmentation with appearance of the somites, and (4) secondary neurulation (caudal cell mass).

The first stage of gastrulation occurs during the second or third week of embryonic development and involves conversion of the embryonic disk from a bilaminar disk (ectoderm and endoderm) to a trilaminar disk composed of ectoderm, mesoderm, and endoderm. Ectodermal cells glide between the ectoderm and endoderm; most of the ectodermal cells migrate laterally to form the mesoderm, and those that remain in the midline migrate along the craniocaudal axis of the primitive streak to form the notochordal process. At 20 days of life, resorption of the floor of the notochordal process results in the definitive notochord. The definitive notochord defines the primitive axis and skeleton of the embryo and is eventually replaced by the vertebral column.

The second stage of primary neurulation occurs during the third or fourth week of embryonic development. The notochord induces the transformation of the overlying ectoderm into neuroectoderm with formation of the neural plate signaling the onset of primary neurulation. The neural plate transforms to a neural groove, bends, and folds to form the neural tube, which then closes. During the closure of the neural tube, the overlying neuroectoderm progressively detaches from the adjacent surface ectoderm. This process is known as disjunction. Surface ectoderm closes and covers the neural tube. Simultaneously, cells at the border of the neuroectoderm and ectoderm detach and form the neural crests. The neural crests subsequently fragment and give rise to the primordia of the ganglia, which again give rise to the sensory nerves. The corresponding level of the neural tube and later the spinal cord furnishes the motor nerves. Primary neurulation is responsible for the development of the brain and upper 90% of the spinal cord.

The third stage of embryonic development involves forming a somite plate on each side of the neural tube. At the end of the fifth week of gestation, 42 pairs of somites are formed. The somites further differentiate into sclerotomes, dermatomes, and myotomes.

The fourth or final stage is secondary neurulation, which occurs between the fifth and sixth week of embryonic life during which the lower 10% of the spinal cord and filum terminale develop. A portion of the neural tube also known as the secondary neural tube develops from the caudal cell mass to the posterior neuropore. The caudal cell mass is derived from the caudal end of the primitive streak. The caudal cell mass is initially solid but subsequently undergoes a process of cavitation and canalization, eventually forming the tip of the conus medullaris and filum terminale by a process called *retrogressive differentiation.*

DEVELOPMENTAL ABNORMALITIES

A malformation is defined as a congenital morphologic anomaly of a single organ or body part caused by an alteration of the primary developmental program. Based on the normal processes of development of the spinal canal and its contents, malformations can be classified as: (1) disorders of primary neurulation, (2) disorders of secondary neurulation, or (3) anomalies of notochordal development.

Disorders of Primary Neurulation

From a clinical and embryologic perspective, disorders of primary neurulation can be divided into (1) open spinal dysraphism, (2) closed spinal dysraphism, and (3) dorsal dermal sinus. In an open spinal dysraphism, there is a defect in the overlying skin, and the neural tissue is exposed to the environment. In closed spinal dysraphism, the malformed neural tube is covered by mesodermal (subcutaneous fat) and ectodermal (skin) elements.

Open (Non–Skin–Covered) Spinal Dysraphism

Myelomeningocele and Myelocele. Incomplete or defective closure of the neural tube results in a neural placode that fails to detach from the adjacent surface ectoderm, a process termed nondisjunction. Consequently, a flattened midline neural placode is either flush with the cutaneous surface (myelocele-MC) or is pushed above or dorsal to the adjacent skin (myelomeningocele-MMC). MMC accounts for more than 98% of open spinal dysraphism. The prognosis of MMC and MC is worse than that of a skin-covered spinal dysraphism. MMC and MC have a significant impact on the quality of life. All children with an open spinal dysraphism have an associated Chiari II hindbrain malformation [**Fig. 9.1**]. It is hypothesized that the chronic leakage of CSF at the level of the neural placode during the intrauterine development of the fetal brain results in an incomplete or defective expansion of the rhombencephalic vesicle. This in turn prevents normal growth of the skull base causing a small posterior fossa with herniation of hindbrain elements into the upper cervical spinal canal. Varying degrees of central canal dilation or frank hydromyelia may be present in the spinal cord in patients with MMC or MC. These malformations can be diagnosed by ultrasound during fetal life and confirmed by fetal MRI.

Hemimyelomeningocele and Hemimyelocele. Hemimyelomeningoceles and hemimyeloceles are rare and are associated with diastematomyelia (cord splitting), and occur when one hemicord fails to undergo primary neurulation.

Closed (Skin-Covered) Spinal Dysraphism

Lipomyelomeningocele and Lipomyelocele. Lipomyelomeningoceles (LMMC) and lipomyeloceles (LMC) have a significantly better neurologic prognosis than open neural tube defects, presumably because the neural placode is covered and protected by skin and subcutaneous tissue. LMMC and LMC are typically not associated with Chiari II malformation. Premature disjunction of the neural tube from the adjacent surface ectoderm before closure of the neural tube results in mesenchymal elements having access to the neural groove and ependymal lining of the grove. It is hypothesized that the interaction of mesenchymal elements with the inner lining of the neural tube induces an

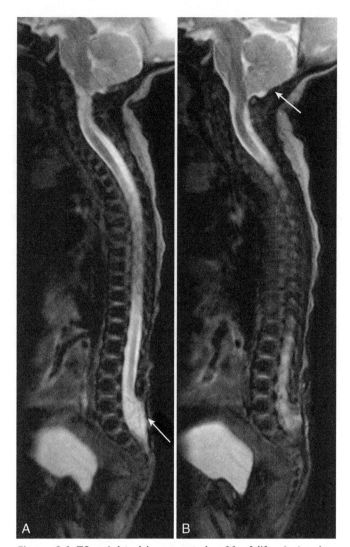

Figure 9.1 T2-weighted images at day 11 of life. A, Lumbar open myelomeningocele status post intrauterine closure (*arrow*). **B,** Chiari II hindbrain malformation (*arrow*).

excess production of fat. On imaging, in lipomyeloceles, the neural tissue is flush with the spinal canal; in lipomyelomeningoceles, the neural tissue is pushed outside of the spinal canal with expansion of the subarachnoid space [**Fig. 9.2**]. Large lipomas typically cover the neural placode and may extend from the subcutaneous region into the widened spinal canal.

Dorsal Dermal Sinus

Dorsal dermal sinuses are a distinct group of malformations that are classified as an intermediate between open and closed spinal dysraphisms. They are epithelial-lined fistulae or tracts connecting the skin surface with neural tissue or meninges. They are believed to result from a focal incomplete disjunction of the neuroectoderm from the surface ectoderm. Physical examination reveals a midline dimple or pinpoint ostium and may also reveal an associated hairy nevus, hyperpigmented patch, or capillary hemangioma. CSF may intermittently leak out of the ostium. The sinus tract may represent a port of entry for infections and may result in meningitis or abscess formation. The fistulous tract is well demonstrated on thin-slice, high-resolution T1- or T2-weighted sagittal images as a T1 hypointense, T2 hypointense, or hyperintense linear streak extending from the cutaneous dimple to the spinal canal [**Fig. 9.3**]. The malformation may

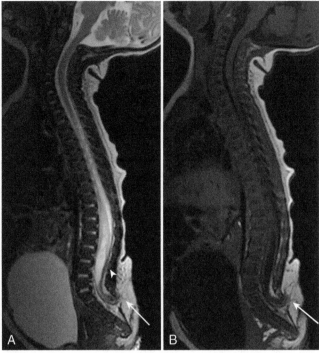

Figure 9.2 Lipomyelomeningocele with neural placode extending outside the spinal canal to terminate in a lipoma which is skin covered (*arrow*) and a caudal hydromyelia (*arrowhead*) on sagittal T2- (**A**) and T1-weighted (**B**) images. Note the normal posterior fossa in this skin-covered spinal dysraphism.

result in a low-lying spinal cord (ie, below the L2-3 disk level) and spinal cord tethering.

Disorders of Secondary Neurulation

Secondary neurulation is responsible for formation of the lowest part of the spinal cord including the conus medullaris and filum terminale. Secondary neurulation disorders include: (1) fibrolipoma of the filum terminale, (2) tight filum terminale syndrome, (3) caudal regression syndrome (CRS), and (4) sacrococcygeal teratoma (SCT).

Fibrolipoma of the Filum Terminale

Fibrolipomatous thickening of the filum terminale is referred to as a filar lipoma. However, filar thickening may be exclusively fibrous. Filar thickening, with or without fat, is a frequent normal finding on autopsy studies (4%–5%) and is only relevant if spinal cord tethering occurs. Tethered-cord syndrome is a clinical syndrome characterized by progressive neurologic abnormalities in the setting of traction on a low-lying spinal cord and conus medullaris. On imaging, a filar lipoma appears as a hyperintense strip or dot of signal on sagittal and axial T1-weighted images, respectively, within a thickened filum terminale [**Figs. 9.4** and **9.5**]. Axial T2-weighted imaging is generally required to demonstrate fibrous thickening of the filum.

Tight Filum Terminale

Tight filum terminale syndrome is characterized by hypertrophy and shortening of the filum terminale. This condition causes tethering of the spinal cord and impaired relative ascent of the conus medullaris during development. The conus medullaris is low lying relative to its normal position, above the L2-L3 disk level [**Fig. 9.6**].

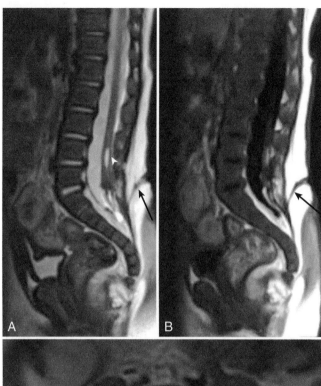
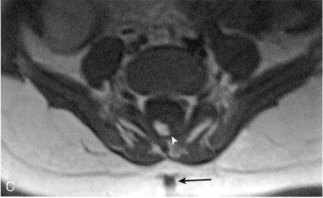

Figure 9.3 Dorsal dermal sinus. Sagittal T2- (**A**) and T1-weighted (**B**) images demonstrate a dorsal dermal sinus (*arrows*), low-lying conus with a tethered cord, and caudal hydromyelia (*arrowhead*). Axial T1-weighted image (**C**) shows filar lipoma (*arrowhead*) and dorsal dermal sinus (*arrow*).

Caudal Regression Syndrome

CRS is a spectrum of anomalies that have in common partial absence of lower vertebral elements and caudal spinal cord. CRS is associated with anorectal, lower-limb, and genitourinary malformations. In addition, CRS may be seen as part of the OEIS association (omphalocele, exstrophy, imperforate anus, spinal defects). The characteristic imaging findings are lack of the most distal segments of the spinal cord and matching musculoskeletal elements. Typically the spinal cord abruptly terminates with a club- or wedge-shaped inferior border [**Fig. 9.7**]. The sacrum and coccyx are typically absent. The malformation can be categorized into two types depending on position and configuration of the conus medullaris: high and abrupt (type I) or low and tethered (type II).

Sacrococcygeal Teratoma

SCTs are the most frequently encountered large, congenital tumors in neonates and arise from the pluripotent cells of the caudal cell mass. SCTs occur more often in girls than in boys (3 : 1 ratio). SCTs are classified as types I to IV depending on the

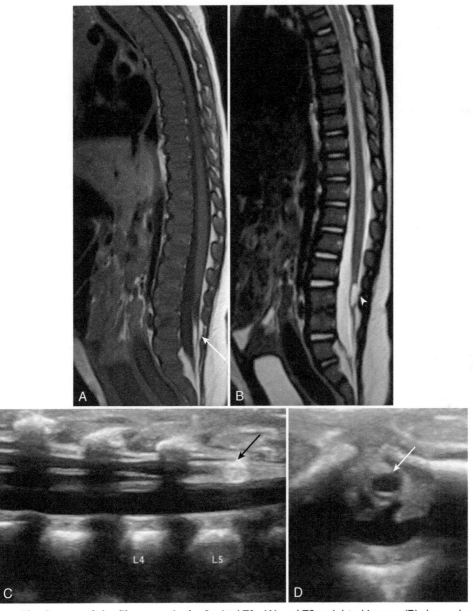

Figure 9.4 Fibrolipoma of the filum terminale. Sagittal T1- (**A**) and T2-weighted images (**B**) show a low-lying conus medullaris with thickening of the filum, lipoma (*arrow*). In addition, there is cystic dilatation (*arrowhead*) of the terminal ventricle. Sagittal (**C**) ultrasound image demonstrates a low-lying conus with a lipoma at the L5 level (*arrow*). Axial ultrasound image (**D**) at the L4 level shows the dilatation of the terminal ventricle (*arrow*).

location of the mass. In type I the lesion is exclusively outside the pelvis, whereas in type IV it is entirely inside the pelvis. Prenatal ultrasound and fetal MRI allow identification and characterization (cystic vs. solid) of SCT [**Fig. 9.8**]. Postnatal MRI is essential in the preoperative diagnostic workup to delineate the extension of tumor into the pelvis and degree of displacement or infiltration of pelvic structures.

Anomalies of Notochordal Development

Anomalies of notochordal development represent a complex dysraphism. These malformations may partially overlap with disorders of secondary neurulation (eg, CRS). These include the following entities: (1) split notochord syndrome, also known as diastematomyelia; (2) neurenteric fistula and (3) segmental

disorders of notochordal development resulting in the previously described spectrum of CRSs; and (4) segmentation and formation anomalies of the vertebral column.

Diastematomyelia

The splitting of the spinal cord into two hemicords is referred to as diastematomyelia. The hemicords may be separated by either a membranous septum or a bony spur. Ectodermal cells that are encoded to glide between the ectoderm and endoderm do not remain in the midline but form two more laterally positioned hemi-notochords, which in turn induce the formation of two separate neuroectodermal layers resulting in two hemicords. Each hemicord has one ventral and one dorsal nerve root and one central canal. In addition, the two hemicords may

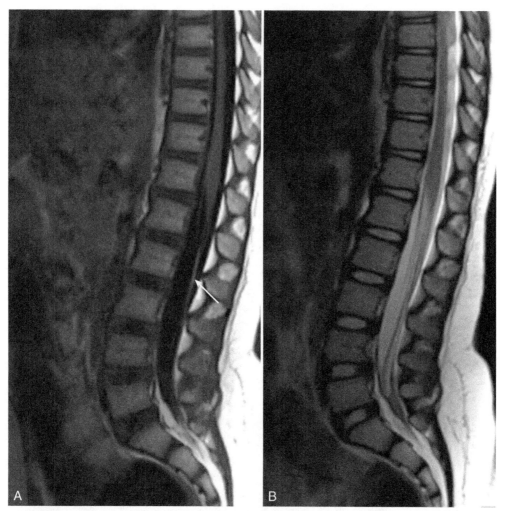

Figure 9.5 Filar lipoma (*arrow*) with normal position and configuration of the conus medullaris is shown on sagittal T1- (**A**) and T2-weighted (**B**) images.

either be located either within a single shared dural sac or in two distinct dural sacs [**Fig. 9.9**]. Diastematomyelia is associated with formation and segmentation anomalies of the vertebral bodies. It is a skin-covered defect with associated cutaneous stigmata in 50% to 70% of patients. Up to 90% of patients have symptoms related to spinal cord tethering. The diagnosis should be made using fetal ultrasound or MRI. Postnatal MRI evaluates the spinal cord anatomy in detail. CT is especially helpful in the identification of a bony spur, if present.

Neurenteric Fistula

Neurenteric fistula is a rare malformation resulting from a persistence of the notochordal process. Consequently, there is a direct connection between derivates of the endoderm and the neuroectoderm resulting in a fistulous connection between the skin surface and bowel. Neurenteric cysts represent a more localized form of a neurenteric fistula and extend anteriorly.

Segmentation and Formation Anomalies of the Spinal Column

A spectrum of segmentation and formation anomalies may be recognized (1) as an incidental finding, eg on a plain radiograph of the chest or abdomen, with no neurologic compromise, (2) during the workup of scoliosis, and (3) as part of various

syndromes and associations (eg, Klippel-Feil, VACTERL). Vertebral abnormalities result from a segmental derangement of the musculoskeletal somites. In addition to evaluating the bony anatomy, the contents of the spinal canal should be studied using MRI.

Other Developmental Abnormalities

Myelocystocele

Myelocystocele is an occult, skin-covered spinal dysraphism where the spinal cord with a dilated central canal and arachnoid protrude dorsally through a bony spine defect. Terminal myelocystoceles are believed to result from an abnormality of secondary neurulation, with an inability of CSF to exit from the early neural tube causing ballooning of the terminal ventricle of the conus placode into a cyst [**Fig. 9.10**]. Nonterminal myelocystoceles result from partial failure of primary neurulation, with the presence of spinal cord parenchyma distal to the CSF-filled cyst, and frequently occur in the cervical or cervicothoracic regions.

Meningocele

Meningocele is an uncommon entity with herniation of a CSF-filled sac lined by dura and arachnoid matter beyond the spinal canal. No neural tissue is included in the meningocele [**Fig. 9.11**]. The extension may be dorsal, lateral, or ventral.

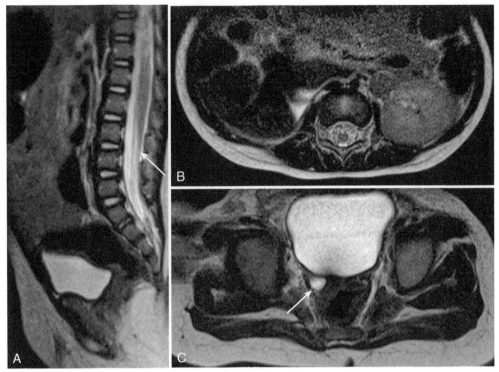

Figure 9.6 Tight filum terminale syndrome. Sagittal T2-weighted image (**A**) demonstrates a low-lying spinal cord with conus medullaris terminating at L3-L4 and mild hypertrophy of the filum terminale (*arrow*). In addition, axial T2-weighted images showing absence of the right kidney (**B**) and right-sided seminal vesicle cyst (*arrow*) (**C**), which may indicate Zinner syndrome.

Spondylodysplasias

Spondylodysplasia refers to any developmental abnormality of the bony spinal column. This category includes idiopathic scoliosis, congenital scoliosis and kyphosis, Scheuermann disease, and the skeletal dysplasias (eg, neurofibromatosis type 1 [NF-1], mucopolysaccharidoses [MPSs], spondyloepiphyseal dysplasia [SED], achondroplasia, and Down syndrome). An abnormality of the spinal curvature is a common presentation, based on clinical examination and CR, and includes scoliosis (lateral curvature), kyphosis (posterior angulation), and lordosis (increased anterior angulation). Skeletal dysplasias are a heterogeneous group of disorders in which there is abnormal cartilage and bone formation, growth, and remodeling. Compromise of the spinal canal/neural foramina and craniocervical instability, which may cause mechanical compression of the neural axis, are of major concern in skeletal dysplasias. CR, CT, and MRI play important roles in the evaluation of spondylodysplasias.

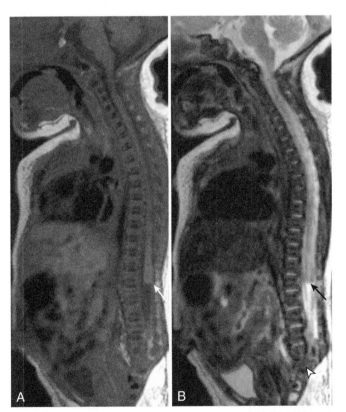

Figure 9.7 Caudal regression syndrome. Sagittal T1- (**A**) and T2-weighted (**B**) images show dysplasia of the distal spinal cord (*arrows*) and lumbosacral dysgenesis (*arrowhead*). The spinal cord stops abruptly as if it has been cut off.

Idiopathic Scoliosis

Scoliosis is defined as a lateral curvature of the spine greater than 10 degrees on radiography and is typically associated with trunk rotation. The two major categories of scoliosis are idiopathic scoliosis and nonidiopathic scoliosis. Nonidiopathic scoliosis can be classified as (1) congenital scoliosis caused by malformation of vertebrae-like hemivertebra or block vertebra; (2) neuromuscular scoliosis caused by insufficiency of active muscular stabilizers of the spine, as in cerebral palsy, spinal muscular atrophy, spina bifida, muscular dystrophies, or spinal cord injuries; and (3) mesenchymal scoliosis caused by insufficiency of passive stabilizers of the spine, as in Marfan syndrome, mucopolysaccharidosis, or osteogenesis imperfecta. The diagnosis of an idiopathic scoliosis is made if a nonidiopathic cause has been excluded.

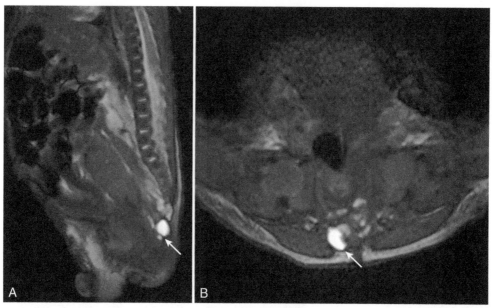

Figure 9.8 Sacrococcygeal teratoma. Sagittal (**A**) and axial (**B**) T2-weighted images demonstrate a multiseptate cystic mass (*arrows*) arising from coccyx with an intrapelvic component.

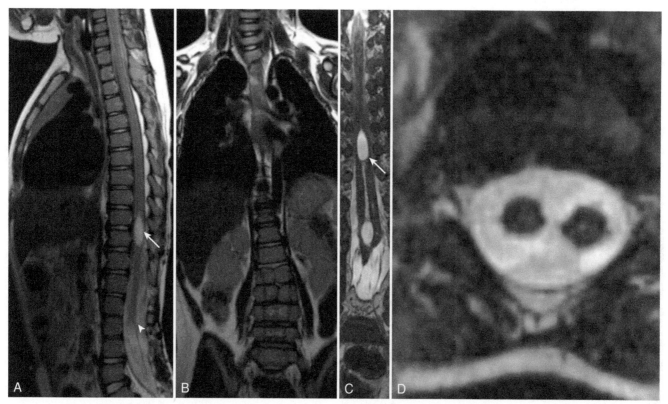

Figure 9.9 Diastematomyelia. Sagittal (**A**) and coronal (**B**) T2-weighted images showing hydromyelia of lower thoracic spinal cord (*arrow*), truncation of the conus medullaris (*arrowhead*), and segmentation anomalies of the lumbar spine. Coronal (**C**) and axial (**D**) constructive interference in steady-state images demonstrates splitting of the spinal cord into two hemicords below the thoracic hydromyelia (*arrow*).

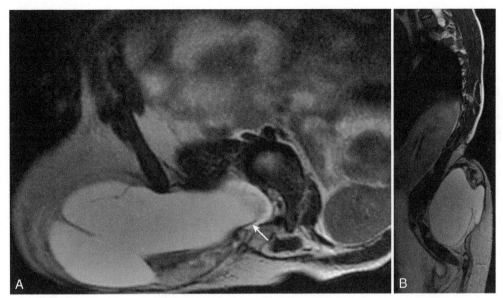

Figure 9.10 Terminal myelocystocele. Axial (**A**) and sagittal (**B**) T2-weighted images demonstrate cystic dilatation of the central canal with stretching and thinning of the distal posterior spinal cord parenchyma (*arrow*).

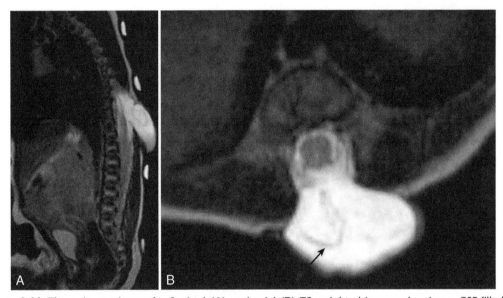

Figure 9.11 Thoracic meningocele. Sagittal (**A**) and axial (**B**) T2-weighted images showing a CSF-filled sac lined by dura and arachnoid. The meningocele contains thin septations (*arrow*) but no neural tissue.

Idiopathic scoliosis (IS) is divided into three subcategories based on patient age: (1) infantile onset IS affects patients younger than 3 years; (2) juvenile onset IS occurs in children between 3 and 10 years of age, and (3) adolescent onset IS occurs in skeletally immature patients older than 10 years. Adolescent onset IS accounts for approximately 90% of cases of idiopathic scoliosis in children. The complications of IS include curve progression, cardiopulmonary compromise, painful curves, cosmetic deformity, neurologic dysfunction, and degenerative joint disease. Curve progression usually occurs during periods of growth acceleration. Treatment may be required and involves bracing or surgical instrumentation and fusion (eg, Harrington rods).

CR represents the gold standard in confirming the diagnosis and surveillance of IS. CT may be required for a preoperative evaluation [**Fig. 9.12**]. The prevalence rate of CNS abnormalities in patients with IS is between 2% and 4%. The presence of an atypical curve pattern (left thoracic, absence of thoracic apical segment lordosis), abnormal neurologic finding (hyperreflexia, asymmetric deep tendon reflexes, urinary dysfunction, diminished rectal tone, or skin lesions over the lower back), and infantile or juvenile onset of scoliosis should prompt evaluation with MRI. MRI can show underlying abnormalities such as hydrosyringomyelia, tumor, cyst, or skin-covered spinal dysraphisms.

Congenital Scoliosis and Kyphosis

Congenital scoliosis occurs because of the presence of an underlying vertebral malformation. Vertebral malformations include hemivertebrae, vertebral bar (an abnormality of vertebral separation during development), butterfly vertebrae, and wedge-shaped vertebrae. Vertebral malformations may (1) present as an isolated finding; (2) occur in association with renal, cardiac, or spinal cord malformations; or (3) occur as part of an underlying

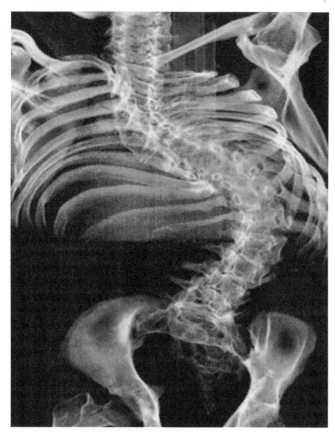

Figure 9.12 Idiopathic scoliosis. CR image shows severe S-shaped scoliosis and resultant chest cage deformity.

syndrome or chromosomal abnormality [**Fig. 9.13**]. Common syndromes associated with vertebral malformations are summarized in **Table 9.1**. Other causes of kyphosis and kyphoscoliosis in childhood are postural, Scheuermann disease, neuromuscular disorder, trauma, inflammation, surgery, radiation therapy, metabolic disorders, arthritis, and tumor.

Scheuermann Disease

Scheuermann disease occurs in adolescents, is characterized by painful, fixed, dorsal kyphosis, and consists of wedged vertebrae with disturbances of the vertebral endplates. Typical radiographic findings are vertebral wedging, irregular vertebral endplate, and Schmorl nodes (intraosseous disk herniation). The kyphosis commonly occurs in the midthoracic spine.

Neurofibromatosis Type 1

NF-1 is an autosomal dominant condition caused by heterozygous mutations of the *NF1* gene. Scoliosis is present in approximately 10% to 20% of children with NF-1. Scoliosis has been postulated to occur because of mesodermal dysplasia. Spinal lesions that may occur in NF-1 include spinal meningoceles, dural ectasia, and tumors (isolated and plexiform neurofibromas) [**Fig. 9.14**]. Other anomalies include cervical kyphosis, hypoplasia of the spinous process, transverse process, or pedicle, and twisted-ribbon ribs.

Achondroplasia

Achondroplasia is a skeletal dysplasia caused by gain-of-function mutations in the *FGFR3* gene. The phenotype is characterized

by disproportionately short stature with rhizomelic shortening of the extremities and results from defective formation of endochondral bones. Macrocephaly, hydrocephalus, and craniocervical junction (CCJ) compression are the major neurologic complications in children with achondroplasia. Spinal stenosis is a frequent finding in achondroplasia [**Fig. 9.15**]. Premature fusion of the ossification centers of the vertebral bodies and posterior neural arches results in laminae and pedicles that are short and thick. In addition, the reduced vertebral body height, vertebral body scalloping, and reduced interpedicular distance may cause narrowing of the spinal canal or neural foramina. Scoliosis, kyphosis, or kyphoscoliosis occurs in about one-third of patients with achondroplasia. Other craniocervical abnormalities include odontoid hypoplasia, AA instability, basilar impression, and occipitalization of the atlas.

Mucopolysaccharidosis

MPSs are a group of metabolic disorders characterized by the accumulation of glycosaminoglycans (GAGs), caused by enzyme deficiencies in the lysosomal metabolism of these normal cellular by-products. Spinal cord compression at the occipitocervical junction is common in MPS. Spinal stenosis results from GAG accumulation behind the odontoid process, dural thickening, and C1 ring hypoplasia. In addition, GAG accumulation in soft tissues may facilitate AA instability [**Fig. 9.16**]. Skeletal features include pectus carinatum, thoracolumbar kyphosis, scoliosis, genu valgus, platyspondyly, anterior vertebral body beaking, flaring of the ribs, and joint hypermobility.

Down Syndrome

Down syndrome, caused by trisomy of chromosome 21, is the most common inherited chromosomal disorder, with an estimated incidence of 1 in 700 live births. AA instability is frequently encountered in children with Down syndrome and is postulated to be related to excessive ligamentous laxity of the transverse ligaments at the C1-C2 articulation. In addition, osseous abnormalities such as os odontoideum, odontoid hypoplasia, ossiculum terminale, or rotary AA subluxation are common and can contribute to instability as well [**Fig. 9.17**]. The atlantodens interval (ADI) is measured between the posterior surface of the anterior arch of C1 and the anterior surface of the dens. In healthy children, an ADI of 4 to 5 mm is considered the upper limit of normal. Screening for cervical instability may be performed with CR. If the ADI is greater than 5 mm on cervical CR, MRI should be obtained to assess for evidence of spinal cord injury.

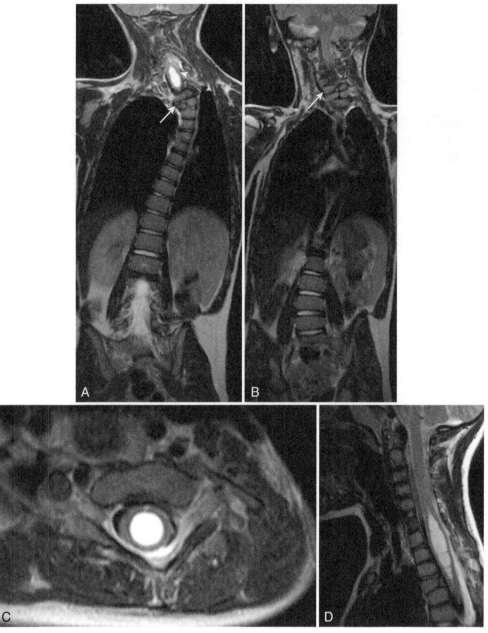

Figure 9.13 Congenital scoliosis. Coronal T2-weighted images (**A, B**) of the spine demonstrate formation and segmentation anomalies with butterfly vertebrae (*arrows*) and hydromyelia (*arrowhead*). Axial and sagittal T2-weighted images (**C, D**) of the cervical spine demonstrate hydromyelia.

Spondyloepiphyseal Dysplasia

SED is characterized by abnormal growth of the spinal vertebrae and epiphysis. There are two major types: congenita and tarda. In the congenita form there is dwarfism, thoracolumbar kyphosis, lumbar lordosis, platyspondyly, and odontoid hypoplasia with AA instability [**Fig. 9.18**]. The tarda form of SED consists of platyspondyly, dwarfism, and early degenerative spine and hip disease.

Craniocervical Junction Anomalies

The CCJ consists of the complex articulation of the atlas (C1), occiput, and axis (C2), established by the atlantooccipital (AO) and AA joints. Imaging evaluation of this region typically requires

CR including flexion-extension radiographs and is supplemented as needed by fluoroscopy, CT, and MRI.

A number of landmarks may be helpful in evaluating the CCJ. Chamberlain's line extends from the posterior margin of the hard palate to the opisthion (posterior margin of the foramen magnum). The tip of the odontoid process normally lies below Chamberlain's line. The predental space or atlantodental distance in infants and young children (anterior atlas–dens gap) varies from 3 to a maximum of 5 mm in flexion with a 2-mm excursion from extension to flexion. The gap is normally less than 3 mm in adolescents and adults. The postdental space (dens–posterior atlas gap or dens–posterior foramen magnum gap) is at least 15 mm in children and 19 mm in adults. The dens tip should align with tip of the clivus (basion), and these two structures should not be separated by more than 1 cm.

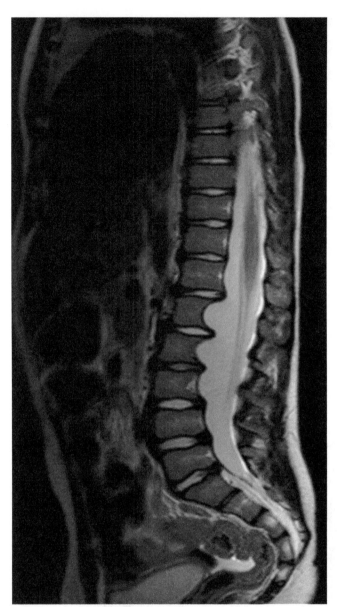

Figure 9.14 Neurofibromatosis type I. Lumbar dural ectasia with dorsal scalloping of multiple vertebral bodies.

Common anomalies of the CCJ include basiocciput hypoplasia, occipitalization of the atlas, Klippel-Feil anomaly, odontoid anomalies, and CCJ instability. CCJ anomalies may manifest clinically with torticollis, craniofacial or craniocervical dysmorphism, limitation of motion, headache, or neck pain.

Basiocciput Hypoplasia

Basiocciput hypoplasia, also referred to as "basilar invagination" or "short clivus," is the superior displacement of the odontoid relative to Chamberlain's line. Basiocciput hypoplasia may be associated with occipital condyle hypoplasia [**Fig. 9.19**]. Basilar invagination may be (1) primary (ie, developmental) and associated with other craniocervical anomalies or syndromes, or (2) secondary (ie, basilar impression) and associated with osteochondral dysplasias or metabolic disorders (eg, rickets, fibrous dysplasia, achondroplasia, the MPSs, osteogenesis imperfecta, osteomalacia, cleidocranial dysplasia). Vascular or neural compromise may occur depending on the severity of basilar invagination.

Occipitalization of the Atlas

The failure of segmentation between the fourth occipital sclerotome and the first cervical sclerotome results in atlanto-occipital (AO) nonsegmentation/assimilation or fusion, also known as occipitalization of the atlas. The fusion may be limited to the anterior arch, the posterior arch, the lateral masses, or a combination of all three. The lack of mobility at the AO junction related to abnormal fusion results in the C1-2 articulation becoming the sole mobile segment of the upper cervical spine. C1-2 instability occurs in 50% of patients. Fusion between the anterior atlas arch and the clivus or opisthion often results in a characteristic "comma-shaped" configuration. Basilar invagination and dorsal displacement of the odontoid process typically occurs resulting in a decreased anterior-posterior dimension of the foramen magnum and compression of the underlying cervicomedullary junction.

Klippel-Feil Syndrome and Segmentation Anomalies

The triad of clinical findings in Klippel-Feil syndrome (KFS) consists of short neck, low hairline, and limited neck mobility. KFS results from failure of segmentation and manifests as bony fusion of the cervical spine at one or more levels [**Fig. 9.20**]. Other CCJ anomalies including basilar invagination, odontoid hypoplasia, AO assimilation, and platybasia are often present. In addition, cardiovascular, genitourinary, and other congenital anomalies may be associated with KFS and may result in significant morbidity.

Odontoid Anomalies

Odontoid anomalies include aplasia, hypoplasia, and os odontoideum. Odontoid hypoplasia is uncommon and has been reported in association with SED, MPS, Down syndrome, and metatropic dwarfism. Odontoid aplasia is rare. The absence of apical and alar ligaments in odontoid hypoplasia and aplasia predisposes to severe AA instability and resultant cervical cord compression.

The term *os odontoideum* refers to an independent proatlas remnant/ossicle located cephalad to the body of the axis [**Fig. 9.21**]. One theory for the development of an os odontoideum is underrecognized cervical trauma between 1 and 4 years of age. In os odontoideum there is odontoid hypoplasia, with an ossicle located between the dens tip and the basion. The interspace between the ossicle and the axis body extends above the level of the superior articular facets, resulting in incompetence of the cruciate ligament, and AA instability is common. The os may be discovered incidentally or associated with symptoms of CCJ compression. The nature and degree of instability must be carefully assessed with flexion and extension examinations. The osseous relationships are best demonstrated using flexion and extension plain radiographs or CT while the effect of instability on the cervicomedullary junction is best assessed with MRI. There is an increased incidence of os odontoideum in association with Down syndrome, MPS, SED, and KFS.

Craniocervical Junction Instability

CCJ instability includes translational or rotary AA instability and AO instability. CCJ instability often results from ligamentous deficiency or insufficiency (eg, transverse ligament in AA instability). Odontoid anomalies are commonly associated with CCJ instability. AA and AO instabilities most commonly occur with Down syndrome. Other common causes are the skeletal dysplasias (eg, Morquio syndrome or SED), rheumatoid arthritis, and trauma. Rotary AA instability includes displacement, subluxation, or dislocation and produces torticollis [**Fig. 9.22**]. Rotary instability may be spontaneous or related to trauma, infection, or CCJ anomalies (eg, odontoid anomalies or Klippel-Feil anomaly).

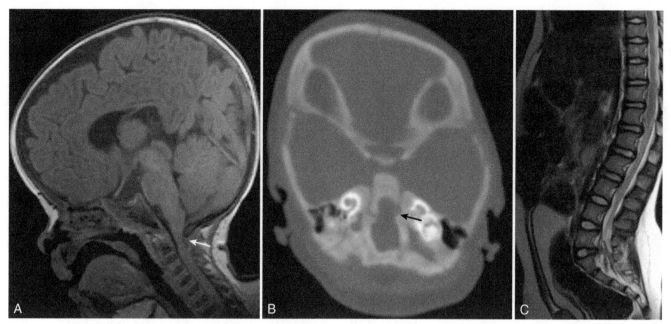

Figure 9.15 Achondroplasia. Macrocephaly, foramen magnum and upper cervical spinal canal stenosis, and cervicomedullary compression (*arrow*) are shown in the sagittal T1-weighted image (**A**). Axial computed tomography image (**B**) demonstrates narrowing of the foramen magnum (*arrow*), and sagittal T2-weighted image of thoracolumbar spine (**C**) shows mild spinal canal stenosis with scalloping of the posterior aspect of the vertebral bodies.

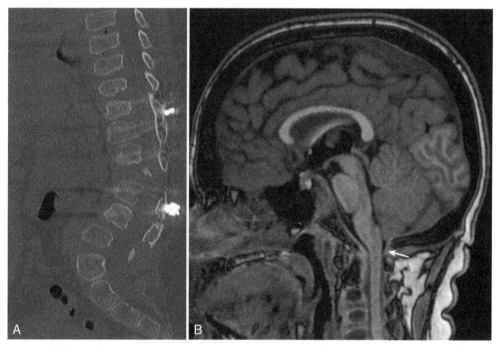

Figure 9.16 Hurler syndrome. A, Sagittal multiplanar reconstruction computed tomography image in bone kernel demonstrates flattened appearance with inferior beaking of multiple lumbar vertebral bodies and a focal gibbus deformity that has required posterior spinal fusion. **B,** Sagittal T1-weighted image shows narrowing of the craniocervical junction (*arrow*).

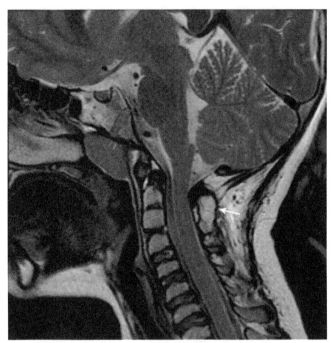

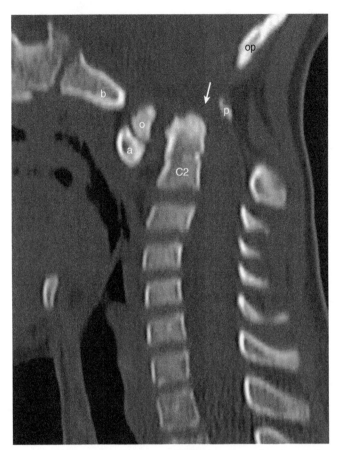

Figure 9.17 Down syndrome. Sagittal computed tomography image demonstrates odontoid hypoplasia (*C2*), os odontoideum (*o*) and marked spinal canal stenosis at C1-C2 (*arrow*). *a*, anterior arch of atlas; *b*, basion; *op*, opisthion; *p*, posterior arch of atlas.

Spinal Vascular Anomalies

Vascular anomalies include vascular tumors, such as hemangioma and vascular malformations. Vascular malformations are categorized based on their hemodynamics into "high flow" and "low flow" lesions. High flow lesions include arteriovenous fistula (AVF) in which there is a direct connection between an artery and a vein and arteriovenous malformation (AVM) in which there is a tangle of dysplastic vessels, termed the "nidus" interposed between the supplying artery and draining vein. Low-flow lesions include venous, lymphatic and capillary malformations.

Spinal arteriovenous lesions are rare in children and are often congenital or associated with underlying genetic disorders. Several classification systems have been proposed. Location and shunt morphology have the greatest influence on treatment implications. AVF and AVM may be associated with genetic conditions such as hereditary hemorrhagic telangiectasia (HHT) and nonhereditary conditions, such as Parkes Weber syndrome, neurofibromatosis I, and Ehlers-Danlos syndrome type IV.

In AVF and AVM the abnormal communication may occur within the substance of the spinal cord (intramedullary), along the surface of the spinal cord (perimedullary), or within the dura (dural) or may involve all layers of a spinal segment (metameric). Metameric lesions without soft tissue overgrowth are seen in patients with Cobb syndrome. Segmental vascular anomalies, including both AVM and lymphatic, or capillary malformation may be seen in patients with Congenital Lipomatous Overgrowth, Vascular Malformations, Epidermal Nevi, and Scoliosis/Skeletal anomalies (CLOVES) syndrome. The initial imaging

Figure 9.18 Spondyloepiphyseal dysplasia. Sagittal T2-weighted image of the cervical spine showing odontoid hypoplasia, platyspondyly, and posterior fusion of C1-C3 vertebral bodies (*arrow*).

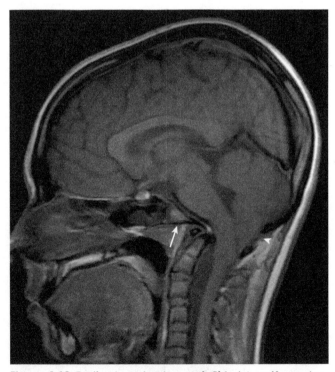

Figure 9.19 Basilar invagination and Chiari I malformation. Sagittal T1-weighted image showing a horizontal short clivus (*arrow*), superiorly displaced odontoid process (above Chamberlain's line), and inferior cerebellar tonsillar descent (*arrowhead*).

evaluation of spinal vascular anomalies is often with MRI. Prominent and tortuous flow voids representing congested dilated veins are seen on standard spin-echo and high-resolution steady-state Constructive Interference in Steady State (CISS)/Fast Imaging Employing Steady State Acquisition (FIESTA) pulse sequences [**Fig. 9.23**] in high flow anomalies. In addition, the

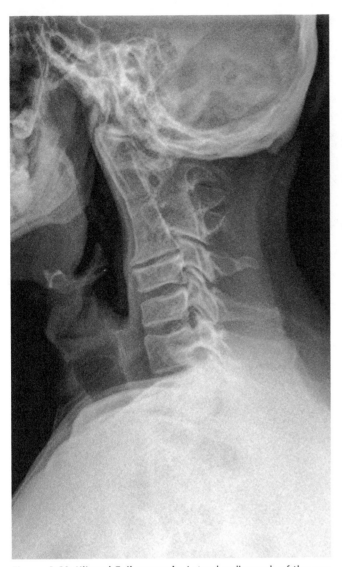

Figure 9.20 **Klippel-Feil anomaly.** Lateral radiograph of the cervical spine showing fusion of the C1-C3 vertebral bodies and basilar invagination.

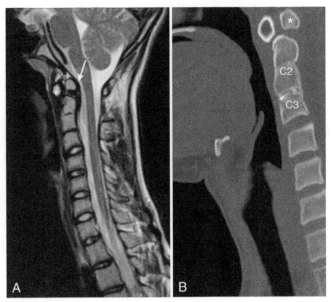

Figure 9.21 **Os odontoideum.** Sagittal T2-weighted image (**A**) of the cervical spine shows ossicle cephalad to C2 vertebral body (*arrow*), and corresponding CT image (**B**) demonstrates a well-corticated ossicle (*asterisk*). Incidental note is made of partial fusion of C2 and C3 vertebral bodies.

spinal cord parenchyma should be assessed for presence of edema related to venous hypertension or hemorrhage on the T1- and T2-weighted images. Spinal angiography is considered the gold standard diagnostic imaging modality for high flow vascular lesions of the spine and may also be performed with the intent of endovascular treatment of the anomaly. Selective injections of all feeding pedicles and analysis of the draining veins is essential in the assessment and treatment planning of AVMs.

TRAUMA

Spinal trauma in children is different from that seen in adults for several reasons. The immature spine contains regions of unossified cartilage and lax ligaments which results in less frequent vertebral body fractures and more frequent dislocations, ligamentous injuries, and epiphyseal detachments than are seen in adults. In addition, the disproportionately large head to torso ratio in infants and young children, shallow occipital condyles, and relatively horizontal orientation of the facet joints render the CCJ and upper cervical spine more vulnerable to sudden acceleration and deceleration forces. Pediatric spinal injury occurs most often in the cervical spine. In children younger than 8 years, the C1, C2, and C3 vertebral bodies are the most

often involved. The fulcrum of flexion shifts caudally from C2/3 to C5/6 as the child ages. After the age of 10 years, an adult distribution of injury is noted, affecting predominantly the cervicothoracic junction. Also in older children, similar to in adult patients, the thoracic spine is less frequently affected due to the stabilizing effects of the adjacent rib cage. Hyperflexion, hyperextension, axial compression, distraction, and translational or rotation forces are potential mechanisms in isolation or combination for causing spinal injury. In a child presenting with spine injury, CR may be performed initially with the patient properly immobilized. CT with sagittal and coronal reformatting is often helpful to further assess the injury. MRI is used to assess for ligamentous injury, intraspinal hematoma, or spinal cord injury. Occasionally, it may be difficult to differentiate between an anterior wedging of the vertebral bodies as a normal developmental variant especially at the thoracolumbar junction and a wedge compression fracture. When an acute wedge fracture cannot be distinguished from a normal variant on CR or CT, an MR showing bone marrow edema and/or paravertebral soft tissue edema can confirm acute injury.

Spine Fractures

Cervical Spine

A Jefferson fracture is a burst fracture of C1 resulting from an axial compression from a fall onto the head (eg, diving accidents), whereas anterior and posterior arch fractures of C1 typically result from C1/2 hyperextension. Fractures of C2 include the Anderson fracture which typically occurs after hyperflexion and a "hangman" fracture that results from hyperextension [**Figs. 9.24** and **9.25**]. Compression fractures (C3-C7) typically result from hyperflexion and present with anterior wedging of the vertebral bodies.

Thoracic and Lumbar Spine

In children older than 10 years, the predominant location of spinal injuries is in the thoracic and lumbar spine. Fractures are typically seen at the thoracolumbar junction and in the region of the lumbar spine. Thoracic and lumbar fractures include (1) lateral

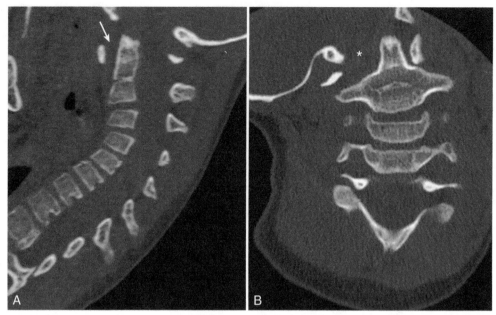

Figure 9.22 Severe torticollis. Sagittal reformatted computed tomography (CT) image of the cervical spine in bone kernel (**A**) shows widening of the atlantodens interval (*arrow*) and atlantooccipital distance. Coronal CT reformat (**B**) shows widening of the space (*asterisk*) between the right lateral mass of C2 and the odontoid process.

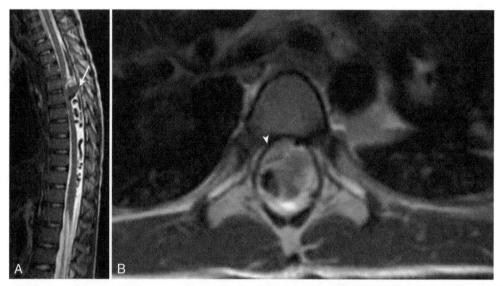

Figure 9.23 Dorsal perimedullary arteriovenous fistula. Sagittal T2-weighted (**A**) and axial T2-weighted (**B**) images of the thoracic spine showing prominent flow voids dorsally in the thecal sac (*arrow*) with anterior and right lateral displacement of the thoracic spinal cord (*arrowhead*).

shear-translation fractures; (2) compression fractures (typically from falls); (3) burst fractures; (4) Chance fracture (flexion-distraction injury); and (5) focal, direct impact fractures. Compression fractures are characterized by a wedge-shaped deformity of the involved vertebral body with interruption of the anterior vertebral contour and are typically stable if they involve the anterior column only. Burst fractures may occur from a combination of axial, flexion, or lateral forces resulting in a fracture of both the anterior and the posterior aspect of the vertebral body. Burst fractures may be unstable when there is posterior column disruption and may cause compromise of the spinal canal and compression of the spinal cord. Chance fracture in the lumbar region is characterized by a transverse or oblique fracture with involvement of all three longitudinal vertebral columns. Chance fracture results from a combined flexion-distraction mechanism around a

fulcrum, most commonly a seat belt, and is consequently also known as seat belt or lap belt fracture. The anterior vertebral body is typically compressed, whereas the posterior vertebral body height is increased by the distraction component of the injury [**Fig. 9.26**]. The posterior distracting forces increase the interspinous distance and widen the facet joints. Additional injuries to abdominal structures may occur including pancreatic fracture, duodenal wall hematoma, or stomach rupture and may be partially included on imaging directed to the spine.

Spine Ligamentous Injury

On CR and CT, spinal alignment may be preserved in mild injuries even with stretched or torn ligaments occurring as a result of both accidental and inflicted trauma. Alternatively, CR

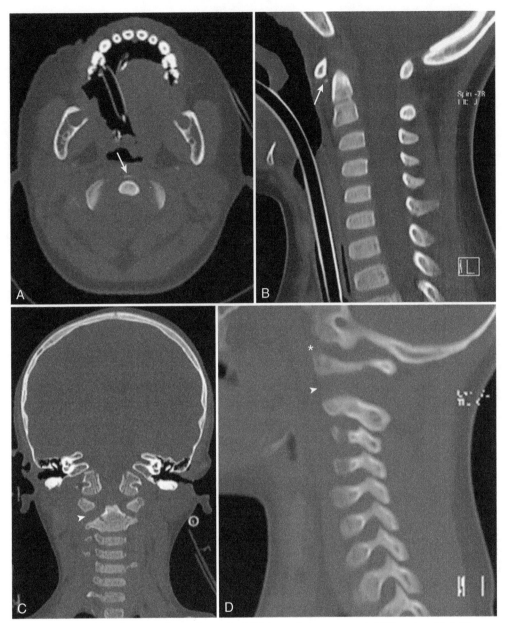

Figure 9.24 Small avulsion fracture of anterior arch of C1 (*arrow*) shown on axial (**A**) and sagittal (**B**) computed tomography (CT) images. Coronal (**C**) and sagittal (**D**) CT images demonstrate associated widening of the right atlantooccipital (*asterisk*) and atlantoaxial (*arrowheads*) articulations.

and CT may demonstrate straightening of the physiologic cervical lordosis (guarding) and mild paravertebral edema or an epidural, retroclival, or intraspinal hematoma [**Fig. 9.27**]. MRI may show increased signal due to edema within the injured ligaments on both T2-weighted and STIR imaging. A high-resolution 3D T2-weighted CISS sequence may directly show the interruption/disruption of the injured ligaments and is particularly useful in evaluating the soft tissue structures at the craniocervical and C1-2 junction (eg, transverse, alar and apical ligaments). These high resolution sequences are also useful in identifying individual nerve root injuries when present. Due to the high mobility and flexibility of the pediatric spine, subluxation of the facet joints may be transient, and evidence of injury may be lacking on CR and CT. MRI is extremely helpful in this scenario in demonstrating the soft tissue and ligamentous injury that is not evident on CR and CT.

In more severe injury to the cervical spine, axial dislocation of C1 in relation to the occiput (atlanto-occipital dislocation) or

between C1 and C2 (atlanto-axial dislocation) may occur (see **Fig. 9.24**). Anterior dislocations are more common than posterior dislocations. The facets as well as the occipital condyles should be carefully evaluated for fractures associated with the dislocation. The most severe form of significant axial/vertical AO dislocation is known as AO dissociation [**Fig. 9.28**]. AO dissociation typically occurs in high-speed motor vehicle accidents and is characterized by a complete rupture of the ligaments between the occiput and C1/C2 with "separation" of the spinal column from the skull. The spinal cord is usually severely injured or may even be transected in these patients.

Spinal Cord Injury

SCIWORA (spinal cord injury without radiographic abnormality) is defined as objective signs of spinal cord injury without evidence of ligamentous injury or fractures on CR or CT. The presence of neurologic deficit should prompt an evaluation with MRI

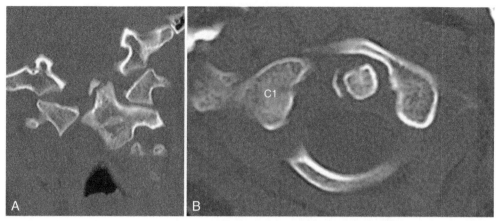

Figure 9.25 Odontoid fracture with rotatory subluxation of C1 on C2 is demonstrated on coronal (**A**) and axial (**B**) computed tomography images.

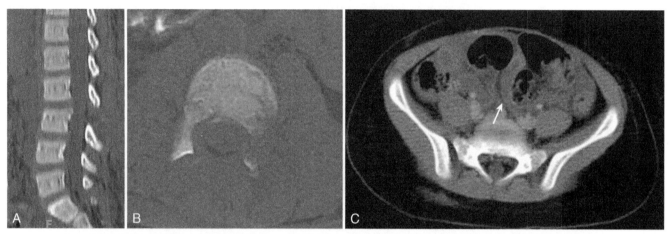

Figure 9.26 Chance fracture. Sagittal reformatted (**A**) and axial (**B**) computed tomography (CT) images demonstrate a fracture of the L3 with compression of the vertebral body and distraction of the posterior elements consistent with a Chance fracture. Axial CT image of the abdomen (**C**) in soft tissue window demonstrates a bowel wall hematoma (*arrow*).

to search for evidence of spinal cord injury. Acute spinal cord injury includes contusion, hemorrhage, edema, avulsion, and transection. Chronic sequelae, such as a posttraumatic cyst, syringomyelia, or myelomalacia, are also best evaluated with MRI.

Spondylolysis and Spondylolisthesis

The most common causes of back pain in children over the age of ten years are spondylolysis and spondylolisthesis. Spondylolysis is a defect in the pars interarticularis, and most commonly affects the L5 or less often L4 or higher level. Spondylolysis is more common in boys. Most cases in children are believed to be due to a fatigue or stress fracture of the pars interarticularis. Spondylolysis is especially common in athletes participating in sports involving repetitive extension, flexion, and rotation. Spondylolisthesis, or the displacement of one vertebral body relative to another, occurs in the presence of bilateral pars defects and is characterized by the anterior translation of the rostral vertebra over the next caudal segment. The extent of slippage may be assigned as Meyerding grade 1 (up to 33%), grade 2 (up to 66%), grade 3 (up to 99%), or grade 4 (100% with spondyloptosis). CR may establish the diagnosis of spondylolysis, especially on oblique views that show the typical "Scottie dog" with the collar sign. However, the pars interarticularis may lie oblique to the obtained planes, and the fracture may not be apparent on a plain

radiograph. CT readily demonstrates the fracture line, and sagittal reconstructions show the presence or absence of spondylolisthesis [**Fig. 9.29**]. Due to concerns about the potential deleterious effects of ionizing radiation, MRI is often used to assess for evidence of acute injury to the pars which is apparent as marrow edema in the pars and adjacent pedicle. The fracture line of spondylolysis is usually more difficult to reliably demonstrate with MRI than with CT although MRI is especially helpful in showing exiting nerve root compression due to disk uncovering in cases with associated spondylolisthesis.

Lumbar Disk Herniation

Lumbar disk herniation is extremely uncommon prior to adolescence and usually results from trauma (eg, athletic activity). Children with disk herniation may have minimal back pain and may not have a radiculopathy. MRI is the imaging modality of choice in symptomatic patients. Lumbar disk herniation associated with a slipped vertebral apophysis is best demonstrated by CT [**Fig. 9.30**].

INFECTION

Infection may involve the intervertebral disk, vertebral body, paravertebral soft tissues, epidural space, meninges, or spinal neuraxis.

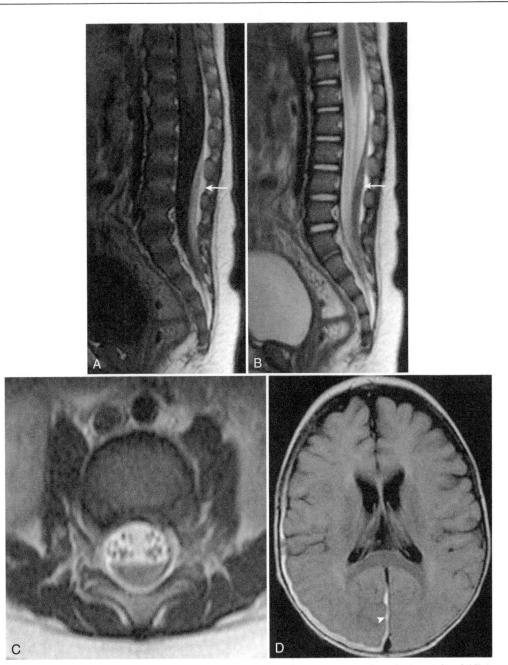

Figure 9.27 Neonate with nonaccidental injury. Sagittal T1- (**A**), T2- (**B**), and axial T2-weighted (**C**) images of the lumbar spine showing T1 hyperintense (*arrow*) and T2 hypointense (*arrow*) hemorrhage within the dorsal, dependent lower part of the thecal sac. **D,** Axial fluid-attenuated inversion recovery image of the brain shows a hyperintense right panhemispheric subdural hematoma (*arrowhead*).

Infectious Diskitis, Spondylitis, or Spondylodiskitis

Spondylodiskitis most often affects children between the age of two and eight years and typically involves the lumbar or lumbosacral spine. The predominant source of spinal infection in children is hematogenous dissemination (arterial or venous, via the paravertebral Batson plexus). Direct inoculation (postsurgical) or spread from contiguous structures is less frequent. Intervertebral disks are highly vascularized in children and, therefore, susceptible to hematogenous spread of infection. The portion of the disk adjacent to the vertebral body endplates may be the first to be inflamed. *Staphylococcus aureus* is the most common organism. Isolated vertebral osteomyelitis in children is relatively rare, however, accompanying vertebral end plate involvement

(ie, osteomyelitis or spondylodiskitis) in the setting of diskitis is common. CR has a very low sensitivity and specificity for diagnosis of early diskitis. MRI is the imaging modality of choice. The intervertebral disk is hyperintense on T2-weighted images due to inflammatory edema. The bone marrow is also typically edematous as evidenced by T1 and T2 prolongation [**Fig. 9.31**]. Fat suppressed T2-weighted or STIR images show the marrow edema to good advantage. The utilization of gadolinium contrast further improves the visualization of the affected vertebral endplates, disk, and paraspinal soft tissues. There may be an associated epidural or paraspinal abscess.

Granulomatous spondylitis usually results from *Mycobacterium tuberculosis,* relatively uncommon in North America and Europe, but more common in other regions of the world. Thoracolumbar involvement is common and may be primary or

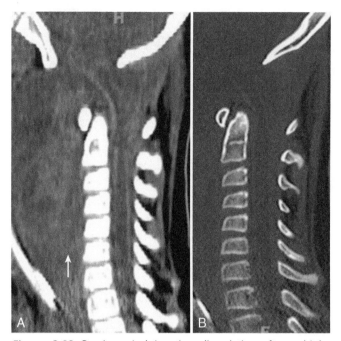

Figure 9.28 Craniocervical junction dissociation after a high-speed motor vehicle accident. Sagittal computed tomography images in soft tissue (**A**) and bone (**B**) kernels demonstrate marked separation of the craniocervical junction and a large prevertebral hematoma (*arrow*).

secondary (spread from other organs). Insidious onset and gradual progression are characteristic. Imaging may show anterior vertebral erosion or extensive vertebral destruction, with or without disk loss, paraspinal masses (granuloma or abscess), and calcification. Progression to kyphosis with gibbus deformity may also occur.

Epidural Abscess

Spinal epidural abscess is a rare condition in children that is most frequently caused by *Staphylococcus aureus,* and is most often hematogenous in origin, although it may arise from direct extension of suppurative spondylitis. MRI is the imaging modality of choice and shows a collection that is T2 hyperintense and T1 hypointense with rim enhancement [**Fig. 9.32**]. Diffusion weighted imaging shows decreased diffusion within the abscess. Paravertebral soft tissue edema and enhancement may extend over several segments. Diffuse homogeneous enhancement suggests phlegmon.

Meningitis

Bacterial, fungal, viral, or parasitic organisms may cause meningitis. The majority of cases are bacterial. MRI may demonstrate nonspecific, linear, or nodular gadolinium enhancement of the meninges, spinal cord, or nerve roots.

Arachnoiditis

Arachnoiditis may occur after infection, subarachnoid hemorrhage, intraspinal injection (eg, for anesthesia or chemotherapy),

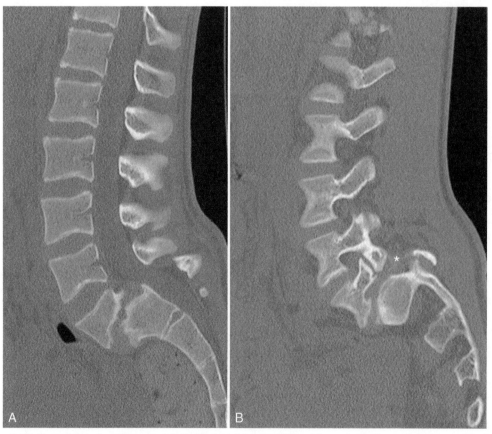

Figure 9.29 Spondylolysis with spondylolisthesis. Midsagittal (**A**) and parasagittal computed tomography (**B**) images in bone kernel demonstrate grade 3 spondylolisthesis of L5 over S1 with a pars interarticularis defect (*asterisk*).

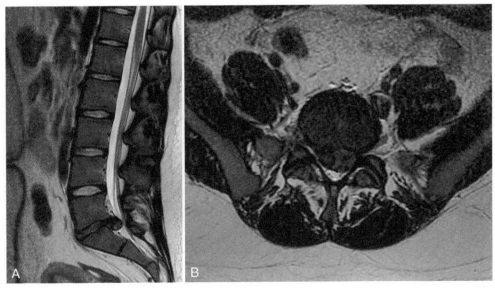

Figure 9.30 Lumbar disk herniation. Sagittal (**A**) and axial T2-weighted (**B**) images demonstrate a disk extrusion at L5-S1 level with near-complete infilling of bilateral lateral recesses, left greater than right, and effacement of the thecal sac.

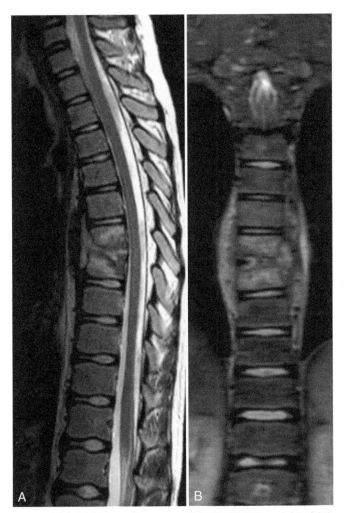

Figure 9.31 Diskitis and osteomyelitis. Sagittal T2-weighted (**A**) and coronal short tau inversion recovery (**B**) images demonstrate destruction of T7-T8 intervertebral disk with abnormal marrow signal in the adjacent vertebral bodies and associated paravertebral soft tissue phlegmon.

surgery, or trauma. MRI shows nerve root thickening, often with enhancement, and occasionally a mass-like lesion due to nerve root clumping.

Myelitis or Infectious Myelopathy

Viral or bacterial infection of the spinal cord is rare in the immunocompetent host. Viruses associated with myelitis include herpesvirus, coxsackievirus, poliovirus, and human immunodeficiency virus (HIV) [**Fig. 9.33**], West Nile virus, human T-cell lymphotropic virus, and enteroviruses. MRI findings include intramedullary T2 hyperintensity, spinal cord expansion, and enhancement.

INFLAMMATION

Inflammatory immune-mediated disorders of the spinal cord include idiopathic isolated transverse myelitis (TM), neuromyelitis optica (NMO), and multiple sclerosis (MS). Postinfectious inflammation may present as TM following the resolution of active infection.

Idiopathic Acute Transverse Myelitis

The diagnosis of acute transverse myelitis (ATM) requires both the presence of spinal cord inflammation, as defined by CSF pleocytosis, elevated CSF IgG index, or gadolinium enhancement on a spinal MRI, and the absence of an identified CNS infection. Idiopathic TM also requires exclusion of acute myelopathy secondary to a known underlying disease (MS, NMO, infectious, vascular, or connective tissue disease) or from a compressive myelopathy. MRI demonstrates focal or extensive regions of increased signal on T2-weighted or fluid-attenuated inversion recovery images. Following contrast administration, enhancement may be present. MRI of the brain is required during the initial evaluation to search for clinically silent lesions of MS.

Multiple Sclerosis

Spinal cord involvement may be present in children with polyfocal deficits as their first MS manifestation. MS relapses involving

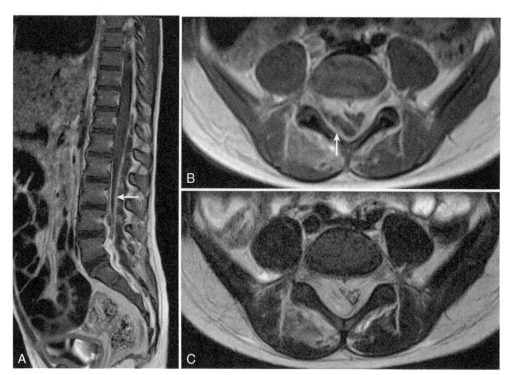

Figure 9.32 Epidural abscess. Sagittal (**A**) and axial (**B**) T1 postcontrast images of the thoracolumbar spine show a peripherally enhancing collection in the epidural space (*arrows*). In addition, axial T2-weighted image (**C**) shows edema and fluid in the epidural space and erector spinae muscles.

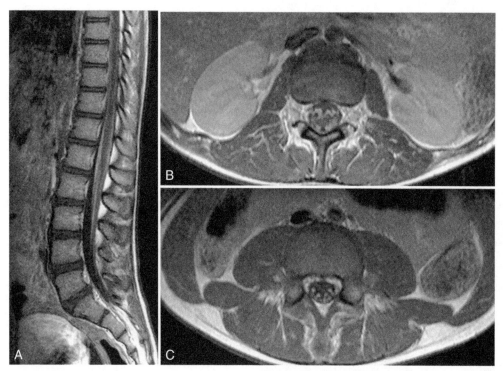

Figure 9.33 HIV polyradiculitis. Sagittal (**A**) and axial (**B, C**) postcontrast T1-weighted images of the lumbar spine demonstrate diffuse smooth thickening and enhancement of the cauda equina nerve roots.

the spinal cord occur in most children and adolescents with active MS. Posterior involvement of the spinal cord or partial myelitis is a typical finding in MS when reviewing the axial plane on MRI [**Fig. 9.34**]. Focal lesions involving fewer than three vertebral body segments in rostral-caudal length are more typical of MS than monophasic idiopathic TM.

Neuromyelitis Optica

NMO is defined by monophasic or recurrent inflammatory demyelination of the optic nerves and spinal cord. The revised criteria for diagnosis now require optic neuritis and TM, as well as two of the following: (1) longitudinally extensive lesions (LETMs);

(2) initial brain MRI nondiagnostic for MS; and (3) seropositivity for NMO IgG. LETMs are defined as lesions extending more than the rostral-caudal length of three spinal vertebral bodies. MRI of the spine typically demonstrates LETMs with T2 hyperintense signal. MRI of the orbits may demonstrate T2 hyperintense signal

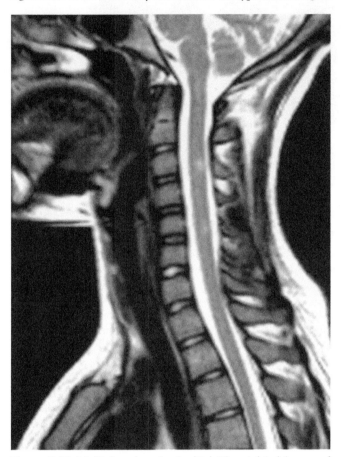

Figure 9.34 Multiple sclerosis. Sagittal T2-weighted image of the cervical spine showing T2 hyperintense lesions at the C3 and C5 levels, consistent with demyelination.

of the optic nerves or chiasm. MRI of the brain may show clinically silent or symptomatic lesions in the hypothalamus, thalamus, peritrigonal white matter, and brainstem.

GUILLAIN BARRE SYNDROME

Guillain Barre Syndrome is an autoimmune disorder resulting in demyelination of peripheral nerves. The cause is unknown although the disorder may occur following viral or bacterial infection. Affected children typically present with muscle weakness and tingling that may progress to disordered breathing and abnormal heart rate. MRI may be useful in aiding in the diagnosis. Noncontrast imaging is most often normal, but the nerve roots of the cauda equine are seen to enhance following the administration of gadolinium.

TUMORS

Spinal tumors may be classified by location as extradural (eg, bone, paraspinal, or parameningeal), intradural extramedullary, or intramedullary (ie, spinal cord).

Extradural

Extradural, or parameningeal, tumors arise from the spinal column or paraspinal soft tissues. These tumors may spread to the spinal canal directly, by epidural venous extension, or by hematogenous, lymphatic, or CSF dissemination. Extradural tumors include benign and malignant primary bone and soft tissue tumors, metastases, and tumor-like conditions of mesenchymal, neural crest, primitive neuroepithelial, origins.

Benign Tumors of Mesenchymal Origin

Osteoid osteoma is a benign tumor with an osteoid matrix and a fibrovascular nidus. Approximately 10% of osteoid osteomas are found in the spine, most frequently within the lumbar spine, and usually, though not exclusively, arise in the posterior elements. CT is the imaging modality of choice. On CT osteoid osteomas present as a well-circumscribed radiolucency with a central calcified nidus and surrounding sclerosis [**Fig. 9.35**]. Osteoid osteoma typically measures less than 2 cm. Increased

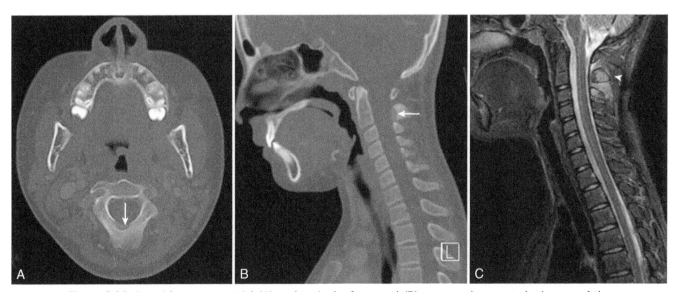

Figure 9.35 Osteoid osteoma. Axial (**A**) and sagittal reformatted (**B**) computed tomography images of the cervical spine in bone kernel demonstrate a well-circumscribed lytic lesion in the right lamina of C2 (*arrows*) with surrounding sclerosis. Sagittal short tau inversion recovery image (**C**) demonstrates edema (*arrowhead*) in the spinous processes of C2 and C3.

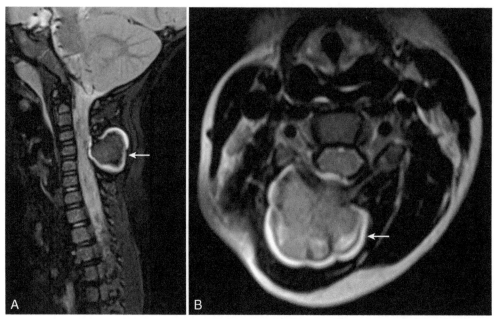

Figure 9.36 Osteochondroma. Sagittal short tau inversion recovery (**A**) and axial T2-weighted (**B**) images of the cervical spine showing a lobulated mass with a hyperintense rim representing the cartilage cap (*arrows*).

radionuclide uptake is seen on bone scan. MRI may show extensive bone edema (T1 hypointense, T2 hyperintense), sclerosis or calcification (T1 and T2 hypointense), and the nidus (T1 isointense to hypointense, T2 hypointense or hyperintense, variable gadolinium enhancement). The lesion may be treated by surgical excision or interventional ablation.

Osteoblastoma, also known as giant osteoid osteoma (>2 cm), has a fibrovascular matrix with sclerotic osteoid mesenchyme and giant cells. Approximately 40% of osteoblastomas arise in the spine (eg, cervical). On CT, the nidus is generally larger than 2 cm. Osteoblastoma typically has less surrounding host bone sclerosis than osteoid osteoma and may have an aggressive appearance, with cortical disruption and soft tissue extension.

Osteochondroma is a benign osteocartilaginous exostosis that occurs rarely in the spine (eg, cervical or thoracic posterior elements). Osteochondromas are usually solitary lesions but may be multiple (eg, hereditary multiple osteochondromas). CR or CT of osteochondroma shows a bony projection with cartilaginous cap. MRI shows associated T1 isointensity or hyperintensity and T2 hyperintensity [**Fig. 9.36**]. Treatment is primarily surgical. Malignant degeneration (eg, osteosarcoma or chondrosarcoma) is indicated by additional soft tissue mass, marrow involvement, a disorganized cap, or increased size or enhancement.

Aneurysmal bone cyst (ABC) is primarily a lesion of the immature skeleton comprised of large blood-filled cavities lined by fibrous components, inflammatory cells, and islands of bone. ABC may occur in other precursor entities (giant cell tumor, fibrous dysplasia, osteoblastoma, chondroblastoma, nonossifying fibroma, or fibrous dysplasia). ABC can be locally aggressive. About 20% of ABCs arise in the spine, where they typically involve the posterior elements of the cervical or thoracic spine. CR or CT shows an expansile lytic lesion with peripheral shell-like calcification and fluid–fluid levels [**Fig. 9.37**]. MRI demonstrates multiple internal septations, fluid–fluid levels, and hemorrhage of varying ages within the mass.

Giant cell tumor is an osteoclastoma composed of multinucleated giant cells, a fibroblastic stroma, and prominent vascularity. It rarely occurs in the spine but may arise in the sacrum. CR or CT shows a lytic, expansile bone lesion breaking through the

cortex. MRI of the mass may demonstrate T1 isointensity or hypointensity, T2 isointensity or hyperintensity, associated hemorrhage or cysts, and gadolinium enhancement.

Malignant Tumors of Mesenchymal Origin

Malignant tumors of mesenchymal origin broadly include the malignant "round cell tumors" of childhood that primarily or secondarily involve the reticuloendothelial system (eg, leukemia, lymphoma, rhabdomyosarcoma, Ewing sarcoma, primitive neuroectodermal tumor, neuroblastoma). Malignant small round cell tumors are characterized by small, round, and relatively undifferentiated cells.

Lymphoma and leukemia represent 40% of pediatric malignancies but have relatively infrequent spinal involvement. Bone marrow infiltration may be focal or diffuse. Chloromas are solid leukemic masses arising from myelogenous stem cells that invade the epidural fat and are usually found in children with acute myelogenous leukemia. CT may demonstrate diffuse bone marrow infiltration as osteopenia, permeative lytic destruction, lucent bands, patchy sclerosis, or a densely sclerotic "ivory" vertebra. MRI shows hypercellular marrow infiltration as T1-hypointensity and T2-hyperintensity with respect to adjacent disks and demonstrates gadolinium enhancement within involved regions. In younger patients, it may be difficult to distinguish tumor infiltration of marrow from hematopoietically active red marrow (also T1 hypointense, T2 isointense to hyperintense, and enhancing) [**Fig. 9.38**]. Marrow invasion may be more reliably determined by MR in older children in whom fatty marrow would normally be present and in children with fatty marrow replacement from radiotherapy. A mottled marrow pattern may represent combined tumor and treatment effects. Fat-suppressed T2-weighted or STIR imaging and fat suppressed, gadolinium-enhanced T1-weighted sequences increase sensitivity and specificity for tumor (ie, marked enhancement).

Rhabdomyosarcoma, one of the most common solid tumors of childhood, frequently occurs in the first decade. This tumor may primarily involve the paraspinal soft tissues or spinal column or may result from lymphatic or hematogenous metastasis to the vertebrae. CR, CT, and MRI findings are similar to those for other round cell tumors.

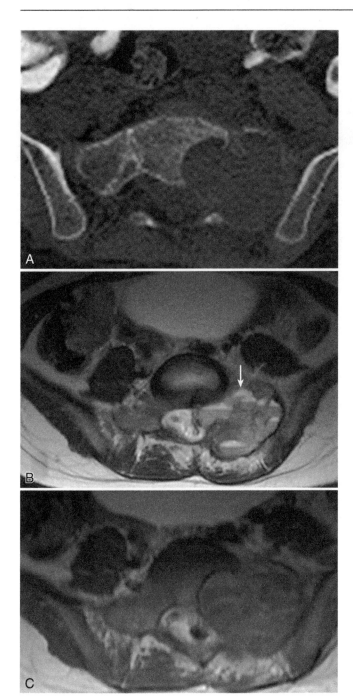

Figure 9.37 Aneurysmal bone cyst. Axial computed tomography image of the sacrum (**A**) in bone kernel demonstrates an expansile lytic lesion centered in the left sacral alum with cortical disruption. Axial T2 (**B**) and T1 postcontrast images (**C**) demonstrate a multilobulated mass with internal fluid levels (*arrow*) and heterogeneous enhancement.

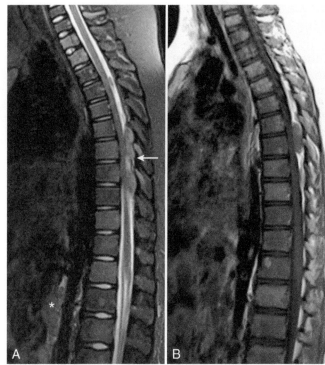

Figure 9.38 Burkitt lymphoma. Sagittal short tau inversion recovery (STIR) (**A**) and T1 postcontrast (**B**) images of the thoracic spine show diffuse replacement of normal marrow with hyperintense signal on STIR and hypointense signal on T1 weighted imaging. The soft tissue epidural mass centered at T7 (*arrow*) causes partial spinal cord compression. There is lymphadenopathy in the paraaortic region (*asterisk*).

Ewing sarcoma is the most common primary malignant spinal bone tumor in children, with up to 10% of all Ewing sarcoma cases presenting as primary spine tumors. However, metastases to spine are more common than is a primary sarcoma of the spine. Ewing frequently presents in the first and second decades of life. The tumor may arise from the bone or from the epidural or paraspinal soft tissues [**Fig. 9.39**]. CR and CT demonstrate permeative and lytic bone destruction. MRI readily defines the extent of the soft tissue component. Ewing sarcoma is typically hypointense on T1-weighted images,

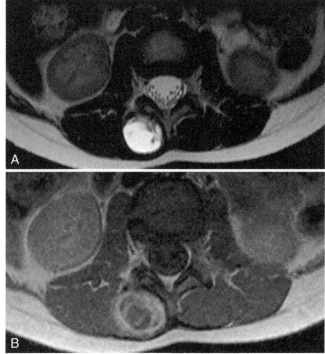

Figure 9.39 Ewing sarcoma. Axial T2 (**A**) and T1 postcontrast (**B**) images showing a hyperintense solid mass with heterogeneous enhancement in the right paraspinal soft tissues.

is hyperintense on T2-weighted images, and demonstrates contrast enhancement.

Other "Malignant" Tumors of Mesenchymal Origin

Osteosarcoma is an osteoid forming neoplasm that is extremely rare in the spine in children. Osteosarcoma of the spine is most often due to metastatic disease. Subtypes include osteoblastic, chondroblastic, telangiectatic, and fibroblastic osteosarcoma. CR or CT may show a lytic, sclerotic, or mixed lesion. MRI is particularly helpful in the evaluation of nonossified soft tissue components, which are typically T1-hypointense and T2-hyperintense. Osseous components are hypointense on most pulse sequences.

Chondrosarcoma is a neoplasm of cartilage origin that may originate de novo or from an existing lesion (eg, osteochondroma). CR or CT typically shows lytic involvement with calcific rings or nodules. MRI may show a heterogeneous pattern of T1 and T2 signal and enhancement.

Chordomas arise from notochordal remnants and most commonly occur in the clivus and sacrum. They are uncommon in the spine in children. CR or CT shows a lytic lesion with calcification and a soft tissue mass. MRI demonstrates T1 isointensity or hypointensity, T2 hyperintensity, and enhancement.

Tumors of Neural Crest Origin

Neuroblastoma is the most common extracranial solid malignancy in infancy and childhood. It arises from neural crest cell derivatives (neuroblasts) of the sympathetic nervous system (eg, paraspinal sympathetic chain, adrenal medulla, carotid body, aortic bodies, and organ of Zuckerkandl). A paraspinal location in the abdomen with epidural and transforaminal extension leading to spinal cord compression is typical in the pediatric population. Spinal osseous involvement is usually attributable to lymphatic or hematogenous seeding. CR or CT may show paraspinal masses often with calcification and bony destruction [**Fig. 9.40**]. MRI may show varying signal intensities related to calcification, hemorrhage, edema, and necrosis and gadolinium enhancement. Radionuclide imaging is also important in defining the extent of disease as neuroblastoma tends to have avid uptake of MIBG (iodine-131-meta-iodobenzylguanidine). Chemotherapy, radiotherapy, and surgical decompression with laminectomy are effective therapeutic options in the treatment of spinal cord compression.

Ganglioneuroblastoma is intermediate in malignancy. It contains both mature ganglion cells and immature neuroblast cells. Its behavior may be similar to that of neuroblastoma, including both metastases and spinal canal extension.

Ganglioneuroma is a benign tumor that consists of mature ganglion cells. It commonly originates in the posterior mediastinum as a paraspinal mass. CR, CT, or MRI show a calcified paraspinal mass with enhancement.

Intradural and Extramedullary

Lesions in an intradural/extramedullary location characteristically displace and compress the spinal cord, expand the ipsilateral thecal sac, and form a "meniscus" sign or interface with the adjacent spinal cord on myelography.

Nerve sheath tumors include neurofibromas and schwannomas. These are benign tumors which are typically associated with neurofibromatosis (NF) 1 (neurofibromas) and NF 2 (schwannomas). CT findings include expansion of the involved neural foramen, osseous erosion, and vertebral body scalloping. On MRI, both schwannomas and neurofibromas are usually T1 isointense and T2 hyperintense, and both demonstrate avid contrast enhancement [**Figs. 9.41** and **9.42**]. Neurofibromas, especially plexiform neurofibromas, may have a T2 hypointense central portion, an imaging finding known as the "target sign."

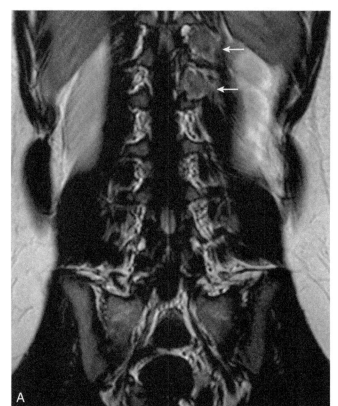

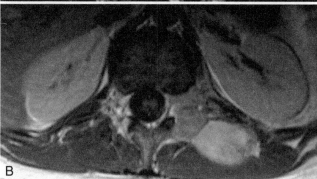

Figure 9.40 Neuroblastoma. Coronal T2 (**A**) and axial T1 postcontrast (**B**) images of the lower thoracic spine demonstrate lobulated soft tissue masses arising from the left T10/T11 and T11/T12 neural foramina (*arrows*) extending to the paraspinous soft tissues.

Meningiomas are rare in pediatric and adolescent patients. NF-2 patients and patients with a history of prior radiation are at increased risk for spinal meningioma. On MRI, meningiomas are most commonly T1 and T2 isointense to spinal cord parenchyma and demonstrate avid, homogenous contrast enhancement.

Myxopapillary ependymoma is considered a benign (World Health Organization grade 1) ependymoma. Myxopapillary ependymomas constitute about 13% of all spinal ependymomas in children and are more common in males. These tumors typically arise from the ependymal glia of the conus medullaris and filum terminale. Depending on the exact location of the tumor, children may present with lower back, leg, or sacral pain muscle weakness, or sphincter dysfunction. Myxopapillary ependymomas typically fill the intradural space, have a lobulated contour, and may result in scalloping of the posterior vertebral bodies. On MRI, they are typically T1 isointense and T2 hyperintense relative to the spinal cord and demonstrate avid enhancement postcontrast [**Fig. 9.43**].

Lipomas and *dermoids* are rare developmental tumors. Lipomas are associated with skin-covered spinal dysraphism, are typically intradural and extramedullary in location, and are located within the dorsal midline lumbosacral spinal canal. Children present with symptoms related to tethering of the spinal cord and a low-lying conus medullaris. On MRI, the signal intensity of a lipoma follows fat on all sequences. Loss of signal on fat suppressed imaging may be helpful in differentiating lipomas from other lesions with intrinsically short T1 such as hemorrhagic or proteinaceous masses which do not lose signal on fat suppressed acquisitions. Dermoids are tumors of ectodermal origin that contain elements of the dermis and epidermis (ie, skin, hair, sweat and sebaceous glands, squamous epithelium). Dermoids are associated with midline closure defects due to ectodermal inclusion at time of closure of the neural tube. They are rare masses that most commonly occur in the lumbosacral region. Dermoids may be associated with dermal sinus tract, spinal cord tethering, abscess, or meningitis. On MRI they may be T1 isointense to hypointense, T2 hyperintense and show decreased diffusion. Occasionally, there is fatlike hyperintensity or calcification. Enhancement may be evident because of inflammation.

Arachnoid cysts are categorized as primary or secondary (eg, postinflammatory). Primary cysts may be intradural or extradural in location, and secondary cysts are usually intradural and associated with arachnoiditis. They usually occur in the thoracic or lumbar region, although they may be seen at any level. There may be scoliosis and spinal canal widening. MRI demonstrates a CSF-intensity cyst that displaces the spinal cord, nerve roots, or epidural fat.

Leptomeningeal metastatic disease commonly occurs with primary CNS neoplasms that are associated with CSF dissemination such as medulloblastoma, ependymoma, choroid plexus tumors, PNET, and high-grade glioma. MRI with gadolinium, the imaging modality of choice, may show single or multiple nodules, diffuse or patchy laminar deposits, irregular nerve root thickening or clumping, or subarachnoid space enhancement.

Intramedullary

Most intramedullary spinal cord neoplasms are glial tumors: astrocytomas (60%) and ependymomas (30%). Nonglial tumors are much less frequent and include a variety of histologic subtypes such as hemangioblastoma, subependymoma, and ganglioglioma.

Spinal cord astrocytomas are the most common spinal cord neoplasm in children. They arise most often in the

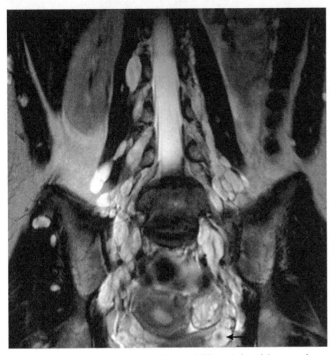

Figure 9.41 Neurofibromas. Coronal T2-weighted image demonstrates multiple neurofibromas along the lumbar and sacral plexus, paravertebral soft tissues, and subcutaneous nerves in this patient with neurofibromatosis type I. Target lesion (*arrow*) with central T2 hypointense component.

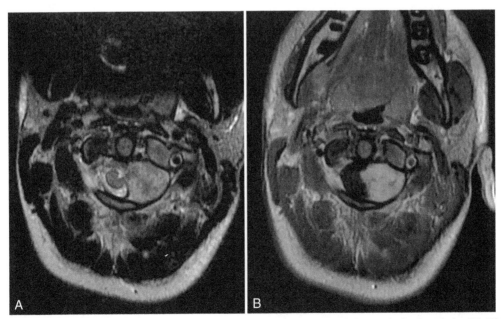

Figure 9.42 Schwannoma. Axial T2 (**A**) and T1 postcontrast (**B**) images of the cervical spine at the C1-C2 level demonstrate a T2 hyperintense lobulated extradural mass with avid enhancement and mass effect on the left lateral aspect of the cervical spinal cord.

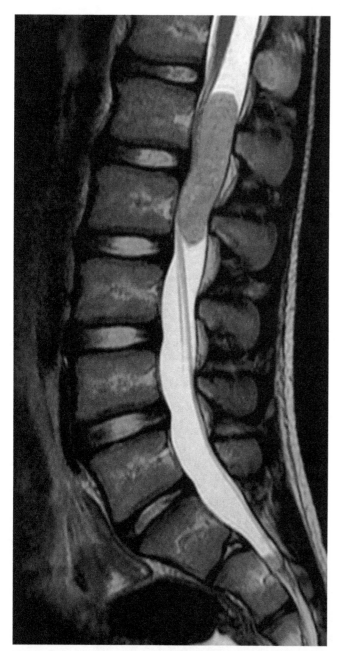

Figure 9.43 Myxopapillary ependymoma. Sagittal T2-weighted image of the lumbar spine demonstrates a well-circumscribed intradural extramedullary mass compressing the nerve roots of the cauda equina.

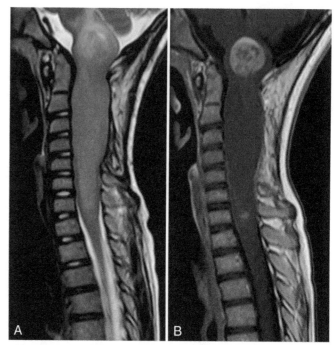

Figure 9.44 Astrocytoma. Sagittal T2 (**A**) and T1 postcontrast (**B**) images of the cervical spine demonstrate an expansile, partially enhancing mass arising from the cervicomedullary junction and involving the entire cervical spinal cord.

cervicothoracic region. Most astrocytomas are World Health Organization grades I and II (75%) and include both pilocytic and fibrillary types. Astrocytomas are typically infiltrative and eccentric in location, resulting in asymmetric spinal cord expansion. Cysts, both polar and intratumoral, are a common feature, occurring in 20% to 40% of pediatric cases. Astrocytomas are typically T2 hyperintense, T1 isointense or hypointense, and they may show patchy, mild-to-moderate contrast enhancement [**Fig. 9.44**]. Enhancement is not always sharply demarcated from the nonenhancing tissue, and tumoral margins may extend beyond the enhancing tissue. Peritumoral edema is common in all glial tumors. Astrocytomas affecting the entire spinal cord from the cervicomedullary junction to the conus have been reported in children, leading to the term *holocord astrocytoma*.

Spinal cord ependymomas occur most often in the cervical region, with 44% involving the cervical cord alone and 23%

extending into the upper thoracic region. These tumors arise from the ependymal cells of the central canal; hence they are located centrally, as opposed to the eccentric location of astrocytomas. Rather than being infiltrative, the tumors are well defined and tend to compress adjacent neural tissue. Most ependymomas are T1 isointense or hypointense and T2 hyperintense relative to the spinal cord. Ependymomas demonstrate stronger and more homogenous enhancement than do astrocytomas. Hemorrhage is common, and the "cap sign," representing a rim of hemosiderin resulting from intratumoral hemorrhage, can often be seen at the cranial or caudal margin of the tumor.

Ganglioglioma/gangliocytomas are low-grade (World Health Organization grade I) tumors composed of well-differentiated ganglion/neuronal cells, with (ganglioglioma) or without (gangliocytoma) a glial component. The tumor typically originates from the sympathetic chain ganglia and is the most benign form of neurogenic tumor. T1 signal can be mixed, possibly secondary to a dual-cell population. T2-weighted images show the tumor to be hyperintense. Surrounding edema is not as frequently seen as with ependymomas or astrocytomas. Patchy enhancement is typical. Tumoral cysts are more common in gangliogliomas than in astrocytomas or ependymomas.

SUGGESTED READINGS

Barkovich AJ, Raybaud C. *Pediatric Neuroimaging*. 5th ed. Philadelphia, PA: Lippincott Williams & Wilkins; 2012.

Huisman TAGM, Rossi A, Tortori-Donati P. MR imaging of neonatal spinal dysraphia: what to consider? *Magn Reson Imaging Clin N Am*. 2012;20:45-61.

Huisman TAGM, Wagner MW, Bosemani T, et al. Pediatric spinal trauma. *J Neuroimaging*. 2015;25:337-353.

Smoker WR, Khanna G. Imaging the craniocervical junction. *Childs Nerv Syst*. 2008;24:1123-1145.

Song D, Maher CO. Spinal disorders associated with skeletal dysplasias and syndromes. *Neurosurg Clin N Am*. 2007;18:499-514.

Studer D. Clinical investigation and imaging. *J Child Orthop*. 2013;7:29-35.

Tortori-Donati P, Rossi A, Biancheri R, et al. Congenital malformations of the spine and spinal cord. In: Tortori-Donati P, ed. *Pediatric Neuroradiology, Head, Neck and Spine*. Berlin, Germany: Springer; 2005.

Verhey LH, Banwell BL. Inflammatory, vascular, and infectious myelopathies in children. *Handb Clin Neurol*. 2013;112:999-1017.

Chapter 10
Head and Neck Imaging

Caroline D. Robson and Amy Juliano

The "head and neck" encompasses extracranial structures from the skull base to the thoracic inlet including the orbits, nasal cavity, paranasal sinuses (PNSs), face, jaws, temporal bones and soft tissues of the neck, oral cavity, and upper aerodigestive tract. In this chapter we describe approaches to imaging, highlighting typical and atypical imaging features and the differential diagnosis for a variety of processes that involve the pediatric head and neck.

IMAGING TECHNQUES AND MODALITIES

The choice of imaging modality depends on the clinical indication, region of interest, patient age, need for sedation or anesthesia, and parental concerns regarding the use of ionizing radiation.

Conventional Radiography

Plain films (PF) or digital radiography is requested for evaluation of osseous structures in trauma, to evaluate the sinuses for suspected sinusitis, and the soft tissues of the neck for airway narrowing caused by adenoidal hypertrophy, laryngotracheobronchitis, or occasionally epiglottitis. Intraoperative or postoperative temporal bone PFs are useful for assessment of the position of cochlear implant arrays. Radiopaque foreign bodies are also well demonstrated by PF or digital radiography. This is of particular importance in assessing patients undergoing magnetic resonance imaging (MRI) where the presence of a ferromagnetic foreign body could contraindicate the examination.

Fluoroscopy

Video fluoroscopy (VF) may be used to assess airway and palatal motion during speech. VF and a barium pharyngogram or esophagogram demonstrate causes of extrinsic airway compression (eg, vascular slings/rings) and intrinsic or mural abnormalities affecting the pharynx or esophagus. A barium pharyngogram can also be used to evaluate for an underlying pyriform sinus tract in a child with recurrent infrahyoid neck infections. This examination should be performed after resolution of infection/inflammation to avoid a false-negative examination from edematous effacement of the tract. Conventional sialography is seldom performed in children but can be used to demonstrate salivary ductal anatomy in sialectasis.

Ultrasonography

Real-time ultrasonography is often the initial mode of evaluation for pediatric neck masses and thyroid and ocular lesions. Ultrasonography helps distinguish between solid versus cystic masses and nodal versus nonnodal neck masses. Cystic masses range from anechoic with increased through transmission to mildly or moderately echoic depending on the presence of hemorrhagic,

proteinaceous, or purulent material. Oscillating compression of the mass with the transducer helps demonstrate the swirling nature of echogenic contents as seen in viscous or solid-appearing cystic masses such as abscess or lymphatic malformation (LM). Doppler ultrasonography provides important information regarding vascularity, direction of flow, and pulsatility. For example, Doppler ultrasonography is used to distinguish venous from arterial flow and helps characterize masses as markedly vascular (eg, proliferating infantile hemangioma [IH]), moderately vascular, or avascular.

Computed Tomography

High-resolution multidetector computed tomography (CT) provides information that is complementary to that provided by ultrasonography and MRI, and is particularly helpful in osseous assessment. CT is also useful for demonstrating calcifications such as phleboliths, tumoral calcification, and sialoliths. Images should be acquired using the lowest dose that provides diagnostic quality images. Axial images are generally acquired or reformatted parallel to the hard palate, with coronal reformatted images perpendicular to the plane of the hard palate. For indications that require contrast, images are obtained only with contrast. CT angiography (CTA) and CT venography (CTV) require the acquisition of images during the administration of a bolus of intravenous contrast, timed to demonstrate the arterial or venous anatomy, respectively.

Neck CT is primarily used for evaluating acute infection, and sometimes characterization of congenital or acquired neck masses. Images are acquired with intravenous (IV) contrast using the "split-dose" technique. After acquiring the scout images, half of the IV contrast dose is administered as a bolus, followed by a 3-minute pause. Helical 3-mm images are then acquired during the rapid administration of the second half of the contrast bolus. This technique allows the contrast to percolate through enhancing lesions while still providing excellent information about neck vasculature. Multiplanar reconstructions (MPRs) are created in soft tissue and bone algorithms.

CT of the orbits, sinuses, nasal cavity, and facial bones is obtained without contrast for evaluating congenital lesions (eg, choanal atresia), trauma, chronic sinus disease, and osseous lesions. Acute complicated sinus and orbital infection, suspected invasive fungal sinusitis, and soft tissue tumors or developmental masses are evaluated with contrast-enhanced CT (CECT). Three-dimensional (3D) images can be created for assessment and follow-up of craniofacial malformations.

Temporal bone CT without contrast is used for evaluation of congenital malformations, chronic infection, cholesteatoma, trauma, and conductive, mixed, or sensorineural hearing loss (SNHL). Depending on the need for sedation, MRI is sometimes preferred for SNHL evaluation. CECT is required for the evaluation of suspected coalescent mastoiditis (CoM) and temporal bone region masses. Temporal bone CT is also useful for the evaluation of local vascular variants.

Radionuclide Imaging

[^{18}F]fluorodeoxyglucose ([^{18}F]-FDG) positron emission tomography (PET)-CT is an extremely useful modality for the diagnosis, staging, and follow-up of malignant head and neck tumors. Radionuclide imaging is helpful in evaluating the pediatric thyroid gland. Iodine 123 (^{123}I) and technetium 99m (^{99m}Tc) pertechnetate are primarily used. Indications for thyroid radionuclide imaging include identification of ectopic thyroid tissue, assessment of congenital hypothyroidism, and evaluation of a solitary thyroid nodule. Metaiodobenzylguanidine labeled with radioactive iodine is used for the assessment, staging, and follow-up of neuroblastoma.

Magnetic Resonance Imaging

MRI provides superior soft tissue characterization that is complementary to that provided by ultrasonography and CT. MRI is indicated for the initial evaluation and follow-up of congenital and acquired masses and for the assessment of complicated sinus, orbital, and temporal bone infections. Pulse sequences typically include multiplanar, high-resolution, fat-suppressed (FS) T2-weighted (T2W) or T2 short tau inversion recovery images, axial diffusion-weighted images (DWI), axial T1-weighted (T1W) images, and gadolinium (Gd)-enhanced FS T1W images. The field of view and slice thickness vary depending on the size of the patient and lesion. Vascular pulsation in the neck produces phase artifact, which should be taken into consideration when selecting the direction of the phase and frequency-encoding steps, to minimize phase artifact through the region of interest. Non-echo-planar DWI images are sometimes acquired to mitigate the geometric distortion caused by susceptibility effects at the skull base. Susceptibility sequences are sometimes required for confirmation of hemorrhage or mineralization. A flow-sensitive gradient echo sequence or 3D time-of-flight MR angiogram (MRA) is useful for evaluating vascular malformations, vascular tumors, and arterial morphology of the neck. Time-of-flight MR venography (MRV) is used for assessment of venous thrombosis or venous anatomy. Gd-enhanced gradient echo images are of use for the depiction of nonocclusive venous thrombi and are a useful adjunct to MRV.

MR of the temporal bones is useful for evaluating SNHL and cranial nerve (CN) palsies. Imaging at 3T with heavily T2W sequences such as axial and oblique sagittal T2 3D Sampling Perfection with Application optimized Contrast using different flip angle Evolutions (SPACE) or Constructive Interference in Steady State (CISS) provide excellent detail of the fluid-containing inner ear structures. These sequences also provide exquisite detail of the globes. Gd-enhanced, thin-section, high-resolution FS T1W images are indicated for acquired SNHL, tumors/masses, and inflammatory conditions involving the temporal bones, PNSs, and orbits. Images can be obtained immediately after the administration of contrast, but delayed (eg, 5 minutes) images may be of use to detect subtle enhancement, for example, if autoimmune labyrinthitis is suspected.

Angiography

Conventional angiography is reserved for detailed assessment of neck vasculature and for endovascular treatment of arteriovenous malformation (AVM) and fistulae (AVFs) and certain vascular tumors (eg, juvenile angiofibroma [JA]).

CONGENITAL AND DEVELOPMENTAL ABNORMALITIES

Orbit and Globe

Normal Development and Anatomy

The eye and orbit develop from neuroectoderm, cutaneous ectoderm, mesoderm, and neural crest cells. The optic primordium gives rise to the optic vesicle and stalk, which become the globe and the optic nerve (ON). A transitory vascular system, the hyaloid artery and its branches, forms the primary vitreous and then involutes. The hyaloid artery and vein ultimately become the central artery and vein of the retina. The globe is located within the orbital fat. The outer layer of the globe is the opaque sclera and translucent cornea; the middle vascular layer is the uvea, which includes the choroid, ciliary body, and iris. The inner layer is the retina, which is continuous posteriorly with the ON. The anterior segment structures lie anterior to the lens. The iris and ciliary body divide the anterior segment into anterior and posterior chambers, both of which contain aqueous humor. The posterior segment structures are posterior to the lens and include the vitreous humor. The lacrimal gland lies in the superolateral orbit; tears drain via the superior and inferior lacrimal canaliculi into the inferomedially located lacrimal sac before coursing into the nasolacrimal duct, which drains into the inferior meatus of the nasal cavity.

The orbit contains orbital fascia, fat, extraocular muscles (EOMs), the globe, lacrimal system, vessels, and nerves. The optic foramen lies at the orbital apex and transmits the ON and ophthalmic artery. The superior orbital fissure lies inferolateral to the optic foramen and transmits CN III and IV, the ophthalmic division of CN V, CN VI, sympathetic nerves, and the superior ophthalmic vein (SOV). The inferior orbital fissure separates the lateral orbital wall and orbital floor and connects posteromedially with the pterygopalatine fossa and posterolaterally with the retromaxillary fissure and infratemporal fossa. Most of the EOMs originate at the orbital apex and insert on the globe, forming a cone about the globe and ON. The EOMs consist of the levator palpebrae superioris the superior, middle, lateral, and inferior rectus muscles and the superior and inferior oblique muscles. The orbital fascia forms the periosteum of the orbit, and its anterior reflection about the globe is termed the *orbital septum*. This septum separates the anterior preseptal space from the posterior postseptal space. The postseptal space is further subdivided by the muscular cone into intraconal and extraconal components. Growth of the orbital cavity is contingent upon normal growth of the globe. The globe is 75% of adult size at birth and is fully grown by age 7 years.

Congenital and Developmental Abnormalities of the Globe

Anophthalmos and Microphthalmos. Anophthalmos or anophthalmia refers to complete absence of the globe, and microphthalmos or microphthalmia refers to ocular hypoplasia [**Fig. 10.1**]. These conditions, which are an important cause of blindness, can be unilateral or bilateral, symmetric or asymmetric in appearance, and syndromic (eg, the holoprosencephaly [HPE] disorders, trisomy 13) or nonsyndromic in nature. Congenital anophthalmos is rare and usually results from a genetic mutation or an insult early during gestation. Anophthalmos can also result from degeneration of the optic vesicle. Imaging of anophthalmos reveals a small orbit and absent globe. Microphthalmos is characterized by a small globe. It is usually associated with a small orbit unless there is an associated large orbital cyst. Microphthalmos can also be seen in association with other ocular abnormalities such as anterior (eg, cataract) or posterior (eg, coloboma) segment dysgenesis.

Macrophthalmos. A large globe is frequently caused by severe myopia that is sporadic or syndromic in nature (eg, Stickler syndrome). Buphthalmos is enlargement of the globe due to increased intraocular pressure, as seen in glaucoma, which may be caused by various factors such as neurofibromatosis type 1 (NF-1). Imaging is helpful in excluding an intraorbital mass and reveals enlargement of the globe [**Fig. 10.1**]. The differential

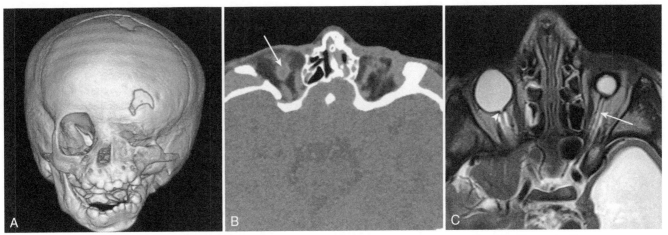

Figure 10.1 Anophthalmos, microphthalmos, and buphthalmos. A, Anophthalmos. Three-dimensional computed tomography (CT) shows a small, deformed left orbit. There is also a left frontal bony defect associated with a cephalocele, and the left nasal cavity is absent. **B,** Anophthalmos and microphthalmos. Axial CT image shows left anophthalmos and right microphthalmos with a small cystic globe remnant (*arrow*). **C,** Microphthalmos and buphthalmos. Axial T2-weighted magnetic resonance shows left microphthalmos and optic nerve hypoplasia (*arrow*). There is mild right buphthalmos and a small optic nerve coloboma or pit (*arrowhead*). The left lateral ventricle is dilated.

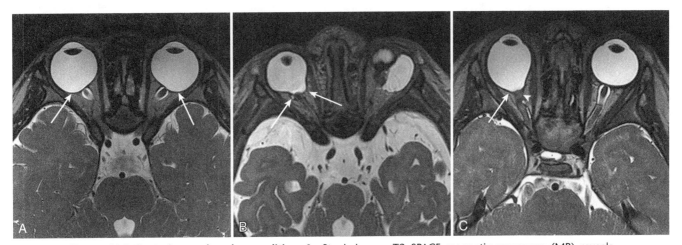

Figure 10.2 Posterior ocular abnormalities. A, Staphylomas. T2 SPACE magnetic resonance (MR) reveals smooth chorioretinal bulging consistent with bilateral staphylomas (*arrows*). **B,** Coloboma in CHARGE syndrome. Axial T2 SPACE MR shows right chorioretinal colobomas (*arrows*). There is left microphthalmos with a left orbital cyst. **C,** Morning glory disc anomaly. Axial T2 SPACE MR shows a funnel-shaped right optic disc defect (*arrow*) with abnormal tissue within the distal optic nerve (ON) with effacement of the adjacent subarachnoid space (*arrowhead*). Compare with the normal left globe and ON.

diagnosis includes congenital cystic eye in which a cystic orbital mass is present without identifiable ocular structures.

Staphyloma. Staphyloma is an ocular outpouching caused by stretching and thinning of the sclera and uvea without an actual focal defect in the layers. Causative factors include prior infection or inflammation, severe axial myopia, glaucoma, trauma, and surgery. On imaging, staphyloma appears as a bulge typically involving the posterior contour of the globe [**Fig. 10.2**].

Coloboma. Coloboma is a congenital ocular defect that results from faulty closure of the embryonic optic fissure producing a notch or gap in the affected part of the iris, retina, choroid, or optic disc. Coloboma can be unilateral or bilateral and may be associated with a normally sized globe, microphthalmos, or glaucoma. Coloboma is often familial and occurs in several syndromes including Treacher-Collins syndrome (TCS), CHARGE,

and trisomies 13 and 18. On ultrasonography, CT, or MR, coloboma appears as a protrusion of vitreous into a chorioretinal gap or into the optic disc [**Fig. 10.2**]. The differential diagnosis for chorioretinal coloboma is staphyloma (acquired bulge lined by retina and choroid). The differential diagnosis for ON head coloboma is the morning glory disc anomaly (MGDA; see later).

Morning Glory Disc Anomaly. MGDA is an uncommon optic disc malformation that resembles a morning glory flower. MGDA is usually unilateral and sporadic but is sometimes associated with cephaloceles, moyamoya disease, and PHACES association (*p*osterior fossa malformations, *h*emangiomas, *a*rterial anomalies, *c*oarctation of the aorta and cardiac defects, *e*ye abnormalities, *s*ternal clefting and *s*upraumbilical abdominal raphe). On funduscopy, there is optic disc excavation with an annulus of chorioretinal pigmentary changes, straightening of retinal vessels, and central glial tissue. On MR, there is a funnel-shaped optic disc defect with elevation of adjacent retinal margins and lack of normal ON head enhancement. There is abnormal tissue within the distal ON with effacement of the adjacent subarachnoid space [**Fig. 10.2**] and sometimes ON atrophy. The funnel-shaped morphology and heaped up margins distinguish MGDA from coloboma.

Malformations of the Orbit

Hypertelorism and Hypotelorism. *Hypertelorism,* referring to an increased distance between the medial orbital walls, is a feature of numerous syndromes and developmental disorders including syndromic craniosynostosis, cephalocele, agenesis of the corpus callosum (ACC), and frontonasal dysplasia [**Fig. 10.3**]. Imaging of hypertelorism demonstrates widely spaced orbits. *Dystopia canthorum* refers to telecanthus in which there is an increased distance between the inner canthi of the eyes with lateral displacement of the lacrimal puncta, as seen in some types of Waardenburg syndrome.

Hypotelorism refers to a decreased distance between the medial orbital walls, as seen in a variety of syndromic and developmental disorders including the HPEs, arrhinencephaly, and premature fusion of the metopic and sagittal sutures. Other manifestations of HPE include *cyclophthalmos* or *cyclopia* (single median eye), *synophthalmos* (partial fusion of the eyes), *ethmocephaly* (hypotelorism with median proboscis), and *cebocephaly* (hypotelorism with rudimentary nose/single nostril). Imaging reveals closely set eyes with normal-sized globes, microphthalmos, or anophthalmos, and sometimes other craniofacial anomalies [**Fig. 10.3**].

Abnormalities of Orbital Size. Orbital enlargement results from bony defects as seen with NF-1-associated sphenoid dysplasia or orbital cephalocele, or arises because of a congenital or acquired intraorbital mass such as an ocular cyst, vascular anomaly, or tumor. A small orbit is a feature of anophthalmos or microphthalmos resulting from malformation or an early insult (eg, infection, ocular enucleation, or orbital irradiation) [**Fig. 10.1**]. *Exorbitism* referring to shallow orbits with ventral protrusion of the globes as seen in syndromic craniosynostosis (eg, Apert and Crouzon syndromes) [**Fig. 10.3**] should not be mistaken for proptosis in which ocular protrusion occurs from orbital mass effect caused by tumor, inflammation, or thyroid

ophthalmopathy. Enlargement of the optic canal occurs because of ON tumor and/or dural ectasia, as seen in NF-1. A small optic canal accompanies ON hypoplasia and disorders such as osteopetrosis and fibrous dysplasia.

Optic Nerve Hypoplasia. ON hypoplasia is a developmentally small ON. This anomaly can be unilateral or bilateral and isolated or syndromic. Numerous syndromes, many with well-characterized underlying genetic mutations, are associated with ON hypoplasia, perhaps the best known being septooptic dysplasia (absent septum pellucidum, midline forebrain anomalies, and pituitary hypoplasia). On MR, the affected ONs, chiasm, and tract(s) appear diminutive [**Fig. 10.1**]. The differential diagnosis is ON atrophy.

Persistent Hyperplastic Primary Vitreous. Persistent hyperplastic primary vitreous (PHPV) results from failure of the normal process of embryonic hyaloid vasculature regression, with persistence of hyperplastic primary vitreous and the capillary vascular network overlying the lens. PHPV is usually unilateral and associated with microphthalmos, cataract, and leukocoria. Bilateral PHPV is seen in various syndromic disorders such as trisomy 13 and Walker-Warburg disease. PHPV is characterized by a triangular morphology of the lens, which "points" toward a linear density (on CT) or hypointensity (T2W MR) representing retrolental fibrovascular tissue and the persistent hyaloid remnant of Cloquet canal [**Fig. 10.4**]. Abnormal vitreous density or signal intensity reflects hemorrhage and layering debris. Complications include glaucoma and progressive retinal hemorrhage leading over time to phthisis bulbi. The differential diagnosis includes Coats disease, retinopathy of prematurity (ROP), retinal detachment, and retinoblastoma (RB).

Coats Disease. Coats disease results from defective retinal vascular development, leading to retinal telangiectasias with leaky vessels, subretinal exudates, and retinal detachment. Coats disease is usually unilateral and presents with leukocoria and strabismus. On CT, Coats disease appears as a hyperdense exudate, usually without calcification [**Fig. 10.4**]. On MR, the subretinal exudate appears hyperintense on T1W and T2W images. The differential diagnosis includes RB, but RB presents as a mineralized mass with or without retinal detachment.

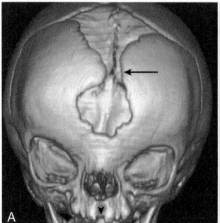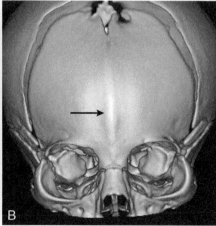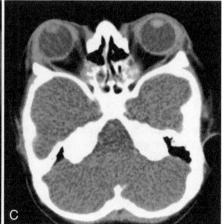

Figure 10.3 Hypertelorism, hypotelorism, and exorbitism. A, Hypertelorism in frontonasal dysplasia. Three-dimensional (3D) computed tomography (CT) image reveals marked hypertelorism. The metopic suture is abnormally widened (*arrow*), the nasal root is broad, and there is splaying of the central incisor teeth (*arrowhead*). **B,** Hypotelorism and trigonocephaly. 3D CT shows hypotelorism and premature fusion of the metopic suture (*arrow*). **C,** Hypertelorism with exorbitism in syndromic craniosynostosis. Low-dose preoperative axial CT image reveals hypertelorism with shallow orbits resulting in exorbitism with ocular protrusion beyond the orbital margins.

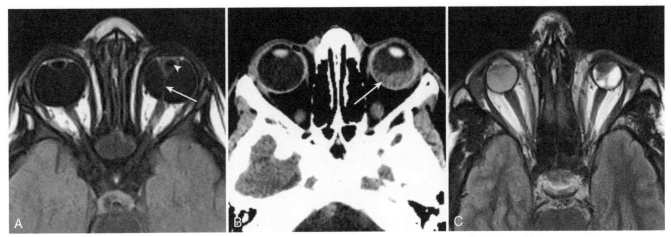

Figure 10.4 Retinal and vitreous abnormalities. A, Persistent hyperplastic primary vitreous. Axial fluid attenuation inversion recovery (FLAIR) magnetic resonance (MR) reveals a triangular morphology of the lens (*arrowhead*) that points toward the linear persistent hyaloid remnant of Cloquet canal (*arrow*). **B,** Coats disease. Axial computed tomography image shows the hyperdense exudate without mineralization. **C,** Retinopathy of prematurity. Axial FLAIR MR demonstrates bilateral microphthalmos with abnormal vitreous signal intensity caused by prior retinal detachment and fibrovascular organization of the vitreous.

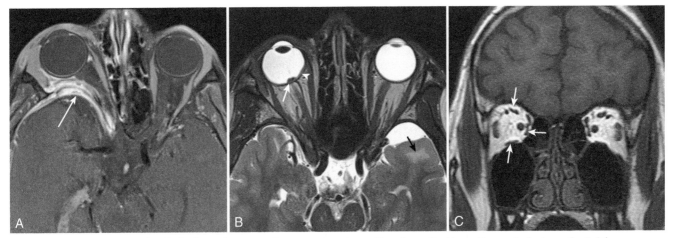

Figure 10.5 Orbital findings in central nervous system disorders. A, Neurofibromatosis type 1. Axial gadolinium-enhanced fat-suppressed T1-weighted (T1W) magnetic resonance (MR) shows deficiency of the right sphenoid bone with the defect filled by enhancing fibrovascular tissue (*arrow*). There is resultant deformity of the right orbit. **B,** Tuberous sclerosis. Axial T2-weighted MR reveals a hypointense optic disc retinal hamartoma (*white arrow*), with an associated retinal detachment (*arrowhead*). A left temporal lobe tuber (*black arrow*) and small arachnoid cyst are also seen. **C,** Congenital cranial dysinnervation disorders. Coronal T1W MR demonstrates small superior, medial, and inferior rectus muscles (*arrows*) attributable to bilateral CN3 aplasia (not shown).

Retinopathy of Prematurity. ROP or retrolental fibroplasia is attributed to excessive oxygen therapy in premature, low-birth-weight infants, but is now relatively uncommon. ROP manifests as fibrovascular organization of the vitreous sometimes resulting in retinal detachment, microphthalmos, and blindness. On CT the globes appear small and hyperdense, sometimes with dystrophic mineralization. The differential diagnosis includes prior infection (eg, cytomegalovirus [CMV]) and RB (calcified mass, normal-sized globe). MR shows abnormal signal intensity caused by subretinal hemorrhages [**Fig. 10.4**].

Ocular and Orbital Abnormalities Associated With Craniofacial and Central Nervous System Malformations

Ocular and orbital anomalies are seen in numerous craniofacial disorders. *Cephaloceles* and *nasal dermoids* are variably associated with widening of the nasal bridge, hypertelorism, and sometimes intracranial anomalies (eg, ACC, polymicrogyria). The *syndromic craniosynostoses* are associated with hypertelorism, exorbitism, midfacial hypoplasia, and occasionally cleft lip and palate (CLCP). Hypertelorism is a feature of *frontonasal dysplasia* with broadening of the nasal bridge and a bifid nose [**Fig. 10.3**]. *HPE* disorders are associated with hypotelorism, microphthalmia, nasal anomalies (eg, pyriform aperture stenosis or more severe manifestations), and sometimes central megaincisor. *Septooptic dysplasia* is associated with optic hypoplasia.

NF-1 is characterized by sphenoid bone deficiency with pulsatile proptosis and orbital deformity [**Fig. 10.5**], buphthalmos, ON glioma, nerve sheath tumors, and rarely rhabdomyosarcoma (RMS). Orbital manifestations of *Sturge-Weber syndrome* include buphthalmos, glaucoma, venous dysplasia, and venous hypertension. Retinal neuroglial hamartomas appearing as small, hypointense retinal nodules on T2W MR are a feature of *tuberous*

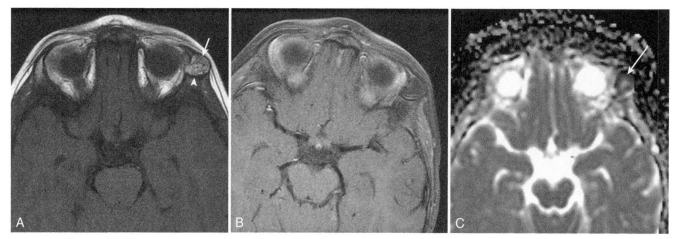

Figure 10.6 Dermoid. A, Axial T1-weighted (T1W) magnetic resonance imaging (MRI) shows an ovoid, heterogeneous, partly hyperintense lesion (*arrow*) involving the superolateral margin of the left orbit. There is sharply defined bony erosion with hypointense corticated margins (*arrowhead*). **B,** Axial fat-suppressed gadolinium-enhanced T1W MRI demonstrates fat suppression within the nonenhancing lesion. **C,** Axial diffusion-weighted imaging apparent diffusion coefficient map shows decreased diffusivity within the dermoid (*arrow*).

sclerosis [**Fig. 10.5**]. Enhancing retinal hemangioblastomas occur in *von Hippel-Lindau disease.*

Joubert syndrome is characterized by absent cerebellar vermis, abnormal eye movements, and sometimes retinal abnormalities with chorioretinal coloboma. *Walker-Warburg syndrome* and the *congenital muscular dystrophies* feature ocular abnormalities such as cataracts and other anterior segment anomalies, microphthalmos, PHPV, retinal detachment, vitreous hemorrhage, coloboma, and ON hypoplasia. *Aicardi syndrome* (X-linked, affects females) is characterized by ACC, polymicrogyria, choroid plexus tumors, and chorioretinal lacunae. Ocular manifestations include microphthalmos, retinal detachment, coloboma, staphyloma, and cataract.

The *congenital cranial dysinnervation disorders* are characterized by abnormal development of cranial motor nuclei and absence or hypoplasia of affected CNs, leading to fibrosis of the affected EOMs (previously known as congenital fibrosis of the EOMs). Clinical signs depend on the affected CNs and include strabismus, gaze limitation or ophthalmoplegia, ptosis, and poorly reactive pupils. On high-resolution MR there is absence or hypoplasia of the affected CNs, and the affected EOMs appear small [**Fig. 10.5**].

Developmental Masses and Anomalies

Malformation or maldevelopment of orbital tissues can create a variety of masses. The more frequently encountered lesions are described in the following subsections. Vascular malformations and lipoma are considered in a later section.

Dermoid and Epidermoid. Dermoids are common congenital masses thought to arise from epithelial rests sequestered in bony sutures. A dermoid usually presents as a small, firm nodule, often along the lateral orbital rim. Dermoids (and less common epidermoids) are composed of cysts lined by keratinized, stratified squamous epithelium. Dermoids also sometimes contain hair and sebaceous glands. On CECT, dermoid/epidermoid appears as a well-defined, low-density mass with minimal, if any, peripheral enhancement. Bone remodeling or erosion is sharply defined and well corticated. Thick, irregular peripheral enhancement and irregular osseous destruction suggests inflammation/infection. Sometimes fatty density is seen within the cyst. On MR, dermoid/epidermoid appears rounded and sharply circumscribed, usually with high signal intensity on T2W images,

decreased diffusivity, low signal intensity on T1W images, and minimal, if any, peripheral Gd enhancement. Fat content produces high signal intensity on T1W imaging that suppresses with FS techniques [**Fig. 10.6**]. Imaging does not reliably distinguish between dermoid and epidermoid.

Nasolacrimal Duct Cyst. Congenital nasolacrimal duct cyst (NLDC) or mucocele is a common anomaly thought to arise due to failure of canalization of the distal NLD at the valve of Hasner beneath the inferior turbinate on one or both sides. Clinical signs and symptoms include a cystic medial canthal swelling and/or neonatal nasal obstruction and respiratory distress. On imaging, NLDC appears as a cystic structure that is tubular on coronal images [**Fig. 10.7**]. It extends inferiorly from the medial canthus and protrudes inferior to the inferior turbinate, sometimes with lacrimal sac enlargement. The differential diagnosis includes meningocele and cystic neuroglial heterotopia (NGH); unlike NLDC, these entities project superior to the inferior turbinate.

Lacrimal Gland Anomalies. Lacrimal gland anomalies are uncommon and include ectopic or absent lacrimal tissue. Neoplastic transformation of ectopic lacrimal tissue is rare, especially in children.

Nasal Cavity, Paranasal Sinuses, Face, and Mandible

Normal Development and Anatomy

The facial structures develop from mesenchymal primordia surrounding the stomodeum (primitive mouth). The nasomedial processes create the philtrum of the lip, the premaxillary portion of the upper jaw, and the primary palate. The forehead, nose, and nasal septum derive from the frontonasal prominence. Portions of the upper lip, maxilla, and secondary palate derive from the maxillary processes. The nasolacrimal groove is located between the maxillary process and the nasal primordium and gives rise to the NLD and lacrimal sac. The mandible, lower lip, chin, and lower cheek arise from paired mandibular prominences. The muscles of mastication (first arch derivatives, innervated by CN V) and the muscles of facial expression (second arch derivatives, innervated by CN VII) are derived from mesodermal cells of the pharyngeal arches. The nasal cavities communicate with the nasopharynx and oral cavity after rupture of the oronasal membrane at the choanae. PNSs form as diverticula

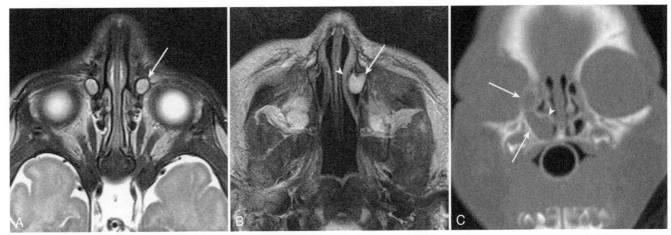

Figure 10.7 Nasolacrimal duct cyst (NLDC). A, Axial T2-weighted (T2W) magnetic resonance imaging (MRI) shows bilateral hyperintense NLDC (*arrow*). **B,** Axial T2W MRI shows a left NLDC (*arrow*) projecting inferolateral to the inferior turbinate (*arrowhead*). **C,** Reformatted low-dose coronal computed tomography shows a right NLDC (*arrows*) extending from the medial canthus to the nasal cavity inferior to the inferior turbinate (*arrowhead*).

of the nasal cavity walls, and subsequently pneumatize with progressive development through childhood. Specialized olfactory epithelium develops along the roof of each nasal cavity and connects with the olfactory bulbs. The nasal cavity and PNSs are lined with respiratory epithelium.

At birth, the face is relatively small compared with the head, and this craniofacial proportion alters as the face enlarges during childhood. The neonate is an obligate nose breather. The nasal airway consists of the pyriform apertures anteriorly, the nasal cavities divided by the cartilaginous and bony nasal septum, and the posterior nasal choanae. The paired inferior, middle, superior, and sometimes supreme turbinates are located along the lateral nasal cavity. The cribriform plate and fovea ethmoidalis form the roof of the nasal cavity and ethmoid air cells, respectively, on each side. The U-shaped hard palate forms the nasal cavity floor. The developing teeth are closely related to the alveolar recesses of the maxillary antra. The pterygoid plates arise from the sphenoid bone and lie posterior to the maxillary antra. The pterygopalatine fossae, located between the maxillary antra and the pterygoid plates, communicate with the masticator spaces and inferior orbital fissures. The thin lamina papyracea separates the ethmoid air cells from the orbit and the orbital floor is formed by the roof of the maxillary antrum.

The maxillary sinuses and ethmoid air cells are present at birth and attain adult size by about 10 to 12 years. The sphenoid sinuses develop at about 2 years of age, converting from hematopoietic to fatty marrow before pneumatization. The sphenoid sinus attains adult size by about 14 years of age. The frontal sinuses develop toward the end of the first decade of life. Each frontal sinus drains through an ostium into the frontal recess and ultimately into the middle meatus. The anterior ethmoid air cells drain into the hiatus semilunaris and middle meatus. The maxillary sinus also drains into the middle meatus via the maxillary ostium and infundibulum. The ostiomeatal unit consists of the infundibulum, uncinate process, hiatus semilunaris, ethmoid bulla, and middle meatus. The posterior ethmoid air cells and sphenoid sinus drain into the sphenoethmoidal recess and superior meatus. The sphenoid sinuses are close to the ONs, pituitary gland, cavernous sinuses, and internal carotid arteries (ICAs).

Developmental Sinonasal Variants

The turbinates are convex toward the nasal cavity. Turbinates with *paradoxical curvature* are concave toward the nasal

cavity. *Concha bullosa* or middle turbinate pneumatization is a common anatomic variant that can cause nasal septal deviation [**Fig. 10.8**] if unilateral or asymmetric. Nasal septal deviation with or without a septal spur can be developmental (eg, in association with unilateral cleft palate) or acquired (eg, post trauma). Underpneumatization or hyperpneumatization of the PNS can occur [**Fig. 10.8**]. The maxillary sinuses often contain septations and frequently have accessory ostia. Ethmoid air cell variations include infraorbital extension (Haller cells), extension ventral to the NLD (agger nasi cells), supraorbital air cells, and sphenoethmoidal air cells (Onodi cells). Sometimes the ethmoid bulla is quite large. It is not unusual to see thinning or even apparent dehiscence of the lamina papyracea. Not infrequently, developmental variants occur in the sphenoid bone that may be mistaken for a dermoid or tumor; however, the hallmark of the developmental lesion is a corticated lucency on CT [**Fig. 10.8**], facilitated diffusion with fluid or fatty signal intensity on MR, and no Gd enhancement.

Congenital Nasal Malformation

Nasal agenesis with complete absence of the nose and nasal cavity is uncommon and is usually a manifestation of a craniofacial syndrome. Midnasal cavity stenosis and midface hypoplasia is seen in a variety of craniofacial disorders, especially the syndromic craniosynostoses.

Pyriform aperture stenosis is an uncommon congenital narrowing of the anterior nasal apertures that presents as neonatal airway obstruction. On CT or MR, there is narrowing of the anterior nasal apertures associated with a triangular hard palate morphology [**Fig. 10.9**]. Pyriform aperture stenosis is sometimes associated with a solitary central megaincisor (SCMI) [**Fig. 10.9**]. Pyriform aperture stenosis and SCMI sometimes occur with HPE. Therefore an infant with pyriform aperture stenosis and SCMI should undergo brain MRI to assess for HPE. Other facial features of HPE include a small/absent nose, hypotelorism, and midline cleft palate.

Choanal atresia is congenital posterior choanal obstruction. Bilateral choanal atresia causes neonatal airway obstruction. Unilateral atresia is more common and presents later with unilateral nasal stuffiness. CT or MRI shows thickening of the posterior vomer and medial deviation of the lateral wall(s) of the nasal cavity and pterygoid plates [**Fig. 10.9**]. The anomaly is either bony (lateral wall meets thickened vomer) or part bony and part

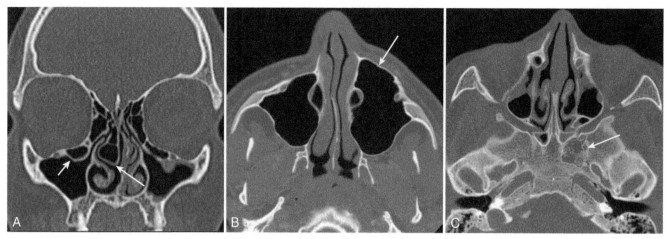

Figure 10.8 Sinonasal variants. A, Concha bullosa. Reformatted coronal computed tomography (CT) shows a markedly enlarged, pneumatized right middle turbinate (*long arrow*), resulting in mild leftward nasal septal deviation. There is infraorbital extension of right ethmoid air cells (*short arrow*; Haller cells). **B,** Pneumosinus dilatans. Axial CT shows a hyperpneumatized left maxillary antrum (*arrow*) resulting in facial asymmetry. **C,** Benign marrow variant. Axial CT shows a well corticated lucency within the left sphenoid bone (*arrow*) in an asymptomatic patient.

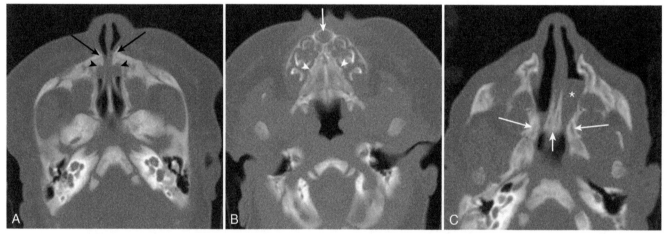

Figure 10.9 Nasal obstruction. A, Pyriform aperture stenosis. Axial computed tomography image shows narrowing of the anterior nasal apertures (*long arrows*) resulting in PAS, compounded by bilaterally prominent nasolacrimal ducts (*arrowheads*). **B,** A more caudal image (same patient) shows a central megaincisor (*short arrow*) and triangular morphology of the hard palate (*arrowheads*). **C,** Choanal atresia in CHARGE syndrome. There is medial deviation of the lateral nasal cavity walls (*long arrows*) and thickening of the vomer (*short arrow*). There is pooling of secretions within the nasal cavity (*asterisk*). These features are consistent with bilateral bony and membranous choanal atresia.

membranous, with pooling of nasal secretions. Bilateral choanal atresia is typically associated with CHARGE syndrome (*c*oloboma, *h*eart defect, *a*tresia choanae, *r*etarded growth and development, *g*enital hypoplasia, and *e*ar anomalies). Other imaging features of CHARGE include CLCP, skull base anomalies (constricted clivus), olfactory bulb hypoplasia/aplasia, pituitary and pontine hypoplasia, and hypoplasia of the vestibules with absent/hypoplastic semicircular canals (SCCs).

Congenital Nasal Masses

Congenital nasal masses include NLDC (discussed earlier), disorders resulting from defective neural tube closure, vascular malformations (discussed later), and congenital tumors (eg, teratoma, hemangioma, and juvenile xanthogranuloma; see later). Disorders resulting from defective neural tube closure include cephalocele, neuroglial heterotopia (NGH), dermoid, and dermal sinus

tract (DST). Development of the nasofrontal region results in transient nasofrontal structures termed the fonticulus frontalis (separating the nasal and frontal bones) and prenasal space (between the nasal bones and the underlying nasal capsule) that involute in early gestation. Usually the only remnant is the foramen cecum, ventral to the crista galli, containing fibrous tissue and sometimes a small emissary vein. Persistence of these primitive structures may be associated with a dural diverticulum and protrusion of intracranial contents as a nasofrontal or nasoethmoidal cephalocele. Partial or complete obliteration of the intracranial connection results in sequestered NGH ("nasal glioma"). NGH can be extranasal (faulty fonticulus frontalis closure) or intranasal (faulty prenasal space closure). With dural diverticulum regression, incorporation of surface ectoderm may form a DST and/or dermoid along the nasal dorsum, sometimes extending from the nasal bridge through the nasofrontal suture into the anterior cranial fossa, or extending along the nasal

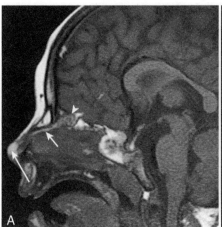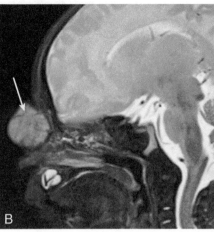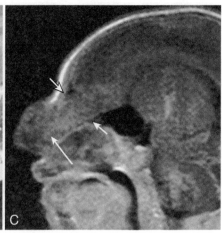

Figure 10.10 Lesions resulting from defective nasofrontal closure. A, Nasal dermoid. Sagittal T1-weighted (T1W) magnetic resonance imaging (MRI) shows an ovoid high signal intensity nasal dermoid (*long arrow*) at the tip of the nose. It is connected by a thin high signal intensity tubular dermal sinus tract (*short arrow*) to an ovoid dermoid located in the foramen cecum (*arrowhead*). **B,** Neuroglial heterotopia (NGH). Sagittal fat-suppressed T2-weighted MRI shows a rounded NGH overlying the nasal bridge. It is isointense with cortex and, unlike a cephalocele, does not have an intracranial connection. **C,** Frontonasal cephalocele. Sagittal T1W contrast-enhanced MRI shows a large defect in the frontal calvarium (*short arrows*) with herniation of dysplastic frontal lobes into the frontonasal cephalocele (*long arrow*). There is a subfrontal arachnoid cyst.

septum and sometimes through the foramen cecum to the anterior cranial fossa. Nasal dermoid can occur alone or with a DST.

The clinical presentation of children with congenital nasal masses includes respiratory distress caused by nasal obstruction or a visible mass. The presence of a nasal pit, hairy tuft, or small midline nasal nodule suggests a diagnosis of nasal dermoid. A bluish mass suggests venous malformation (VM); a strawberry-red mass is characteristic of IH, or occasionally NGH. Yellowish discoloration suggests juvenile xanthogranuloma. On CECT a dermoid appears rounded and hypodense with minimal, if any, peripheral enhancement. DST appears similar with a tubular morphology. Bone erosion is smoothly marginated and corticated, sometimes appearing as a "gap" at the nasofrontal suture or as scalloping of the affected bone. Enlargement of the foramen cecum greater than 2 mm suggests intracranial extension; however, the foramen cecum is not fully ossified at younger than 2 years of age. For this reason it is helpful to obtain CECT to delineate the enhancing cartilaginous anterior skull base. NGH may appear isodense with brain, or cerebrospinal fluid (CSF), or may have a combination of two densities, and typically appears as a teardrop-shaped mass within the anterior nasal cavity extending from an intact anterior cranial fossa into the nasal cavity, superior to the inferior turbinate. Cephaloceles (meningocele, encephalocele) appear similar to NGH but communicate with intracranial CSF (meningocele) or contain herniated dysplastic brain and CSF (encephalocele).

More frequently, MRI alone is performed to avoid ionizing radiation, with CT reserved for osseous assessment if indicated. Dermoid and DST usually appear hyperintense on thin-section high-resolution FS T2W MRI. DWI characteristically reveals decreased diffusivity; non-echo-planar imaging technique with imaging in the coronal plane is preferred because of decreased susceptibility effects at the skull base compared with the echo planar imaging technique or imaging in the axial plane, thereby improving diagnostic sensitivity. The signal intensity of dermoid on T1W images is variable depending on lipid content, which can render a lesion inconspicuous on all FS sequences [**Fig. 10.10**]. There is usually minimal, if any, peripheral Gd enhancement on FS T1W images. NGH appears isointense with CSF or brain, or there may be a combination of two signal intensities [**Fig. 10.10**]. Although usually nonenhancing, mild

enhancement is occasionally observed. Sometimes a small fibrous tag extending toward foramen cecum renders distinction from a cephalocele challenging. Cephaloceles contain CSF and sometimes dysplastic brain with intracranial communication through a nasofrontal or nasoethmoidal bone defect [**Fig. 10.10**].

Fissural Cysts

Fissural cysts arise along lines of embryologic fusion and include nasolabial (along the base of nasal ala and anterior nasal fold), nasopalatine (incisive canal), and median palatal (midline hard palate) cysts. On CT, these cysts appear lucent with smooth bone remodeling.

Facial and Mandibular Anomalies

Cleft Lip and Palate. Clefts arise from abnormal fusion or maldevelopment of facial structures. CLCP are unilateral or bilateral, and complete (separated margins) or incomplete (partially opposed margins). The most common CLCP is off midline, resulting from failure of fusion of nasomedial and maxillary processes. Syndromic association is highest with bilateral CLCP, is next highest with unilateral CLCP, and seen least often with unilateral cleft lip. CLCP is well seen on fetal ultrasonography/MRI particularly when complete. Bilateral CLCP results in a protruding premaxillary segment [**Fig. 10.11**]. Determining the extent of hard palate involvement can be challenging. True midline/median CLCP is rare; associated hypertelorism should prompt a search for cephalocele and ACC. Hypotelorism with midline CLCP suggests HPE.

Isolated secondary cleft palate may result as follows: micrognathia → glossoptosis (tongue pushed up and back) → failure of apposition of secondary palatal shelves → U-shaped cleft palate [**Fig. 10.11**]. The triad of micrognathia, glossoptosis, and postnatal feeding difficulty is termed *Pierre Robin sequence.* This descriptive term encompasses many syndromes (eg, 22q11del, Stickler, and TCS). Micrognathia should prompt a search for isolated cleft secondary palate which appears on sagittal fetal ultrasonography/MRI as a shortened hard palate with glossoptosis. Oblique (medial canthus to nose) and transverse

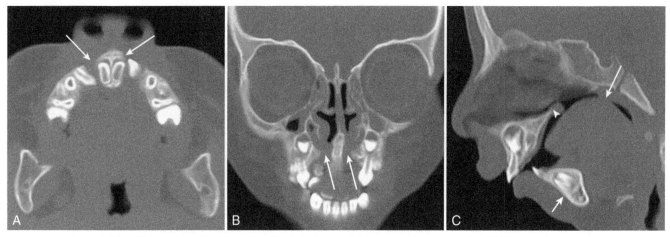

Figure 10.11 Cleft palate. A, Bilateral cleft palate. This axial computed tomography (CT) image demonstrates bilateral bony defects (*arrows*) affecting the maxillary alveolar margins and primary palate. **B,** The coronal reformatted image shows parallel bony clefts (*arrows*) affecting the hard palate. **C,** Cleft secondary palate. Sagittal reformatted CT in this patient with Pierre Robin sequence reveals micrognathia (*short arrow*) that has led to glossoptosis (*long arrow*) that has in turn prevented apposition of the palatal shelves leading to a palatal deficiency (*arrowhead*) with a cleft of the secondary palate.

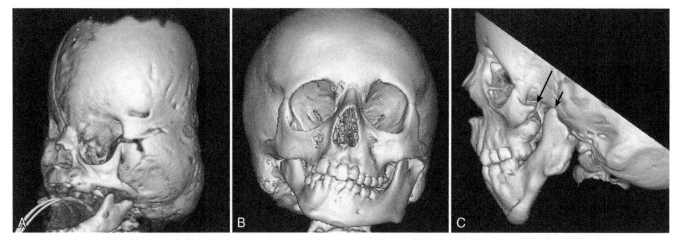

Figure 10.12 Craniofacial syndromes. A, Pfeiffer syndrome. Three-dimensional (3D) computed tomography (CT) image reveals a Kleeblattschädel or cloverleaf skull caused by premature fusion of the coronal, squamosal, and lambdoid sutures. The metopic and sagittal sutures are widely patent. Note the shallow anterior cranial fossa and midface hypoplasia. **B,** Hemifacial microsomia. 3D CT image demonstrates asymmetric hypoplasia of the right hemimandible. **C,** Treacher Collins syndrome. 3D CT image shows micrognathia with a prominent coronoid process (*short arrow*) and absence of the mandibular condyle and ramus. The zygomatic arch is deficient (*long arrow*). There is also malar flattening.

facial clefts (laterally from mouth) are rare. Facial clefting can also result from amniotic bands.

Preoperative imaging of cleft palate with cone beam CT may be obtained to assess the bone over the roots of teeth along the cleft margins to determine the feasibility of successful bone grafting. Complications of CLCP include dental crowding, abnormal dental eruption, oronasal/oroantral fistulae, maxillary retrusion, midface hypoplasia, and nasal septal deviation, with disruption of speech, feeding, and Eustachian tube function.

Craniofacial Syndromes. The *syndromic craniosynostoses* are characterized by premature fusion of coronal and other sutures. Many of these disorders (eg, Crouzon and Apert syndromes) also have hypertelorism, exorbitism, midface hypoplasia, and maxillary retrusion. Midface underdevelopment causes upper airway narrowing that is compounded by adenotonsillar hypertrophy. Fusion of multiple sutures produces a *cloverleaf*

or "kleeblattschädel" skull deformity [**Fig. 10.12**]. The hallmark of Apert syndrome is bicoronal craniosynostosis with wide patency of metopic and sagittal sutures, polysyndactyly, and malformed horizontal SCC.

Micrognathia is a small mandible and *retrognathia* is posterior mandibular positioning. Micrognathia (with retrognathia) can be sporadic or inherited, isolated or syndromic, and results in airway narrowing and sometimes obstruction. Numerous syndromes are associated with micrognathia. Images should be assessed for symmetry and facial malformation to determine the most likely causative factor. *Unilateral micrognathia* is the hallmark of *hemifacial microsomia* (HFM), a heterogeneous group of conditions of uncertain cause that involve the first and second brachial apparatus and neural crest derivatives [**Fig. 10.12**]. There are also ipsilateral congenital external and middle ear anomalies, facial hypoplasia, hypoplasia of muscles of mastication and parotid gland, zygomatic arch hypoplasia, and sometimes transverse facial clefts. The *Goldenhar* HFM pheno-type is characterized by epibulbar lipodermoids and vertebral and renal anomalies. *Bilateral asymmetric micrognathia* is seen in *branchio-oto-renal syndrome* (BOR). BOR is also associated with branchial cleft anomalies (eg, cysts or sinus tracts), characteristic temporal bone anomalies, and renal findings (eg, cysts). *Bilateral symmetric micrognathia* is a feature of *TCS* and *Nager syndrome*. TCS features marked micrognathia, sometimes with absent mandibular condyles, deficient zygomatic arches, posterior malar slanting, downward slanting palpebral fissures, coloboma, and severe bilateral temporal bone anomalies [**Fig. 10.12**]. As mentioned earlier, *Pierre Robin sequence* refers to the clinical triad of micrognathia, glossoptosis (leading to U-shaped cleft palate), and feeding difficulty, featured in a variety of syndromes. Preoperative imaging of craniofacial disorders, before reconstructive surgery, requires low-dose CT with creation of MPRs and 3D images.

Ear and Temporal Bone

Normal Development and Anatomy

The external and middle ear are derived from branchial apparatus, and the internal ear is derived from neurectoderm. The first branchial cleft gives rise to the external auditory canal (EAC); the first branchial pouch forms the Eustachian tube and middle ear cavity (MEC). The auricles develop from the first and second branchial arches. The ossicles grow and ossify during fetal life. The malleus and incus are derived from the first and second branchial arches. The stapes suprastructure and tympanic segment of CN VII derive from the second branchial arch; the stapes footplate partly arises from otic capsule. MEC and mastoid antrum pneumatization commences in the fetus; aeration occurs after birth. Mastoid air cell pneumatization continues during childhood. The inner ear structures develop in the fetus; the cochlea and endolymphatic sac and duct are the last to differentiate.

The temporal bone comprises the squamosal, mastoid, tympanic, and petrous portions and the styloid process. The EAC is part cartilaginous and part bony (tympanic plate), bounded medially by the tympanic membrane (TM), which is attached to the tympanic plate, and scutum. The MEC is bounded laterally by the TM and medially by the cochlear promontory. On coronal CT images, the MEC is divided into the hypotympanum (below TM level), mesotympanum (at TM level), and epitympanum or attic (above TM). The tegmen tympani forms the MEC roof and continues laterally as the mastoid tegmen. Prussak space is located between the scutum, the TM pars flaccida, the lateral malleal ligament, and the malleus neck. The oval window is located over the vestibule, above the cochlear promontory. The carotid canal (CC) lies inferior to the cochlea. The internal jugular vein (IJV) lies inferior to the vestibule.

On axial images the anterior wall of the MEC includes the CC, Eustachian tube, and the semicanal for the tensor tympani tendon which attaches to the malleus. The posterior wall of the MEC has two recesses and an intervening bony protrusion, forming a W-shape in the axial plane. This consists of the sinus tympani (medially) separated by the pyramidal eminence from the facial recess (laterally). The stapedius tendon arises from the pyramidal eminence and attaches to the stapes. The round window niche overlies the cochlear basal turn. The MEC contains the ossicles: malleus, incus, and stapes. The malleus attaches to the TM and articulates with the incus in the attic, resembling an ice cream cone. The incus then curves downward and medially (long and lenticular processes) to articulate with the stapes. The stapes has two crura and a footplate attached to the oval window.

The inner ear is located in the petrous portion of the temporal bone (often simply referred to as the petrous bone) and consists of the cochlea, vestibular aqueduct (which contains the endolymphatic sac and duct), vestibule, SCC (superior, posterior, and lateral), cochlear aqueduct, facial nerve canal (FNC), and internal auditory canal (IAC), mostly enclosed within dense otic capsule bone. The cochlea consists of $2\frac{1}{2}$ to $2\frac{3}{4}$ turns, separated by the shelflike interscalar septum and a central conical bony projection (modiolus), and containing a wafer-thin osseous spiral lamina. The IAC transmits CNs VII and VIII; the medial IAC opening is the porus acusticus; the fundus is lateral. The crista falciformis (a horizontal bony plate) and Bill's bar (a vertical crest) divide the IAC into quadrants: CN VII is located in the anterosuperior quadrant; CN VIII trifurcates into the anteroinferiorly located cochlear nerve and posteriorly located superior and inferior vestibular nerves. The cochlear nerve travels through the cochlear aperture into the modiolus. CN VII enters the labyrinthine FNC, forms an anterior genu where the geniculate ganglion is located, then travels posteriorly along the medial MEC in the tympanic FNC, passing beneath the lateral SCC and above the oval window. Next, CN VII forms the posterior genu, then courses inferiorly in the mastoid FNC. CN VII exits the stylomastoid foramen before entering the parotid gland. The chorda tympani branches off the mastoid segment of CN VII and courses toward the MEC. The exiting CN VII is prone to birth injury before mastoid process development.

Developmental Variants

On CT images obtained in the first few years of life, it is normal to see a thin pericochlear lucency (*cochlear cartilaginous cleft*); this ossifies over time and should not be mistaken for cochlear otospongiosis [**Fig. 10.13**]. Under age 2 years the posterior petrous bone is not fully ossified, with a small depression adjacent to the vestibular aqueduct and thin bone over the SCC. It is important to bear these developmental variants in mind in order not to misdiagnose large vestibular aqueduct (LVA) or SCC dehiscence, respectively. In infancy there is also transient prominence of the subarcuate canal that travels between the superior SCC limbs; this should not be mistaken for bone erosion caused by an underlying mass [**Fig. 10.13**].

Congenital External and Middle Ear Malformations

Because the external and middle ear structures are both derived from branchial apparatus, congenital external ear malformations are invariably associated with malformed middle ear structures. Clinical presentation includes microtia (small auricle), anotia (absent auricle), abnormally shaped or low-set ears, EAC atresia or stenosis, periauricular tags, pits or masses, craniofacial malformation, and conductive hearing loss (CHL) or mixed hearing loss. EAC malformations may be unilateral or bilateral (symmetric or asymmetric) and isolated or syndromic. Pointers to a syndromic cause or teratogenic insult include micrognathia, bilateral congenital external and middle ear malformation (CEMEM), and associated inner ear malformation. Micrognathia is associated with a low-set auricle; normal fetal mandibular growth is required for the auricle to ascend to its normal location.

EAC atresia is characterized by absence of the EAC and tympanic plate. Coronal CT images show a thick or thin bony and sometimes partly membranous plate at the expected location of the TM [**Fig. 10.14**]. *EAC stenosis* is a narrowed EAC with a hypoplastic tympanic plate [**Fig. 10.14**]. A stenotic EAC tends to trap debris that can, over time, lead to paradoxical EAC widening because of scalloping or erosion from keratosis obturans or EAC cholesteatoma, respectively. EAC atresia and stenosis are associated with deficiency of the manubrium of the malleus, the malleus being fused laterally to the atresia plate in EAC atresia. There is also variable malformation of the incus and stapes, sometimes with additional sites of ossicular fixation. The MEC ranges from near normal to severely hypoplastic. Congenital

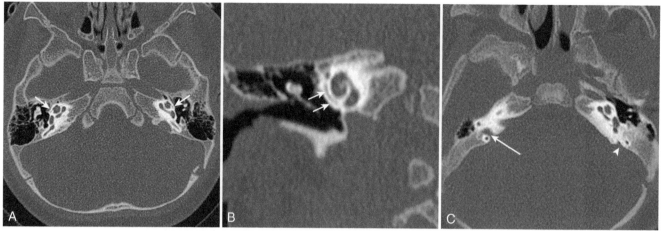

Figure 10.13 Developmental variants of the inner ears in infants. Cochlear cartilaginous cleft. A, Axial and **(B)** coronal computed tomography (CT) images show bilateral, linear perichlear lucencies (*arrows*) that will gradually disappear over time and should not be mistaken for cochlear otospongiosis. **C,** Unossified subarcuate canal and pseudoenlarged vestibular aqueduct. This axial CT demonstrates a prominent right subarcuate canal (*arrow*) traveling between the limbs of the superior SCC. This canal will ossify over the ensuing year, leaving a submillimeter diameter vascular channel. On the left there is incomplete ossification of the posterior petrous bone that simulates the large vestibular aqueduct (LVA; *arrowhead*). Unlike the LVA this normal depression does not connect with the vestibule.

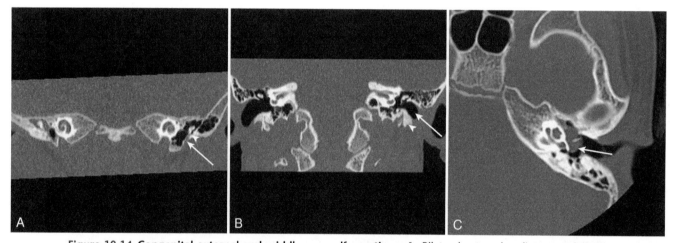

Figure 10.14 Congenital external and middle ear malformations. A, Bilateral external auditory canal (EAC) atresia. Coronal reformatted computed tomography (CT) image reveals that the EACs and tympanic plates are absent. There is a thin bony atresia plate (*long arrow*) on each side. The malleus is ankylosed to the atresia plate (*arrowhead*) with deficiency of the manubrium. The right middle ear cavity is opacified and mastoid pneumatization is poor. **B,** Left EAC stenosis. Coronal reformatted CT image shows narrowing of the EAC (*arrow*). The tympanic plate is mildly misshapen (*arrowhead*). **C,** Congenital cholesteatoma. Axial CT image shows a rounded opacity (*arrow*) surrounding the malleus and abutting the cochlear promontory. This appearance and location is characteristic of congenital cholesteatoma.

MEC cholesteatoma may occur in association, and results in a clinically occult erosive MEC opacity. It is also important to look for *oval window stenosis or atresia,* associated with stapedial malformation and an abnormal course of the FNC tympanic segment, coursing between the stapedial crura over the atretic oval window, over the promontory, or over the MEC floor. The mastoid FNC also descends more ventrally, sometimes over the atresia plate or into the temporomandibular joint (TMJ). Additional malformations include mastoid bone hypoplasia/decreased pneumatization, micrognathia/absent mandibular condyle, and hypoplastic zygomatic arches (eg, TCS, HFM).

Temporal bone findings in *TCS* (see micrognathia) include bilateral EAC atresia/stenosis, severe MEC hypoplasia/aplasia, rudimentary ossicles, oval window atresia, and poor/absent mastoid pneumatization. Variable inner ear malformations

include flattened cochlear turns and malformed vestibules/SCCs. CEMEM occurs in a variety of other syndromes; CEMEM is unilateral in HFM, and bilateral and asymmetric in BOR (with anomalous dilated, Eustachian tubes).

Minor MEC and ossicular anomalies without EAC malformation occur less frequently. Isolated ossicular anomalies include alteration in size, shape, orientation, fusion, and/or fixation. A *monopod stapes* has a single strut in place of two crura. Congenital fusion of the malleus to the attic is termed a *malleus bar*. Isolated oval window stenosis or atresia is associated with stapedial and FNC anomalies as mentioned earlier. FNC dehiscence permits CN VII to protrude into the MEC. CN VII aplasia/hypoplasia is associated with various syndromes (eg, Moebius, CHARGE, and HFM). *Congenital MEC cholesteatoma* appears as a rounded white mass behind an intact TM. CT reveals a rounded mass ventral to or surrounding the malleus and abutting the promontory [**Fig. 10.14**]. Bone erosion and growth into surrounding structures characterizes advanced disease. Congenital EAC cholesteatoma appears as a rounded erosive mass lateral to the TM.

Inner Ear Malformations

Inner ear anomalies present with SNHL, mixed hearing loss, disturbed balance, or with syndromic features affecting other organs. Genetic disorders are a significant cause of SNHL, as are CMV infection and prematurity (multifactorial). Imaging is sometimes helpful in suggesting a genetic or syndromic etiology and provides information that is useful for surgical planning and counseling. Following is a descriptive classification of inner ear malformations.

Vestibular Aqueduct Malformation

1. LVA; large endolymphatic sac anomaly (LESA): usually with cochlear incomplete partition type II (IP-II) or modiolar deficiency

Cochlear Malformations

1. Complete labyrinthine aplasia (Michel anomaly): absent inner ear structures
2. Cochlear aplasia: absent cochlea, normal or malformed vestibule and SCC
3. Cochlear hypoplasia: a small cochlea, usually less than turns, ± internal structure
4. Common cavity malformation: cystic cavity (cochlea + vestibule + SCC)
5. Cystic cochleovestibular malformation: globular cochlea, no internal architecture—IP-I; cochlea, vestibule, and lateral SCC form a bilobed cyst
6. Cochlear IP-I: no internal cochlear architecture; normal or malformed vestibule and SCC
7. Cochlear IP-II (Mondini anomaly): normal cochlear basal turn, deficient septation between plump middle and apical turns, deficient modiolus, LVA
8. Cochlear modiolar deficiency: deficient cochlear modiolus, ± LVA
9. Cochlear nerve and cochlear nerve aperture aplasia or hypoplasia: cochlear nerve canal < 0.7 mm wide or atretic; variable modiolar thickening; cochlear nerve hypoplasia/aplasia

Vestibular and Semicircular Canal Malformations

1. Complete labyrinthine aplasia (Michel deformity): as described earlier

2. Common cavity malformation: as described earlier
3. Cystic cochleovestibular malformation: as described earlier
4. Vestibular hypoplasia with SCC aplasia/hypoplasia: small vestibule; small/absent SCC
5. Vestibule-SCC globular anomaly: dilated vestibule and lateral SCC form a single space
6. SCC small bone island: small bone island between lateral SCC and vestibule

Internal Auditory Canal Malformations

1. IAC aplasia: absent IAC; absent CNs VII and VIII
2. IAC stenosis: narrowed IAC; variable CNs VII and VIII hypoplasia or aplasia
3. IAC enlargement: large IAC; CNs VII and VIII usually normal
4. IAC duplication: variable CNs VII and VIII hypoplasia or aplasia

Perilymph Fistula

1. Communication between inner ear and middle ear cavity at the round or oval window

Genetic or Syndromic Inner Ear Anomalies. *LVA* is the most common inner ear malformation. Clinical presentation is fluctuating, progressive SNHL sometimes following relatively mild head trauma. Children with LVA are advised to avoid contact sports. CT reveals the flared LVA with a midpoint width of ≥1 mm and an opercular width ≥2 mm [**Fig. 10.15**]. On reformats parallel to the plane of the superior SCC long axis, the LVA measures ≥1 mm in width. On thin-section, heavily T2W MR images, there is enlargement of the endolymphatic sac and duct lateral to the dura [**Fig. 10.15**]. There is usually associated cochlear modiolar deficiency or IP-II (the cochlea resembles a *baseball cap*) with variable enlargement of the vestibule and lateral SCC [**Fig. 10.15**]. LVA is associated with a heritable genetic mutation that encodes for the pendrin protein, sometimes resulting in *Pendred syndrome* (LVA with thyroid organification defect leading to hypothyroidism and sometimes goiter).

BOR has a characteristic cochlear anomaly; the basal turn is tapered and the middle and apical turns are hypoplastic and offset anteriorly (*unwound* appearance) [**Fig. 10.16**]. There is also a funnel-shaped LVA, posterior SCC malformation, large/anomalous Eustachian tubes, and CEMEM. *CHARGE* syndrome (see choanal atresia) is characterized by hypoplasia of the vestibule and SCC hypoplasia/aplasia [**Fig. 10.16**]. Other temporal bone findings include oval window atresia, ossicular malformation, absence/flattening of the apical/middle cochlear

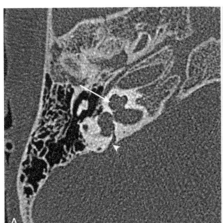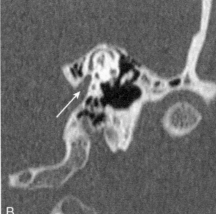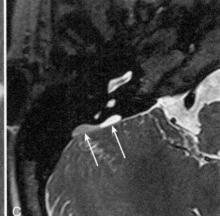

Figure 10.15 Large vestibular aqueduct (LVA) and cochlear incomplete partition type II as seen in Pendred syndrome. A, Axial computed tomography image shows the flared morphology of the LVA (*arrowhead*) extending from the posterior surface of the petrous bone to the vestibule. There is deficient septation between the apical and middle cochlear turns (*arrow*) which appear plump. The modiolus is absent. The cochlear resembles a baseball cap in shape. **B,** The LVA (*arrow*) is well demonstrated on this oblique reformatted image. **C,** Axial T2 SPACE magnetic resonance image showing enlargement of the endolymphatic sac (*arrows*) containing a fluid–fluid level.

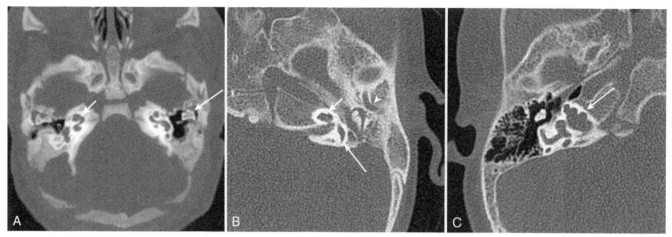

Figure 10.16 Syndromes with characteristic inner ear findings. A, Branchio-oto-renal syndrome. Axial computed tomography (CT) image shows tapered cochlear basal turns with anteriorly offset middle and apical turns producing an "unwound appearance" of the cochlea (*short arrow*). The middle ear spaces are misshapen and partly opacified, and the ossicles are malformed (*long arrow*). **B,** CHARGE syndrome. Axial CT image reveals hypoplasia of the vestibule (*long arrow*) with absent SCC. The cochlea consists of a single turn without internal structure (*short arrow*). The cochlear aperture is stenotic. The MEC is opacified. There is a prominent, anomalous emissary vein coursing along the MEC (*arrowhead*). **C,** X-linked stapes gusher. Axial CT image demonstrates a corkscrew-like appearance of the cochlea (*arrow*) which lacks internal structure with widening of the cochlear aperture. The lateral half of the IAC is dilated.

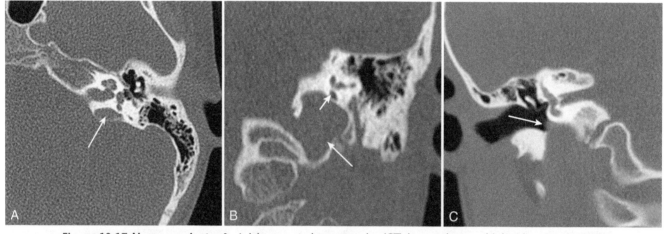

Figure 10.17 Venous variants. A, Axial computed tomography (CT) image shows a high riding jugular bulb (*arrow*) that should not be mistaken for large vestibular aqueduct. **B,** Reformatted coronal image demonstrates the high riding jugular bulb (*long arrow*) in close proximity to the vestibule (*short arrow*). **C,** Dehiscent jugular bulb. Coronal reformatted CT shows deficiency of the bony covering of the jugular bulb (*arrow*) permitting the internal jugular vein to protrude into the middle ear space.

turns, atresia/stenosis of the cochlear nerve aperture, and funnel-shaped LVA. MRI shows variable deficiency of CNs VII and VIII. X-linked mixed hearing loss with stapes gusher affects boys and is associated with an increased risk for CSF gusher during attempted stapedectomy or cochleostomy. Imaging reveals a malformed, *corkscrew-shaped* cochlea without internal structure, with enlargement of the lateral IAC, and sometimes the vestibule and SCC [**Fig. 10.16**]. SCC malformations most frequently involve the lateral SCC, may be isolated or syndromic, and are common in trisomy 21 and Apert syndrome, in which there is a small bone island and globular lateral SCC, or a lateral SCC-vestibule common cavity. Posterior SCC anomalies are seen in a subtype of Waardenburg syndrome and in Alagille syndrome.

Vascular Variants

The IJVs are often asymmetric in size, with the right side larger than the left. A *high-riding jugular bulb* is diagnosed on coronal CT images when its superior aspect protrudes above the IAC floor and is visible on axial images at the level of the cochlear basal turn [**Fig. 10.17**]. A *dehiscent jugular bulb* can produce pulsatile tinnitus and appears as a bluish retrotympanic mass. On CT the jugular bulb protrudes through a bone defect into the posteroinferior MEC [**Fig. 10.17**]. *Jugular venous stenosis/atresia* is associated with some craniofacial disorders such as syndromic craniosynostosis and achondroplasia. In these syndromes, regional emissary veins enlarge and provide collateral venous drainage. An *aberrant ICA* occurs because of segmental aplasia of the extracranial ICA, which is reconstituted by the external carotid artery (ECA) branches before rejoining the horizontal petrous ICA. Clinical presentation is pulsatile tinnitus with a red retrotympanic mass. The aberrant ICA courses lateral to the IJV and lies exposed within the MEC. A *persistent stapedial artery* arises from the petrous ICA, courses in proximity to the stapes, and enters the FNC before reconstituting the middle meningeal artery. The foramen spinosum is absent.

Neck and Oral Cavity

Normal Development and Anatomy

Head and neck structures arise from the branchial apparatus, consisting of paired branchial arches, branchial (or pharyngeal) pouches, branchial clefts (grooves), and branchial membranes. The branchial arches form along the lateral primitive pharynx. Each arch consists of a mesenchymal core (containing neural crest cells and arterial, neural, cartilaginous, ligamentous, and muscular elements). The arches are covered externally by ectoderm and internally by endoderm, and are separated from each other by the branchial clefts externally and the branchial pouches internally. The primitive mouth (stomodeum) arises from surface ectoderm in contact with the amniotic cavity externally. The oral tongue arises primarily from paired lingual mesenchymal proliferations derived from the first branchial arches. The foramen cecum is located in the midline along the posterior third of the tongue. The salivary glands begin as solid proliferations from epithelial buds.

The thyroid primordium is a focal endodermal thickening that arises between the first and second branchial pouches at the site that will become the foramen cecum. The primordium elongates caudally along a diverticulum that continues to develop into a long tract, termed the thyroglossal duct (TGD), and the caudally migrating primordial cells eventually divide into what will become the thyroid lobes and isthmus, with cells contributed from surrounding endoderm. The TGD (and thus path of migration of thyroid primordia) originates in the midline posterior tongue at a point termed the foramen cecum, continues caudally ventral to the hyoid bone, and then transiently loops just posterior to the body of the hyoid before continuing further inferiorly to the thyroid bed. The TGD normally involutes; however, the distal half of the TGD may persist, with the primordial thyroid cells in that location eventually becoming the pyramidal lobe. The thymus and inferior parathyroid glands originate from the third branchial pouch. The superior parathyroid glands arise from the fourth branchial pouch. The laryngotracheal groove and tracheoesophageal folds become the ventral laryngotracheal lumen and dorsal esophagus.

The neck is divided by the hyoid bone into suprahyoid and infrahyoid compartments. Two layers of fascia encompass the neck: the superficial and deep cervical fasciae. The deep cervical fascia in turn consists of superficial, middle, and deep layers. The fascial layers divide the suprahyoid neck into eight compartments (parapharyngeal, pharyngeal mucosal, masticator, parotid, carotid, retropharyngeal (RP), danger, and perivertebral spaces). The sternocleidomastoid muscle (SCM) divides the infrahyoid neck into anterior and posterior triangles. The layers of the deep cervical fascia further subdivide the infrahyoid neck into five major spaces that are continuous with corresponding spaces in the suprahyoid neck (carotid, visceral, posterior cervical, RP, and perivertebral spaces).

The lymphatic system of the neck consists of lymph nodes (LNs) and lymphoid tissue in the Waldeyer ring (the nasopharyngeal adenoid, paired palatine tonsils, and lingual tonsillar tissue). The adenoid becomes prominent within the nasopharynx by 2 to 3 years of age, then regresses during adolescence. If no adenoidal tissue is seen in a young child without prior adenoidectomy, the possibility of immunodeficiency should be considered. The cervical LNs occur in contiguous groups and are classified according to various systems. Parotid, RP, facial, and occipital LNs are named according to location. Level IA is submental LNs; level IB is submandibular LNs. Level II, III, and IV nodes are jugular chain LNs (cranial to caudal). Level V nodes are posterior triangle spinal accessory LNs; level VI nodes are infrahyoid LNs medial to the carotid arteries. Normal LNs are homogeneous, have a fatty hilum, and are oval.

The major head and neck vessels include the common carotid arteries (CCAs), each of which bifurcates into the external carotid artery (ECA) and ICA, and the external, anterior, and IJVs. The IJVs are often asymmetric, right larger than left, sometimes with ectasia in the supine position. The pterygoid venous plexus is sometimes prominent and larger on one side. Medialization of one or both ICAs may occur as an isolated or syndromic finding (eg, 22q11 deletion or velocardiofacial syndrome). This finding is important if pharyngeal or neck surgery is planned. The major nerves traversing the neck include CNs IX through XII, the sympathetic chain, and CN VII and branches of CN V.

The oral cavity contains the tongue, teeth, portions of the mandible, and the floor of the mouth inferiorly, which is bounded by the paired mylohyoid muscles. The mylohyoid muscles form a sling when viewed in the coronal place. Resting within the sling are the left and right sublingual spaces (within the floor of mouth); lateral and external to the sling are the left and right submandibular spaces (outside of the floor of mouth). Thus each sublingual space and the ipsilateral submandibular space are separated by the mylohyoid muscle. The major salivary glands consist of paired parotid, submandibular, and sublingual glands. Minor salivary glands also exist in many locations in the head and neck, including on the oral mucosa, in the floor of mouth, along the palate, and even in the sinonasal cavity. Most muscles of the suprahyoid neck attach to the mandible. The maxilla contains the maxillary sinuses.

Tornwaldt Cyst

Tornwaldt cyst is a developmental nasopharyngeal cyst that is usually an incidental finding. On imaging, it is sharply circumscribed, thin-walled, and located in the midline along the posterior nasopharynx. It is typically hyperintense on T2W MR, variable in signal on T1W MR, and does not enhance [**Fig. 10.18**].

Branchial Apparatus Anomalies

Branchial anomalies are thought to arise due to remnants or incomplete obliteration of the branchial apparatus, or due to

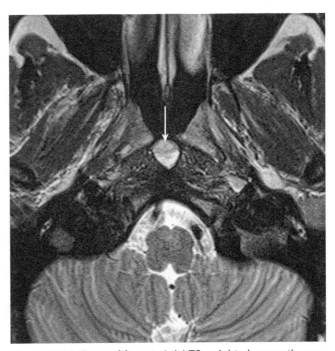

Figure 10.18 Tornwaldt cyst. Axial T2-weighted magnetic resonance image shows a sharply circumscribed ovoid lesion (*arrow*) nestled between the prevertebral muscles, posterior to the adenoid.

trapped epithelial rests. Branchial apparatus anomalies include cysts, sinus tracts (ectodermal or endodermal opening), fistulae (both openings) and aberrant tissue, and are classified according to the arch, cleft, or pouch of origin. Fistulae and sinuses, usually identified at birth because of drainage, are best imaged by CT, sometimes with a contrast-enhanced fistulogram. Branchial apparatus cysts (BAC) are more frequently diagnosed in older children and adults. Ultrasonography reveals an anechoic or hypoechoic thin-walled cyst. CT and MRI show an oval or round cyst with minimal, if any, peripheral enhancement. Wall thickening, enhancement, and surrounding edema suggest superimposed inflammation.

First BAC locations include the parotid region, periauricular soft tissues, EAC, MEC, or nasopharynx. A *Work type I* BAC is periauricular and *Work type II* is periparotid [**Fig. 10.19**]. The differential diagnosis of first BAC includes dermoid cyst, LM, and necrotic adenopathy (eg, nontuberculous mycobacterial infection). The *second BAC* is the most common branchial anomaly. The usual location is at the mandibular angle, posterior to the submandibular gland, lateral to the ICA/IJV, and anterior to SCM (type II second BAC) [**Fig. 10.19**]. Type I second BAC is deep to platysma, lateral to SCM. Type III second BAC protrudes between the ICA and ECA, and may extend to the lateral pharyngeal wall or skull base. Type IV (second pouch anomaly) is adjacent to the lateral pharyngeal wall. The differential diagnosis includes dermoid, LM, necrotic adenopathy, and laryngocele. The *third BAC* is in the upper posterior cervical space or lower anterior neck. Recurrent infrahyoid neck abscess or suppurative thyroiditis, particularly if it contains air, should raise the possibility of an underlying pyriform sinus tract [**Fig. 10.20**]. This anomaly is thought to arise from the embryonal thymopharyngeal duct of the third branchial pouch. After resolution of inflammation, a contrast swallowing study may demonstrate the sinus tract. Other branchial anomalies include thymic [**Fig. 10.21**] and parathyroid anomalies such as aberrant cervical thymus, thymic cysts, parathyroid cysts, aberrant parathyroid tissue, and thyroid anomalies (see later).

Thyroid Anomalies

TGD cyst is common and arises from TGD remnants. TGD cyst occurs in the midline from the foramen cecum to the hyoid bone or off midline in the infrahyoid neck. Ultrasonography,

CT, and MRI reveal a circumscribed rounded, ovoid, or elliptical cyst, often in proximity to the hyoid bone or in association with the strap muscles [**Fig. 10.22**]. TGD cyst is anechoic or hypoechoic on ultrasonography, hypodense on CT, hyperintense on T2W MRI, and variable in signal on T1W MRI with minimal, if any, peripheral contrast enhancement. Irregularity, thickening, and enhancement of the cyst wall occurs because of inflammation. TGD cyst may contain ectopic thyroid tissue; however, mineralization in the cyst or necrotic adenopathy in the neck suggests development of malignancy (usually papillary carcinoma), which occasionally occurs in children. The differential diagnosis includes vallecular cyst, foregut duplication cyst (FDC), dermoid, LM, and BAC. *Thyroid gland anomalies* include complete or hemiagenesis and ectopic thyroid [**Fig. 10.23**]. The most common location of ectopic thyroid is the *lingual thyroid,* located in the midline at the tongue base. Ectopic thyroid may occur elsewhere in the neck, analogous to the locations of TGD cyst. The ectopic thyroid may be the only functioning thyroid tissue; therefore imaging should include a search for orthotopic thyroid especially if surgical removal of the ectopic thyroid tissue is planned. Thyroid scintigraphy is useful for assessing functioning thyroid tissue. CT reveals the hyperdense ectopic thyroid tissue, which is less readily appreciated on MRI. Hypothyroidism should prompt a search for ectopic thyroid.

Laryngocele

An aerated or fluid-filled (saccular) laryngocele results from obstructive dilatation of the laryngeal ventricle appendix. A laryngocele may be internal, external, or translaryngeal. Complications include infection and airway compromise. The appearance on imaging varies with air and fluid content. Coronal images are useful for showing its relationship to the larynx. The differential diagnosis includes TGD cyst, LM, and FDC.

Anomalies of the Oral Cavity, Tongue, and Salivary Glands

TGD cyst, lingual thyroid, and BAC are discussed earlier. Other congenital cystic lesions of the tongue and oral cavity may present as a mass or airway obstruction and must be

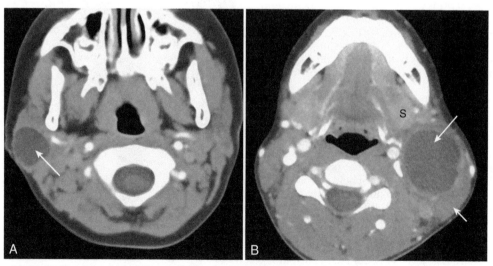

Figure 10.19 A, First branchial cleft cyst (BCC). Axial contrast-enhanced computed tomography (CECT) shows a sharply circumscribed, nonenhancing, low-attenuation right parotid cyst (*arrow*). **B,** Second BCC. CECT image reveals a rounded low-attenuation, nonenhancing cyst (*long arrow*) located posterior to the submandibular gland (*S*), lateral to the carotid sheath, and anteromedial to the SCM muscle (*short arrow*).

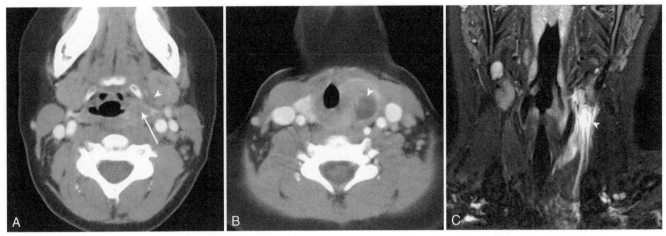

Figure 10.20 Pyriform sinus tract. A, Axial contrast-enhanced computed tomography (CECT) shows mucosal swelling with effacement of the left pyriform sinus (*arrow*). There is mild adjacent edema (*arrowhead*). **B,** CECT more caudal image demonstrates low attenuation with peripheral enhancement intimately involving the left lobe of the thyroid gland (*arrowhead*), consistent with suppurative thyroiditis caused by an underlying pyriform sinus tract. **C,** Coronal T2 short tau inversion recovery magnetic resonance image reveals mucosal swelling surrounding the left pyriform sinus and linear high signal intensity in the adjacent soft tissues (*arrowhead*). The presence of infrahyoid neck infection, typically left-sided should raise concern for an underlying branchial pouch anomaly.

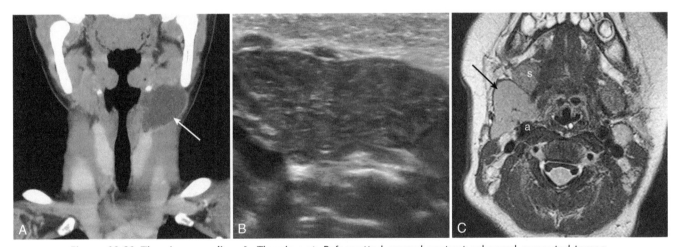

Figure 10.21 Thymic anomalies. A, Thymic cyst. Reformatted coronal contrast-enhanced computed tomography (CECT) shows an ovoid submandibular cyst (*arrow*) with peripheral enhancement and a pointed inferior margin. It extends toward the superior pole of the thyroid gland. The differential diagnosis primarily includes a thyroglossal duct cyst [see **Fig. 10.22C**] or branchial cleft cyst. **B,** Ectopic thymus. Ultrasound of this solid neck mass reveals a lesion that is isoechoic with thymus. **C,** On T2-weighted MRI there is a solid triangular mass (*arrow*) located posterior to the submandibular gland (*s*) and ventral to the common carotid artery (*a*). This location and triangular morphology is characteristic of cervical thymus.

differentiated from TGD cyst, such as FDC, dermoid, and vallecular cyst. All appear hypodense on CT, hyperintense on T2W MRI, and of variable signal on T1W MRI, with little, if any, peripheral Gd enhancement [**Fig. 10.24**]. Dermoid and FDC are usually midline; FDC most commonly occurs in the anterior third of the tongue, whereas dermoid is sublingual. FDC is rounded, ovoid, or tubular with facilitated diffusion on MRI, whereas dermoid is rounded or ovoid, but usually with decreased diffusivity on MR. Vallecular cyst arises in the vallecula and abuts the epiglottis. Salivary gland agenesis is rare, causes xerostomia, and may be associated with lacrimal gland aplasia. Unilateral parotid hypoplasia is associated with HFM. Failure of canalization of the distal salivary duct leads to a salivary mucocele.

Vascular Anomalies

Vascular anomalies include malformations and true tumors (eg, IH; see section in tumors). Vascular malformations are divided into low-flow lesions such as LM and VM, and high-flow lesions such as AVM and AVF. Vascular malformations are present at birth, grow commensurately with patient growth, and manifest as a mass and/or alteration in function. Clinically occult lesions may present later because of sudden enlargement from intercurrent hemorrhage or infection (LM), or painful thrombophlebitis (VM). Neonatal proptosis or sudden onset of proptosis (other than from complicated sinusitis) should prompt a search for orbital LM/VM or AVM/AVF.

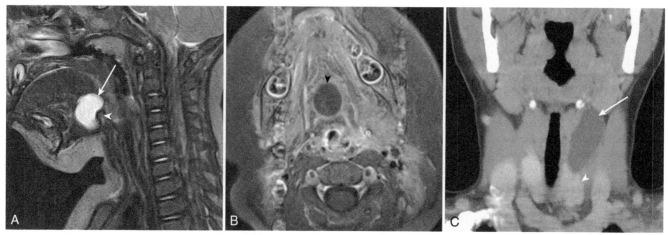

Figure 10.22 Thyroglossal duct cyst (TGDC). A, Sagittal T2-weighted magnetic resonance imaging (MRI) demonstrates a midline, sharply defined cystic-appearing lesion (*arrow*) abutting the ventral aspect of the hyoid bone (*arrowhead*), an appearance that is typical for TGDC. **B,** Axial gadolinium-enhanced fat-suppressed T1-weighted MRI shows that the hypointense TGDC (*arrowhead*) has only minimal peripheral enhancement. **C,** Coronal reformatted contrast-enhanced computed tomography (CECT) shows an off-midline infrahyoid TGDC (*arrow*) indenting the superior pole of the left lobe of the thyroid gland (*arrowhead*). Note the similarity to a thymic cyst [see **Fig. 10.21A**].

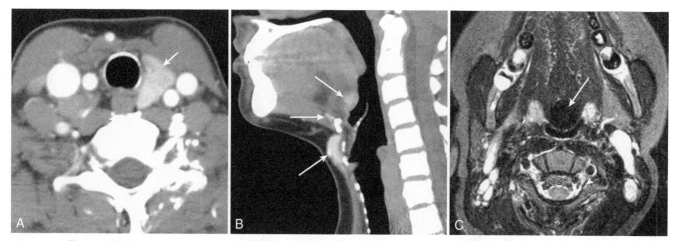

Figure 10.23 Thyroid hemiagenesis with ectopic thyroid tissue. A, Axial contrast-enhanced computed tomography (CECT) image demonstrates only a left lobe of thyroid (*arrow*). The right lobe is absent. **B,** The sagittal reformatted CECT image (same patient) shows that there are three midline foci of ectopic thyroid tissue (*arrows*) located at the base of the tongue, and ventral and inferior to the hyoid bone. **C,** Lingual thyroid tissue. This axial fat-suppressed T2-weighted magnetic resonance image reveals a nodule of lingual thyroid tissue (*arrow*) that is minimally hypointense compared with muscle, located between the lingual tonsillar tissue along the posterior aspect of the tongue.

LMs consist of dysplastic lymphatic channels and appear unilocular or multilocular and microcystic and/or macrocystic [**Figs. 10.25** and **10.26**]. On ultrasonography, LMs range from hypoechoic to echogenic because of infection/hemorrhage [**Fig. 10.25**]. On CT and MR, *fluid–fluid* levels are characteristic of LM [**Fig. 10.26**]. Uncomplicated LM appears hypodense on CT, hyperintense on T2W MRI, and usually hypointense on T1W MRI. Adjacent veins are sometimes dilated. Increased CT density, high or low signal on T2W, and high signal on T1W imaging occurs because of hemorrhage [**Fig. 10.26**]. Infection causes stranding of adjacent fat. Contrast-enhanced images show septal enhancement only—the lymph fluid does not enhance. Enhancement of fluid may reflect the presence of a mixed LM-VM. Orbital LM or LM-VM is strongly associated with intracranial developmental venous anomalies, cavernous

malformations, and occasionally AVF/AVM. Multiple LMs with osseous involvement leading to demineralization is a feature of Gorham-Stout syndrome. The differential diagnosis depends on location and size, and includes VM, dermoid, BAC, TGDC, ranula, teratoma, and plexiform neurofibroma.

VMs consist of dysplastic venous channels. VMs enlarge with Valsalva maneuver or dependent positioning and appear bluish if superficial or involving skin. The imaging hallmark of VMs is phleboliths, which are small, rounded, and mineralized [**Figs. 10.27** and **10.28**]. Although similar to LM on nonenhanced images, fluid–fluid levels are not usually seen and the venous blood within the VM usually enhances gradually on CECT and MRI [**Figs. 10.27** and **10.28**]. Midline facial VM may be associated with transcalvarial venous connections (sinus pericranii) and intracranial developmental venous anomalies. Multiple VMs

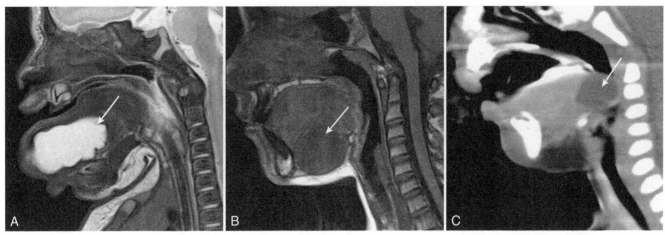

Figure 10.24 Developmental tongue cysts. A, Foregut duplication cyst (FDC). Sagittal T2-weighted magnetic resonance (MR) image shows a lobulated, midline, cystic lesion (*arrow*) in the anterior half of the tongue. The cyst is more ventrally located than a TGDC. The differential diagnosis includes a lymphatic malformation. **B,** Dermoid. Sagittal T1-weighted MR imaging reveals a sharply circumscribed, midline oval lesion (*arrow*) in the floor of the mouth. It is mildly hypointense compared with muscle. The lesion is more inferiorly located than would be typical for FDC and more ventrally located than TGDC. Decreased diffusivity (not shown) supports the diagnosis of dermoid. **C,** Vallecular cyst. Reformatted sagittal contrast-enhanced computed tomography (CECT) shows a cyst (*arrow*) located superior to the epiglottis and protruding into the vallecula, with mass effect on the airway. Although the differential diagnosis includes TGDC, TGDC is located slightly more anteriorly and does not usually protrude into the vallecula in this fashion.

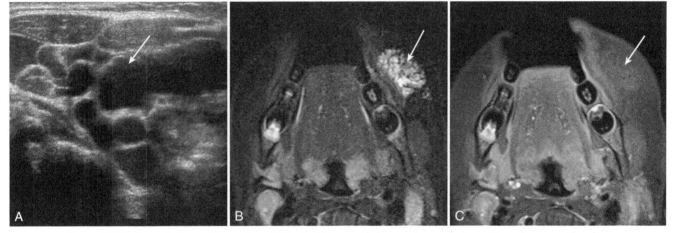

Figure 10.25 Lymphatic malformation (LM). A, Ultrasound shows a hypoechoic cystic neck mass with echogenic septations (*arrow*), consistent with a macrocystic LM. **B,** Axial T2 short tau inversion recovery magnetic resonance (MR) image reveals a left buccal microcystic lesion (*arrow*). **C,** Axial gadolinium-enhanced fat-suppressed T1-weighted MR image (same patient) shows that the cyst (*arrow*) contents do not enhance, distinguishing this LM from a venous malformation.

are a feature of *blue rubber bleb nevus syndrome.* Extensive cutaneous capillary-venular malformation in the distribution of the trigeminal nerve is a feature of Sturge-Weber syndrome. Dilated orbital venous structures may be seen because of VM, secondary to AVM or AVF, or because of IJV obstruction.

AVMs and AVFs may produce a bruit and sometimes hyperemia and overgrowth of the affected part. Ultrasonography, CT, and MRI reveal enlarged arterial feeders and draining veins. AVM has a mesh of intervening vessels known as a nidus [**Fig. 10.29**]. Wyburn-Mason syndrome (an example of a cerebrofacial metameric or segmental syndrome) is characterized by orbital, maxillary, and diencephalic AVMs. Carotid cavernous fistula (CCF) may be congenital or acquired (posttraumatic or iatrogenic) [**Fig. 10.30**]. In addition to CTA and MRA, conventional catheter angiography, which provides temporal information in addition

to the anatomic information available on cross-sectional imaging, may be required to diagnose and differentiate AVM and AVF and/or to deliver endovascular treatment [**Figs. 10.29** and **10.30**].

TRAUMA

Orbit and Globe

Orbital injuries are common, are usually due to blunt or penetrating trauma, and include corneal laceration, traumatic hyphema (bleeding into the anterior chamber), vitreous hemorrhage, globe rupture, lens rupture/dislocation, ocular detachments (retinal, choroidal, or vitreous), foreign body, ON injury, orbital hematoma, and fracture. Unexplained retinal hemorrhage in an infant should prompt a search for abusive head trauma. Globe

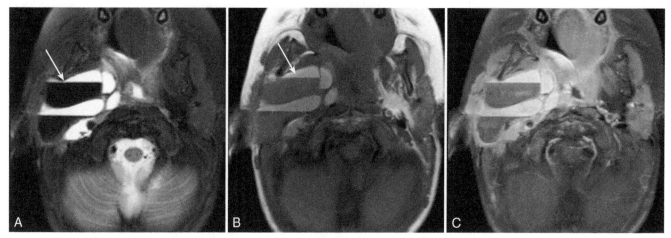

Figure 10.26 Lymphatic malformation (LM) complicated by hemorrhage. A, T2 short tau inversion recovery magnetic resonance (MR) image shows a macrocystic LM within the right parapharyngeal space. The fluid–fluid levels (*arrow*), a characteristic finding for LM, are due to hemorrhage. **B,** Axial T1-weighted (T1W) MR image demonstrates that the ventral component of the fluid is hyperintense relative to muscle (*arrow*). **C,** Axial gadolinium-enhanced fat-suppressed T1W MR image shows that the fluid does not enhance per se. It is important to review the unenhanced T1W images so as not to misinterpret the ventral high signal intensity as enhancement, as would be seen in a venous malformation.

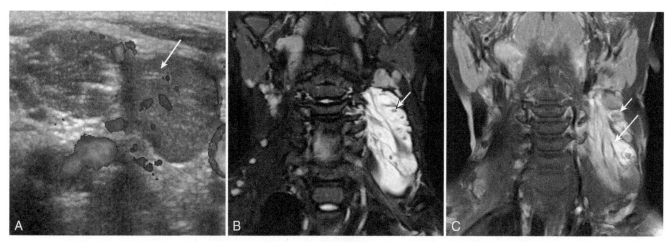

Figure 10.27 Venous malformation (VM). A, Ultrasonography shows a lobulated mass (*arrow*) with moderately echogenic contents and increased through-transmission. **B,** Coronal T2 STIR magnetic resonance (MR) image reveals a septated cystic neck mass containing small, rounded, hypointense foci (*arrow*), due to phleboliths, as are characteristic of VM. **C,** Coronal gadolinium-enhanced fat-suppressed T1-weighted MR image shows that, unlike LM, the fluid within the VM enhances (*long arrow*). The phleboliths are again demonstrated (*short arrow*).

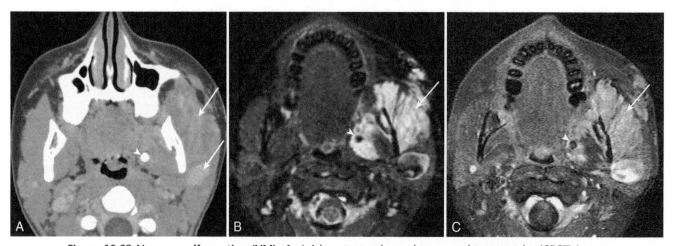

Figure 10.28 Venous malformation (VM). A, Axial contrast-enhanced computed tomography (CECT) image demonstrates heterogeneous enhancement (*arrows*) in a left masticator space VM. A phlebolith (*arrowhead*) is present in the deeper component along the pterygoid muscles. **B,** Axial T2 short tau inversion recovery magnetic resonance (MR) image shows that the cheek and masticator space VM (*arrow*) is isointense with CSF. The phlebolith appears as a rounded signal void (*arrowhead*). **C,** Gadolinium-enhanced fat-suppressed T1-weighted MR image showing that the VM enhances (*arrow*). The phlebolith is again seen (*arrowhead*).

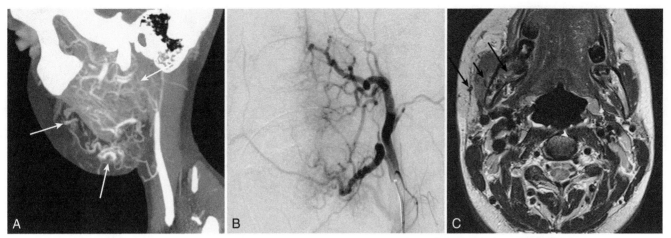

Figure 10.29 **Arteriovenous malformation (AVM). A,** Sagittal reconstructed maximum intensity projection computed tomography angiography image demonstrates a right masticator and buccal space AVM (*arrows*) with arterial supply from multiple external carotid artery (ECA) feeders. **B,** Lateral projection from the conventional angiogram, right ECA injection, shows a capillary blush with arterial supply from branches of the internal maxillary and facial arteries. **C,** Axial T2-weighted magnetic resonance image shows prominent signal voids due to vessels within the mildly swollen right masseter muscle and cheek (*short arrows*). Venous drainage is primarily to the retromandibular vein. Note the asymmetric low signal intensity and prominent vascular flow voids due to mandibular involvement (*long arrow*).

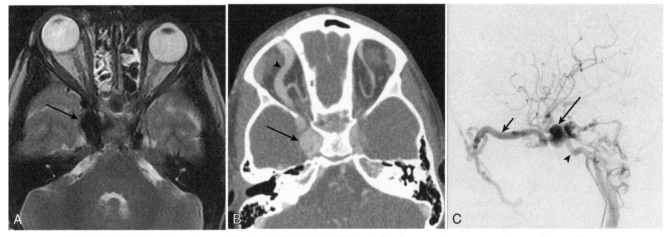

Figure 10.30 **Carotid-cavernous fistula (CCF). A,** Axial T2-weighted magnetic resonance image shows a large, asymmetric right cavernous sinus (CS) vascular flow void (*arrow*). **B,** Axial computed tomography angiography image demonstrates a right CCF (*arrow*) with drainage primarily via a large superior ophthalmic vein (SOV; *arrowhead*). **C,** Conventional catheter angiogram right internal carotid artery (ICA) (*arrowhead*) injection confirms the CCF with brisk filling of the distended CS (*long arrow*) via a defect in the cavernous segment of the right ICA with rapid drainage into an enlarged SOV (*short arrow*).

rupture constitutes an emergency with the risk for unilateral or bilateral blindness. Imaging features include volume loss or irregularity of the globe, intraocular gas, or ocular foreign body [**Fig. 10.31**]. The presence of an orbital ferromagnetic foreign body is an absolute contraindication to MRI.

Orbital fractures may be isolated or accompany other facial and calvarial fractures. *Orbital roof fracture* poses a risk for CSF leak, meningitis, and traumatic cephalocele. A depressed fracture fragment may impinge upon the globe. An *orbital blow-out fracture* results from direct blunt injury producing an orbital floor fracture (inferior blow-out; most common), lamina papyracea fracture (medial blow-out), or both. Displaced bone fragments result in herniation of orbital fat and sometimes herniation or entrapment of the inferior rectus with or without the inferior oblique (inferior blow-out; herniates into maxillary antrum) or medial rectus muscles (medial blow out; herniates

into ethmoid air cells). Thin-section helical CT with submillimeter MPRs demonstrates the fracture(s), sometimes with herniated fat and muscle [**Fig. 10.32**]. Orbital gas points to an underlying fracture, and the affected sinus usually contains an air–fluid level because of hemorrhage. Clinical signs of entrapment include diplopia, numbness in the distribution of the inferior orbital nerve, and gaze limitation. Enophthalmos is a late complication. A *tripod fracture* results from a malar blow and comprises fractures of the orbital floor/rim and maxillary antrum, zygomatic arch, and the lateral orbital wall or zygomaticofrontal suture. Greater wing of sphenoid fracture involves the lateral orbital wall. Severe trauma resulting in anterior and central skull base fracture may extend to the orbital apex and/or involve the optic strut/ON canal with potential ON contusion or laceration. CTA may be required to diagnose vascular complications including CCF.

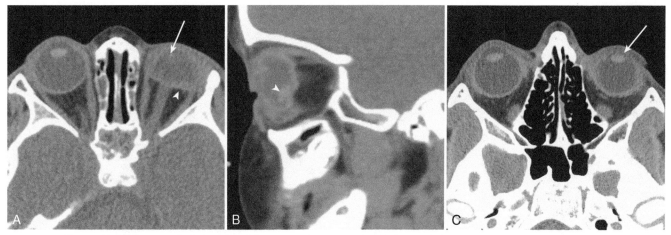

Figure 10.31 Ruptured globe. A, Axial computed tomography (CT) image shows irregularity of contour of the left globe which appears smaller than the right with flattening posteriorly (*arrowhead*). Only a small fragment of the lens is present (*arrow*). **B,** Reformatted sagittal CT image (same patient) demonstrates the irregular contour of the ruptured globe which contains high attenuation material because of vitreous hemorrhage, lens material, or both (*arrowhead*). **C,** Axial CT image shows subtle flattening of the anterior chamber of the globe (*arrow*) and the smaller ruptured left globe.

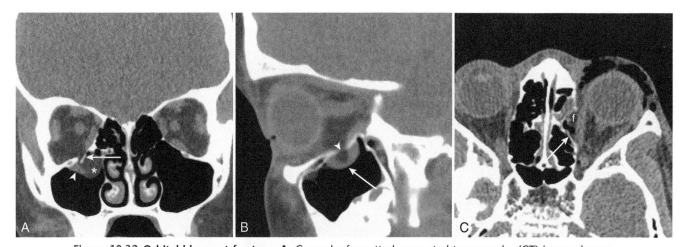

Figure 10.32 Orbital blow-out fracture. A, Coronal reformatted computed tomography (CT) image demonstrates a comminuted inferior blow-out fracture with a displaced angulated fracture fragment (*arrow*), and herniation of the inferior rectus muscle (IRM; *arrowhead*) and orbital fat (*asterisk*) into the maxillary antrum. **B,** Sagittal reformatted CT image (same patient) shows the herniated, trapped IRM (*arrow*) and fat (*arrowhead*). **C,** Axial CT image reveals a medial blow-out fracture caused by a comminuted, angulated lamina papyracea fracture (*arrow*). There is herniation of extraconal fat (*f*) into the adjacent ethmoid air cell. There is extensive preseptal gas and the lens is not seen, consistent with ocular injury.

Nasal Cavity, Paranasal Sinuses, and Face

The nose is a favorite hideout for inserted or expectorated foreign bodies, often without a preceding history in a young child. CT or MRI demonstrates a variable-density/intensity and sometimes air-containing foreign object in the nasal cavity, often with sharply defined contours [**Fig. 10.33**]. Rhinoliths are mineralized concretions. Complications include irritation and sinonasal infection. Facial fractures are uncommon in young children but tend to occur as the sinuses pneumatize. Thin-section helical CT with submillimeter MPRs is used to diagnose the site and evaluate for displacement and complications of fractures. Le Fort type fractures are not prevalent in young children compared with older children and adults. Nasal fractures are often comminuted or bilateral and may be associated with nasal septal fracture, deviation, and hematoma [**Fig. 10.33**]. Involvement of the NLD leads to complications such as obstruction and epiphora. Mandibular fractures are often bilateral with condylar and

tympanic plate fractures resulting from a blow to the chin [**Fig. 10.34**]. Mandibular neck, coronoid process, or symphyseal fractures also occur, sometimes involving the teeth. Complications include TMJ subluxation or dislocation and, later, TMJ ankylosis.

Ear and Temporal Bone

Temporal bone fractures result from severe temporoparietal impact (resulting in longitudinal fractures) or frontooccipital impact (resulting in transverse fractures). Fractures are traditionally classified according to the fracture trajectory with respect to the petrous bone and more recently according to whether the otic capsule is fractured (otic capsule-violating) or not (otic capsule-sparing). Longitudinal fractures are parallel and transverse fractures are perpendicular to the petrous bone long axis; in reality, mixed (oblique) fractures are common in children.

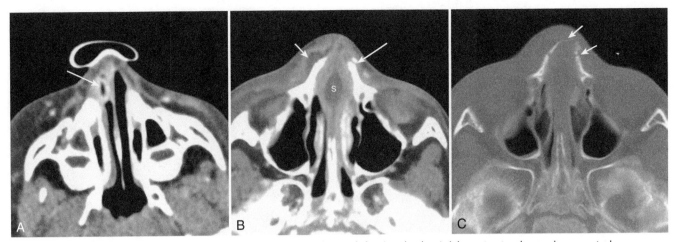

Figure 10.33 Nasal foreign body and injury. A, Nasal foreign body. Axial contrast-enhanced computed tomography (CECT) image shows a sharply defined, centrally hypodense, ovoid structure (*arrow*) within the right nasal vestibule. A lima bean was subsequently extracted. **B,** Nasal fracture. Axial CECT demonstrates an elliptical rim-enhancing subperiosteal fluid collection along the right nasal bone (*short arrow*) and a low-density focus within the nasal septum (*s*) consistent with infected hematomas in this patient with nasal bone fractures (*long arrow*). **C,** Bone window computed tomography (same patient) shows comminuted, displaced nasal bone fractures (*arrows*).

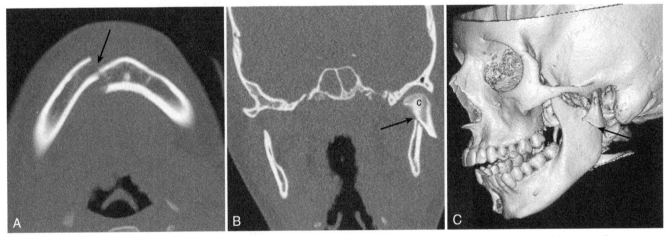

Figure 10.34 Mandibular fractures. A, Axial computed tomography (CT) image shows a displaced fracture of the anterior right mandibular body (*arrow*). **B,** Coronal reformatted CT and (**C**) three-dimensional CT demonstrate a displaced, angulated left mandibular neck/ramus fracture (*arrow*) with overlapping fracture fragments.

Imaging requires subaxial temporal bone CT with submillimeter MPRs. Foci of subcutaneous and/or intracranial gas and MEC/mastoid air cell opacification caused by hemotympanum and mastoid blood are usually seen. *Longitudinal fractures* are more likely to be *otic capsule-sparing*, and course through the mastoid air cells and middle ear, with a tendency to cause ossicular fracture, dislocation, or subluxation, with ossicular fragmentation, displacement, and/or joint diastasis [**Fig. 10.35**]. Tegmen fracture is best diagnosed on coronal views. The fracture then courses anteriorly, sometimes involving the proximal tympanic FNC/anterior genu, Eustachian tube, and the CC. Further imaging with MRI/MRA and/or CTA may be indicated to assess for ICA dissection if the CC is fractured. Fracture of the jugular foramen may be associated with IJV thrombosis. Complications include CHL, CN VII palsy, Eustachian tube dysfunction, CSF leak, meningitis, vascular complications, posttraumatic cephalocele, and pars tensa cholesteatoma. *Transverse fractures* are more likely to be *otic capsule-violating* [**Fig. 10.35**]. The fracture may traverse any inner ear structure. Otic capsule bone is extremely hard and has a poor osteogenic response leading to

a high incidence of fibrous union or nonunion [**Fig. 10.35**]. Pneumolabyrinth may occur with or without fracture. The labyrinthine segment of the FNC is sometimes fractured. Complications include SNHL, vertigo, facial nerve palsy, labyrinthitis ossificans, perilymph and/or CSF leak, and meningitis.

Oral Cavity and Neck

The oral cavity and neck may be injured by a variety of mechanisms. Toddlers who fall with objects (such as toothbrushes or lollipops) in their mouths are at risk for *oropharyngeal perforation.* CT reveals mucosal swelling and extraluminal gas. Vascular complications are uncommon and include IJV thrombosis, arterial dissection, contusion, laceration, or pseudoaneurysm. *Foreign body impaction* (eg, fish or chicken bone, ingested coin) is sometimes detectable on PF or CT. Complications include airway perforation and infection [**Fig. 10.36**]. CT manifestations of blunt or penetrating neck trauma include swelling, hematoma, soft tissue emphysema (from penetrating airway injury or laceration), airway compromise, and vascular injury.

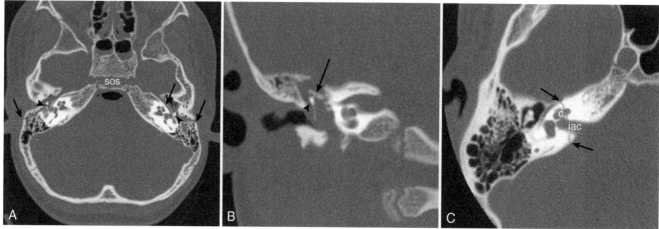

Figure 10.35 Temporal bone fractures. A, Longitudinal fracture. Axial computed tomography (CT) image shows bilateral diastatic longitudinal temporal bone fractures (*arrows*). The middle ear cavities (MECs) and mastoid air cells are opacified. The head of the left malleus (*arrowhead;* "ice cream") is dislocated and displaced against the tympanic segment of the facial nerve canal. There is also dislocation and displacement of the right incudomalleal joint (*arrowhead*). Pneumocephalus is present, and there is diastasis of the sphenooccipital synchondrosis (*sos*). **B,** Tegmen tympani fracture. Coronal reformatted CT demonstrates a comminuted tegmen tympani fracture with inferior displacement of the fracture fragment (*arrow*) and ossicles (*arrowhead*). There is extensive MEC and mastoid opacification. Fracture complications include cerebrospinal fluid leak, meningitis, and posttraumatic cephalocele. **C,** Transverse temporal bone fracture. Axial CT image shows an otic capsule-violating transverse fracture (*arrows*) traversing the internal auditory meatus (*iac*) and middle turn of the cochlea (*c*) leading to sensorineural hearing loss.

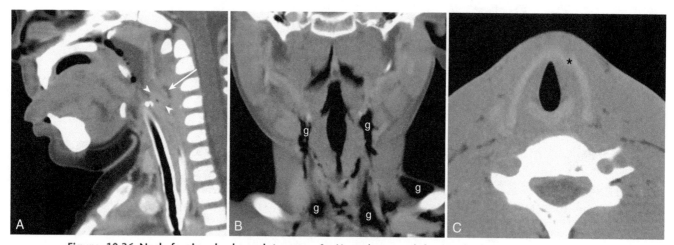

Figure 10.36 Neck foreign body and trauma. A, Hypopharyngeal foreign body. Reconstructed sagittal contrast-enhanced computed tomography (CECT) image shows retropharyngeal swelling and a small low-density fluid collection (*arrow*) caused by infection secondary to a retained hypopharyngeal foreign body (*arrowheads*). **B,** Soft tissue emphysema. Reformatted coronal CECT demonstrates extensive gas (*g*) within the soft tissues of the neck caused by airway laceration from blunt trauma. **C,** Laryngeal fracture. Axial computed tomography image shows a displaced fracture (*asterisk*) of the left thyroid cartilage.

Vascular complications also include transection, AVF, and thrombosis. Fracture of the hyoid bone and laryngeal or thyroid cartilages may occur, and contrast-enhanced thin-section CT is useful for assessment of unossified cartilage in children [**Fig. 10.36**].

INFECTION AND INFLAMMATORY PROCESSES

Orbit and Globe

Orbital infection is common. Imaging is warranted when there are symptoms or signs such as periorbital swelling, proptosis, painful ophthalmoplegia, diplopia, and blurred or decreased vision. In the acute setting, if there is suspected bacterial infection (eg, orbital complications of acute sinusitis), CECT (or CT venography) is obtained with soft tissue and bone MPRs. MR is preferred for the assessment of visual symptoms and to assess for intracranial complications. Ocular infections are not usually imaged acutely. However, infection with toxocariasis and CMV can result in ocular scarring with mineralized microphthalmos seen on CT and MRI.

Suppurative Infection

Suppurative infection is usually caused by bacteria (eg, staphylococcus, streptococcus, or pneumococcus). *Preseptal cellulitis* produces periorbital and preseptal soft tissue thickening of the

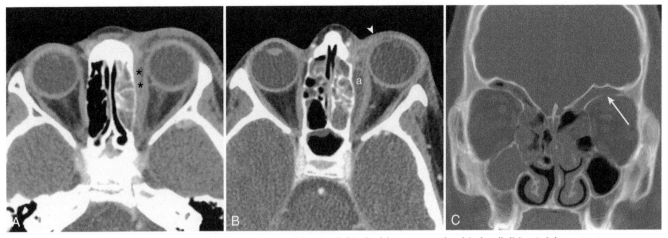

Figure 10.37 **Orbital complications of sinusitis. A,** Orbital phlegmon and orbital cellulitis. Axial contrast-enhanced computed tomography (CECT) shows left preseptal periorbital soft tissue swelling (STS) and left ethmoid air cell opacification. There is increased density of the left medial extraconal orbital fat (*asterisks*), consistent with phlegmon. The adjacent medial rectus muscle is thickened. There is subtle increased density of the intraconal orbital fat, consistent with orbital cellulitis. **B,** Orbital subperiosteal abscess. Axial CECT shows preseptal periorbital STS (*arrowhead*), extensive left ethmoid air cell opacification, and an elliptical low-density, peripherally enhancing, medial subperiosteal abscess (*a*). **C,** Reformatted coronal image in a patient with a superior subperiosteal abscess (not shown) shows opacification of paranasal sinuses with subtle erosion of the left orbital roof (*arrow*), consistent with osteomyelitis.

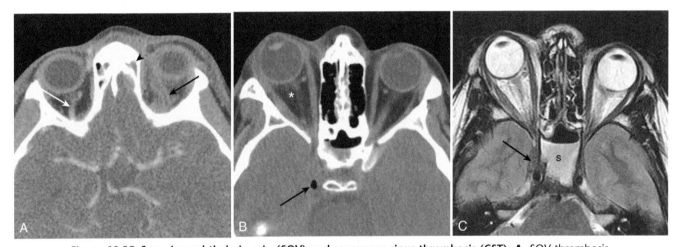

Figure 10.38 **Superior ophthalmic vein (SOV) and cavernous sinus thrombosis (CST). A,** SOV thrombosis. Axial contrast-enhanced computed tomography (CECT) shows opacification of the partially visualized paranasal sinuses (*arrowhead*). There is a tram-track sign due to lack of enhancement of the thrombosed left SOV (*black arrow*). Compare with the normally enhancing right SOV (*white arrow*). **B,** CST. Axial computed tomography image demonstrates a sphenoid sinus air–fluid level caused by sphenoid sinusitis. Gas is present within the right cavernous sinus (*arrow*) due to CST. There is resultant right ocular proptosis with minimal reticulation of the right intraconal orbital fat (*asterisk*). **C,** Axial T2-weighted magnetic resonance (same patient) shows low signal intensity within the right cavernous sinus with lateral convexity of its lateral margin (*arrow*), consistent with CST. Note the sphenoid sinus air–fluid level (*s*).

soft tissues anterior to the orbital septum. When preseptal cellulitis occurs in isolation, the orbital septum serves as an excellent barrier to the postseptal spread of infection. *Postseptal infection* usually results from acute complicated sinusitis and occurs in proximity to the inciting infected PNS. It is most commonly medial (from ethmoid sinusitis), but can be inferior (from maxillary sinusitis) or superior (from frontal sinusitis). Spread occurs directly through infected bone or via emissary veins. On CECT, phlegmonous change results in extraconal soft tissue thickening with increased density of the affected extraconal fat [**Fig. 10.37**]. This can progress to an elliptical ring-enhancing subperiosteal abscess with associated local EOM swelling [**Fig.**

10.37]. Increased density of the intraconal fat occurs because of intraconal orbital cellulitis, SOV thrombosis, or cavernous sinus thrombosis (CST), or a combination of these causes [**Figs. 10.37** and **10.38**]. Other causes of infection include penetrating trauma, seeding from systemic infection, NLD infection, and surgery.

Venous complications of orbital infection include SOV thrombosis, CST, or both. On CECT and Gd-enhanced FS T1W MRI there is a "tram-track" appearance of the SOV which fails to enhance [**Fig. 10.38**]. Gas may be seen in an abscess, thrombosed SOV, or CST. CST is suggested by asymmetric convexity of the affected cavernous sinus with or without enhancement [**Fig. 10.38**]. The CST appears isointense or hyperintense on

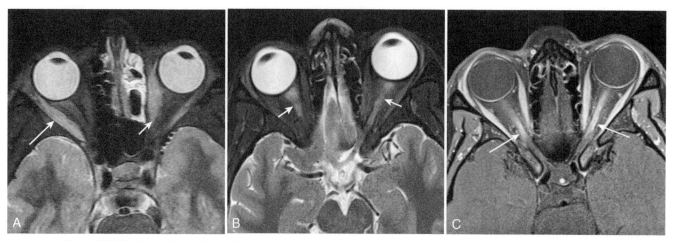

Figure 10.39 Idiopathic orbital inflammatory syndrome (IOIS) and optic neuritis. A, Idiopathic orbital inflammatory syndrome. Axial fat-suppressed (FS) T2-weighted (T2W) magnetic resonance imaging (MRI) shows swelling and high signal intensity of the muscle bellies and anterior tendinous portions of the right (*long arrow*) greater than left lateral rectus muscles and the left medial rectus muscle (*short arrow*). **B,** Optic neuritis. Axial FS T2W MRI reveals high signal intensity and poorly defined margins of both optic nerves (*arrows*). **C,** Gadolinium-enhanced FS T1-weighted MRI (same patient) shows enhancement of the affected optic nerves (*arrows*).

T1W images and hypointense on T2W images; nonenhancing areas may reflect thrombus, purulent material, or both. Arterial complications include spasm, stenosis, and thromboembolic infarction. Intracranial complications also include epidural empyema, subdural empyema, cerebritis, meningitis, brain abscess, venous sinus thrombosis, and venous infarction. Spread of inflammation and/or swelling at the orbital apex can affect the ON, leading to visual impairment. On MR, the affected ON appears hyperintense on T2W FS images, with loss of definition of the surrounding ON sheath with subsequent ON atrophy.

Idiopathic Orbital Inflammatory Syndrome (Pseudotumor)

Idiopathic orbital inflammatory syndrome (IOIS), or orbital pseudotumor, is a benign, steroid-responsive inflammatory disease of unknown cause. IOIS can be unilateral or bilateral, and is uncommon in children. Clinical signs and symptoms include pain, swelling, erythema, proptosis, diplopia, painful ophthalmoplegia, and sometimes visual impairment. IOIS is a diagnosis of exclusion, based on history, physical examination, and response to steroids. IOIS may be classified into different types, based on the location of the inflammatory manifestations, including focal or diffuse orbital inflammation, myositis, perineuritis, an inflammatory masslike lesion, and lacrimal adenitis. As such, the CT and MR appearances can be highly variable and include preseptal swelling, orbital fat stranding, an enhancing orbital mass, EOM enlargement (including tendinous insertions), scleral thickening, and periscleral and/or perineural stranding, lacrimal gland enlargement/enhancement, or orbital apex and cavernous sinus soft tissue thickening [**Fig. 10.39**]. Tolosa-Hunt syndrome is considered a subtype of IOIS involving the orbital apex back to the cavernous sinus, the hallmark of which is painful ophthalmoplegia due to inflammation of the orbital apex, superior orbital fissure, and cavernous sinus. Differential diagnosis of IOIS includes infection, tumor such as lymphoma or RMS, sarcoidosis, and granulomatous polyangiitis (Wegener granulomatosis). Biopsy should be considered for atypical cases or if tumor is suspected.

Other Inflammatory Processes

Less common infections include orbital fungal disease resulting from fungal infection (eg, mucormycosis, aspergillosis), notably in immunocompromised patients. Vascular complications (venous and arterial) can be catastrophic in aggressive fungal infection.

Ocular and Optic Inflammatory Processes

Toxocara canis infestation causes granulomatous uveitis leading to sclerosing endophthalmitis. Chorioretinitis leads to high density within the vitreous on CT and abnormal signal intensity on MR, with retinal detachment and ultimately ocular calcification. The differential diagnosis includes Coats disease. *TORCH infections* (eg, CMV) also cause chorioretinitis and may appear similar. Thyroid-associated orbitopathy due to Graves disease is uncommon in children. Coronal CT or MR images show swelling of the bellies of the EOMs (tendon-sparing) and an increase in orbital fat. The differential diagnosis includes IOIS and myositis caused by infection. *Optic neuritis* may be unilateral or bilateral. Clinical signs and symptoms include decreased vision, painful eye movements, dyschromatopsia (colors appear "washed-out"), afferent pupillary defect, and disc swelling. Causative factors include viral infection, postviral acute disseminated encephalomyelitis (ADEM), IOIS, vasculitis, leukemia, granulomatous disease, neuromyelitis optica, clinically isolated demyelinating syndrome, and juvenile multiple sclerosis. Coronal FS T2W MRI shows hyperintensity of the affected nerve, ON enhancement, and ON swelling [**Fig. 10.39**]. Elevation of the optic papilla and loss of definition of the ON sheath may also be seen. It is important to also image the brain and spine to look for other evidence of demyelinating disease.

Nasal Cavity, Paranasal Sinuses, and Face
Acute Sinusitis

Acute inflammatory changes of the PNS are common and result from numerous causes such as allergy, viral upper respiratory tract infection, bacterial infection (including dental infection), and fungal infection (especially in immunocompromised patients). Acute nonfungal rhinosinusitis is diagnosed clinically and treated without imaging, unless the patient is immunocompromised. Inflammatory or congestive mucosal thickening is commonly seen as an incidental finding on CT and MR. The inflamed and/or edematous mucosa appears hyperintense on T2W MRI and enhances, and there may be underlying nonenhancing submucosal edema. Mucosal thickening and sinus fluid

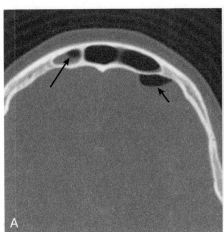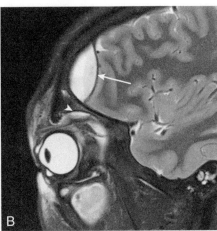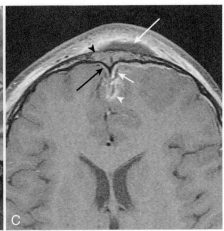

Figure 10.40 Acute complicated sinusitis. A, Frontal sinusitis and epidural abscess. Axial computed tomography image shows a frontal sinus air–fluid level (*long arrow*). There is also an intracranial air–fluid level associated with an epidural abscess (*short arrow*). **B,** Frontal sinusitis, epidural abscess, and orbital abscess. Sagittal fat-suppressed (FS) T2-weighted magnetic resonance (MR) image demonstrates a biconvex epidural abscess (*arrow*) containing a sediment level. There is also a small superior extraconal subperiosteal abscess (*arrowhead*). Periorbital STS is present, and there are secretions within the maxillary antrum. **C,** Pott puffy tumor, frontal osteomyelitis, and subdural empyema. Axial gadolinium-enhanced FS T1-weighted MR image shows frontal scalp swelling ventral to an elliptical low signal intensity, peripherally enhancing, frontal subperiosteal abscess (*long white arrow*). There is enhancement of the subjacent frontal bone, consistent with osteomyelitis (*black arrowhead*). There is also dural enhancement (*black arrow*) and a small left frontal interhemispheric subdural empyema (*short white arrow*) with subtle enhancement of the adjacent frontal leptomeninges and cortex caused by meningitis and cerebritis (*white arrowhead*).

is common in children; it is nonspecific and does not distinguish between acute, subacute, and chronic inflammatory or congestive causative factors. Acute bacterial sinusitis is suggested by longer symptom duration (>10 days), and severe or worsening symptoms, such as headache, facial tenderness, fever, and purulent nasal discharge. The hallmark of acute sinusitis is air–fluid levels [**Figs. 10.38** and **10.40**].

Other than in immunocompromised patients, imaging is usually reserved for evaluation of suspected *acute complicated sinusitis* as suggested by development of facial/periorbital swelling, proptosis, worsening headache, diplopia, ophthalmoplegia, or neurologic symptoms. Proptosis is a good predictor for the development of orbital complications. Orbital complications (detailed earlier) include periorbital and/or orbital cellulitis, extraconal phlegmon, extraconal subperiosteal abscess, SOV thrombosis, and rarely, optic neuritis [**Figs. 10.37** and **10.38**]. Purulent sinus secretions exhibit decreased diffusivity on DWI. Osteomyelitis, complicating sinusitis (frontal > sphenoid), is best diagnosed on MRI [**Figs. 10.37** and **10.40**]. FS T2W images reveal high signal intensity in affected bone, with enhancement. CT reveals demineralization of normally sharply corticated sinus margins [**Fig. 10.37**]. Over time, bone erosion becomes more apparent on CT, even as the patient improves clinically in response to treatment. Spread of infection to frontal soft tissues from frontal sinusitis results in soft tissue thickening and phlegmon, sometimes with a frontal subperiosteal abscess or *Pott puffy tumor* [**Fig. 10.40**]. Intracranial complications (see Chapter 8), caused by spread via bone or emissary veins, include subdural empyema, epidural or brain abscess, meningitis, cerebritis, dural, cortical, or even jugular venous thrombosis, venous infarction, CST, and ICA spasm with thromboemboli and arterial infarction [**Figs. 10.38, 10.40,** and **10.41**]. Spread of infection via emissary veins may produce complications that are remote from the initiating sinus infection. CST most frequently complicates sphenoid sinusitis; a sphenoid sinus air–fluid level in a patient with headaches should be considered a significant finding [**Figs. 10.38** and **10.41**].

Subacute and Chronic Sinonasal Infection

Chronic rhinosinusitis is diagnosed if symptoms persist for at least 12 consecutive weeks. CT is reserved for preoperative evaluation and reveals mucosal thickening, sometimes with lobulated sinonasal polyps protruding into the nasal cavity. Other features of chronicity include indistinct mucoperiosteal margins, bone demineralization or dehiscence, and/or reactive hyperostosis and marginal sclerosis. The sinus drainage pathways should be carefully assessed for opacification or anatomic variation. Occlusion of a sinus ostium results in a *mucocele,* or *mucopyocele* if infected, with complete opacification and expansion of the affected sinus [**Figs. 10.42** and **10.43**]. Over time, progressive expansion results in thinned or eroded bone margins. Ruptured mucocele or mucopyocele is rare in children [**Fig. 10.43**]. On T2W MRI, mucocele is usually hyperintense with variable signal on T1W images depending on the amount of inspissation or proteinaceous content. Decreased diffusivity is seen with inspissation or purulence. Gd-enhanced T1W MRI shows peripheral enhancement that distinguishes mucocele from neoplasm. Occlusion of the maxillary infundibulum, with negative pressure in the antrum, results in inward bowing of the maxillary sinus walls, including the orbital floor and the uncinate process, resulting in a hypoplastic, opacified maxillary antrum [**Fig. 10.44**]. This entity is also known as the *silent sinus syndrome* and over time can result in ipsilateral enophthalmos.

Ovoid or rounded *mucous retentions cysts* are frequently seen within the PNS and are not considered clinically significant [**Fig. 10.44**]. *Antrochoanal polyp* arises in the maxillary antrum and usually protrudes via an accessory ostium into the middle meatus, sometimes extending posteriorly into the pharynx [**Fig. 10.44**]. *Sinonasal polyposis* results from lobulated inflammatory mucosal swelling that protrudes from the sinuses into the nasal cavity [**Fig. 10.45**]. Sinonasal polyposis occurs in patients with allergy, asthma, Samter triad (asthma, aspirin/nonsteroidal anti-inflammatory drug sensitivity, chronic rhinosinusitis/sinonasal polyps), primary ciliary dyskinesia, and cystic fibrosis. CT

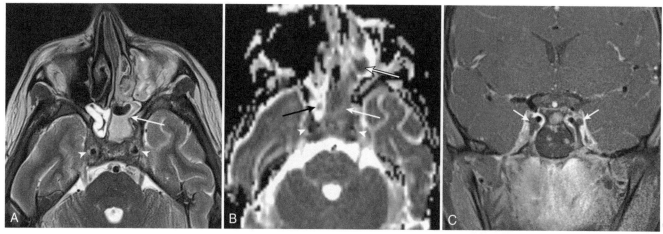

Figure 10.41 Cavernous sinus thrombosis (CST) complicating acute sinusitis. A, Axial T2-weighted magnetic resonance imaging (MRI) shows extensive sinus disease with a left sphenoid sinus air–fluid level (*white arrow*). There is abnormal hypointense signal within the cavernous sinus bilaterally with high signal intensity of the walls of the internal carotid arteries (*arrowheads*). **B,** Diffusion-weighted imaging apparent diffusion coefficient map shows decreased diffusivity within the left sphenoid sinus and posterior ethmoid air cells and the left maxillary antrum caused by purulent secretions (*white arrows*). The contralateral sinus secretions exhibit facilitated diffusion (*black arrow*). There is also decreased diffusivity within the cavernous sinuses (*arrowheads*). **C,** Coronal gadolinium-enhanced fat-suppressed T1-weighted MRI demonstrates abnormal low signal intensity (*arrows*) within the cavernous sinuses due to cavernous sinus thrombosis or thrombophlebitis.

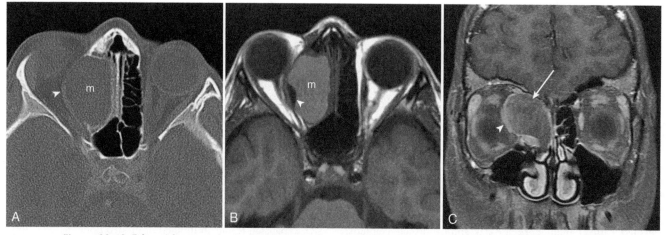

Figure 10.42 Ethmoid mucocele. A, Axial computed tomography image demonstrates an opacified, expanded right ethmoid air cell (*m*), with markedly thinned bony margins (*arrowhead*). **B,** Axial T1-weighted (T1W) magnetic resonance imaging (MRI) shows the sharply circumscribed homogeneous mucocele (*m*) that is mildly hyperintense compared with muscle, because of proteinaceous content. There is mild right proptosis. A small lateral inspissated component is shown (*arrowhead*). **C,** Coronal gadolinium-enhanced fat-suppressed T1W MRI demonstrates characteristic peripheral enhancement (*arrow*). Note displacement of the medial rectus muscle (*arrowhead*).

features of cystic fibrosis include chronic sinusitis with high attenuation, inspissated secretions, and sinonasal polyposis [**Fig. 10.45**]. Inspissated secretions appear markedly hypointense on T2W MRI. Other than inspissation, the differential diagnosis for high-density material within the sinuses includes hemorrhage, allergic mucin, and fungal colonization with hyphae. Granulomatous polyangiitis (Wegener granulomatosis) is an uncommon cause of chronic sinonasal inflammation with polypoid lesions and nasal septal destruction.

Fungal Sinus Disease

Fungal sinus disease has the following manifestations: acute, granulomatous or chronic invasive fungal rhinosinusitis, allergic

fungal rhinosinusitis, and fungus ball (mycetoma; rare in childhood). *Acute invasive fungal rhinosinusitis* is usually due to mucor or aspergillus and occurs in immunocompromised patients. CT reveals unilateral nasal soft tissue thickening, sometimes with decreased turbinate enhancement, sinus opacification (most common in ethmoid and maxillary sinuses), bone destruction, periantral fat infiltration, and sometimes complications such as CST and arterial and other intracranial complications [**Fig. 10.46**]. Increased density caused by fungal elements is a feature of *chronic fungal rhinosinusitis* with a greater predilection for ethmoid and sphenoid sinuses. Fungal elements may appear markedly hypointense on T2W MRI simulating sinus aeration. Acute invasive fungal sinusitis has a high mortality. *Allergic fungal sinusitis* is a form of chronic

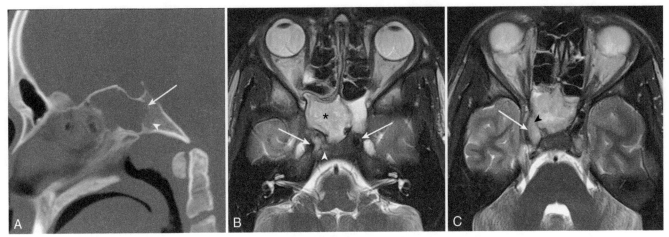

Figure 10.43 Ruptured mucopyocele with osteomyelitis. A, Reformatted sagittal computed tomography shows complete opacification of the right sphenoid sinus. There is loss of cortical definition of the posterior margin of the right sphenoid sinus (*arrow*), and basisphenoid demineralization (*arrowhead*) consistent with osteomyelitis. **B,** Axial T2-weighted (T2W) magnetic resonance imaging (MRI) shows high signal intensity material filling the right sphenoid sinus (*asterisk*), with mucoperiosteal thickening. Note the difference in signal intensity between secretions in the right and left sphenoid sinuses. There is leftward bowing of the sinus septum. There is right basisphenoid high signal intensity consistent with osteomyelitis (*arrowhead*). Note the asymmetric internal carotid artery signal voids (*arrows*) with spasm present on the right. **C,** Axial T2W MRI shows dehiscence of the lateral sinus wall (*black arrowhead*) with extruded material medial to the cavernous sinus caused by mucopyocele rupture (*white arrow*).

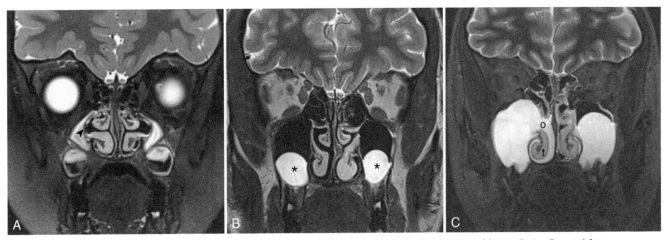

Figure 10.44 Antral hypoplasia, retention cysts, and antrochoanal polyp. A, Antral hypoplasia. Coronal fat-suppressed (FS) T2-weighted (T2W) magnetic resonance (MR) image shows small maxillary antra filled with high signal intensity material. Note the lateral convexity of the medial antral walls (*arrowhead*). **B,** Antral retention cysts (*asterisks*). Coronal FS T2W MR image demonstrates homogeneous, rounded, hyperintense lesions along the inferior aspects of both maxillary antra—a common incidental finding. **C,** Antrochoanal polyp. Coronal FS T2W MR image shows a right antrochoanal polyp that protrudes into the nasal cavity via an accessory ostium (*o*) located between the inferior (*t*) and middle turbinates. On the left there is either a large retention cyst or polyp.

rhinosinusitis in which allergic eosinophil-rich mucin is produced in response to fungal hyphae. Affected patients are immunocompetent. CT reveals pan-sinonasal or hemisinonasal opacification with increased density material [**Fig. 10.46**]. MRI shows marked hypointensity on T2W images. Mycetoma or fungus ball is uncommon in children and appears as a hyperdense mass on CT, sometimes with punctate calcifications.

Ear and Temporal Bone

Acute Infection

Acute otitis media (OM) is diagnosed clinically and treated without imaging. Nonerosive MEC and mastoid air cell

opacification on CT, with high signal intensity on T2W MRI and facilitated diffusion on DWI, is frequently seen in children imaged for other reasons, often with adenoidal hypertrophy or other cause of Eustachian tube dysfunction/obstruction. These findings do not necessarily infer "mastoiditis." Imaging is reserved for worsening symptoms, such as otalgia, persistent otorrhea, and/or signs suggestive of *acute CoM*. Acute CoM refers to the development of mastoid osteomyelitis heralded by retroauricular pain, tenderness, erythema, and/or swelling. Subacute or chronic CoM has been attributed to antibiotic usage that masks typical acute CoM symptoms leading to more indolent disease. The hallmark of CoM on CT is MEC and mastoid air cell opacification with mastoid bone erosion [**Fig. 10.47**]. Because mastoid air

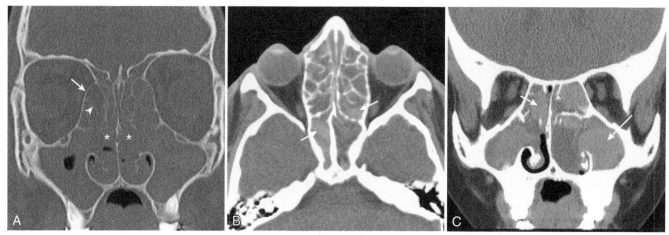

Figure 10.45 Chronic rhinosinusitis with sinonasal polyposis. A, Samter triad. Coronal computed tomography (CT) demonstrates near-total paranasal sinus opacification with polypoid opacities protruding into the nasal cavity (*asterisks*). The sinuses are expanded with lateral bowing of the lamina papyracea on each side (*arrow*). There are postoperative changes after functional endoscopic sinus surgery consisting of bilateral uncinectomy, middle turbinectomy, and ethmoidectomy. The residual ethmoid septations are demineralized (*arrowhead*). **B,** Axial CT (same patient) reveals increased density within sinus secretions (*arrows*) caused by "allergic" mucin. The differential diagnosis for this appearance includes inspissated secretions (as seen in cystic fibrosis), fungal hyphae, and hemorrhage. **C,** Cystic fibrosis. Coronal CT showing postoperative changes and pan sinus opacification with polypoid opacities extending into the nasal cavity and increased density of sinus secretions because of inspissation (*arrows*).

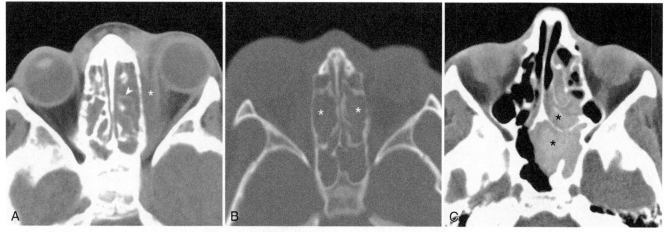

Figure 10.46 Fungal sinus disease. A, Invasive fungal sinusitis. Axial contrast-enhanced computed tomography (CECT) image shows pan sinus opacification. The ethmoid septations are demineralized (*arrowhead*). There is medial extraconal phlegmon (*asterisk*) with thickening of the medial rectus muscle and mild preseptal periorbital swelling. **B,** Invasive fungal sinusitis. Axial computed tomography (CT) shows marked demineralization of ethmoid septations (*asterisks*). There is associated right preseptal periorbital swelling. **C,** Allergic fungal sinusitis. Axial CT image demonstrates localized left ethmoid air cell and sphenoid sinus opacification with increased density secretions (*asterisks*).

cells are often asymmetric, it can be difficult to diagnose erosion of intramastoid septa. CoM is readily diagnosed when there is erosion of the lateral retroauricular cortex, sinus plate, and/or tegmen [**Fig. 10.47**]. MRI shows MEC and mastoid fluid signal with decreased diffusivity from pus. Lateral spread of infection causes retroauricular phlegmon or subperiosteal abscess, and less often periauricular or preauricular abscess. Inferior spread to the upper neck deep to the SCM may produce a *Bezold abscess.*

Intracranial complications are best diagnosed with MRI and include epidural, cerebellar, or temporal lobe abscess, subdural empyema, meningitis, cerebritis, compression and/or thrombosis of the sigmoid sinus, thrombosis of the transverse sinus and IJV (sometimes with otitic hydrocephalus), and venous infarction. Infection spreads to the posterior fossa either directly via bone or via emissary veins. Epidural abscess usually occurs adjacent to the proximal sigmoid sinus. It can be challenging to distinguish between epidural abscess compressing the sinus (sometimes with downstream sigmoid/IJV thrombosis) and sigmoid sinus thrombosis; often both are present. On CT an epidural abscess is hypodense; a thrombosed sinus does not enhance normally but is denser than an abscess [**Fig. 10.47**]. Coronal CT reformats or MR images are helpful; an epidural abscess appears elliptical and sinus thrombosis appears tubular [**Fig. 10.48**]. On T2W MRI an epidural abscess is usually hyperintense, whereas acute thrombus is usually hypointense but without a signal void [**Fig. 10.47**]. Both epidural abscess and sinus thrombus demonstrate decreased diffusivity and peripheral

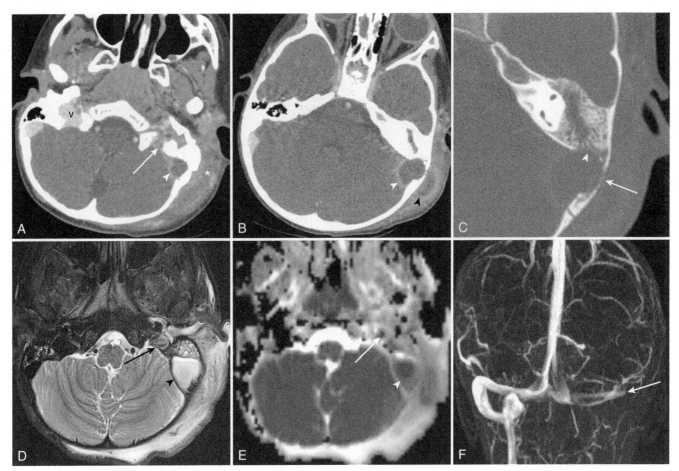

Figure 10.47 Coalescent mastoiditis and complications. A, Epidural abscess and internal jugular vein (IJV) thrombosis. Axial contrast-enhanced computed tomography (CECT) image reveals a low-density left epidural abscess (*arrowhead*) compressing the sigmoid sinus. There is intermediate density thrombosis within the non-dominant left IJV (*arrow*). Note the normally enhancing right IJV (*v*). There is extensive left occipitomastoid scalp swelling (*asterisk*). **B,** A more cephalad image (same patient) shows opacified left mastoid air cells, a large epidural abscess (*white arrowhead*), and a lateral retroauricular subperiosteal abscess (*black arrowhead*). **C,** Bone windows (same patient) reveal erosion of the lateral retroauricular cortex (*arrow*) and the posterior mastoid cortex (*arrowhead*) consistent with coalescent mastoiditis. **D,** Axial T2-weighted MR (same patient) shows the high signal intensity epidural abscess (*arrowhead*) compared with the low signal intensity IJV thrombus (*arrow*). There is extensive mastoid air cell fluid signal and soft tissue swelling. **E,** Diffusion-weighted imaging apparent diffusion coefficient image shows decreased diffusivity within the abscess (*arrowhead*) and the IJV thrombus (*arrow*). **F,** Two-dimensional time-of-flight MR venography coronal maximum intensity projection image shows the proximal nondominant left transverse sinus (*arrow*) and absence of flow-related enhancement within the distal left transverse sinus, sigmoid sinus, and IJV.

enhancement. MRV may not reliably distinguish between sinus compression and thrombosis. Gd-enhanced flow-sensitive T1W sequences (eg, magnetization prepared rapid acquisition gradient-echo [MPRAGE], fast spoiled gradient echo [FSPGR]) may help discriminate between venous compression and occlusive and nonocclusive thrombus [**Fig. 10.48**]; however, chronic thrombus may enhance. Occasionally otitic venous thrombosis occurs without radiographic evidence of CoM, presumably because of spread of thrombophlebitis via emissary veins. Suppurative labyrinthitis and CN VII palsy attributable solely to CoM occasionally occur and result in labyrinthine and/or CN VII enhancement on MRI.

Petrous apex infection usually accompanies MEC and mastoid infection. *Gradenigo triad* refers to petrous apicitis, CN V irritation with deep facial pain, and CN VI palsy. However, children do not always manifest all of these symptoms and the diagnosis of petrous apex infection may be missed or overlooked. Imaging findings depend on whether the petrous apex is pneumatized (petrous apicitis or apical petrositis) or not (petrous apex

osteomyelitis). *Petrous apex osteomyelitis* is suggested by narrowing of the petrous ICA on CT. Bone destruction is unusual at the time of presentation. FS T2W MR images reveal marrow edema with enhancement. *Petrous apicitis* is characterized by opacified, fluid-containing petrous apex air cells with bone destruction; pus causes decreased diffusivity on DWI [**Fig. 10.49**]. ICA narrowing with decreased flow-related enhancement on MR accompanies petrous apex infection. Complications are as for CoM and also include CST, ICA stenosis, thromboembolism, and arterial infarction.

The differential diagnosis for CoM and petrous apex infection is cholesteatoma, cholesterol granuloma (CG), and erosive tumor, occurring alone or with CoM. Ossicular, FNC, and/or otic capsule erosion are uncommon features of acute CoM and should prompt a search for underlying obstructing cholesteatoma or occasionally tumor. CoM bone defects tend to seal with granulation tissue; therefore CSF leak in association with CoM should prompt a search for coexistent pathology. Hypointense signal on T2W MRI or a defined area of rounded enhancement

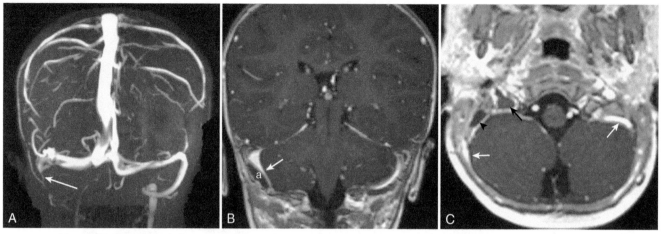

Figure 10.48 Epidural abscess and internal jugular vein (IJV) thrombosis. A, Two-dimensional time-of-flight magnetic resonance (MR) venography coronal maximum intensity projection image shows absent flow-related enhancement beyond the proximal sigmoid sinus (*arrow*). **B,** Coronal gadolinium-enhanced T1 fast spoiled gradient echo MR (same patient) shows an elliptical epidural abscess (*a*) compressing the proximal sigmoid sinus (*arrow*). **C,** Reconstructed axial image (same patient) demonstrates the patent, enhancing right transverse and left sigmoid sinuses (*white arrows*), right IJV thrombus (*black arrow*), which is isointense with brain, and a hypointense perisinus epidural abscess (*arrowhead*).

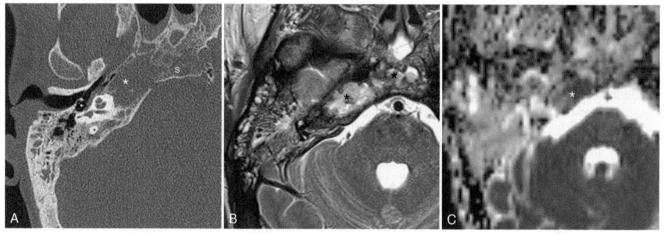

Figure 10.49 Petrous apicitis. A, Axial temporal bone computed tomography demonstrates opacification and erosion of the right petrous apex (*asterisk*) and erosion of the sphenoid bone (*s*). **B,** Axial T2-weighted magnetic resonance image (same patient) shows high signal intensity in the right petrous apex and sphenoid bone (*asterisks*), and extensive fluid in the mastoid air cells. **C,** Diffusion-weighted imaging apparent diffusion coefficient image shows corresponding decreased diffusivity (*asterisk*) caused by pus.

suggest tumor. The differential diagnosis includes unilateral or bilateral Langerhans cell histiocytosis (LCH), metastatic disease (eg, neuroblastoma), and primary tumor (eg, RMS).

Acute otitis externa is a superficial infection that is infrequently imaged. By contrast, *malignant otitis externa* is an aggressive, necrotizing infection that is rare in childhood and affects immunocompromised patients. CT and MRI are obtained to define the extent of infection which may cause extensive bone erosion. *Acute labyrinthitis* results from hematogenous, meningogenic, or tympanogenic spread of infection. Symptoms include rapidly progressive SNHL and vertigo/disturbed balance. Bacterial meningitis (eg, from *Streptococcus pneumoniae, Haemophilus influenza*) predominates as a cause of childhood acquired profound bilateral SNHL. In the acute phase, high-resolution thin-section Gd-enhanced FS T1W MRI reveals labyrinthine (cochlear, vestibular, and SCC) enhancement [**Fig. 10.50**]. *Labyrinthine fibrosis* rapidly ensues, leading to a

loss of labyrinthine fluid high signal intensity on heavily T2W MRI [**Fig. 10.50**]. Over weeks, *labyrinthitis ossificans* ensues, appearing similar to fibrosis on T2W MRI (loss of fluid signal). On CT it initially appears as subtle haziness within the cochlear basal turn near the round window (cochlear ossification). Progressive ossification of the vestibule, cochlea, and SCC may occur [**Fig. 10.50**]. Labyrinthitis is an important diagnosis to make; profound SNHL may necessitate cochlear implantation for which timing is critical. Cochlear implantation has a greater chance of success when performed before florid ossification.

Chronic Otitis Media

Chronic OM results in MEC/mastoid fluid and granulation tissue. Symptoms include otorrhea, TM perforation, and CHL. CT reveals decreased MEC/mastoid pneumatization and aeration with surrounding sclerosis [**Fig. 10.51**]. Chronic inflammation

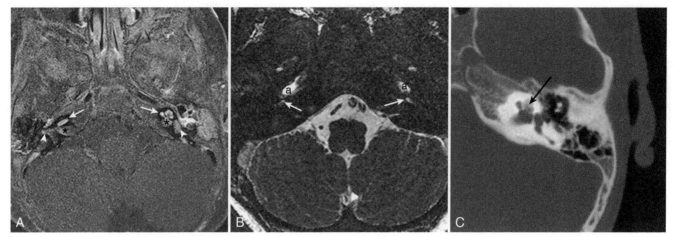

Figure 10.50 Labyrinthitis. A, Acute labyrinthitis associated with pneumococcal meningitis. Axial gadolinium-enhanced fat-suppressed T1-weighted magnetic resonance (MR) image shows diffuse cochlear enhancement (*arrows*) and enhancement within the right SCC (*arrowhead*) and left vestibule (*arrowhead*). Faint enhancement is also seen within the internal auditory canals bilaterally (*asterisks*). **B,** Labyrinthine fibrosis versus ossification. Axial fast imaging employing steady-state acquisition (FIESTA) image shows near-complete loss of the usual high signal intensity labyrinthine fluid. Only minimal fluid is seen within the cochleae (*arrows*) located posterolateral to the internal carotid arteries (*a*). This finding occurs with labyrinthine fibrosis or ossification, or both. **C,** Cochlear ossification. Axial computed tomography image demonstrates increased density (*arrow*) due to ossification within the cochlea.

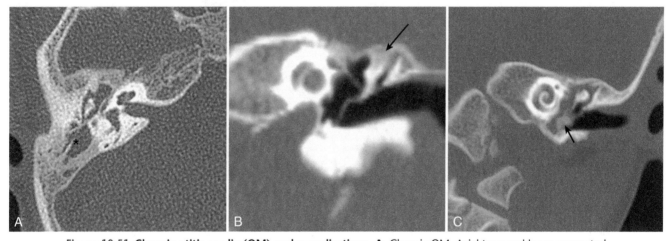

Figure 10.51 Chronic otitis media (OM) and complications. A, Chronic OM. Axial temporal bone computed tomography (CT) shows poor mastoid pneumatization and absent aeration with sclerosis surrounding the opacified middle ear cavity (MEC) and mastoid antrum (*asterisk*). **B,** Chronic OM with postinflammatory ossicular fixation. Reformatted coronal CT image demonstrates ankylosis of the malleus to the tegmen tympani by ossific material (*arrow*) with a small amount of adjacent epitympanic opacification. **C,** Tympanosclerosis. Reformatted coronal CT image shows ill-defined mineralization (*arrow*) along the tympanic membrane, projecting into the MEC. There is extensive MEC opacification and absent mastoid pneumatization.

leads to TM retraction, thickening, mineralization (myringosclerosis), and/or perforation. Additional features include ossicular erosion, typically involving the long/lenticular process of the incus and postinflammatory ossicular fixation [**Fig. 10.51**]. Tympanosclerosis refers to the presence of postinflammatory fibrous, calcific, or ossified foci within the MEC [**Fig. 10.51**].

Acquired Cholesteatoma

Acquired cholesteatoma is a pearly-white, stratified, epithelium-lined sac containing desquamated keratin debris. It is frequently seen within the MEC where it is termed pars flaccida (most common) or pars tensa cholesteatoma. Other sites include the EAC, mastoid, and petrous apex air cells. The exact cause of *pars flaccida cholesteatoma* is unknown; a popular theory is

Eustachian tube dysfunction → MEC ventilatory disturbance → to pars flaccida retraction/pocket → cholesteatoma. Cholesteatoma enlarges over time and produces proteolytic enzymes that erode bone. Symptoms are indistinguishable from chronic OM. CT reveals an opacity involving Prussak space with variable atticoantral extension. There is erosion/blunting of the scutum and medial ossicular displacement and erosion [**Fig. 10.52**]. *Pars tensa cholesteatoma* is attributed to traumatic or iatrogenic causes; pars tensa perforation leads to implantation or migration of TM epithelial cells into the MEC, which form a cholesteatoma nidus. CT shows MEC opacity with lateral ossicular displacement and erosion. The differential diagnosis of cholesteatoma is granulation tissue, chronic OM with ossicular erosion, CG (often coexists with cholesteatoma), and tumor. Cholesteatoma characteristically exhibits decreased diffusivity on DWI (preferably

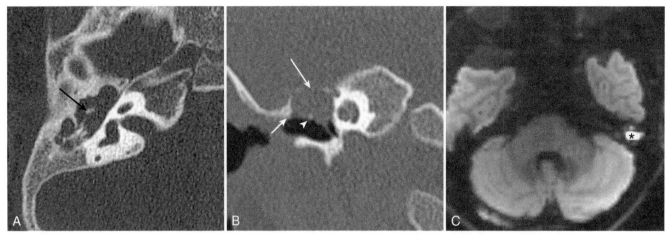

Figure 10.52 Cholesteatoma. A, Axial temporal bone computed tomography (CT) shows middle ear cavity (MEC) opacification, expansion of the attic, and ossicular erosion. Only a small remnant of malleus (*arrow*) is shown. **B,** Reformatted coronal CT image (same patient) shows erosion of the tegmen tympani (*long arrow*) and malleus (*arrowhead*) with blunting of the scutum (*short arrow*) because of pars flaccida cholesteatoma. **C,** Recurrent cholesteatoma. Axial nonecho planar imaging diffusion-weighted imaging trace image shows high signal intensity (*asterisk*) within the MEC with low signal intensity on the apparent diffusion coefficient image (not shown) consistent with decreased diffusivity in recurrent cholesteatoma.

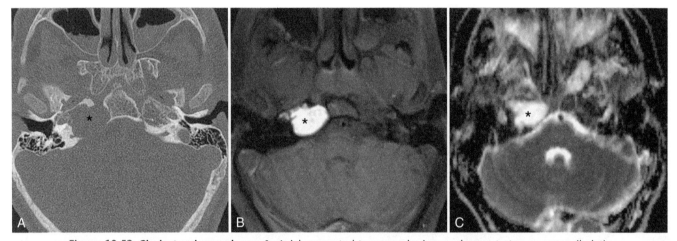

Figure 10.53 Cholesterol granuloma. A, Axial computed tomography image demonstrates an expansile lytic lesion with sharply defined margins involving the right petrous apex (*asterisk*). **B,** Axial fat-suppressed T1-weighted magnetic resonance image shows the hyperintense lesion (*asterisk*). **C,** Diffusion-weighted imaging apparent diffusion coefficient image shows facilitated diffusion in the lesion (*asterisk*).

performed with nonecho planar imaging technique) [**Fig. 10.52**] and appears hypointense on T1W MR, mildly hyperintense on T2W, and is nonenhancing. Complications include FNC erosion, otic capsule erosion leading to labyrinthine fistula, and tegmen erosion and cephalocele.

Cholesterol Granuloma

CG arises as follows: (1) negative pressure in an air space → blood vessel rupture → red blood cell/tissue breakdown → cholesterol release → foreign body giant cell reaction → CG; or (2) cholesteatoma rupture → cholesterol release → foreign body giant cell reaction → CG. CG occurs in the MEC (Eustachian tube dysfunction, ruptured cholesteatoma), in a pneumatized petrous apex air cell (obstructed drainage), or in a mastoidectomy cavity. The imaging appearance is attributed to cholesterol elements, blood products, or both. CG results in smoothly marginated expansile bony scalloping or erosion, characteristically appears

hyperintense on FS T1W MRI, and does not enhance [**Fig. 10.53**]. The differential diagnosis includes cholesteatoma, fat, and granulation tissue. Mixed features may occur if CG and cholesteatoma coexist.

Mastoidectomy

A canal wall-up mastoidectomy refers to resection of mastoid air cells with EAC preservation (eg, for CoM). A canal wall down mastoidectomy entails resection of part of the posterior EAC wall and mastoid air cells with variable ossicular resection, and sometimes ossicular reconstruction or insertion of a total or partial ossicular reconstruction prosthesis. Postoperative imaging is indicated if there is concern for residual disease or recurrence. CT is used for bone assessment; MRI may help distinguish residual/recurrent cholesteatoma (decreased diffusivity, nonenhancing) from granulation tissue (facilitated diffusion, enhancement) [**Fig. 10.52**].

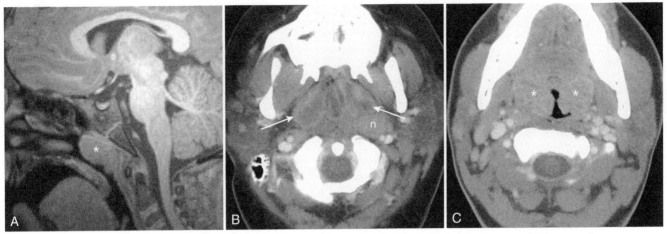

Figure 10.54 Adenoidal hypertrophy and adenotonsillitis. A, Adenoidal hypertrophy. Sagittal T1 magnetization prepared rapid acquisition gradient-echo MR image demonstrates marked adenoidal hypertrophy (*asterisk*) with mass effect on the airway. **B,** Adenotonsillitis. Axial contrast-enhanced computed tomography (CECT) image shows severe edema and swelling of the nasopharyngeal adenoid (*arrows*) with effacement of the nasopharynx. There is also an enlarged lateral retropharyngeal lymph node (*n*) displacing the carotid sheath posteriorly. **C,** A more caudal axial CECT image shows marked enlargement of the palatine tonsils (*asterisks*) with streaky enhancement, and mass effect on the oropharynx. This appearance is typically seen with EBV or streptococcal infection.

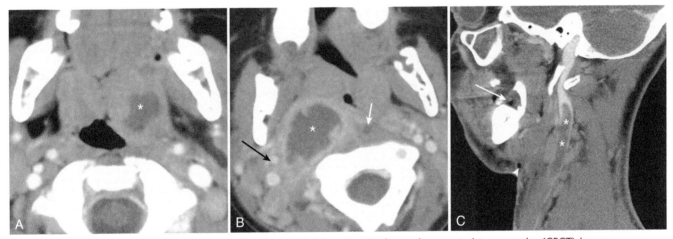

Figure 10.55 Abscess. A, Peritonsillar abscess. Axial contrast-enhanced computed tomography (CECT) image shows an irregular, low-attenuation focus within the asymmetrically enlarged left palatine tonsil (*asterisk*), consistent with a crypt abscess. Pus was drained at surgical exploration. **B,** Retropharyngeal abscess (RPA). Axial CECT image reveals an irregular low-density and peripherally enhancing right RPA (*asterisk*), with mass effect on the airway that is compounded by enlarged palatine tonsils. There is midline retropharyngeal edema (*white arrow*), posterolateral displacement of the right carotid sheath, and mild attenuation of the right internal carotid artery (*black arrow*). **C,** Lemierre syndrome. Reformatted sagittal CECT image shows thrombus (*asterisks*) within the internal jugular vein associated with infection after dental extraction (*arrow*). There is submandibular subcutaneous gas and phlegmonous change.

Neck, Oral Cavity, and Jaw
Adenotonsillar Hypertrophy, Inflammation, and Peritonsillar Abscess

Adenotonsillar hypertrophy is common in young children and peaks during the first decade of life [**Fig. 10.54**]. Adenotonsillar hypertrophy may cause or exacerbate Eustachian tube dysfunction and/or result in airway obstruction with sleep apnea that is particularly problematic for children with midface hypoplasia (eg, craniosynostosis, trisomy 21) or micrognathia. A lateral neck PF may be obtained to assess symptomatic children. *Adenoidal retention cysts* and *adenotonsillar calcified concretions* are often seen as incidental findings. *Acute adenotonsillitis,* pharyngitis, and lymphadenitis are frequent manifestations of acute viral

and bacterial infection. On CECT, there is marked edematous adenotonsillar enlargement with streaky enhancement that should not be mistaken for abscess formation [**Fig. 10.54**]. There is often mass effect on the airway. Enlarged, enhancing LNs are also seen. Infection is usually due to Epstein-Barr virus (EBV) or streptococcal infections, which appear indistinguishable on imaging. Tonsillitis may be complicated by development of a *peritonsillar* or *crypt abscess.* Symptoms include persistent or worsening fever, sore throat, dysphagia, drooling, and marked enlargement of one tonsil. CT shows marked asymmetric tonsillar enlargement with peripherally enhancing low-attenuation change in/around the palatine tonsil and mass effect on the airway [**Fig. 10.55**]. The RP soft tissues are not thickened unless there is concurrent RP adenopathy. In young children,

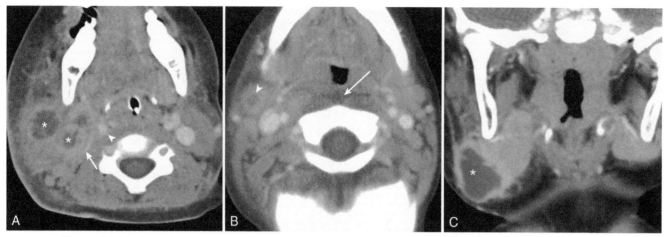

Figure 10.56 Necrotic or suppurative adenopathy. A, Methicillin-resistant staphylococcal infection. Axial contrast-enhanced computed tomography (CECT) image shows enlarged lymph nodes (LNs) with nodal necrosis (*asterisks*). There is extensive stranding of the adjacent subcutaneous fat with ill-defined phlegmonous change. There is medial deviation of the right carotid artery (*arrowhead*) and attenuation of the right internal jugular vein (*arrow*). **B,** Kawasaki disease. Axial CECT image reveals retropharyngeal edema (*arrow*). There are mildly enlarged cervical LNs and a focus of nodal necrosis is present (*arrowhead*), with stranding of the surrounding fat. **C,** Nontuberculous mycobacterial infection. Reformatted coronal CECT image shows a conglomerate mass of enlarged submandibular LNs with necrotic material (*asterisk*) extruding into the subcutaneous tissues. Unlike acute inflammatory disorders, there is negligible stranding of subcutaneous fat.

Kawasaki disease should be considered in the differential diagnosis for intense adenoidal enhancement and enlargement, RP low-density edema, and enlarged, enhancing/edematous cervical LNs. The differential diagnosis for adolescent adenotonsillar enlargement includes lymphoid hyperplasia, other lymphoproliferative disorders (eg, posttransplant lymphoproliferative disorder), lymphoma, and nasopharyngeal carcinoma (NPC), particularly if asymmetric.

Retropharyngeal Inflammation and Abscess

Suprahyoid medial and lateral RP LNs enlarge in response to upper respiratory tract and/or temporal bone infection. RP abscess arises from infected medial or lateral RP LNs. Symptoms suggestive of RP abscess include fever, sore throat, dysphagia, drooling, stiff neck, and torticollis. CT shows linear low-density *RP edema* crossing the midline, extending into the infrahyoid neck and sometimes the mediastinum. *RP cellulitis* is less common. RP LNs are enlarged and appear enhancing or edematous, or hypodense with peripheral enhancement (suppurative LN/intranodal abscess). *RP abscess* arising from *suppurative LNs* is suggested by low attenuation with peripheral enhancement and irregular margins [**Fig. 10.55**]. PF reveal widening of the prevertebral/RP soft tissues. Airway compromise is an important consideration if the patient requires sedation, which may precipitate overt airway obstruction. CT is highly sensitive in depicting infection but lacks specificity in distinguishing between edematous or suppurative LNs and RP abscess. There is often mass effect on and attenuation of the adjacent ICA and IJV that usually resolves without consequences [**Fig. 10.55**]. RP abscess (off-midline) must be distinguished from midline periverterbral infection resulting from vertebral or clival osteomyelitis. Complications of RP abscess include airway compromise, torticollis, and vascular sequelae. Torticollis, caused by spasm of prevertebral muscles, is usually transient and alleviated by analgesia and treatment of the infection. Occasionally, true rotary subluxation ensues, termed *Grisel syndrome*. Arterial complications are uncommon and include ICA pseudoaneurysm and rupture. Venous thrombosis is a complication of *Fusobacterium necrophorum* infection. *Lemierre syndrome* refers to neck

infection, venous thrombophlebitis, and septic pulmonary emboli [**Fig. 10.55**].

Lymphadenitis and Abscess

Enlarged cervical LNs are frequently seen in children. Acutely inflamed LNs enhance. Nodal necrosis is usually due to acute bacterial infection or granulomatous disease, but can also occur with Kawasaki disease [**Fig. 10.56**]. *Acute abscess* (eg, staphylococcal) tends to arise in jugulodigastric LNs with a differential diagnosis of infected second BAC. Rupture of an abscess simulates infected LM. Ultrasonography after resolution of infection may be of use to exclude an underlying congenital lesion. Nodal necrosis is also a feature of subacute and chronic granulomatous disorders. *Cat scratch disease* is suggested by a conglomerate necrotic nodal mass sometimes with stranding of surrounding fat. *Nontuberculous mycobacterial* infection occurs in 2- to 5-year-old immunocompetent children and presents as a nontender or mildly tender mass with violaceous skin discoloration. CT shows a periparotid or submandibular necrotic nodal mass, sometimes with punctate calcifications [**Fig. 10.56**]. Necrotic material tends to extrude out toward the skin. Stranding of surrounding fat is usually minimal or absent. In the parotid region, the differential diagnosis is an inflamed first BAC. *Tuberculosis* tends to cause bilateral necrotic and sometimes calcified cervical LNs in a systemically unwell child with night sweats and a cough. Enlarged LNs and enlarged salivary glands are a feature of HIV/AIDS, sarcoidosis, and autoimmune disorders (eg, Sjögren syndrome). Enlarged LNs without typical signs or symptoms of infection have a broad differential diagnosis that includes lymphoma and other lymphoproliferative disorders. Nodal necrosis can occur due to malignancy metastatic to LNs (eg, from papillary thyroid carcinoma or squamous cell carcinoma) but is far less common in children than in adults.

Soft Tissue Inflammation, Cellulitis, and Necrotizing Fasciitis

Soft tissue inflammation and sometimes cellulitis occur due to a variety of causes including infected skin lesions, infected

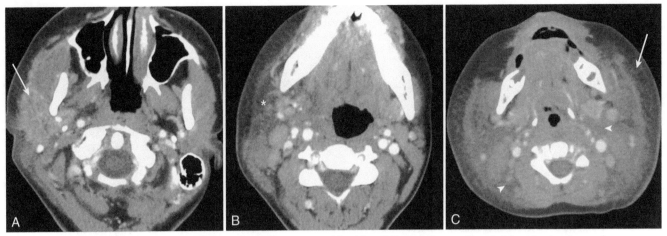

Figure 10.57 Soft tissue inflammation. A, Acute parotitis with soft tissue inflammation. Axial contrast-enhanced computed tomography (CECT) image shows enlargement and prominent enhancement of the right parotid gland (*arrow*), with stranding of the adjacent subcutaneous fat. **B,** More caudal image (same patient) demonstrates phlegmonous change (*asterisk*) extending inferior to the parotid tail and deep to the platysma muscle with extensive stranding of the right facial subcutaneous fat. There are also enlarged right cervical LNs. **C,** Necrotizing fasciitis. Axial CECT image shows generalized stranding of the subcutaneous fat (*arrow*). There is multifocal phlegmonous change (*arrowheads*) and loss of distinction of muscle borders.

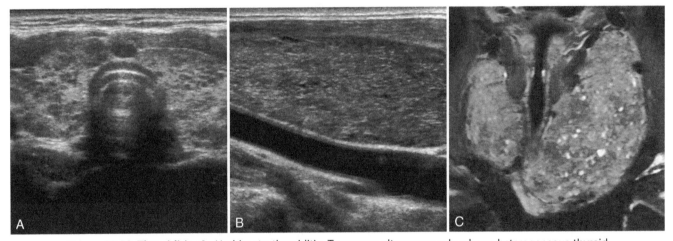

Figure 10.58 Thyroiditis. A, Hashimoto thyroiditis. Transverse ultrasonography shows heterogeneous thyroid gland enlargement. **B,** Graves disease with multinodular goiter. Longitudinal ultrasonography image and (**C**) coronal fat-suppressed T2-weighted magnetic resonance image show heterogeneous thyroid gland enlargement with small cysts.

piercings, trauma, sinusitis, dental infection, and parotitis. CT demonstrates soft tissue swelling, stranding of the subcutaneous fat, and sometimes nonenhancing edema that should not be mistaken for an abscess [**Fig. 10.57**]. Necrotizing fasciitis is a fulminant infection typically caused by alpha-hemolytic streptococci. CT reveals extensive soft tissue swelling of the neck, stranding of subcutaneous and deeper fat, ill-defined muscle borders, and nonenhancing low-density fluid collections due to edema/phlegmon [**Fig. 10.57**]. The differential diagnosis includes edema due to other causes (eg, venous thrombosis/obstruction); thus a diagnosis of necrotizing fasciitis requires clinical correlation.

Thyroid Inflammation

Perithyroidal inflammation or suppurative thyroid infection, particularly on the left, should raise concern for an underlying pyriform sinus tract (see earlier). Infectious thyroiditis is otherwise uncommon in children. Hashimoto thyroiditis is the most

common acquired thyroid disorder of childhood. Imaging shows diffuse homogeneous or heterogeneous thyroid enlargement [**Fig. 10.58**]. Multinodular goiter is of mixed echogenicity, density, and intensity on ultrasonography, CT, and MRI, respectively [**Fig. 10.58**].

Salivary Gland Inflammation

Acute viral or bacterial sialadenitis usually affects the parotid glands. *Acute bacterial parotitis* occurs because of stasis and ascending bacterial infection. Predisposing factors include dehydration, decreased salivary flow, and/or salivary duct obstruction. Symptoms include unilateral facial pain, tenderness, and swelling. CT reveals enlargement and increased enhancement of the affected parotid gland with overlying cellulitis and edema deep to the platysma muscle [**Fig. 10.57**]. Abscess formation is uncommon. Neonatal suppurative parotitis caused by *Staphylococcus aureus* is uncommon. Submandibular sialadenitis usually results from *sialolithiasis,* which is most common within the

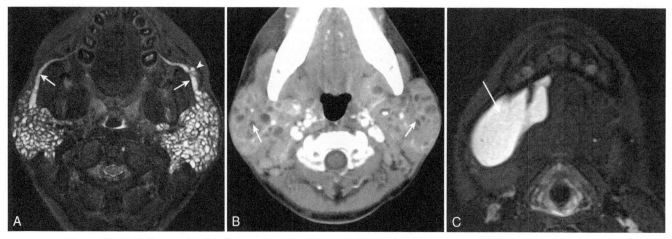

Figure 10.59 Salivary gland inflammation. A, Sjögren disease. Axial fat-suppressed T2-weighted magnetic resonance (MR) image shows parotid enlargement with innumerable small cysts, also present in accessory parotid tissue (*arrowhead*). There is dilatation of the parotid ducts (*arrows*). **B,** Lymphoepithelial cysts in HIV/AIDS. Axial contrast-enhanced computed tomography (CECT) image reveals enlarged parotid glands that contain numerous cysts of varying size (*arrows*). **C,** Plunging ranula. Axial T2 short tau inversion recovery MR image shows an elliptical high signal cystic intensity lesion (*arrow*) extending into the submandibular space.

submandibular duct. Ultrasonography shows the echogenic calculus, which may be visible on CT if radiopaque. *Sialodochitis* usually affects Stensen or Wharton ducts due to ductal obstruction. The inflamed duct appears dilated with enhancing walls, sometimes with strictures. *Chronic recurrent parotitis* of childhood is a bilateral disease characterized by intermittent recurrent, sometimes unilateral acute exacerbations. Ultrasonography, CT, and MRI reveal numerous bilateral small parotid cysts caused by sialectasis. The imaging appearance is indistinguishable from *Sjögren syndrome* [**Fig. 10.59**]. Multiple parotid and submandibular *lymphoepithelial cysts* are seen in *HIV/AIDS* [**Fig. 10.59**]. A *ranula* is a pseudocyst thought to result from sublingual gland or duct obstruction or trauma, leading to fluid accumulation in the sublingual space above the mylohyoid muscle (*simple ranula*) or extending around or through the mylohyoid muscle into the submandibular space (*diving or plunging ranula*). CT and MRI reveal a well-defined, thin-walled, nonenhancing elliptical or lobulated cystic sublingual lesion lateral to genioglossus (simple ranula) or lateral to the mylohyoid extending into the submandibular space (diving or plunging ranula) [**Fig. 10.59**]. Cyst contents vary in signal intensity depending on prior hemorrhage or infection. The differential diagnosis includes dermoid and LM.

Osteomyelitis

Acute mandibular osteomyelitis may result from trauma, foreign body, surgery, hematogenous spread (eg, distant infection, vascular catheter), or contiguous spread (eg, dental or sinus infection). Imaging features include permeative bone destruction, soft tissue edema, cellulitis, and abscess. Chronic nonbacterial osteomyelitis usually affects the mandible. This sterile inflammatory osteitis can affect any bone or multiple bones, manifesting as chronic recurrent multifocal osteomyelitis. Chronic recurrent multifocal osteomyelitis has been linked to various chronic autoinflammatory disorders. CT reveals chronic lamellated periosteal reaction, bone sclerosis, and lucency, with avid uptake on ^{99m}Tc isotope bone scan [**Fig. 10.60**].

NEOPLASMS AND TUMOR-LIKE CONDITIONS

Following is a description of head and neck tumors that can occur throughout the head and neck or in multiple locations.

This is followed by a description of additional region-specific tumors.

Infantile Hemangioma

IH is an extremely common benign tumor that most often arises during infancy, proliferates during the first year of life, and then involutes over the ensuing several years. IH is more common in girls; multiple lesions occur in up to 20% of cases. Congenital IH is uncommon and manifests as a rapidly involuting congenital hemangioma or noninvoluting congenital hemangioma. Cutaneous IH produces plaquelike, red skin discoloration or a bosselated strawberry-red mass. Symptoms depend on site and extent. Large regional craniofacial, midline, or beardlike IH are a feature of PHACES association (*p*osterior fossa malformations, *h*emangiomas, *a*rterial anomalies, *c*oarctation of the aorta and cardiac defects, *e*ye abnormalities, and *s*ternal clefting and *s*upraumbilical abdominal raphe). IH is usually managed expectantly, anticipating involution; treatment (eg, propranolol) is reserved for IH that interferes with vital functions (eg, vision, breathing, and feeding). Subglottic IH may be treated with laser therapy to prevent airway obstruction. Imaging with ultrasonography or MR is indicated to evaluate the extent of known IH, for diagnostic purposes such as evaluation of symptoms (eg, proptosis) or a deep-seated mass, and to assess for possible PHACES in some cases. Ultrasonography reveals a bosselated, moderately echogenic tumor containing prominent vessels. On CT, IH enhances intensely. On T2W MRI, proliferating IH is solid, sharply circumscribed with lobulated borders, and isointense with gray matter. *Prominent vascular flow voids* and *intense, homogeneous enhancement* are key imaging features, considered pathognomonic for IH [**Fig. 10.61**]. Involution results in a decrease in size, vascularity, and enhancement with increasing fibrofatty matrix. Favored sites include the cheek, parotid, orbit, periorbital soft tissues, neck, and larynx. Atypical features that should prompt consideration of a tumor other than IH include poorly defined margins, less-than-avid enhancement, heterogeneous enhancement, and lack of prominent vascularity. The differential diagnosis varies by location and includes other infantile tumors, such as kaposiform hemangioendothelioma (KHE), LCH (in the case of an intraosseous IH), congenital fibrosarcoma, rhabdomyoma, and schwannoma (in the case of an IAC or cavernous sinus IH).

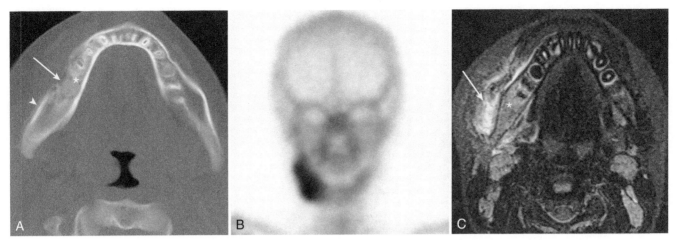

Figure 10.60 Chronic nonbacterial osteomyelitis of the mandible. A, Axial computed tomography image demonstrates cortical destruction of the body of the mandible (*arrow*) with sclerosis of the medullary cavity (*asterisk*) and adjacent periosteal reaction (*arrowhead*). This characteristic appearance should not be misinterpreted as a neoplasm. **B,** Technetium 99m (⁹⁹ᵐTc) methylene diphosphonate isotope bone scan demonstrates corresponding increased uptake of radiotracer in the right mandibular body. **C,** Axial T2 short tau inversion recovery magnetic resonance image shows abnormal high signal intensity within the medullary space of the right mandible (*asterisk*) with swelling of the muscles of mastication (*arrow*).

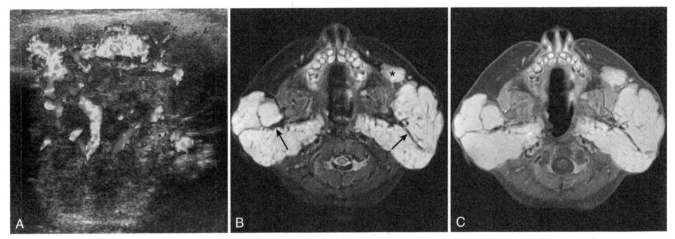

Figure 10.61 Proliferating infantile hemangioma (IH). A, Ultrasonography color Doppler image reveals a lobulated mass with very prominent high-flow vascularity. **B,** Axial T2 short tau inversion recovery magnetic resonance (MR) image shows bilateral parotid hemangiomas which are sharply defined, lobulated, and hyperintense relative to muscle and contain prominent signal voids due to vessels (*arrows*). A smaller left cheek IH is present (*asterisk*). **C,** Axial gadolinium-enhanced fat-suppressed T1-weighted MR image demonstrates intense, homogeneous enhancement of the IHs.

KHE is an uncommon vascular tumor that is associated with severe and sometimes fatal consumptive coagulopathy known as Kasabach-Merritt phenomenon. On T2W MRI, KHE has irregular, poorly defined margins and contains small foci of hypointensity caused by hemosiderin from platelet trapping. There is moderate enhancement; prominent vascularity is not a feature.

Teratoma

Teratoma contains multiple tissue types derived from all three germ cell layers. Congenital teratoma is usually benign and typically arises in the infrahyoid neck where it is intimately related to the thyroid gland. Other locations include the orbit, sinuses, and infratemporal fossa (sometimes with skull erosion). *Epignathus* is an uncommon midline teratoma arising from the oral cavity or pharynx and associated with other midline anomalies. Key ultrasonography, CT, and MR features include a cystic and solid mass, sometimes with calcific and fatty foci, with enhancing solid components on CT and MR [**Fig. 10.62**]. When infrahyoid, the ipsilateral thyroid gland may be inapparent, or there may be a *claw sign* with the thyroid gland draped around the tumor periphery. Detection of a fetal neck mass should prompt assessment for fetal airway obstruction. Classic imaging features are diagnostic of teratoma. By contrast, LM appears purely cystic, envelops the thyroid gland, and is not calcified. The differential diagnosis for nasal teratoma includes nasal *chondromesenchymal hamartoma,* a rare cystic and solid nasal mass with an increased incidence in patients with pleuropulmonary blastoma.

Lipoma

As seen elsewhere in the body, lipoma appears as a bland rounded or oval fatty mass without other distinguishing

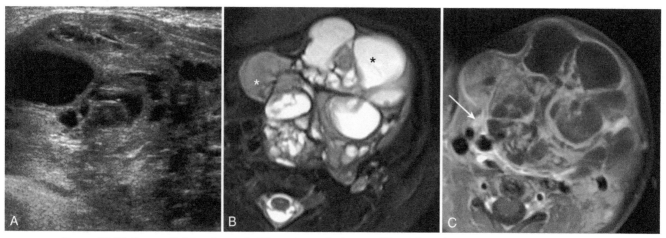

Figure 10.62 Congenital teratoma. A, Ultrasonography image. **(B)** Axial T2 short tau inversion recovery magnetic resonance (MR) image and **(C)** axial gadolinium-enhanced fat-suppressed T1-weighted MR image demonstrate a solid (*white asterisk*) and cystic (*black asterisk*) left neck mass. **C,** There is enhancement of the solid components and cyst walls. The enhancing right lobe of the thyroid gland is visible (*arrow*), but the left lobe is not clearly seen.

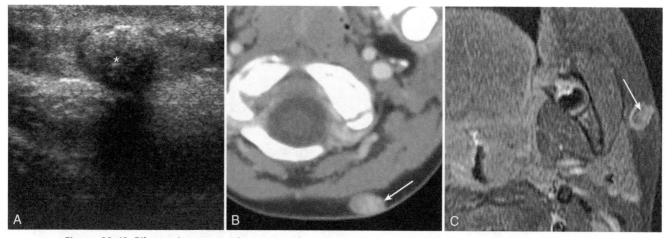

Figure 10.63 Pilomatrixoma. A, Ultrasonography image reveals a small, subcutaneous mass (*asterisk*) containing echogenic foci with acoustic shadowing, consistent with mineralization. **B,** Axial contrast-enhanced computed tomography (CECT) image shows a small, hyperdense, ovoid nodule (*arrow*) within the subcutaneous fat, extending to the skin. **C,** Axial gadolinium-enhanced fat-suppressed T1-weighted magnetic resonance image demonstrates a small, hypointense, peripherally enhancing, preauricular subcutaneous mass (*arrow*).

characteristics. Soft tissue or enhancing foci, pain, or rapid growth are atypical and should prompt an alternative diagnosis such as *lipoblastoma.*

Pilomatrixoma (Calcifying Epithelioma of Malherbe)

Pilomatrixoma (PMX) is a common tumor arising from hair follicles. PMX presents as a small, hard, cutaneous or subcutaneous mass, sometimes with skin discoloration. Although usually diagnosed clinically, imaging is sometimes obtained or PMX may be seen as an incidental finding on imaging performed for other reasons. Ultrasonography reveals an echogenic subcutaneous nodule with posterior acoustic shadowing [**Fig. 10.63**]. On CT, PMX appears as a small, often preauricular, subcutaneous, densely mineralized nodule with extension to the skin [**Fig. 10.63**]. On MRI, typical PMX appears hypointense on all sequences with minimal peripheral enhancement [**Fig. 10.63**]. Although the typical imaging features of PMX are characteristic, the differential diagnosis includes first BAC and nontuberculous mycobacterial infection.

Nerve Sheath Tumors

Benign nerve sheath tumors include plexiform neurofibroma, solitary neurofibroma, and schwannoma (see also temporal bone tumors). Neurofibroma and plexiform neurofibroma are characteristic of NF-1. Schwannoma not infrequently occurs as an isolated tumor or may occur in association with NF-2. Nerve sheath tumors arise along CNs, peripheral nerves, or both. Symptoms include a mass, deformity, and/or functional impairment. On CT and MRI, plexiform neurofibroma resembles a bag of worms, with tumor extending along nerves producing a heterogeneous, so-called target appearance [**Fig. 10.64**]. Imaging of solitary neurofibroma and schwannoma reveals a rounded or oval mass that is hypodense or isodense on CT with variable signal on T2W MRI [**Fig. 10.64**]. Low signal intensity is attributable to fibrous tissue (in neurofibroma) or high cellularity (in schwannoma). Tumors enhance homogenously unless there is cystic change. Rapid increase in size and/or development of pain suggest transformation to *malignant peripheral nerve sheath tumor* [**Fig. 10.64**]. Malignant peripheral nerve sheath tumor can also arise de novo.

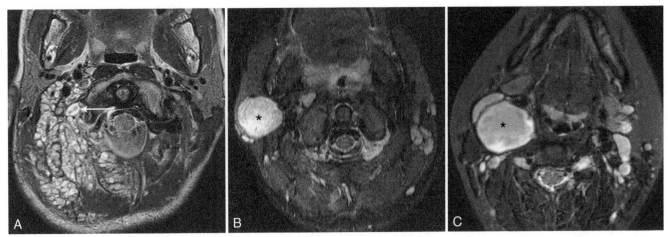

Figure 10.64 Nerve sheath tumors. A, Plexiform neurofibroma in a patient with neurofibromatosis type 1 (NF-1). Axial T2-weighted magnetic resonance (MR) image shows a lobulated right posterior neck mass consisting of rounded foci of high signal intensity, with central hypointense foci, known as the "target sign" (*arrow*). **B,** Sporadic schwannoma. Axial T2 short tau inversion recovery (STIR) MR image reveals a homogeneous, oval right parotid mass (*asterisk*) that appears hyperintense relative to muscle. Although parotid pleomorphic adenoma and mucoepidermoid carcinoma occur more commonly, the homogeneous signal characteristics and lack of a pseudocapsule favor schwannoma. **C,** Malignant peripheral sheath tumor in a patient with NF-1. Axial T2 STIR MR image shows an ovoid mass (*asterisk*) that is isointense with other smaller NFs. There is peripheral high signal intensity with slightly lower central signal intensity, as may be seen in benign NFs because of fibrous content. Pain and a rapid increase in size heralded the onset of malignant degeneration.

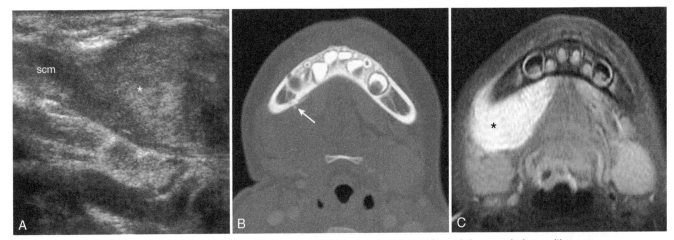

Figure 10.65 Fibrous lesions. A, Fibromatosis colli. Ultrasonography reveals a solid, expanded, masslike appearance of the involved portion of the sternocleidomastoid muscle (*scm*) with heterogeneous echogenicity (*asterisk*). **B,** Desmoid tumor. Axial contrast-enhanced computed tomography (CECT) image bone window shows a subtle spiculated periosteal reaction on the lingual surface of the right mandibular body (*arrow*). **C,** Axial gadolinium-enhanced fat-suppressed T1-weighted magnetic resonance image (same patient) demonstrates that the associated submandibular mass enhances homogeneously (*asterisk*).

Fibrous Tumor-Like Conditions and Fibroblastic Tumors

Fibroblastic or myofibroblastic tumors include benign tumors or tumor-like lesions, intermediate locally aggressive tumors, intermediate rarely metastasizing tumors, and malignant tumors (predominantly in adults). Benign lesions include fibromatosis colli, nodular fasciitis, myositis ossificans, and fibroma (as seen in Gardner syndrome). Intermediate locally aggressive tumors include desmoid. Intermediate rarely metastasizing tumors include infantile fibrosarcoma. *Fibromatosis colli* (SCM pseudotumor) is a benign, congenital, fibrous, masslike lesion of uncertain etiology, possibly caused by birth trauma; venous obstruction leads to edema, SCM muscle fiber degeneration,

and fibrosis. Affected infants present with torticollis and a firm mass involving the distal third of the SCM. Ultrasonography reveals a solid, expanded, masslike appearance of the involved portion of the SCM with variable echogenicity, or diffuse SCM enlargement [**Fig. 10.65**]. CT and MRI show an isodense/isointense SCM mass, sometimes with hemorrhage, calcification, or both. Most cases resolve with conservative therapy; however, facial and calvarial deformity may occur. *Desmoid tumor* has a predilection for the submandibular space. CT reveals an isodense tumor arising along the mandibular body with focal bone erosion and minimal spiculated periosteal reaction. MRI shows an ovoid mass that is hypointense on T2 with mild-to-moderate homogenous contrast enhancement [**Fig. 10.65**].

Fibroosseous, Chondroid, and Osseous Tumors and Tumorlike Conditions

Fibrous dysplasia (FD) is a fibroosseous bone disorder that affects a single bone (monostotic) or multiple bones (polyostotic). Polyostotic FD with premature puberty is termed McCune-Albright syndrome. Symptoms of FD or other fibroosseous lesions include overgrowth of the affected part, cosmetic deformity, and alteration of function. On CT, the hallmark of FD is ground-glass opacification with expansion of affected bone, sometimes with lucent areas [**Fig. 10.66**]. On T2W MRI, FD is markedly hypointense, other than cystic areas which appear hyperintense, and sometimes enhance after contrast [**Fig. 10.66**]. *Ossifying fibroma* usually involves the jaws. Imaging reveals an expansile lucent mass with sclerotic foci, often located in the maxilla. *Giant cell lesion* and *aneurysmal bone cyst* tend to involve the PNSs or bony orbit. Imaging reveals an expansile lesion with thinned cortical margins and characteristic

fluid–fluid levels [**Fig. 10.67**]. Multiple giant cell lesions are a feature of Noonan syndrome. *Cherubism* is a benign hereditary condition that appears between 2 and 5 years of age, progresses until puberty, and then regresses. Children present with mandibular enlargement. CT reveals multiple expansile, lucent, fibroosseous mandibular and maxillary lesions [**Fig. 10.67**]. *Osteoma* is a benign tumor usually in the frontal and ethmoid sinuses, appearing as a small sclerotic focus. *Exostoses* are broad-based sessile lesions. Exostoses and osteomas tend to involve the EAC. Gardner syndrome is characterized by multiple osteomas, dental abnormalities, and desmoid tumors. *Osteochondroma* is a developmental lesion consisting of a bony projection with an overlying cartilaginous cap; multiple osteochondromas occur in hereditary multiple exostoses. CT demonstrates the bony projection, and MRI is used to detect the cartilaginous cap. Malignant transformation to chondrosarcoma or osteogenic sarcoma can occur. *Chordoma* is a rare tumor that arises from intraosseous notochordal remnants in the skull base, near

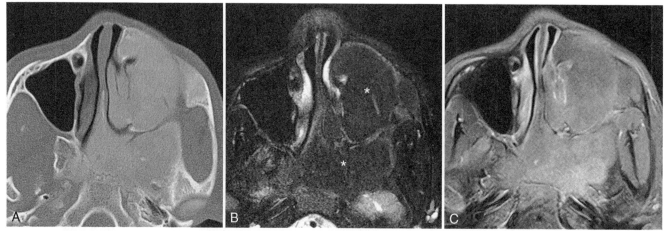

Figure 10.66 Fibrous dysplasia. A, Axial computed tomography image shows characteristic ground-glass opacification and expansion of the left maxilla, adjacent nasal turbinate, and sphenoid bone. **B,** Axial fat-suppressed (FS) T2-weighted magnetic resonance (MR) imaging demonstrates that the lesion is extremely hypointense (*asterisks*) because of fibrous content. **C,** Axial gadolinium-enhanced FS T1-weighted MR image shows mild enhancement in portions of the lesion.

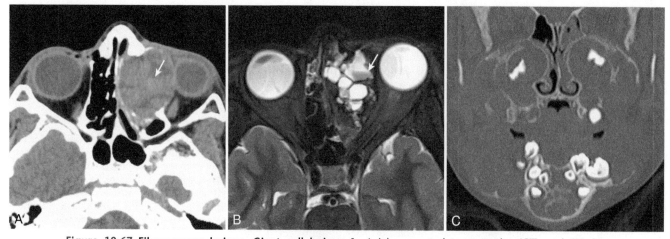

Figure 10.67 Fibroosseous lesions. Giant cell lesion. A, Axial computed tomography (CT) and (**B**) fat-suppressed T2-weighted magnetic resonance imaging show an expansile left ethmoid mass containing numerous fluid–fluid levels (*arrows*). Although the differential diagnosis of an expansile lesion with thinned bony margins includes mucocele, the presence of fluid–fluid levels is helpful in diagnosing a giant cell lesion or aneurysmal bone cyst. **C,** Cherubism. Reformatted coronal CT image demonstrates innumerable maxillary and mandibular expansile, lucent fibroosseous lesions.

midline synchondroses. These tumors are locally invasive, destroy bone, and may metastasize. Chondroid chordoma may be indistinguishable from chondrosarcoma on imaging.

Langerhans Cell Histiocytosis and Other Histiocytoses

LCH is a reticuloendothelial disorder of unknown etiology, characterized by tissue infiltration with reticulum cells, histiocytes, plasmocytes, and leukocytes. LCH can occur as a solitary mass (eosinophilic granuloma), multiple masses, or disseminated disease with cutaneous, visceral, and bone involvement. Symptoms include a mass, secondary effects of a mass (eg, proptosis, otorrhea), pain, or alteration of function. Sites of predilection include the superolateral orbit, temporal bones (bilateral or unilateral), and frontal bones. CT usually shows isodense-to-hyperdense or occasionally hypodense masses that enhance. LCH produces characteristic sharply defined bone destruction with "punched-out" or beveled edges [**Figs. 10.68** and **10.69**]. On

MRI, LCH is of intermediate to low signal intensity on T2W images with moderate or marked homogeneous or heterogeneous enhancement [**Fig. 10.69**], often with epidural extension if involving the calvarium. Disseminated disease may involve the marrow, and intracranial involvement may also occur. The differential diagnosis depends on location and includes other fibro-osseous lesions, lymphoma, sarcoma, and metastatic disease. Temporal bone LCH must be distinguished from cholesteatoma, CG, CoM, RMS, and metastasis (eg, neuroblastoma). *Juvenile xanthogranuloma* is a non-Langerhans histiocytic cutaneous lesion that peaks in infancy. Large or deep-seated lesions appear similar to LCH. A key distinguishing feature is hyperintensity on T1 precontrast MR.

Rhabdomyosarcoma

RMS is the second most common head and neck malignancy after lymphoma. RMS peaks during the first decade of life, typically involving the masticator space and orbit, and is the most

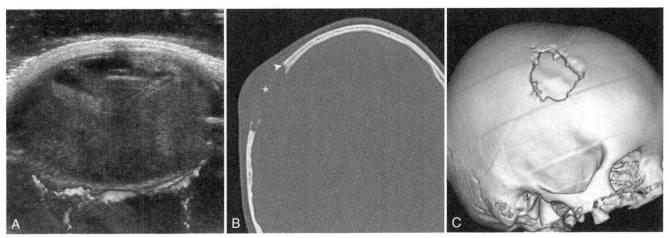

Figure 10.68 Langerhans cell histiocytosis. A, Ultrasonography with color Doppler reveals a relatively avascular scalp mass. **B,** Axial computed tomography image and (**C**) three-dimensional model show the associated sharply defined calvarial erosion (*asterisk*). Note the characteristic beveled edges of the involved bones (*arrowhead*).

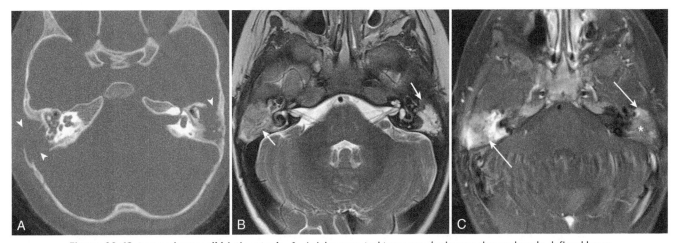

Figure 10.69 Langerhans cell histiocytosis. A, Axial computed tomography image shows sharply defined bony erosion (*arrowheads*) of the mastoid portions of the temporal bones with destruction of mastoid septations. There is associated extensive mastoid and middle ear cavity (MEC) opacification. **B,** Axial T2-weighted magnetic resonance (MR) helps distinguish the hypointense LCH (*arrows*) from hyperintense trapped secretions and/or inflammatory change. **C,** Axial gadolinium-enhanced fat-suppressed T1-weighted MR image shows that the right mastoid and MEC and anterior left mastoid LCH enhance intensely (*arrows*), in contrast with the mildly enhancing inflammatory tissue on the left (*asterisk*).

common primary temporal bone malignancy. A second peak occurs in teenagers with increased sinonasal involvement. Parotid and nasopharyngeal RMS also occur. An increased incidence of RMS occurs in NF-1, Li-Fraumeni syndrome, and hereditary RB. RMS also occurs as a second malignancy after radiation therapy. Symptoms of RMS include a mass, mass effect (eg, proptosis), pain, CN palsies, epistaxis, and obstructive symptoms (eg, nasal stuffiness, snoring, otalgia, or otorrhea). Embryonal and alveolar subtypes predominate in children; the alveolar subtype has a worse prognosis. Prognosis also depends on molecular subtype, presence of parameningeal disease, and tumor stage. Prognosis is best for localized fully resected disease.

CT, MR, and PET-CT are used for RMS evaluation and staging. On CT, RMS is usually isodense to muscle with variable enhancement. Bone remodeling and aggressive, defined or permeative, lytic destruction occurs [**Figs. 10.70** and **10.71**]. Masticator space RMS usually arises in the pterygoid muscles and remodels and erodes the mandible (with TMJ subluxation or dislocation) and maxillary antrum. Eustachian tube obstruction results in ipsilateral MEC and mastoid air cell opacification [**Fig. 10.70**]. Tumor may extend superiorly, widening foramen ovale, resulting in parameningeal disease with cavernous sinus involvement [**Fig. 10.70**]. Orbital RMS usually occurs along extraconal muscles with orbital remodeling, erosion, or both. Sinonasal RMS erodes/remodels the PNS, resulting in trapped secretions

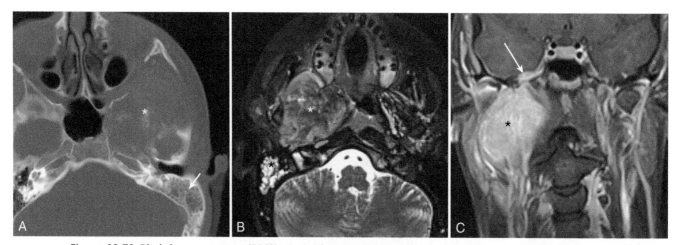

Figure 10.70 Rhabdomyosarcoma (RMS). A, Axial computed tomography image demonstrates lytic destruction of the left sphenoid bone (*asterisk*) due to a destructive masticator space RMS that obstructs the left Eustachian tube. Note opacified left mastoid air cells (*arrow*). **B,** Axial T2 short tau inversion recovery magnetic resonance (MR) image shows a large, heterogeneous masticator space RMS (*asterisk*) that is isointense with brain parenchyma. Fluid is again seen in the ipsilateral mastoid air cells. **C,** Coronal gadolinium-enhanced fat-suppressed T1-weighted MR image demonstrates that the enhancing masticator space RMS (*asterisk*) has spread directly through foramen ovale into the epidural space (*arrow*) and base of the right cavernous sinus, consistent with parameningeal disease.

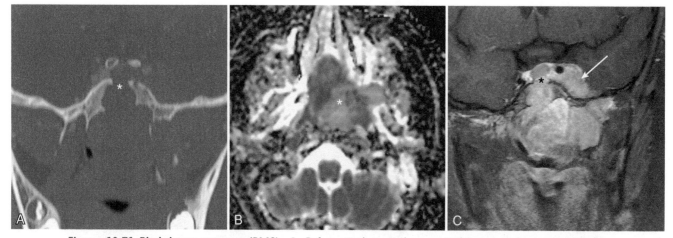

Figure 10.71 Rhabdomyosarcoma (RMS). A, Reformatted coronal computed tomography image demonstrates sharply defined lytic destruction of the body of the sphenoid bone associated with a central skull base and nasopharyngeal RMS (*asterisk*). **B,** Axial diffusion-weighted imaging apparent diffusion coefficient magnetic resonance (MR) shows that the tumor (*asterisk*) has decreased diffusivity consistent with the high nuclear-to-cytoplasmic ratio of RMS tumor cells. **C,** Coronal gadolinium-enhanced fat-suppressed T1-weighted MR image shows the heterogeneously enhancing RMS centered on the sphenoid bone and nasopharynx. Note the erosion of the sella turcica (*asterisk*) and extension of tumor inferior to the pituitary gland and left internal carotid artery into the left cavernous sinus (*arrow*), consistent with parameningeal disease.

with parameningeal disease if tumor breaches the skull base [**Fig. 10.71**]. Temporal bone RMS can compress or invade the IJV. Nodal enlargement may occur because of metastasis but is not usually a feature of orbital RMS. MR distinguishes tumor from trapped sinus secretions and demonstrates parameningeal disease. The tumor usually (but not invariably) appears isointense or hypointense compared with cerebral cortex on T2W images with decreased diffusivity on DWI [**Fig. 10.71**]. Enhancement is variable—mild, moderate, or marked, and homogeneous or heterogeneous, depending on the presence of tumoral necrosis. Parameningeal disease occurs because of intracranial extension through foreman ovale or via skull base erosion resulting in a cavernous sinus or epidural mass with dural enhancement, occasionally with leptomeningeal dissemination and/or parenchymal involvement [**Figs. 10.70** and **10.71**]. Metastatic disease is best assessed with [¹⁸F]-FDG PET-CT.

The differential diagnosis depends on the appearance and location of tumor. Masticator space RMS is often quite characteristic; Ewing sarcoma and desmoid tumor may appear similar. Localized orbital RMS resembles lymphoma or pseudotumor. The differential diagnosis for sinonasal and nasopharyngeal RMS includes metastatic disease (eg, neuroblastoma or leukemia), chloroma, lymphoma, carcinoma, esthesioneuroblastoma (ENB), juvenile angiofibroma (JA; seen in boys), and other sarcomas. The differential diagnosis for temporal bone RMS includes infection, cholesteatoma, LCH, atypical teratoid rhabdoid tumor (seen in infants), and metastases (eg, neuroblastoma). Sharp osseous margins sometimes help distinguish LCH and JA from RMS; however, bone erosion in RMS is variable, sometimes appearing sharply marginated or more permeative in appearance. Unlike JA, RMS does not appear fibrous or hypervascular. Lymphoma appears more homogenous than RMS on MRI.

Other Sarcomas, Neuroepithelial, and Neurogenic Tumors

Other sarcomas include infantile fibrosarcoma, synovial sarcoma, PNET/Ewing sarcoma, chondrosarcoma, and osteogenic sarcoma. CT of maxillary or mandibular *PNET/Ewing sarcoma* shows a soft tissue mass with aggressive bone destruction with a spiculated periosteal reaction. Soft tissue characteristics on MR of Ewing sarcoma, fibrosarcoma, and synovial sarcoma resemble RMS. Fibrous tissue contributes to low signal on T2W MR. *Melanotic neuroectodermal tumor of infancy* is rare, benign but locally aggressive, and involves the maxilla or occipitomastoid bones, the latter associated with florid osseous sclerosis and spiculated new bone formation with large epidural and external soft tissue components [**Fig. 10.72**]. Melanin may cause high signal intensity on unenhanced T1W MRI. *Chondrosarcoma* may arise de novo, from a preexisting osteochondroma, or after radiation therapy. Chondroid matrix (calcific "rings-and-arcs") is characteristic on CT but is not always seen. *Osteosarcoma* appears as an aggressive osseous and soft tissue mass with florid new bone formation [**Fig. 10.72**]. Nodal and hematogenous metastatic disease is common with many of these tumors.

Lymphoma

Lymphoproliferative disorders include reactive lymphoid hyperplasia, posttransplant lymphoproliferative disorder, Castleman disease, and lymphoma. The major types of lymphoma are Hodgkin lymphoma (HL) and non-HL (NHL). HL predominates in the head and neck, is primarily nodal, and presents as a painless enlarging mass or masses. Disease spreads to nodal groups in a contiguous fashion. Imaging reveals enlargement of involved LNs, which appear homogeneous without appreciable enhancement. CT and [¹⁸F]-FDG PET-CT are used for staging (neck, chest, and abdomen) [**Fig. 10.73**]. The differential diagnosis includes infectious lymphadenopathy (eg, EBV infection), lymphoid hyperplasia, Castleman disease, sarcoidosis, and massive lymphadenopathy with sinus histiocytosis (Rosai-Dorfman disease). Nodal necrosis and fat stranding is uncommon in untreated lymphoma.

NHL tends to involve the extranodal tissues of Waldeyer ring, may be EBV related, and therefore has a high incidence in regions endemic with EBV (eg, endemic Burkitt lymphoma in equatorial Africa), and occurs in immunocompromised and/or immunodeficient patients. Endemic NHL peaks in the first decade and nonendemic NHL peaks in the second decade of life. NHL sites include the adenoid, palatine and lingual tonsils, oral cavity, nasopharynx, PNSs, orbit, thyroid, larynx, and salivary glands. Symptoms are as for RMS. Disseminated disease is more common in NHL.

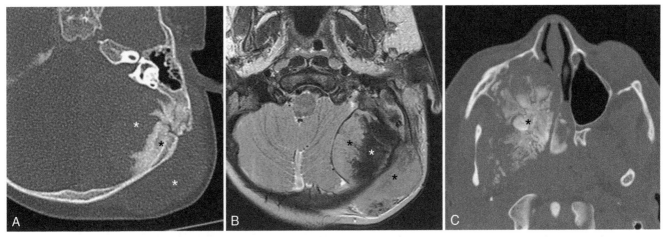

Figure 10.72 Other sarcomas. A, Melanotic neuroectodermal tumor of infancy (MNTI). Axial computed tomography (CT) image shows a tumor straddling the left occipitomastoid suture with exuberant new bone formation (*black asterisk*). Epidural and extracranial soft tissue components of tumor are also present (*white asterisks*). **B,** Axial T2-weighted magnetic resonance (MR; same patient) shows the hypointense new bone formation (*white asterisk*) and soft tissue components of tumor (*black asterisks*). Although MNTI is rare, this imaging appearance in an infant is highly characteristic. **C,** Osteogenic sarcoma. Axial CT image shows a maxillary tumor characterized by florid new bone formation (*asterisk*). The right maxillary antrum is opacified because of trapped secretions.

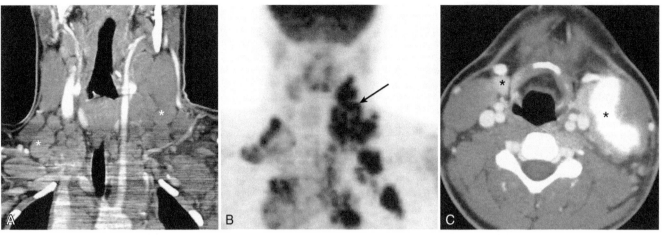

Figure 10.73 Hodgkin lymphoma. A, Reformatted coronal contrast-enhanced computed tomography (CECT) image shows extensive cervical, supraclavicular, axillary, and mediastinal lymphadenopathy (*asterisks*). **B,** Coronal [^{18}F]fluorodeoxyglucose positron emission tomography (PET) image shows intense uptake in the enlarged lymph nodes (LNs) (*arrow*). **C,** Axial PET-computed tomography image shows the intense uptake in affected cervical LNs (*asterisks*).

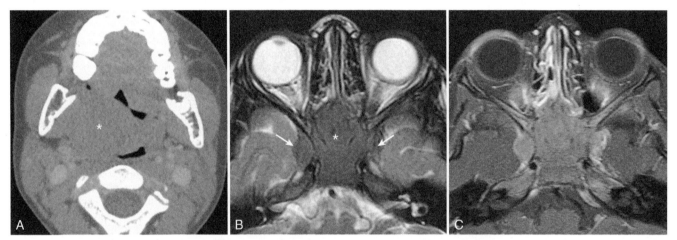

Figure 10.74 Burkitt lymphoma (non-Hodgkin lymphoma). A, Axial contrast-enhanced computed tomography (CECT) image shows marked enlargement of the right palatine tonsil (*asterisk*) with mass effect on the airway. **B,** Axial T2-weighted magnetic resonance (MR) image demonstrates a homogeneous, low signal intensity tumor of the sphenoid bone (*asterisk*) and petrous apices, with extension into the cavernous sinuses (*arrows*). **C,** Axial gadolinium-enhanced fat-suppressed T1-weighted MR image shows mild, homogeneous enhancement of tumor. Although the differential diagnosis includes rhabdomyosarcoma, the homogenous tumor characteristics favor lymphoma.

Imaging features include a tonsillar, nasopharyngeal, orbital, parotid, thyroid, or sinonasal mass, with lytic bone destruction appreciable on CT if adjacent to bone [**Fig. 10.74**]. On MRI, these tumors are characteristically homogeneous and isointense or hypointense relative to cerebral cortex on T2W images, with decreased diffusivity on DWI and mild homogeneous enhancement [**Fig. 10.74**]. The differential diagnosis depends on location and includes RMS, leukemia, ENB, carcinoma (nasopharyngeal and sinonasal), LCH, metastases, sarcoidosis, and granulomatous polyangiitis (Wegener granulomatosis).

Leukemia

Head and neck manifestations of leukemia include extramedullary myeloid sarcoma (also referred to as chloroma and granulocytic sarcoma) or diffuse intramedullary disease [**Fig. 10.75**]. Chloroma tends to involve the orbits and sinonasal regions. CT reveals bone destruction with an isodense, enhancing mass. The

mass appears isointense or hypointense relative to cerebral cortex on T2W MRI, with decreased diffusivity on DWI and moderate to marked Gd enhancement. The differential diagnosis includes RMS or another type of sarcoma, lymphoma, carcinoma, LCH, and metastases.

Carcinoma

Carcinoma is uncommon in childhood; it usually affects teenagers and includes thyroid carcinoma (see later Thyroid Tumors section), parotid mucoepidermoid carcinoma (see parotid tumors), EBV-associated NPC, and nuclear protein in testis (NUT) midline sinonasal or upper aerodigestive tract carcinoma. Symptoms depend on tumor site and include a firm, enlarging mass, sinonasal and airway obstructive symptoms, sequelae of Eustachian tube obstruction, and CN palsies. CT of NPC reveals a nasopharyngeal mass, aggressive skull base bone destruction, and intracranial epidural and cavernous sinus extension. Metastatic

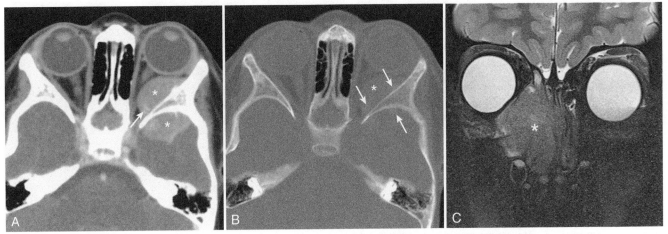

Figure 10.75 Leukemia. A, Axial contrast-enhanced computed tomography (CECT) and (**B**) bone window images show an enhancing mass with soft tissue components in the orbit and middle cranial fossa (*asterisks*). There is an associated spiculated periosteal reaction (*arrows*) with poorly defined permeative destruction of the lateral orbital wall. These leukemic deposits appear indistinguishable from metastatic neuroblastoma. **C,** Extramedullary granulocytic sarcoma associated with leukemia. Coronal fat-suppressed T2-weighted magnetic resonance image shows a homogeneous hypointense right sinonasal tumor (*asterisk*) with extension into the right orbital extraconal space. The appearance is indistinguishable from lymphoma.

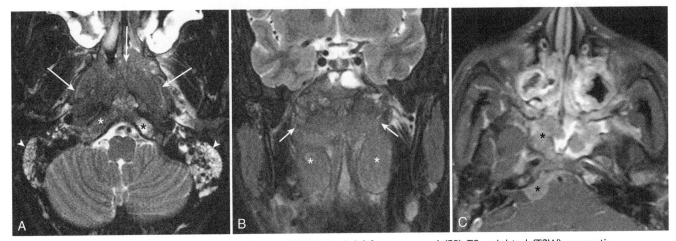

Figure 10.76 Nasopharyngeal carcinoma (NPC). A, Axial fat-suppressed (FS) T2-weighted (T2W) magnetic resonance (MR) image shows a large, mildly heterogeneous, hypointense nasopharyngeal tumor (*arrows*). There is neoplastic invasion of the basiocciput (*white asterisk*), compared with the normal marrow signal on the left (*black asterisk*). NPC obstructs the Eustachian tubes resulting in mastoid air cell secretions (*arrowheads*). There is also maxillary antral mucosal thickening. **B,** Coronal FS T2W MR image shows the NPC (*arrows*) which has spread to retropharyngeal lymph nodes (*asterisks*). Secretions are present in the sphenoid sinus. **C,** Axial gadolinium-enhanced FS T1-weighted MRI shows the mildly enhancing NPC within the sphenoid bone, basiocciput, and posterior fossa (*asterisks*). There is also mucosal enhancement within the paranasal sinuses that should not be mistaken for tumor.

LNs are common at presentation. On MRI, NPC is usually isointense or hypointense relative to cerebral cortex on T2W images, with decreased diffusivity and moderate to marked enhancement [**Fig. 10.76**]. The differential diagnosis includes lymphoma and RMS. NUT midline carcinoma is located in or close to the midline in the larynx, epiglottis, or sinonasal region. This aggressive tumor has similar soft tissue characteristics on MRI to NPC.

Metastatic Disease

Diffuse disseminated metastatic disease most commonly occurs with leukemia and NB. Solitary or multifocal metastases involve bone and/or LNs and occur with a variety of tumors. Metastatic disease is often detected initially on [18F]-FDG PET (or metaiodobenzylguanidine scans for NB) or manifests as a mass, mass

effect, or alteration of function. Disseminated NB involves bone and/or marrow; marrow involvement produces symmetric diploic space expansion. CT of disseminated disease demonstrates aggressive lytic, permeative bone destruction with spiculated periosteal reaction and hyperdense, enhancing soft tissue masses [**Figs. 10.75 and 10.77**]. MRI reveals associated plaque-like or lobulated masses that are isointense or hypointense relative to cerebral cortex on T2W MRI with decreased diffusivity and moderate to marked enhancement [**Fig. 10.77**].

Orbit and Globe

Optic Pathway Glioma

Optic pathway glioma (OPG) is the most common childhood optic pathway tumor, with an increased incidence in NF-1,

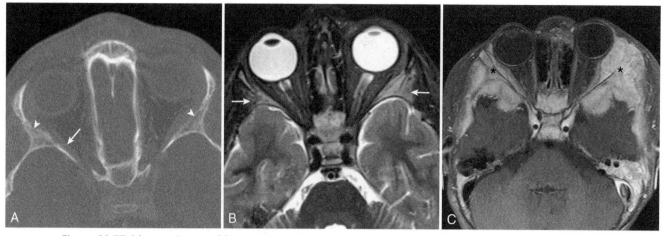

Figure 10.77 Metastatic neuroblastoma (NB). A, Axial computed tomography image shows lytic, permeative destruction of the lateral orbital walls (*arrowheads*) with associated soft tissue thickening (*arrow*). **B,** Axial fat-suppressed (FS) T2-weighted magnetic resonance (MR) imaging (same patient) shows intermediate signal intensity metastatic deposits (*arrows*). **C,** Axial gadolinium-enhanced FS T1-weighted MR image shows florid, enhancing calvarial metastatic deposits (*asterisks*).

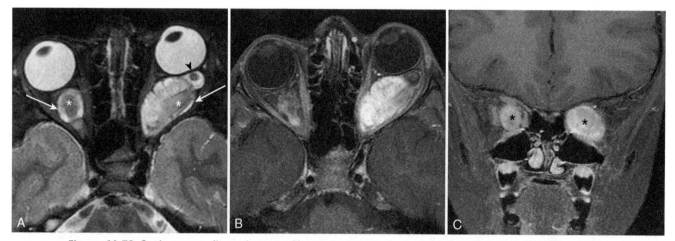

Figure 10.78 Optic nerve glioma in neurofibromatosis type 1. A, Axial fat-suppressed (FS) T2-weighted magnetic resonance (MR) imaging reveals marked enlargement and tortuosity of the optic nerves and optic nerve sheaths (*arrows*) with heterogeneous signal intensity of the optic nerves (*asterisks*). There is flattening of the posterior aspect of the left globe (*arrowhead*). **B,** Axial gadolinium (Gd)-enhanced FS T1-weighted (T1W) MR image shows that the left optic glioma is avidly enhancing, the right less so. **C,** Coronal Gd-enhanced fat-suppressed T1W MR image showing that, unlike meningioma, the nerves (*asterisks*) and nerve sheaths enhance in optic nerve glioma.

especially when bilateral. These low-grade astrocytomas involve the ON(s) and/or chiasm, sometimes extending to the optic tracts or optic radiations. Affected children present with proptosis, visual field abnormalities, or visual impairment. MR features include tubular or ovoid enlargement and sometimes tortuosity of the ON. OPG appears isointense to hyperintense on T2W imaging with facilitated diffusion on DWI and variable, sometimes intense enhancement [**Fig. 10.78**]. Enlargement of the subarachnoid space around the OPG may be seen. The differential diagnosis includes ON meningioma, which demonstrates peripheral enhancement around the affected ON.

Retinoblastoma

RB is a malignant tumor of the immature retina, occurs in the fetus, infant, and young child, and is the most common primary childhood ocular tumor. Sporadic and familial RB is associated with retinal mutations of the RB tumor suppressor gene.

Autosomal dominant familial or hereditary RB has additional germ cell RB mutations and presents at an earlier age with bilateral RB. Familial RB has an increased incidence of second primary neoplasms such as pituitary and/or pineal region tumors (trilateral or quadrilateral RB) and head and neck sarcomas. The classic postnatal presentation of RB is leukocoria. Ocular ultrasonography shows an echogenic, calcified intraocular tumor. CT, although no longer the examination of choice, does reveal a calcified intraocular tumor or multiple tumors within a normal-sized or large globe [**Fig. 10.79**]. On MRI, RB appears markedly hypointense on T2W images and enhances. High-resolution thin-section 3D T2W images can demonstrate small tumor nodules [**Fig. 10.79**]. Retinal detachment may be seen. Tumor extension along the ON produces irregular ON thickening and infiltration of perineural fat. The differential diagnosis of ocular calcific lesions includes *drusen* (calcific focus at the ON papilla), ocular infection (small globe), and ROP (small globe). Coats disease causes leukocoria but does not usually mineralize until late in the disease.

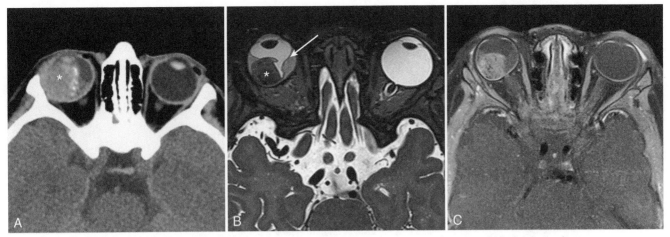

Figure 10.79 Retinoblastoma (RB). A, Axial computed tomography image shows a calcified right ocular tumor (*asterisk*). There is an associated retinal detachment. **B,** Axial T2 SPACE magnetic resonance (MR) image reveals a hypointense right RB (*asterisk*) with an associated retinal detachment (*arrow*). **C,** Axial gadolinium-enhanced fat-suppressed T1-weighted MR image shows the enhancing RB that extends to the optic nerve head.

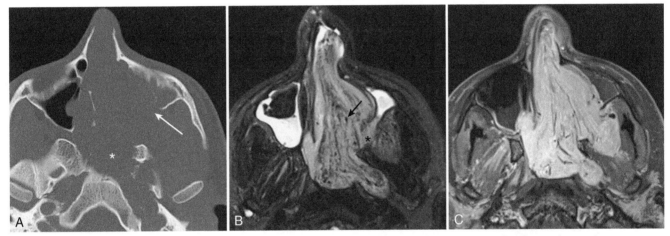

Figure 10.80 Juvenile angiofibroma (JA). A, Axial computed tomography image reveals a large, destructive sinonasal mass with erosion of the sphenoid bone (*asterisk*) and walls of the left maxillary antrum (*arrow*). **B,** Axial fat-suppressed (FS) T2-weighted magnetic resonance (MR) image shows nasal cavity and nasopharyngeal JA, with characteristic extension into the left pterygopalatine fossa (*asterisk*). Although benign, the tumor is isointense with cerebral cortex because of fibrous content. Prominent vascular flow voids are present (*arrow*). **C,** Axial gadolinium-enhanced FS T1-weighted MR image demonstrates that the JA enhances intensely.

Nasal Cavity, Paranasal Sinuses, and Face

Juvenile Angiofibroma

JA is a benign but locally aggressive fibrovascular tumor that typically presents in adolescent boys with epistaxis and nasal stuffiness. CECT reveals an intensely enhancing tumor originating along the lateral nasopharyngeal wall, extending into the ipsilateral nasal cavity and nasopharynx and laterally into the pterygopalatine fossa. Tumor often bows and erodes the posterior wall of the maxillary antrum and erodes the sphenoid sinus, sometimes with intracranial epidural and/or cavernous sinus extension [**Fig. 10.80**]. Involvement of the orbital fissures permits orbital tumor extension. On MRI, JA appears lobulated, markedly hypointense on T2W images (because of fibrous content), and enhances avidly [**Fig. 10.80**]. The internal maxillary, sphenopalatine, and descending palatine branches of the ECA are enlarged, and prominent intratumoral vascular flow voids are seen. MR helps detect intracranial and intraorbital spread of tumor. Both CT and MRI distinguish trapped sinus

secretions from tumor. The differential diagnosis includes sinonasal RMS, which causes lytic permeative bone destruction, does not appear fibrous, and does not exhibit the vascularity of JA. Angiography, performed before preoperative endovascular embolization, reveals a dense tumor blush with arterial supply primarily from ECA branches, sometimes with recruitment of ICA branches.

Esthesioneuroblastoma

ENB or olfactory neuroblastoma is a rare malignant neuroectodermal tumor thought to arise from nasal and cribriform plate olfactory epithelial cells. Clinical symptoms include nasal stuffiness, epistaxis, headache, and hyposmia. CECT reveals a lobulated, enhancing tumor involving the nasal cavity, ethmoid air cells, and maxillary antrum. There is aggressive lytic bone destruction, sometimes with orbital spread and erosion of the cribriform plate with epidural tumor and dural enhancement [**Fig. 10.81**]. Prominent whorls or foci of mineralization may be

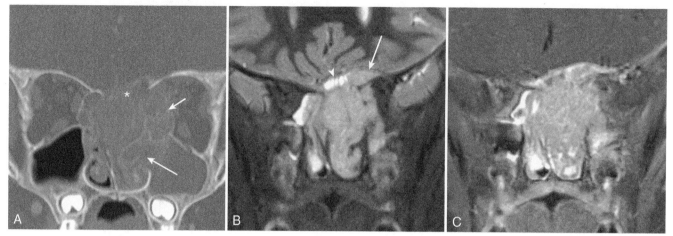

Figure 10.81 Esthesioneuroblastoma. A, Reformatted coronal computed tomography image shows a destructive sinonasal tumor with extensive sinonasal and orbital bony erosion (*arrows*) including erosion of the cribriform plates (*asterisk*). **B,** Coronal fat-suppressed (FS) T2-weighted magnetic resonance (MR) image shows that this cellular tumor is isointense with cerebral cortex and contains small cystic foci along the superior margin (*arrowhead*). The tumor has extended into the epidural space (*arrow*). **C,** Coronal gadolinium-enhanced FS T1-weighted MR image shows moderately intense tumor enhancement.

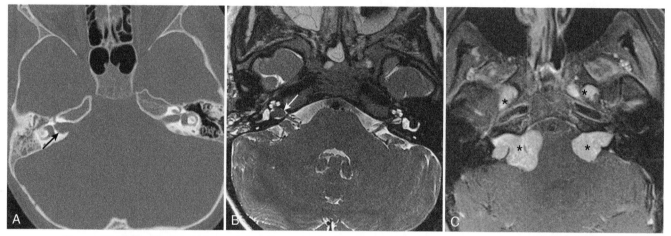

Figure 10.82 Vestibulocochlear schwannoma. A, Axial computed tomography image shows incidental asymmetric widening of the right internal auditory canal (*arrow*) in a patient with a right cholesteatoma. **B,** Axial T2 SPACE magnetic resonance (MR) image (same patient) shows a schwannoma (*arrow*) involving the right vestibulocochlear nerve extending into the cochlear and inferior vestibular divisions. **C,** Multiple schwannomas in NF-2. Axial gadolinium-enhanced fat-suppressed T1-weighted MR image reveals bilateral enhancing vestibular and mandibular nerve schwannomas (*asterisks*).

seen. ENB tends to spread to regional LNs. On MRI, ENB appears isointense to hypointense on T2W images compared with cerebral cortex, with deceased diffusivity and moderate to marked contrast enhancement [**Fig. 10.81**]. Small cysts are sometimes seen along the superior aspect of the tumor, especially with intracranial tumor extension. PET-CT is used for staging and follow-up of ENB. The differential diagnosis includes RMS, lymphoma, sinonasal carcinoma, and inverted papilloma. *Inverted papilloma* is extremely uncommon in children. A convoluted "cerebriform" pattern has been described as a characteristic MRI feature.

Temporal Bone

Schwannoma

Schwannoma occurs as a sporadic or NF-2-associated tumor, typically involving CN VIII (vestibular schwannoma), followed by CN VII and/or CNs in the jugular fossa. CT reveals corticated

expansion of the affected IAC, FNC, or jugular foramen [**Fig. 10.82**]. MR reveals a tumor of variable signal intensity on T2W images (depending on cellularity) with avid enhancement [**Fig. 10.82**]. The differential diagnosis of a small IAC tumor with corticated bone margins includes lipoma (bright on non-FS T1) and IH (seen in infants, prominent vascularity). Paraganglioma is rare except in familial cases and tends to cause irregular "moth-eaten" bone erosion on CT with a salt and pepper appearance on T2W MR images because of intratumoral vascular flow voids.

Oral Cavity and Neck

Thyroid Tumors

Thyroid masses are best assessed with ultrasonography and include hyperplastic and adenomatous nodules, nodules caused by thyroiditis, and multinodular goiter. Thyroid carcinoma occurs in sporadic and hereditary forms (eg, medullary thyroid carcinoma in multiple endocrine neoplasia). Papillary carcinoma

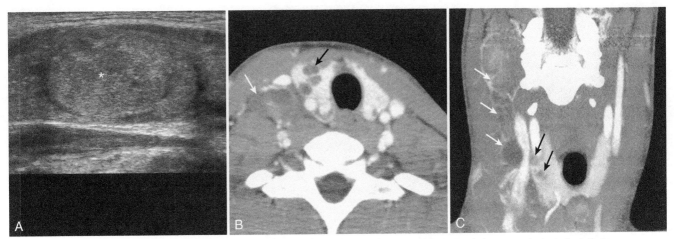

Figure 10.83 Papillary thyroid carcinoma. A, Longitudinal ultrasonography image shows a relatively isoechoic and slightly heterogeneous nodule (*asterisk*). **B,** Axial and (**C**) reformatted coronal contrast-enhanced computed tomography (CECT) images show a hypodense, multinodular right thyroid mass (*black arrow*), with spread to adjacent cervical lymph nodes (*white arrows*). The nodal metastases also appear hypodense.

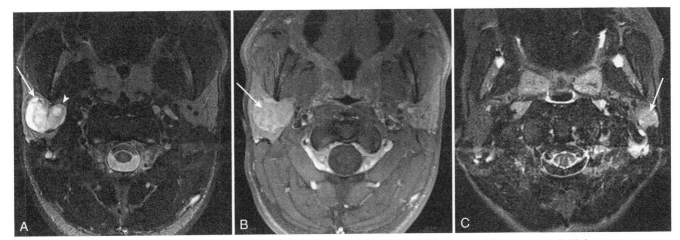

Figure 10.84 Parotid tumors. A, Pleomorphic adenoma. Axial T2-weighted magnetic resonance (MR) image shows a heterogeneous right parotid tumor (*arrow*) that is hyperintense relative to surrounding soft tissues. A sharply defined hypointense peripheral pseudocapsule is present (*arrowhead*). **B,** Axial gadolinium-enhanced fat-suppressed T1-weighted MR image (same patient) shows that the tumor enhances. **C,** Mucoepidermoid carcinoma. Axial T2 short tau inversion recovery MR image shows a small nodule (*arrow*) within the left parotid that is isointense with lymphoid tissue. Note the absence of a hypointense rim.

accounts for most cases of thyroid carcinoma. On ultrasonography, papillary thyroid carcinoma usually appears hypoechoic and may have microcalcifications and internal vascularity. CT reveals a heterogeneous thyroid mass. Cervical nodal metastases are common; the nodes may contain calcifications and may be enhancing or cystic [**Fig. 10.83**]. The differential diagnosis includes follicular thyroid carcinoma and medullary thyroid carcinoma. Children with solitary thyroid nodules are usually evaluated by thyroid scintigraphy using ^{99m}Tc pertechnetate or [123]I. "Hot" nodules that take up ^{123}I are unlikely to be malignant. Cold nodules raise concern for malignancy.

Salivary Gland Tumors

Most salivary gland epithelial tumors arise in the parotid gland. Unusual locations include the submandibular gland or minor salivary gland tissue along the soft palate. Pleomorphic adenoma (benign mixed tumor) and mucoepidermoid carcinoma predominate. CT of pleomorphic adenoma reveals a rounded or lobulated, heterogeneously enhancing, or sometimes cystic tumor.

On MRI, the tumor is usually hyperintense and enhances. A key feature is a hypointense rim or pseudocapsule surrounding the tumor on T2W images [**Fig. 10.84**]. Low-grade mucoepidermoid carcinoma appears similar to pleomorphic adenoma [**Fig. 10.84**]. High-grade mucoepidermoid carcinoma has low to intermediate signal on T2W images because of high cellularity. Parotid tumors in infancy are most likely to be IH; atypical features should prompt consideration of KHE or sialoblastoma.

Cysts and Odontogenic Lesions of the Jaw

Nonodontogenic cysts include fissural (described earlier), hemorrhagic, and Stafne cysts. *Hemorrhagic bone cyst* usually occurs in the mandible and appears on PF as a unilocular, scalloped lucency that is not primarily related to the teeth. *Stafne cyst* is an anatomic variant (related to a focally deep submandibular gland fossa) and also appears as a well-defined, round, or oval lucency near the mandibular angle. Odontogenic lesions arise in association with dentition and include benign cysts, tumorlike lesions, and benign and malignant tumors.

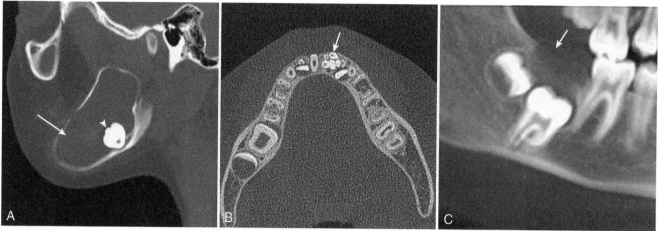

Figure 10.85 Cysts and odontogenic lesions of the jaw. A, Dentigerous cyst. Reformatted sagittal computed tomography (CT) image shows an expansile lucent lesion (*arrow*) associated with the crown of an unerupted molar tooth (*arrowhead*). **B,** Compound odontoma. Axial CT image shows a mass between the incisor teeth containing numerous small "denticles" (*arrow*). **C,** Ameloblastoma. Panorex film shows a lucent, expansile "bubbly" mass (*arrow*) overlying the crowns of the unerupted molar teeth.

These lesions present with facial asymmetry, swelling, dental impaction, malocclusion, or facial pain. Odontogenic cysts appear radiolucent with sharply defined borders on CT or PF. Dentigerous cyst is associated with the crown of an unerupted tooth [**Fig. 10.85**]. Radicular cysts are associated with dental roots and periapical infection. Keratocystic odontogenic tumor (KOT) is a tumor-like condition. KOTs are a feature of basal cell nevus syndrome (Gorlin syndrome). KOT appears as a sharply circumscribed, expansile, lytic lesion arising in proximity to molar teeth. Other odontogenic tumors that occur in childhood include odontoma, cementoblastoma, adenomatoid odontogenic tumor, ameloblastic fibroma, fibroodontoma, and ameloblastoma. Odontoma contains toothlike elements [**Fig. 10.85**]. *Ameloblastic fibroma* and *ameloblastoma* are the most common odontogenic tumors. These benign but locally aggressive tumors appear as a unilocular or multilocular lesion with distinct borders [**Fig. 10.85**]. There may be marginal sclerosis, expansion, a "soap-bubble" appearance, or cortical disruption with a soft tissue mass.

Miscellaneous

Primary head and neck neurogenic tumors include *ganglioneuroma, ganglioneuroblastoma,* and *primary cervical neuroblastoma.* These tumors are uncommon and have a predilection for the carotid sheath. CT and MR reveal an ovoid or elliptical mass of variable density/intensity that enhances, with splaying of the ICA and IJV. *Paraganglioma* is rare in children unless familial. This diagnosis is suggested by a vascular tumor splaying the carotid bifurcation with imaging characteristics as mentioned earlier.

SUGGESTED READINGS

Coley BD, ed. *Caffey's Pediatric Diagnostic Imaging.* 12th ed. St. Louis, MO: Elsevier Saunders; 2013.

Harnsberger HR, Glastonbury CM, Michel MA, et al., eds. *Diagnostic Imaging: Head and Neck.* 2nd ed. Salt Lake City, UT: Amirsys Inc. Lippincott Williams & Wilkins; 2010.

Koch BL. Cystic malformations of the neck in children. *Pediatr Radiol.* 2005;35:463.

Koch BL. Pediatric considerations in craniofacial trauma. *Neuroimaging Clin N Am.* 2014;24:513.

Koenig LJ, ed. *Diagnostic Imaging: Oral and Maxillofacial.* Salt Lake City, UT: Amirsys Inc. Lippincott Williams & Wilkins; 2011.

Lan MY, Shiao JY, Ho CY, et al. Measurements of normal inner ear on computed tomography in children with congenital sensorineural hearing loss. *Eur Arch Otorhinolaryngol.* 2009;266:1361.

Lemmerling MM, De Foer B, Verbist BM, et al. Imaging of inflammatory and infectious diseases in the temporal bone. *Neuroimaging Clin N Am.* 2009;19: 321.

Robson CD. Imaging of head and neck neoplasms in children. *Pediatr Radiol.* 2010;40:499.

Robson CD, Koch BK, Harnsberger HR, eds. *Specialty Imaging: Temporal Bone.* Salt Lake City, UT: Amirsys Inc. Lippincott Williams & Wilkins; 2013.

Som PM, Curtin HD, eds. *Head and Neck Imaging.* 5th ed. Philadelphia, PA: WB Saunders Company; 2011.

Thomas BM, Shroff M, Forte V, et al. Revisiting imaging features and the embryologic basis of third and fourth branchial anomalies. *AJNR Am J Neuroradiol.* 2010;31:755.

Index

Page numbers followed by "*f*" indicate figures, "*t*" indicate tables, and "*b*" indicate boxes.